Ex Libris

Flawlessly yours,

Ultrasonic Testing of Materials

by

J. Krautkrämer H. Krautkrämer

in Collaboration with

W. Grabendörfer L. Niklas

Translation of the
Second Revised German Edition

Springer-Verlag New York Heidelberg Berlin 1969

Josef Krautkrämer
Dr. rer. nat., Cologne

Herbert Krautkrämer
Dr. rer. nat., Cologne

Werner Grabendörfer
Dr. phil., Cologne

Ludwig Niklas
Dr. phil., Cologne

Title of the Original Editon:
Werkstoffprüfung mit Ultraschall

Translated by Dipl.-Ing. B. W. Zenzinger (Pretoria, South Africa)
in Consultation with Dr. J. Krautkrämer

With 456 figures and 10 tables

Printed in Germany
Library of Congress Catalog Card Number: 68-57396

Title No. 1512

Preface

The attempt to write a text-book which deals exclusively with the application of ultrasonics to materials testing seems justified in view of the fact that in the available text-books, which either cover the entire discipline of ultrasonics or the whole field of non-destructive testing of materials, this specialised science is by necessity not dealt with exhaustively enough.

The authors have made a special effort to adapt the standard of this book to the widest possible public. On the one hand it should be useful to the inspector of materials with perhaps only a moderate knowledge of physics and mathematics, while on the other hand the fundamental principles required by the design engineer so as to be able to apply the method to new problems should not be neglected. This is taken care of by the many paragraphs with asterisks and in small print. These can be skipped by the less erudite or less interested reader without the rest remaining incomprehensible.

The presentation of a full list of bibliographic references particularly for the period before 1957, was regarded as unnecessary because the book by L. Bergmann and the supplement to it contain an exceptionally comprehensive collection. Therefore only those publications which have a direct bearing on the text have been listed.

The fact that the authors are also manufacturers of ultrasonic instruments has both advantages and disadvantages. Their own practical participation in this field and their many contacts with instrument users over a period of nearly 18 years have led to a vast accumulation of experience, not previously published in any form and which could now be utilised. Although a conscious effort has been made when describing instruments and methods, to do justice also to the developments pioneered by others, it was inevitable that we should frequently mention our own designs. It is therefore stated here explicitly that wherever an instrument of our own is mentioned, this in no way implies that the results obtainable with other instruments may not be equally good or even better.

It is the pleasant duty of the authors to acknowledge gratefully the assistance rendered by their co-workers of many years standing, and in particular the many experts, named and unnamed, who have made their experiences, testing material or records readily available.

A large portion of the work which went into the preparation of Section 1.6 and the tables and formulas in the appendix was contributed by Dr. A. Lutsch and G. J. Kühn. Their employers, the South African Council for Scientific and Industrial Research, financed their calculations of the transit of sound through interfaces. To Dr. Lutsch we also owe our contact with the translator.

The presentation of the reflection of partially transmissive layers (pp. 253–255) was contributed by Dr. E. Mundry of the Bundesanstalt für Materialprüfung, Berlin.

This first edition of the English translation is based on the unchanged second German edition. Only some errors have been corrected. It has been prepared with great care by Dipl.-Ing. B. W. Zenzinger of Pretoria, to whom the authors are therefore particularly indebted. Due to his sound knowledge of both languages and his early contact with the ultrasonic testing of materials, Mr. Zenzinger, was particularly well qualified to undertake this task. Having already worked in the USA with ultrasonics for non-destructive testing, he was the first to introduce the ultrasonic testing of materials in South Africa at the South African Bureau of Standards and to the local industry in general. In his translation he was assisted with the editing by Dr. O. Brune, former head of the Electrical Engineering Division of the South African Council for Scientific and Industrial Research (CSIR) and previously instructor at the Massachusetts Institute of Technology (MIT) in Cambridge, Mass.

Finally, we wish to express our gratitude to the publishers for having inspired the writing of this book and for the excellent preparation of the two German and the first English editions.

Cologne, August 1968

J. and H. Krautkrämer

Contents*

---

*The sections marked with an asterisk are less important for beginners.

Introduction

Acoustics, the science of sound, describes the phenomenon of mechanical vibrations and their propagation in solid, liquid or gaseous materials. Empty space knows no sound because it is the particles of matter themselves which vibrate, in contrast, for instance, to the oscillations of light or other electromagnetic waves where the electric and magnetic state of the space oscillates. In air a sound wave moves a discrete volume of air back and forth around its neutral position, whereas a light wave has no influence on its state of rest or motion.

If such mechanical movements in matter repeated regularly, i.e. periodically and for a given length of time, are classified according to their number of cycles per second, a range can be defined in which the human ear can serve as detector: the sound is then audible if it reaches the ear either through the air or through the body. This requires, however, that its frequency be neither too low nor too high: sound below approx. 10 Hz (hertz = cycles per second = c/s) and above approx. 15,000 to 20,000 Hz is inaudible to the human ear. (The first statement is. however, strictly correct only where this concerns sinusoidal oscillations. Other forms of vibrations are resolved by the ear into harmonics, thus making them audible as note or bang sequences.)

Just as in the case of light waves where the higher frequencies which are invisible to the eye, are called ultra-violet, so the sound waves above 20,000 Hz are referred to as ultra-sound or ultrasonics. It has been suggested that sound waves below 10 Hz be called subsonics. This division is purely arbitrary and dependent on the human ear. Completely different demarcations apply in the case of other generating and detecting methods.

Ultrasonic waves are a rather common occurrence in nature and in daily life, and are occasionally of such intensity that we may regard ourselves as very fortunate indeed that our ear is not burdened by them, as for instance in the case of steam whistles. A rotating grindstone when used for grinding a specimen generates in addition to audible noise intense ultrasonic waves with frequencies as high as those used for testing materials, viz. above 100,000 Hz (100 kHz, kilocycles per second) and up to 10,000,000 Hz (10 MHz, megacycles per second).

The numerous technical applications of sound waves and ultrasonics may be divided into two groups: as in medicine where X-rays are used for two completely different purposes, viz. therapeutically for their action on tissue (cancer irradiation) and diagnostically for studying certain conditions (radioscopy of lungs), so sound can likewise be used firstly for acting on a given material, and secondly for revealing its physical condition. In the first case the energy of the sound wave is used, for instance, for ejecting particles of dirt from fabrics during washing, for detaching foreign bodies from a given surface during cleaning, for removing chips during drilling, for overcoming surface tension during emulsification, for mixing, and for many other applications of mechanical energy. This concerns the exploitation of sound energy.

In other cases the energy of the sound wave is utilized only to the extent required for transmitting a sufficiently clear signal, e.g. in public address systems, for locating ships at sea, for sounding ocean depths, locating shoals of fish, and for checking the condition of materials, e.g. regarding mechanical flaws, their thickness, and their elastic and metallurgical properties. All these are diagnostic applications, in regard to which this book will discuss only the testing of materials.

To determine the mechanical properties of a given material, the mechanical method is the most direct and ready to hand. To determine whether a shaft is cracked, it can be stressed by tension or bending until the crack manifests itself by an open break. This is a mechanical but unfortunately destructive test. By contrast, sound and ultrasonics furnish, for the same purpose, non-destructive testing methods which basically likewise use mechanical stresses produced by tensile, compressive, shearing or flexural forces but which are of such low intensity as occurs in the various wave modes. This does not imply, however, that an indirect testing method, e.g. a magnetic test which reveals the magnetic field lines produced near a crack, may not at times be more suitable, provided the correlations between the mechanical properties of the specimen concerned and the physical means applied, such as magnetism, electricity, radiation, etc., are unambiguous.

Setting eside the qualification "ultra", sound as such has long been used for testing materials, or rather individual specimens such as for instance forgings or castings, where gross internal defects can be detected by the change in the ringing note when the specimen is struck with a hammer, a method still practised today. Every housewife knows that a cup can be checked for cracks by tapping it. One can therefore with justice maintain that testing by sound is one of the oldest non-destructive methods for detecting hidden defects since it is very probable that the inventors of ceramics would already have put it to use. By the application of modern electronics it has become one of the most recent and most versatile testing tools.

The transition from audible sound to ultrasonic sound has been made possible by modern methods of generation and detection which replace hammer and ear. Whereas the natural vibration produced by a hammer blow depends very little on the hammer but very much on the shape of the specimen and on the striking point (bell), the frequency can be predetermined if electrical sound generators are used. In the case of higher frequencies the wave length of a vibration becomes smaller in inverse proportion and finally even extremely small compared with the dimensions of the specimen concerned. One can then direct a beam of such waves into a specimen without interferences resulting from its shape and dimensions, just as in the case of light from a projector. In this way the specimen is "sounded out", a term already common in popular parlance.

This method was applied by SOKOLOV in 1929 for detecting the presence of defects which revealed themselves by a drop in transmitted sound intensity at such points as compared with points free of defects. In 1942 FIRESTONE was the first to apply the principle of the sonic depth finder, well known from ship locating and depth sounding at sea, to the testing of materials. After 1945, favoured by the increasingly urgent demands for non-destructive testing, this method became generally accepted as a practical tool.

1 Basic Principles of Ultrasonic Testing of Materials

1.1 Oscillations and Waves

Ultrasonic testing of materials makes use of mechanical waves in contrast, for instance, to X-ray techniques which use electromagnetic waves. Any mechanical wave is composed of oscillations of discrete particles of material. The motion carried out by a small mass attached to a spring as shown in Fig. 1.1 if pulled down once and released, is called an oscillation. Left to itself, the mass oscillates about the equilibrium position. The nature of this oscillation is of particular importance inasmuch as it is sinusoidal, the path recorded as a function of time being a sine curve. It is obtained only if the driving force, in this case supplied by the spring, increases proportionally with the displacement. It is then also referred to as elastic force. Furthermore, one can imagine the body to consist of individual particles kept in position by elastic forces. Very much simplified, the model of an elastic body can be visualised as shown in Fig. 1.2, but three-dimensionally. Provided such a body is not stressed by compression or tension beyond its elastic limit, it behaves like this spring model. In it, the particles can perform elastic oscillations. How then does a wave arise from an oscillation?

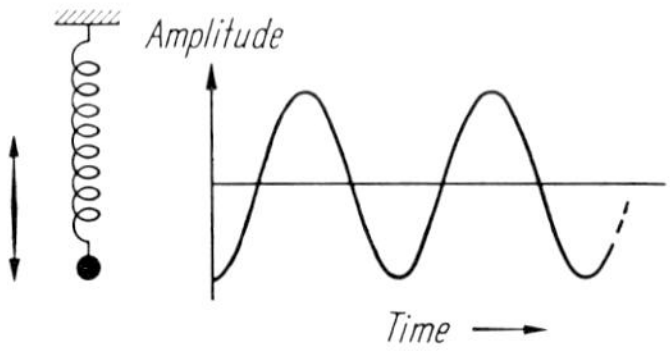

Fig. 1.1 Sinusoidal oscillation of a loaded spring.

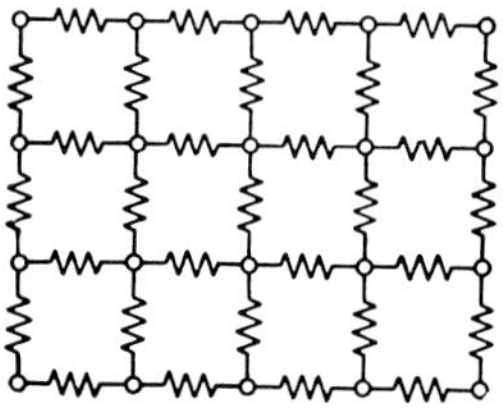
Fig. 1.2 Model of an elastic body.

Let us assume that all material particles on the left side of the model are excited collectively in step with the sinusoidal oscillations, for instance by cementing them to a diaphragm which is made to oscillate by electrical means (loudspeaker). All particles in the first plane are then obliged to oscillate with the same amplitude (width of oscillation) and frequency (number of oscillations per second). The elastic forces transmit the oscillations to the particles in the second plane. When these have started to oscillate, the vibratory movement is transmitted to the third plane, and so forth. If all points were interconnected rigidly, they would all start their movement simultaneously and remain constantly in the same state of motion, i.e. in the same *phase*. In an elastic material this is not the case: the motion requires a certain time to be transmitted and the planes reached later lag in phase behind those first excited. While in a given plane the particles are moving from the right through the point of rest, to the left, the particles in a plane further to the right have only started to move from left to right. Their delay is then exactly one half

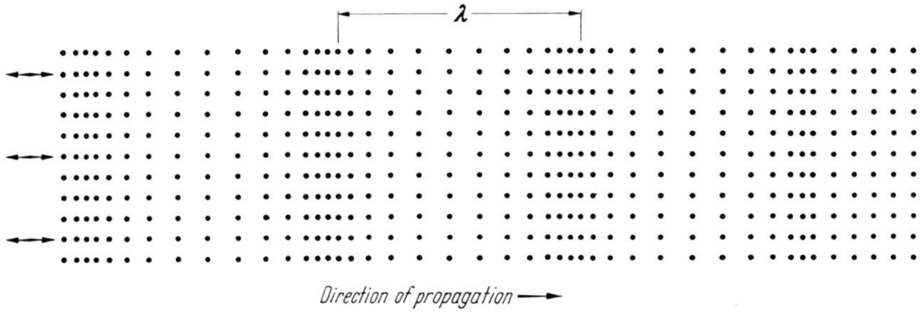

Fig. 1.3 Longitudinal wave.

oscillation. Fig. 1.3 shows the instantaneous picture of a section of the model in which a wave travelling from the left to the right has not yet reached the right edge. It can be seen that the phase shift of the oscillations creates zones where the particles approach each other particularly closely. These compression zones alternate with rarified zones. The chronological pattern of the wave shows that these zones are constantly recreated on the excitation side and that they travel in the body at constant velocity and uniform intervals towards the right. This represents an elastic wave.

Of course, Fig. 1.3 cannot vividly demonstrate the movement of the wave, which could only be done on a cine film. The wave phenomenon as such is, however, well known from another kind of wave, viz. waves in water. A wave crest corresponds to a zone of compression. A naive observer might think that the wave crest transports water, because his eye can follow the wave crest. That this in reality is not the case is borne out by any small body floating on the water, which merely moves up and down. The only thing that travels in the wave is its state, in the case of elastic waves the state of compression and rarefaction. The particles themselves remain in place and merely oscillate about their positions of rest.

Of course, the model of a solid body can be visualised as consisting of many separate particles of material only if it is uniform (homogeneous) throughout and if it shows the same elastic behaviour in all directions (isotropy). Each point shown in Fig. 1.3 then represents the mass of a small cube.

The spring model shown in Fig. 1.2 cannot be applied to liquid or gaseous substances where the individual particles are not tied to a position of rest but where they are free. Nevertheless, these substances too offer a certain resistance when compressed or expanded, as shown for example by an air pump. They can therefore likewise transmit elastic waves.

When visualising the models presented in Figs. 1.3 and 1.4, it should be realised that the plane of dots represents only a section of the three-dimensional body, inasmuch as boundary surfaces would modify the wave process considerably. A wave as depicted in Figs. 1.3 and 1.4 can exist in this way only when remote from any boundaries.

A few parameters of a wave will be defined with the aid of Fig. 1.3: the *frequency* of a wave is the number of oscillations of a given particle per second. Within a given wave it is the same for all particles and it is identical with the frequency of the generator which can be chosen arbitrarily. The *wave length* is the distance between two planes in which the particles are in the same state of motion, i.e. for instance two compression zones. It is inversely proportional to the frequency: high frequencies corresponding to short wave lengths, and vice versa. The *speed of sound* is the velocity of propagation of a given condition, e.g. of a compression zone. This velocity is a characteristic of the material concerned and in general is constant for a given material for any frequency and any wave length. Numerical data and formulas are given in Section 1.4. For us the most important quantity in a given sound field is the *sound pressure*. At points of higher particle density the pressure is likewise higher than the normal pressure, while in the dilated zones it is lower. A very small and inertialess pressure gauge placed in the path of the sound wave would indicate alternately high pressure and low pressure in sinusoidal sequence. This alternating pressure is the sound pressure. It occurs not only in gases, but also in liquid and solid bodies. The maximum deviation from the normal pressure (without sound wave) is called the *amplitude of the sound pressure* which is closely connected to the *amplitude of movement*, i.e. the maximum deflection of the particles from their position of rest.

To indicate shorter wave lengths, in the same way as shown in Fig. 1.3, it would be necessary to choose particles with smaller masses and packed more closely, i.e. to subdivide the material more finely. This has its limits as soon as atomic dimensions are reached. It can then no longer be experted that the masses and forces would be evenly distributed. Elastic waves are therefore possible only in the case of wave lengths which are still very long compared with the distances between atoms or molecules.

1.2 Modes and Forms of Waves

The wave described in par. 1.3, called a *longitudinal wave*, because the oscillations occur in the *longitudinal direction*, i.e. the direction of propagation, is not the only kind of wave although from our point of view it is the most important. Since compressional and dilatational forces are active in it, it is also called a pressure or compression wave, and because its particle density fluctuates it has also been given the name density wave.

This is the real sound wave because it transmits the oscillations of a source of acoustic energy through the air to our ear. Experience shows that the same wave also transmits sound through liquid or solid bodies.

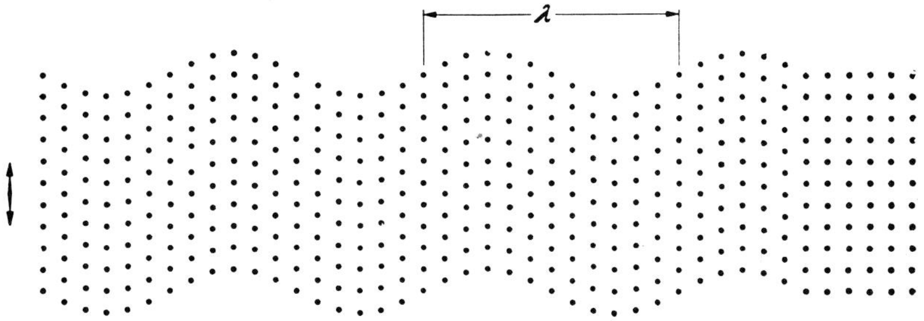

Fig. 1.4 Transverse wave.

However, in solid bodies also another kind of wave can occur, viz. the transverse wave; it is indicated schematically in Fig. 1.4 in the form of an instantaneous picture of the particle motion. It will again be assumed that the wave travels from left to right. It can be seen that in this case the particles no longer oscillate in the direction of propagation but at right angles to it, viz. transverse.

The excitations can be visualised as a motion in which the particles on the left interface of the body are moved sinusoidally up and down by a periodical *shear force*. In solid bodies such a shear force can be transmitted to the particles in the adjacent planes; their transverse oscillations will however show a lag in time, depending on their distance from the plane of excitation. This wave is also called a shear wave. Also in this case the wave length is determined by the distance between two planes in which particles are in a similar state. In Fig. 1.4 the wave length is indicated between two planes in which the particles at this moment pass through their position of rest in a direction from top to bottom.

The sound pressure of the longitudinal wave is in this case replaced by the alternating shear force, but the name "shear of sound" is not used.

The pressure is the force at *right angles* to the unit surface, while the shear force is defined as the force per unit surface, but *parallel* to it. Thus, the only difference between pressure and shear is one of direction. In all other respects these two characteristics are identical. In what follows we shall therefore speak only generally of sound pressure even where this refers to the shear in a transverse wave.

Fig. 1.4 indicates that the shear is greatest where the particles pass through their position of rest because at this point the relative displacement of two consecutive particle planes is greatest. At the points of maximum amplitude the shear is zero. The same has been found in respect of the sound pressure in Fig. 1.3: where the particles oscillate through their position of rest they either come closest to each other or are furthest apart. At these points the sound pressure reaches its maximum (or its minimum) value. The generalized sound pressure and the motion of the particles thus are not *in phase* but transposed a quarter period relative to each other.

Since gases and liquids are practically incapable of transmitting shear (otherwise they could not flow so readily along walls, e.g. through pipes), transverse waves can for the practical testing of materials attain appreciable distances only in solid bodies.

The various *kinds* or *modes* of waves can occur in different wave *forms*, whereby the form of the wave front is meant. Up to now we have described plane waves, i.e. waves in which a given phase of the oscillation is always the same in a given plane. This co-phasal plane is the wave surface which, during propagation, moves parallel to itself. The wave surface need not necessarily be flat and on the contrary is never strictly flat in the case of natural sound generators, but usually of complex curvature. For clearer presentation and to simplify the calculation it is, however, preferable to replace natural sound waves approximately by simple wave forms, e.g. plane, spherical or cylindrical waves.

On a given wave surface, e.g. on a sphere in the case of a spherical wave, only the phase is identical, e.g. the passage through zero at a given moment, but not necessarily the amplitude as well, e.g. the sound pressure. The latter, for instance, may have an appreciable value only within a certain angular sector about a given direction, while in other directions it may disappear completely. This represents a spherical wave beam as produced for instance by directional loud speakers in air, and in most cases also by ultrasonic sound generators in the testing of materials.

To avoid any misunderstanding it should be stated specifically that the description of natural acoustic phenomena by means of such simple wave forms for each case is permissible only within certain limits, e.g. in close proximity to a plane sound generator by plane waves, or at great distance by spherical waves.

In the case of the wave modes discussed above it was always presupposed that these waves are propagated in infinitely large bodies. In limited bodies, e.g. in plates or rods, the propagation is disturbed by refraction or reflection. Furthermore, in the case of reflection longitudinal waves can be transformed into transverse waves and vice versa. Because of these effects it becomes a very complex task to follow the propagation paths of sound even in bodies of relatively simple shape. In order to describe the propagation of sound in finite bodies one usually has to be satisfied with an investigation of the deformation of the surface concerned. This leads apparently to new kinds of waves which are typical for the form and dimensions of the body in which the sound is propagated.

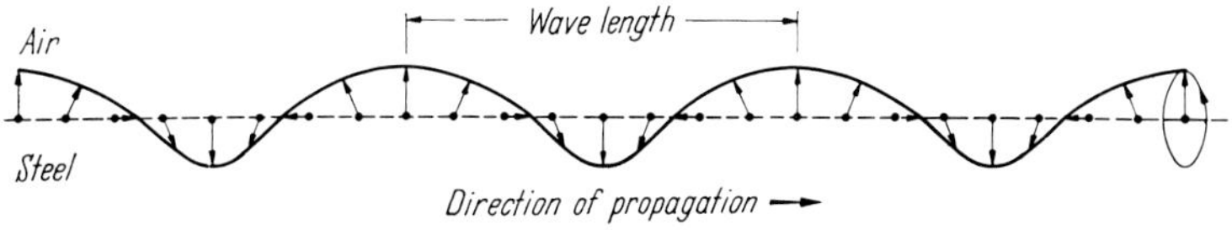

Fig. 1.5 Surface wave on steel; on the right, oscillation ellipse of a particle and sense of rotation (calculated according to [20], ratio of axes 0.44 : 1).

One should, however, very clearly realize that the wave types described in the following only appear to be new and unrelated to the basic longitudinal and transverse types of wave propagation because it had been agreed in advance not to describe in every detail the propagation of the longitudinal and transverse waves in the body concerned.

The *surface wave* which exists on the flat or curved boundary surface of an otherwise "infinite" solid substance, is the *surface or Rayleigh wave*, so called after Lord Rayleigh [18] (see also [67]). Fig. 1.5 shows an instantaneous picture of a surface wave on steel, or more accurately the motion of the top row of particles. The deformation is thus not strictly sinusoidal and is to some extent already known from water waves although the latter are not elastic waves but the result of gravitational forces. For water waves the oscillatory motion of the particles is circular, for Rayleigh waves elliptic, as indicated on the right in Fig. 1.5. At greater depth below the surface the amplitude of the oscillation decreases rapidly so that at a depth of approximately one wave length the particles are practically already at rest.

If the solid substance concerned is still further limited in size, one obtains a plate in which pure surface waves can no longer exist unless their wave length is considerably smaller than the thickness of the plate. This leads to various kinds of *plate waves*. In a given plate there can first of all be a pure transverse wave whose direction of oscillation is parallel to the surface, as shown in Fig. 1.6a (see [20, 129]). For the testing of materials this wave has not yet gained great importance, in contrast to the usual plate waves, also called *Lamb waves* [213, 20, 108] which always contain components of the particle oscillation at right angles to the surface. They occur in two different basic modes (Fig. 1.6b and c), viz. the symmetrical or *dilatational wave* and the asymmetrical or *bending wave*.

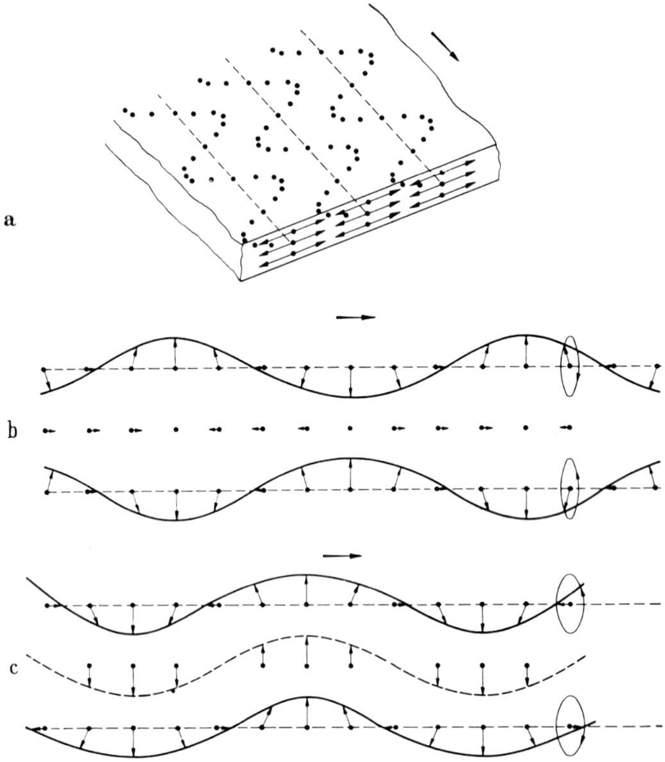

Fig, 1.6 Waves in plates. a) Transverse wave parallel to surface, b) and c) Lamb waves, symmetrical and asymmetrical fundamental waves in aluminium calculated according to [20] (ratio of axes of oscillation ellipses depending on thickness of plate).

The particles of the middle zone, viz. the neutral fibre, perform in the case of the first wave purely longitudinal oscillations, and in the case of the bending wave purely transverse oscillations. The other particles oscillate, in the case of both types, elliptically. For each kind there is an arbitrary number of harmonics which can be characterized briefly by the existence of more than one neutral fibre.

In the case of Lamb waves it is still relatively simple to recognize the basic longitudinal and transverse waves: they represent systems of plane waves reflected along zig-zag paths between the boundaries (see [20, 276, 19, 306]).

In the special case where the plate borders on one side on a different solid body, as in the case of a surface layer, the pure transverse waves (Fig. 1.6a) are called *Love waves* [129].

The plate under discussion is still unlimited in two directions. If still further limited in size, a rod is obtained, e.g. of round or square cross-section. By *rod wave* is usually understood the dilatational wave in a round rod which can be visualized as shown in Fig. 1.6b. In addition there is a great variety of bending waves, torsional waves and radial waves together with their harmonics which up to now have hardly been exploited for the testing of materials.

The discribed wave *forms* in limited bodies, like the plane wave or spherical wave in unlimited bodies, represent only simplified ideal forms of the natural phenomena of sound propagation. The picture of the surface and Lamb waves can be traced back for instance to the reflection of plane waves at the boundaries. In practice plane waves are obtained with good approximation only near sufficiently large, plane sound generators. At greater distances and in the case of small sound generators, the propagation of sound in plates differs considerably from the ideal picture of the Lamb wave.

1.3 Composite and Standing Waves, Interference

So far it has been tacitly assumed that the generating oscillation capable of producing one of the described wave types consists of a single frequency and lasts very long. Complex and brief oscillation phenomena can of course be visualized as consisting of an infinite, or also finite, number of such sinusoidal particle oscillations which differ in their amplitude, frequency and phase. In an elastic medium each such particle oscillation produces its own wave. In the case of longitudinal and transverse waves in a large body all frequencies have practically the same velocity and all component waves travel equally fast, so that each particle carries out the same oscillation. A complex and brief form of oscillation is thus transmitted by these waves unchanged if energy losses are neglected. Absorption or scattering may of course affect the various frequencies differently, as for instance in air where distant thunder appears to have a lower note: the higher frequencies are attenuated more severely.

The undistorted transmission of a signal in the case of the two principal kinds of waves by no means applies generally: in the case of plate waves and rod waves the velocities in general depend on the frequency. A sound pulse, as frequently used for the testing of materials, is thus, in the case of these waves, not sustained over a distance of any length but is dissipated because its component waves travel at different velocities.

Let us now consider two waves of different direction, frequency and amplitude being generated at two different points in a given material, and analyse the movement of a particle which is exposed simultaneously to the action of both waves. Provided both amplitudes do not stress the substance beyond its elastic limit, within the so-called linear range, the motions are added vectorially, i.e. according to a parallelogram and are composed of motions which the particle would carry out alone in each

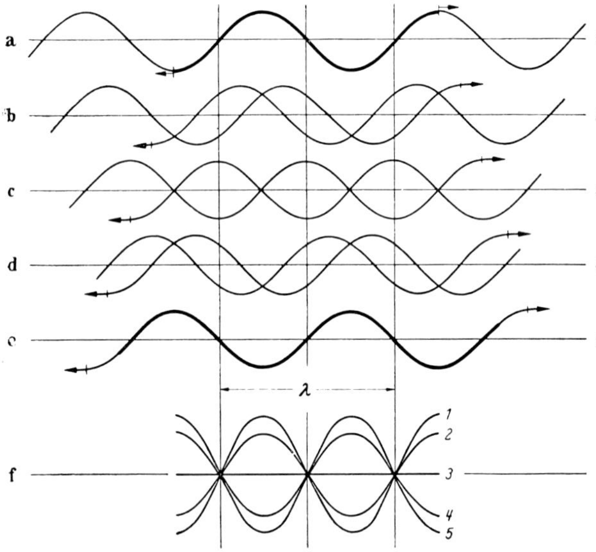

Fig. 1.7 Formation of a standing wave by two waves from opposite directions.

separate wave. In the case of waves of different frequency, the result is in general aperiodic and complex, and therefore of no general interest. In this process however, neither of the waves interferes with the other. For instance, it is possible for one sound beam to penetrate another. The two sound beams then change neither their original direction nor their frequency and amplitude.

In one simple case, however, one obtains an interesting form of the particle oscillations, viz. a *standing wave*. This paradoxical formation (for the essence of a wave is that it travels) results from the superposition of two similar plane waves of identical frequency, amplitude and (in the case of transverse waves) direction of oscillation but different direction of propagation. The special case in which they have exactly opposing directions of propagation is shown in Fig. 1.7 for a transverse wave. The sinusoidal curves represent the connecting lines of a series of particles (of matter) at a given moment. Figs. 1.7a to e show this state for five consecutive moments. Fig. 1.7f is the overall oscillation of the standing wave. The most important fact in this connection is that certain particles constantly remain in a state of rest, which never is the case in an ordinary wave. The points where the two waves constantly cancel each other are called *nodes*, and the points of maximum amplitude between them, *antinodes*.

This form of the wave is generally known from the natural oscillations of taut strings. In the case of the steric standing transverse or longitudinal wave it is, however, necessary to visualize the presentation in Fig. 1.7 supplemented spatially by numerous additional rows of particles. The nodes and antinodes are then located on fixed planes.

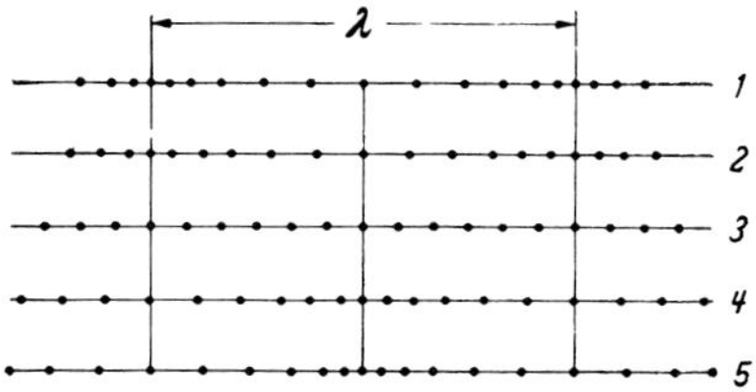

Fig. 1.8 Standing longitudinal wave. Instantaneous pictures at different moments 1 to 5, corresponding to Fig. 1.7. The nodes of the motion are located in planes spaced $\lambda/2$.

It should not be overlooked that the presentation as a standing wave or as the mutual penetration of two opposing waves concerns the same physical fact, as for instance 2 + 2 and 4.

The standing longitudinal wave is derived from the presentation of a standing transverse wave by regarding the amplitudes of the sinusoidal oscillations in Fig. 1.7 as displacements of the particles *in* the direction of wave travel or against it (Fig. 1.8). The points of maximum density and dilution are located in the plane of the nodes spaced one wave length from each other. The nodes of the motion are therefore simultaneously the antinodes of the sound pressure and vice versa, as is readily seen in Fig. 1.8. The nodes of motion and pressure are thus located a quarter wave length from each other.

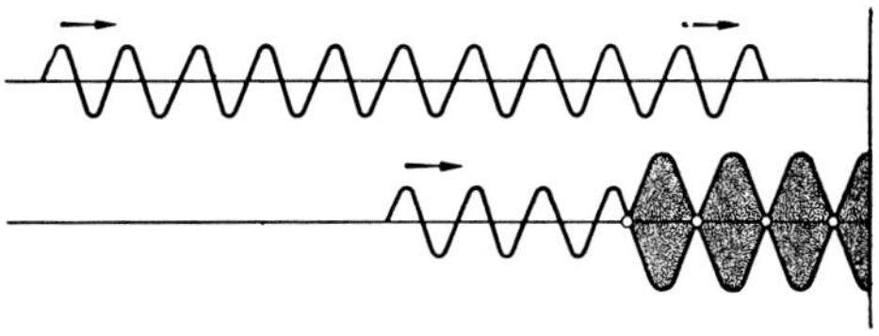
Fig. 1.9 Standing wave through reflection on free wall. Plotted is the amplitude of the particles. At the free wall it has an antinode.

In practical ultrasonics standing waves occur frequently, e.g. if a wave is reflected from a smooth surface. This of course presupposes that the wave, unless it is infinitely long, can still cover itself sufficiently after being reflected. Fig. 1.9 shows the reflection of a short wave train from a wall, resulting in a brief formation of a standing wave over a distance of a few wave lengths.

Fig. 1.9 shows the reflection of a wave on a *free wall*, i.e. at the interface between a given substance and vacuum or air, where the wave is totally reflected. According to the *boundary conditions* the motion of the particles has at that point a maximum, viz. an antinode and the pressure or shear has a node. In Fig. 1.9 is plotted the amplitued of the motion which can be regarded both as longitudinal motion in the case of a pressure wave and as a transverse motion in the case of a shear wave.

Standing ultrasonic pressure waves are produced intentionally when measuring wall thicknesses by the resonance method. In other instances they may, however, cause considerable confusion and should be avoided.

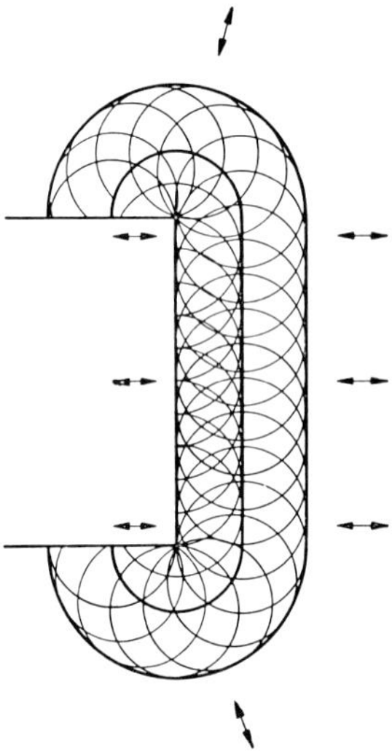

Fig. 1.10 Construction of wave surfaces from elementary waves according to HUYGENS.

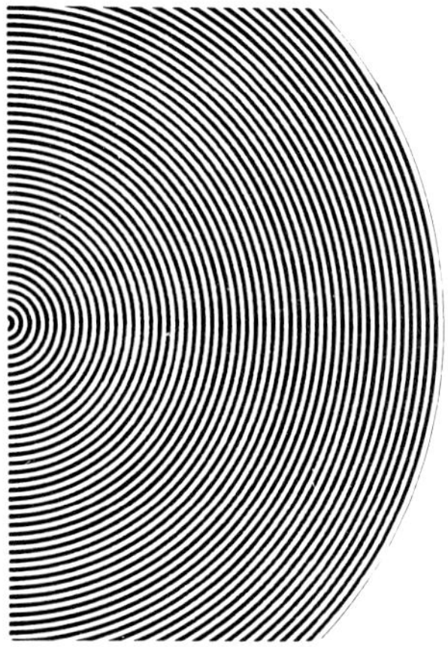

Fig. 1.11 Spherical wave graticule, a device for the construction of simulated wave fields.

The standing wave is a special case of the superposition of different waves of the same frequency, which is generally called interference. This is also the basis of a very vivid method for demonstrating commonly occurring wave forms and wave fields, viz. *Huygens' principle* which will render us good service when explaining the radiation of ultrasonic waves.

Briefly expressed, this principle states that any arbitrary wave form can be constructed from a large number of simple spherical waves of the same frequency, i.e. the so-called elementary waves, which must, however, be chosen correctly regarding origin, phase and amplitude. Every wave surface can be visualized as an envelope of such elementary waves whose origin is located on a preceding wave surface. Fig. 1.10 makes this clear. It shows in cross-section a piston-shaped sound generator with a few wave surfaces constructed according to Huygens' principle. It can be seen that in the centre, in front of the plane sound generator a plane wave surface is formed which at its edge (seen 3-dimensionally) changes into an annular form.

According to the same principle it can also be seen that an impermeable wall produces no sharp shadow in a sound field because its edge can be regarded as the origin of new elementary waves which travel around the wall into the shadow zone.

However, application of this principle cannot yet provide an answer to the question how strong the excitation becomes at a given point of the sound field, e.g. in the shadow of the wall. The solution can only be found by a mathematical treatment, according to FRESNEL (1.8). In some specific cases occurring in practice one can arrive at a vivid construction of wave fields from spherical waves in the following manner. The field of an elementary wave is drawn in the form of a system of black and white rings (Fig. 1.11) reproduced photographically and copied repeatedly superimposed on one another, in which the centres of the individual pictures, each time shifted slightly, are located at uniform distances on a wave surface (POHL [17]). Such a picture discloses the pattern of the wave surfaces and – at least qualitatively – the intensity of the excitation by the mean luminosity of the graticule.

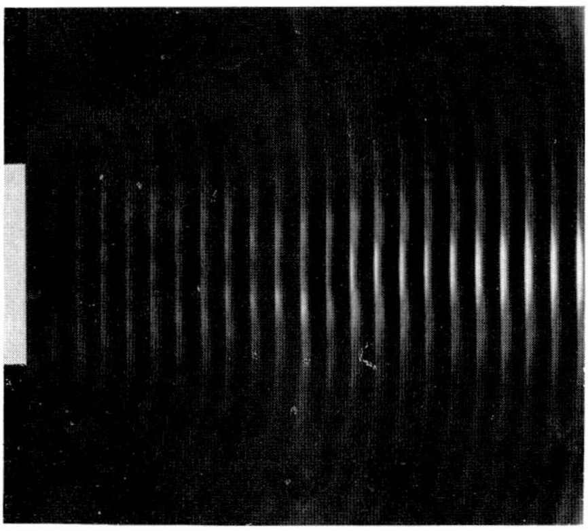

Fig. 1.12 Picture of a simulated sound field in front of a radiator with the diameter to wave length ratio $D/\lambda = 8$.

Fig. 1.12 shows the picture of a sound field in front of a plane oscillator simulated in this manner. It discloses that at greater distances from the radiator the wave surfaces become distinctly spherical. The interesting intensity distribution will be discussed in greater detail in Sec. 1.8.

1.4 Formulas and Numerical Data

Where not stated otherwise, the units of the MKS system are used in the following, viz. the metre (m), the kilogram (kg) and the second (s), furthermore for

Force	1 Newton (N) $= 1$ kgm/s^2 $= 10^5$ dyne
Electrical voltage	1 Volt (V)
Electrical current	1 Ampere (A)
Power	1 Watt (W) $= 1$ Voltampere $= 1$ kgm^2/s^3

In addition the following quantities, designations and units occur:

Density of material	ϱ	kg/m^3
Velocity of sound	c	m/s
Wave length	λ	m
Frequency (or angular frequency $\omega = 2\pi f$)	f	s^{-1} = Hertz (Hz) = cycles/second = c/s
Displacement of a particle (amplitude of its oscillation, maximum displacement from position of rest)	A	m
Sound pressure (amplitude of alternating sound pressure)	P	N/m^2
Sound intensity (energy transfer per second through unit surface of wave surface)	I	W/m^2

The following relation between frequency, wave length and sound frequency is valid for all kinds of waves

$$f\lambda = c. \tag{1.1}$$

Instead of the units Hertz and metre, however, MHz (megahertz or Mc/s) and millimetre are usually used for the frequency and wave length respectively, because this furnishes numerical data of the order 1 which for our purpose are easy to memorise:

$$f \text{ in MHz} \cdot \lambda \text{ in mm} = c \text{ in } 10^3 \text{ m/s or km/s}. \tag{1.2}$$

For general orientation a few rounded-off values of the wave lengths in steel and water in the frequency range from 0.5 to 10 MHz, which are of main interest in the following, are given below.

Table 1.1

Frequency (MHz)	Wave lengths (mm)		
	in steel		in water
	Longitudinal waves ($c_l = 5.9 \cdot 10^3$ m/s)	Transverse waves ($c_t = 3.2 \cdot 10^3$ m/s)	($c = 1.5 \cdot 10^3$ m/s)
0.5	12	6.5	3
1	6	3	1.5
2	3	1.6	0.8
4	1.5	0.8	0.4
6	1	0.6	0.25
10	0.6	0.3	0.15

Table A 1 in the Appendix gives more accurate values of the velocity of sound, and other constants of additional materials. Be it noted here that the most commonly used frequency, 2 MHz in the case of longitudinal waves in steel, the most common material, corresponds to a wave length of approx. 3 mm. This at the same time gives an idea of the dimension of a given flaw which can still be detected reliably when using this frequency. Furthermore it should be kept in mind that for longitudinal waves the ratio of the wave lengths in water and steel is fairly accurately 1 : 4.

In the case of plane and spherical waves sound pressure and particle amplitude are connected to each other by the relation (see [1])

$$P = \varrho\, c\, \omega\, A \quad [\mathrm{N/m^2}],$$
$$= W\, \omega\, A, \tag{1.3}$$

if the product of density and velocity of sound $\varrho c = W$ is abbreviated and called *acoustic impedance* (in the literature also called soundwave impedance or specific acoustic impedance). Materials with high sound resistance are called "sonically hard", in contrast to "sonically soft" materials. Steel with $W = 45 \cdot 10^6$ kg/m²s is sonically harder than water with $W = 1.5 \cdot 10^6$ (see Table A 1).

Although the sound pressure is, from our point of view, the most important quantity of the sound field, the intensity of a wave is nevertheless sometimes also of interest. In the case of plane and spherical waves it is related to the sound pressure or the amplitude as follows:

$$I = \frac{1}{2}\frac{P^2}{W} \quad [\mathrm{W/m^2}], \tag{1.4}$$

$$= \frac{1}{2}\, W \omega^2 A^2 \tag{1.5}$$

The intensity is thus proportional to the square of the amplitude of the sound pressure. All relations apply equally to longitudinal and transverse waves; it is only necessary to insert the applicable value of the acoustic impedance with the correct velocity of sound. For longitudinal waves one derives from (1.3) the sound pressure as force per unit surface at right angles to the wave surface, and for transverse waves as shear force per unit surface parallel to the wave surface.

Sound pressure is here understood to be exclusively the alternating sound pressure. In sound fields there occurs in addition a continuous pressure, the *sound-radiation pressure,* which in the case of liquids for instance produces a flow and which propels suspended particles away from the source of sound. This is of no interest in the testing of materials.

In Fig. 1.3 the amplitude A of the particles has been chosen very large for the sake of clarity, viz. 10% of the wave length. Using formulas (1.3) to (1.5) it is rather interesting to obtain an idea of the values occurring in practice. One thus obtains

$$\frac{A}{\lambda} = \sqrt{\frac{I}{2\pi^2 \varrho c^3}}\,.$$

In air with density 1.3 kg/m³ and the velocity of sound 330 m/s, a value of 10% is reached only at intensities of 10^7 W/m² (1,000 W/cm²), which is among the highest values reached to date for very brief periods only. In liquids and in solid bodies the amplitudes would be much smaller, e.g. in water 0.04% of the wave length. In reality the generation of such high amplitudes is impossible because at the enormous compressional and tensile forces of approx. $6 \cdot 10^6$ N/m² (= 60 atm) cavitation occurs. When testing materials, an intensity of 10 W/cm² is regarded as already very high, but in steel it produces only an amplitude of $1.8 \cdot 10^6$, or approx. 2 millionths of the wave length.

The velocities of the various kinds of sound waves can be calculated from the elastic constants of the material concerned, viz. the modulus of elasticity E (measured in N/m², technically in kp/mm²; for conversion: 1 kp/mm² = $0.98 \cdot 10^7$ N/m²), and Poisson's ratio σ (a dimensionless number).

For longitudinal waves:

$$c_l = \sqrt{\frac{E}{\varrho} \frac{1-\sigma}{(1+\sigma)(1-2\sigma)}}, \tag{1.6}$$

for transverse waves

$$c_t = \sqrt{\frac{E}{\varrho} \frac{1}{2(1+\sigma)}} = \sqrt{\frac{\mu}{\varrho}} \tag{1.7}$$

for surface waves (approximation formula according to BERGMANN [17])

$$c_o = \frac{0.87 + 1.12\,\sigma}{1-\sigma} \sqrt{\frac{E}{\varrho} \frac{1}{2(1+\sigma)}}. \tag{1.8}$$

The various velocities of sound are linked by the following relations

$$c_t = c_l \sqrt{\frac{1-2\sigma}{2(1-\sigma)}}, \tag{1.9}$$

$$c_o = c_t \frac{0.87 + 1.12\,\sigma}{1+\sigma}. \tag{1.10}$$

For all solid materials Poisson's ratio σ lies between 0 and 0.5, so that the value of the expression

$$\sqrt{\frac{1-2\sigma}{2(1-\sigma)}}$$

always lies below 1, or more accurately between 0.7 and 0. In steel and aluminium

$$\sigma = 0.28 \text{ and } 0.34, \text{ respectively.}$$

Therefore

$$\frac{c_t}{c_l} = 0.55 \text{ and } 0.49, \text{ respectively.}$$

Calculated roughly in both substance, the velocity of transverse waves is half that of longitudinal waves.

According to Eq. (1.10) the velocity of the surface waves is always slightly lower than that of the transverse waves, and in the case of steel and aluminium

$$\frac{c_o}{c_t} = 0.92 \text{ and } 0.93, \text{ respectively.}$$

For Lamb waves the velocity of sound cannot be found so easily. It depends not only on the elastic constants of the material, but also on the plate thickness and – in contrast to the longitudinal and transverse waves – on the frequency. In the Appendix the speed of propagation of Lamb waves is shown in the diagram of Table 9. For other materials calculations have been made by Pursey [291], specifically for values of $\sigma = 0.25$; 0.33 and 0.375. For aluminium, Firestone [107] has presented curves determined purely graphically.

The dispersion of the speed of propagation (dependence on the frequency) in the case of Lamb waves has important consequences for the propagation of a limited wave train, viz. a single pulse.

Like the other Tables in the Appendix, the diagram in Table 9 has been calculated on the assumption that purely sinusoidal wave forms are used. A pulse such as shown for instance in Fig. 1.13, however, displays neither uniform height nor uniform length of the individual particle oscillations, and thus lacks the main characteristics of sinusoidal wave motion.

The pulse behaviour can, however, be recognized if a given pulse is visualized as a superposition of purely sinusoidal particle waves with slightly differing frequencies. An example of such a synthesis of a 1 MHz pulse is shown in Fig. 1.14.

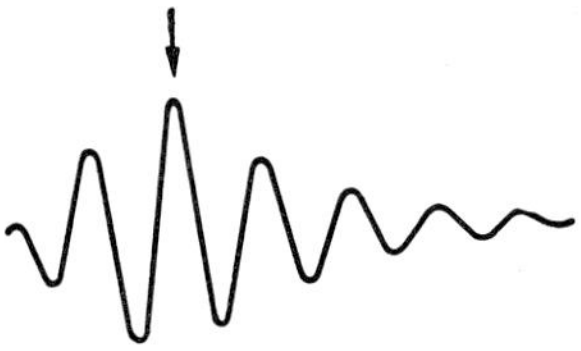

Fig. 1.13 Commonly encountered pulse form when testing materials.

The general rule is that the synthesis of a given pulse requires a greater number of sinusoidal partial waves with frequencies further displaced from the mean frequency, the narrower the pulse. Conversely, an originally narrow pulse is the more deformed (usually broadened), the more the partial waves with frequencies further away from the mean frequency are suppressed, e.g. by unfavourable conditions of propagation. Such a broadening of the pulse also occurs if the partial waves of the pulse have different velocities of propagation, as for example in the Lamb wave. Examples of the "dispersion" of a pulse are shown in Figs. 3.114 and 3.115.

Dispersion phenomena are also evidenced by Love waves if they are propagated in layers whose thickness is of the same order of magnitude as that of the wave length. The dependence of the propagation velocity of plate waves and Love waves on the thickness can be exploited for thickness measurements based on velocity of propagation.

According to [373] surface waves also show dispersion when travelling on curved surfaces. Eq. (1.8) therefore is valid only for plane surfaces. The phase velocity c_0 depends on the ratio of curvature to wave length. For a radius of curvature $R = r\lambda$, c_0 is approximately 10% greater on a convex surface, and lower on a concave surface.

Regarding the velocity of sound as a material constant, it should here also be mentioned that the values given in Table A 1 represent true material constants only for materials having amorphous, vitreous structure. In crystalline materials the elastic properties usually differ in different crystal directions, and therefore also the velocities of sound. The values in the Table are merely mean values for random agglomerations of crystals and therefore in practice deviations from these can easily occur if a given crystal direction is preferred, if the material has a *texture* which can be recognized precisely by the differences in acoustic velocity in different directions of the sample concerned. The elastic anisotropy is particularly pronounced in the case of copper and brass.

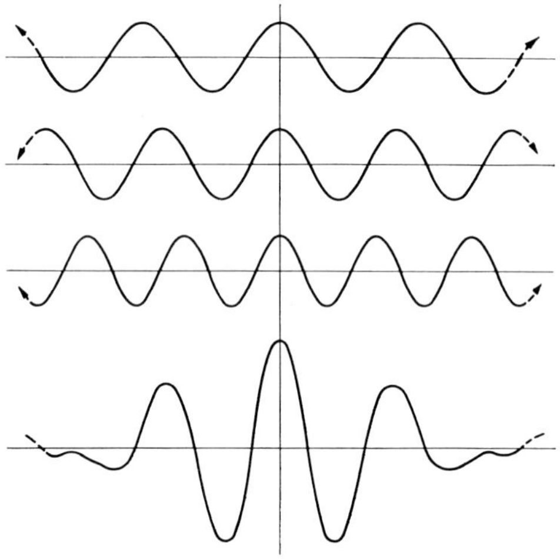

Fig. 1.14 Synthesis of a 1 MHz pulse composed of purely sinusoidal partial waves of 0.85, 1 and 1.21 MHz.

Furthermore, the velocity of sound changes in heterogeneous bodies; usually it is reduced by small admixtures of a foreign substance. A similar effect is produced by pores, e.g. in porcelain where porosity can be detected practically by the reduced velocity of sound.

Finally, the velocity of sound depends on internal and external stresses of the material, which can likewise be measured by this effect (cf. 3.62).

In solid substances the temperature dependence is, for practical purposes, insignificant but it plays a certain role in the case of accurate measurements in liquids.

1.5 Sound Waves on Boundaries at Perpendicular Incidence

1.51 Single, Plane Interfaces

Analysis of a wave in an infinitely extended substance is possible only theoretically because in practice every substance terminates somewhere, i.e. it has a boundary. There the propagation of the wave is disturbed. If the material concerned borders on an empty space, no wave can go beyond this boundary because the transmission of such a wave always requires the presence of particles of material. At such a *free* boundary the wave will therefore return in one form or another. On a smooth boundary one then speaks of reflection, on a rough boundary of scattering. In this connection the roughness, i.e. the irregularities of the boundary, should be measured in terms of the wave length. If another material is behind the boundary, and adheres to the first material so that forces can be transmitted, the wave can be propagated in it, although usually in a more or less changed direction, intensity and mode.

We consider here only the simple case of a plane wave striking a plane and smooth boundary at right angles. For reasons of symmetry only plane waves can then be propagated at right angles from the boundary, viz. a reflected wave which opposes the incident wave, and a transmitted wave.

Let us calculate their sound pressures. For this we require the acoustic impedance of the two materials, W_1 and W_2.

Material 1	Material 2
$W_1 = \varrho_1 c_1$	$W_2 = \varrho_2 c_2$
Incident wave	Transmitted wave
Sound pressure P_e →	Sound pressure P_d →
← Reflected wave	
Sound pressure P_r	

We refer the sound pressures of the reflected and the transmitted waves to the pressure of the incident wave and form the ratios

$$\frac{P_r}{P_e} = R \quad \text{and} \quad \frac{P_d}{P_e} = D .$$

R and D are the coefficients of reflection and transmission, respectively, of the sound pressure; both are dimensionless numerical values.

We then derive (see e.g. Schoch [207]):

$$R = \frac{W_2 - W_1}{W_2 + W_1}, \qquad D = \frac{2 W_2}{W_2 + W_1} . \tag{1.11}$$

As an example we shall calculate R and D on the interface steel/water. According to Table A 1 we have for longitudinal waves

$$W_1 \text{ (steel)} = 45 \cdot 10^6 \text{ kg/m}^2\text{s}, \quad W_2 \text{ (water)} = 1.5 \cdot 10^6 \text{ kg/m}^2\text{s}.$$

Thus

$$R = \frac{1.5 - 45}{1.5 + 45} = -0.935 , \qquad D = \frac{2 \cdot 1.5}{1.5 + 45} = 0.065 .$$

Expressed as percentages the reflected wave has −93.5% of the sound pressure of the incident wave and the transmitted wave 6.5%. The negative sign indicates the reversal of the phase relative to the incident wave: if at a given instant the incident wave has just reached the positive maximum of the sound pressure (excess pressure), the reflected wave has at the same instant its negative maximum (reduced pressure) at this boundary. This case is shown in Fig. 1.15a.

If, in the reverse case the wave coming from water strikes steel, an exchange of W_1 and W_2 furnishes

$$R = +0.935, \quad D = 1.935.$$

Since R is positive, incident and reflected wave are in phase. The transmitted wave has 193.5% of the sound pressure (Fig. 1.15b).

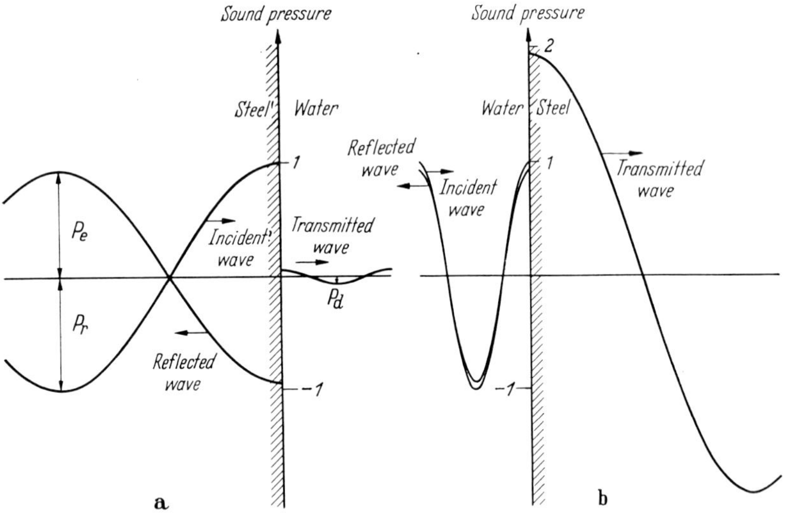

Fig. 1.15 Sound pressure values in the case of reflection on the interface steel/water, incident wave in steel (a) or in water (b).

At first glance a sound pressure exceeding 100% seems paradoxical and one suspects a contradiction of the energy law. However, according to Eq. (1.4) the intensity, i.e. the energy per unit time and unit area, is not calculated from the sound pressure (squared) only but also from the acoustic impedance of the material in which the wave travels. However, since this resistance in steel is very much greater than in water, the calculation shows that the intensity of the transmitted wave is very much smaller there than in water in spite of the higher sound pressure.

The balance expressed in intensities calculated on a given boundary for the case of perpendicular incidence furnishes

$$I_e = I_r + I_d,$$

i.e. the incident intensity appears again in the two emitted intensities, as required for the conservation of energy. However, in the case of sound pressure one has

$$P_e + P_r = P_d \quad \text{or} \quad 1 + R = D,$$

as confirmed when recalculating the above two cases.

Phase reversal, characterized by a negative value of R, always occurs in the case of reflection on the sonically softer material. However, since the phase value is usually of no interest when testing materials, we shall generally omit the negative sign in what follows.

Disregarding the sign, the reflecting power is independent of the sequence of two materials, not, however, their transmittance.

In the literature the coefficients of reflection and transmittance frequently are referred to the intensity (Bergmann [1]) or also to the amplitude of the particle motion (Schoch [207]), which can easily lead to misunderstandings. In this discussion these quantities are exclusively referred to sound pressure.

Table A 2 gives values of the coefficient of reflection for certain interfaces between solid and liquid materials, which are of interest in the testing of materials at perpendicular incidence. When measuring these values, which in this case were calculated from the acoustic impedances, higher figures may be obtained if for instance the two materials do not completely "wet" each other. For instance, mercury does not wet bright steel without taking special precautions (oiling or amalgamating), so that total reflection results.

Compared to liquid and solid materials, gaseous materials have a very low acoustic impedance. For air it is $0.0004 \cdot 10^6$, so that for the interface steel/air the coefficient of reflection differs from the value 1 only by approx. $1 \cdot 10^{-6}$. Where only sound phenomena in liquid or solid materials are considered, boundaries with air can therefore be regarded as boundaries with vacuum, and are called *free* boundaries.

The formulas (1.11) are also valid for transverse waves. Since, however, the velocity of sound in liquids and gases is zero for transverse waves, a transverse wave is always completely reflected (coefficient of reflection = 1) in a solid material on its interface with a liquid or gaseous substance. For transverse waves the formulas are therefore of significance only in the case of solid/solid interfaces.

1.52 Multiple Interfaces, Plate and Gap

In addition to the interface between two materials of large dimensions, the double interface, as in the case of plate and gap, is of interest for the testing of materials, e.g. for the transmission of sound through a sheet immersed in water, or through a crack in a solid body. The wave coming from material 1 reaches the plate consisting of material 2 and is split into a transmitted and a reflected wave. After passing through the plate, the transmitted wave is split again at the second interface, and so forth. The result is a sequence of reflections in both directions inside the plate. On either side a sequence of waves leaves the plate which are superimposed and whose total sound pressure has to be determined. This cannot be done simply by calculating and adding the sound pressure according to Eq. (1.11) for each individual split wave. If the incident wave is of unlimited length, the individual waves are intensified or weakened, depending on the phase position, when they are superimposed, the result being interferences.

Using for the ratio of the two acoustic impedances the abbreviation

$$m = \frac{W_1}{W_2}$$

d for the plate thickness, and λ for the wave length in the plate material 2, one obtains (see also B. BERGMANN [17]):

$$D_{\text{plate}} = \frac{1}{\sqrt{1 + \frac{1}{4}\left(m - \frac{1}{m}\right)^2 \sin^2 \frac{2\pi d}{\lambda}}}\,,$$

$$R_{\text{plate}} = \sqrt{\frac{\frac{1}{4}\left(m - \frac{1}{m}\right)^2 \sin^2 \frac{2\pi d}{\lambda}}{1 + \frac{1}{4}\left(m - \frac{1}{m}\right)^2 \sin^2 \frac{2\pi d}{\lambda}}}\,. \tag{1.12}$$

Because of the sine functions, both expressions are periodical, i.e. their values fluctuate regularly between fixed limits with increasing thickness.

Minima of R and maxima of D occur when $d = 0$, 1/2, 2/2, 3/2 et seq.

and

maxima of R and minima of D occur at $d = 1/4$, 3/4, 5/4 et seq.

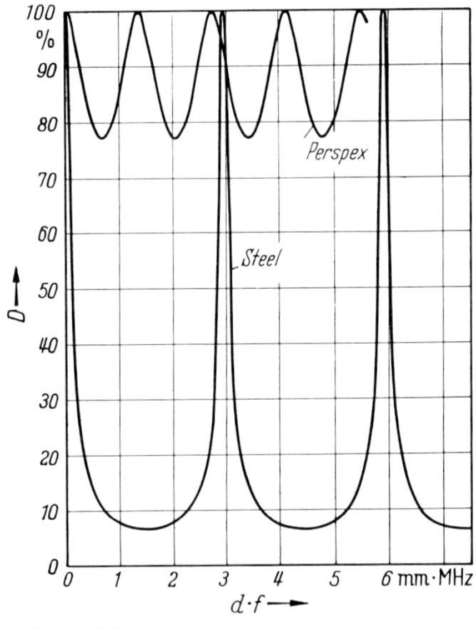

Fig. 1.16 Transmittance D of a steel plate and a perspex plate, respectively, in water, plotted against the product of plate thickness and frequency.

Fig. 1.16 shows the transmittance of a steel plate and a perspex plate in water, plotted over the product of the plate thickness d and the frequency f. At the maxima both plates show complete transmittance and therefore no reflection ($D = 100\%$, $R = 0$).

The presentation of Fig. 1.16 uses the frequency instead of the wave length because usually the former is given when testing materials. For a given frequency the abscissa can be used as a scale of the plate thickness, or alternatively if the thickness is given, as a scale of the frequency. Example: sheet steel of 1 mm thickness transmits completely just at the frequency 2.95 MHz (d in mm, frequency in MHz, $d \cdot f = 2.95$). Or: to permit undisturbed and reflection-free passage of a frequency of 1 MHz, partitions of perspex can be used, having thicknesses of 1.37 mm, 2.74 mm, 4.11 mm.

In the case of steel immersed in water, and similarly for other materials having large acoustic impedance ratios, the transmittance ranges are very small, as in fact Fig. 1.16 shows. At these points even a small change in plate thickness or frequency already produces a pronounced drop in transmittance. This is one of the great difficulties in the testing of materials when using continuous ultrasonic waves.

Since Eq. (1.12) is valid for arbitrary materials 1 and 2, it can also be applied to a sheet of air in a solid body, i.e. an air-filled gap, which in the form of a crack in a given test object plays an important role in the testing of materials. Theoretically the result is a curve of the transmittance similar to that shown in Fig. 1.16 for a steel plate in water, with the difference that the maxima are spaced much more closely, viz. at approx. 1/20 of the distance, and that in addition they are so narrow that on the scale used in Fig. 1.16 they could only be indicated by extremely thin lines on the zero line. Of practical importance is only the drop of the first transmittance maximum at zero in the case of very thin gaps. The remaining maxima could be obtained only with carefully aligned coplanar gap faces at extremely constant frequency.

The result is shown in Fig. 1.17 for the transmittance, and in Fig. 1.18 for the reflection, for a given gap in steel and in aluminium if the gap is filled with air and water, respectively. The scale for the thicknesses is logarithmic so that very thin gaps will be included in the picture. At a frequency of 1 MHz e.g. this scale covers the range from 10^{-8} to 1 mm.

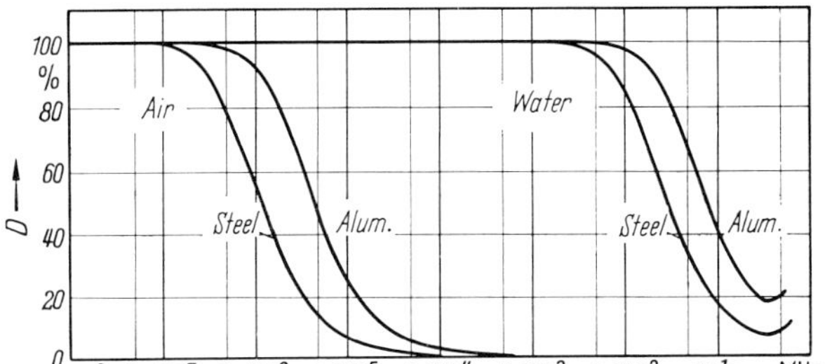

Fig. 1.17 Transmittance of a gap in steel and aluminium when filled with air and water, respectively, plotted against the product of gap thickness and frequency.

First of all, Fig. 1.18 shows that already at 1 MHz a gap of 10^{-8} mm filled with air produces a *reflection* of 1% which is readily measurable. This is the principle of the method for detecting cracks in solid bodies by reflected waves. With such a fine crack however, the *transmittance* could not yet be distinguished from that of a specimen without crack: according to Fig. 1.17 it remains practically unchanged at 100%.

However, an air gap of 10^{-8} mm is purely hypothetical. Even the most accurate end gauges, if pressed together, still have a gap of 10^{-4} to 10^{-5} mm. According to Fig. 1.18 such a gap should reflect almost 100%. However, this is by no means the case because, apparently, a foreign

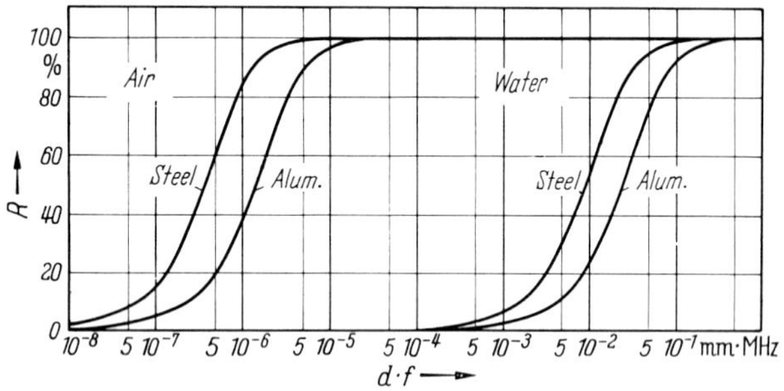

Fig. 1.18 Reflection by a gap as in Fig. 1.17.

layer remains on the surface even if cleaned most carefully, which reduces the reflection and increases the transmission. The pronounced effect of a liquid in the gap is clearly evidenced by Figs. 1.17 and 1.18, which theoretically is equivalent to a reduction of the gap width by 4 orders of magnitude. However, according to [361] even pure air gaps, which can be produced between glass plates and which can be measured very accurately by light interference, transmit even at thicknesses which are several orders of magnitude greater than expected.

Nevertheless, theoretically, a hairline crack of 1 μm in steel and filled with oil can still be expected to reflect 6% at 1 MHz, which would be quite adequate for its detection. (The acoustic impedance of oil is similar to that of water and thus has a similar influence on the reflection). In the materials with an acoustic impedance lower than that of steel the reflection for a given gap is weaker, e.g. in the case of fine gaps in aluminium it is only approx. one third. To counteract this effect it would be necessary to exploit the influence of the frequency: a four-fold frequency would furnish the same value as in the case of steel. In general, therefore, higher frequencies are better suited to the detection of fine cracks.

The above discussions all refer to the reflection and transmission of infinitely long waves, i.e. continuous waves. It is, however, important to have a clear conception of the differences which arise in the case of short wave trains, i.e. so-called pulses of only a few oscillations.

The length of the wave train does not occur in formulas (1.11) for the reflection and transmission at a given interface. It is, however, necessary to ensure that the reflected and the transmitted waves do not later return to the interface after an arbitrary number of reflections and thus disturb the process by interference. In the case of continuous waves this is in fact often not very easy to achieve.

The conditions are quite different, however, for the reflection and transmission in the case of a plate according to (1.12). The interesting behaviour of a plate in an acoustic field depends precisely on these disturbances, viz. the interferences, in a very long wave train. If the wave train is so short that it cannot "bite its own tail" after a single reflection in the plate, no interferences are produced. In this case a given incident pulse is split into a reflected and a transmitted series of completely separate and mutually independent single pulses, each of which can be calculated according to the simple formulas (1.11) by applying them repeatedly to the individual reflection and transmission phenomena. As a result of the repeated splitting, the acoustic pressure of the pulse sequences then decreases continuously, but remains completely independent of the thickness of the plate.

In the transition range between short pulses and continuous waves the wave train partially reaches its tail, resulting in interferences being produced over a certain section of its length. In that case a sequence of connected wave trains with fluctuating amplitude leaves the plate on both sides, the fluctuation in turn depending on the plate thickness and the frequency.

In the case of the above-mentioned thin gaps every pulse, even a short one, is equivalent to a wave train of long duration because the width of the gap is in this case much smaller than one wave length. The results therefore apply also to pulse transmission.

Attention is furthermore drawn to the fact that a smooth transition between the properties of two different materials in a given boundary layer changes the results considerably: reflection may then be completely absent. In the above discussions it was always presupposed that the transition is sharply defined or at least very short compared with one wave length.

1.6 Sound Waves at Interfaces with Oblique Incidence

1.61 The Law of Refraction

If a sound wave strikes a plane interface obliquely, at an angle of incidence α_e to the perpendicular (Fig. 1.19), reflected and transmitted waves arise as in optics. The transmitted waves are also called refracted waves because their direction has changed relative to the direction of incidence. The angles of emergence α_r and α_d depend on the angle of incidence and on the acoustic velocities of the two materials. The acoustic pressures, which in the case of perpendicular incidence could still be determined by relatively simple formulas, have now become functions of the angles, the acoustic velocities and the acoustic impedances. They are tabulated in the Appendix. In contrast to optics, a new phenomenon has now been added according to which one kind of wave can be transformed into another, viz. longitudinal waves into transverse waves and vice versa.

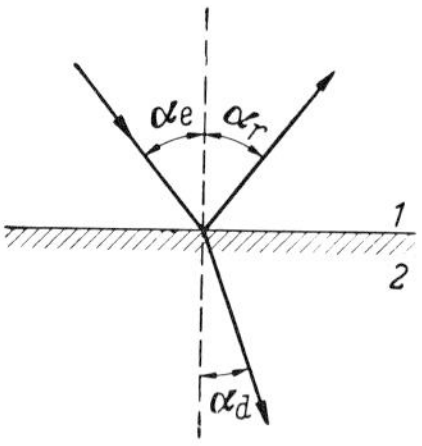

Fig. 1.19 Reflection and refraction of a plane wave on the plane interface between two materials 1 and 2 at oblique incidence.

The directions of the reflected and the transmitted waves are determined by the general law of refraction

$$\frac{\sin \alpha_{\mathrm{I}}}{\sin \alpha_{\mathrm{II}}} = \frac{c_{\mathrm{I}}}{c_{\mathrm{II}}} \tag{1.13}$$

Here I and II are two entirely arbitrary waves linked by a reflection or refraction process, with the acoustic velocities c_{I} and c_{II}. Example: Let I be the incident wave in Fig. 1.19 with α_e and c_1 (in material 1), and let II be the transmitted longitudinal wave with α_d and c_2. Thus

$$\frac{\sin \alpha_e}{\sin \alpha_d} = \frac{c_1}{c_2}$$

With α_e given, α_d is determined by:

$$\sin \alpha_d = \frac{c_2}{c_1} \sin \alpha_e \,.$$

Example: Let (1) be water with $c_1 = 1.5 \cdot 10^3$ m/s, and let (2) be steel with $6 \cdot 10^3$ m/s (rounded off), thus $c_2/c_1 = 4$. At an angle of incidence of 10°, $\sin \alpha_e = 0.17$. Therefore

$$\sin \alpha_d = 4 \cdot 0.17 = 0.68\,,$$

$$\alpha_d = 43°\,.$$

In contrast to Fig. 1.19 the transmitted wave emerges in this case at an angle greater than the incident angle: the greater acoustic velocity is linked to the greater angle. In Fig. 1.19 material 2 has therefore an acoustic velocity less than 1.

If in equation (1.13) waves I and II are considered as incident and reflected waves in the same material and if both are either longitudinal or transverse waves, they will of course have the same acoustic velocity c_1. Consequently

$$\frac{\sin \alpha_e}{\sin \alpha_r} = 1 \quad \text{and} \quad \alpha_e = \alpha_r\,,$$

i.e. the angles of incidence and emergence are identical. However, the reflected wave can also be of a different mode: In that case, although it occurs in the same material as the incident wave, it nevertheless has a different acoustic velocity and therefore also a different angle. The general law (1.13) however, remains valid.

Example: A longitudinal wave in steel strikes a boundary at $\alpha_e = 60°$ with $c_l = c_1 = 6 \cdot 10^3$ m/s. A reflected longitudinal wave has the same angle. Since, however, a transverse wave with $c_t = 3.2 \cdot 10^3$ m/s occurs in steel, a second wave is reflected as a transverse wave according to the law

$$\frac{\sin \alpha_r}{\sin \alpha_r} = \frac{c_t}{c_l} = 0.55 .$$

Therefore

$$\sin\alpha_r = 0.55 \cdot 0.87 = 0.48,$$

$$\alpha_r = 29° .$$

The slower transverse wave has a smaller angle than the longitudinal wave reflected at 60°.

The same applies to the transmitted waves. Provided transverse waves can occur in the material considered, as is the case in all solid bodies, both types of waves are in general obtained at different angles.

1.62 The Acoustic Pressure Values

The law of refraction merely furnishes information regarding the direction of a possibly refracted or transmitted wave but says nothing about its acoustic pressure. A few examples of combinations of different materials will clarify the situation. The description becomes much simpler in the case of gaseous or liquid materials as compared with solid materials because gaseous materials behave in this respect practically like empty space as long as we are interested only in the process in the contiguous liquid or solid material, and because only one kind of wave can occur in liquid materials, viz. the longitudinal wave.

Concerning the state of the two contiguous materials, 4 cases of increasing complexity can be distinguished:

Material 1	Material 2
a) liquid or solid	gaseous (free boundary)
b) liquid	liquid
c) liquid or solid	solid or liquid
d) solid	solid

Case a) liquid or solid free boundary, can quickly be dealt with for *liquid.* There is only one longitudinal wave which for all angles of incidence is totally reflected at the boundary.

Fig. 1.20 shows the case solid/gaseous for an incident longitudinal wave and Fig. 1.21 for a transverse wave. Let us visualize in the left quadrant the incident wave concerned, with the acoustic pressure 1 and angles between 0 and 90°, and in the adjacent quadrant the same kind of wave (i.e. with the same angle) reflected, the curve indicating the magnitude of the acoustic pressure for each angle of incidence. A further quadrant shows the simultaneously reflected other kind of wave. The vectors for one particular example are drawn in each diagram and the correlated angles are shown separately on the right.

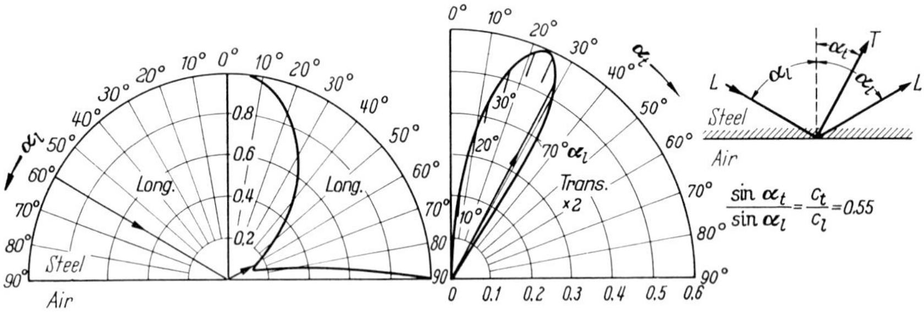

Fig. 1.20 Reflection at the interface solid/gas for an incident longitudinal wave (steel/air).

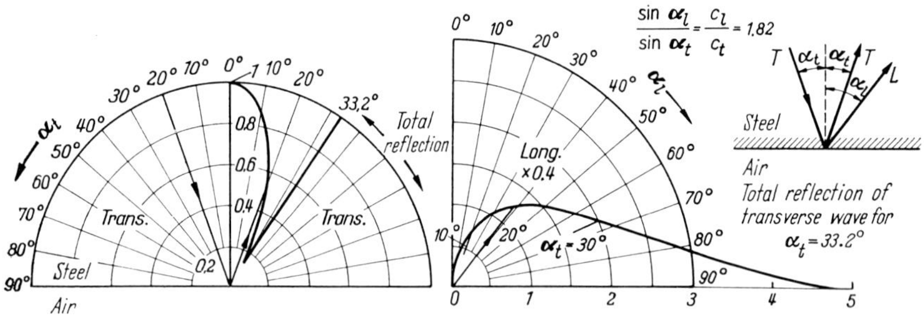

Fig. 1.21 Reflection at the interface solid/gas for an incident transverse wave (steel/air).

For a more quantitative evaluation the curves of the coefficient of reflection are given in the Appendix together with the formulas.

It is worth noting that in Fig. 1.20 the incident longitudinal wave is reflected only very weakly between 60° and 70°. Instead, a strong transverse wave occurs below approx. 30°.

In the case of an incident transverse wave (Fig. 1.21) a similar reflection *gap* occurs at approx. 30°. There one finds a strong longitudinal wave with a broad sector up to 90°. A rather interesting phenomenon occurs immediately beyond the 30° angle of incidence. According to the law of refraction, a value greater than 1 would be obtained for the sine, to which of course no real angle belongs. From our point of view this is merely a warning that the wave concerned ceases to be propagated freely. Consequently, the remaining wave must acquire the full acoustic pressure of the incident wave, i.e. the transverse wave is reflected totally in the sector above 33.2°.

The law of refraction (Fig. 1.21, right) reveals that this can always occur if the acoustic velocity of the reflected (or transmitted) wave is greater than that of the incident wave.

Particular caution is indicated in some cases when interpreting the results of the reflection formulas. For instance, Fig. 1.21 shows that a transverse wave incident at the critical angle 33.2° produces by reflection an approximately 5 times greater longitudinal wave (acoustic pressure), which seems to contradict the law of energy. This reflected longitudinal wave, however, travels at a glancing angle along the interface and, according to Fig. 1.20, is therefore immediately again reflected as a longitudinal wave of equal strength but with a 180° phase shift relative to the incident wave, which is not evident from the diagrams. Incident and reflected waves therefore cancel each other.

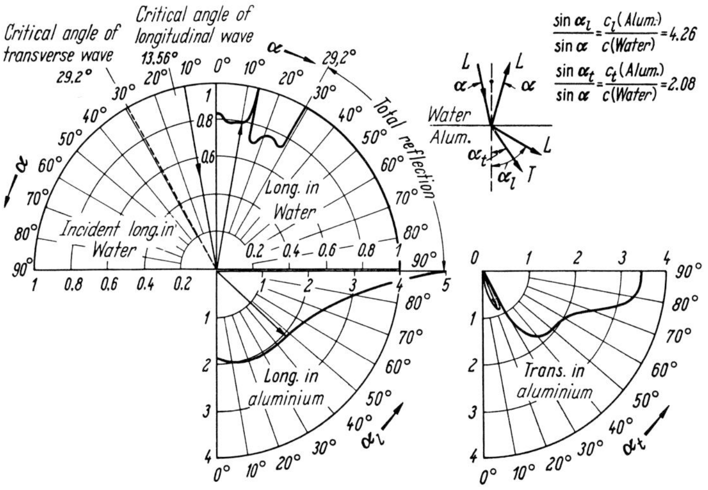

Fig. 1.22 Interface water/aluminium.

Case b) liquid/liquid. The case of two layers of liquid is of no practical importance in the testing of materials and it is therefore not discussed here. Re. formulas see Appendix.

Case c) liquid/solid and solid/liquid is of importance in the practical testing of materials, because when locating defects in solid test specimens, an ultrasonic wave must frequently be beamed into the material at an angle oblique to the surface. To achieve this angle, use is frequently made of the refraction between the material of the test specimen and a liquid. Since in this case, because of the occurrence of transverse waves, the conditions are more complex than for instance in the case of the refraction of light rays in optics, they will be explained in Figs. 1.22, 1.23 and 1.24, using the examples water/aluminium and aluminium/water. The relevant formulas and function tables are found in the Appendix.

In Fig. 1.22 a longitudinal wave emerging from water strikes the interface. At small angles of incidence (compare the drawn path of rays

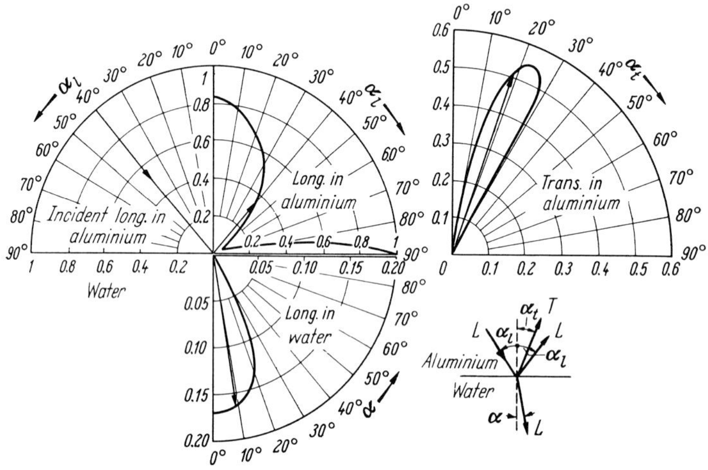

Fig. 1.23 Interface aluminium/water with incident longitudinal wave.

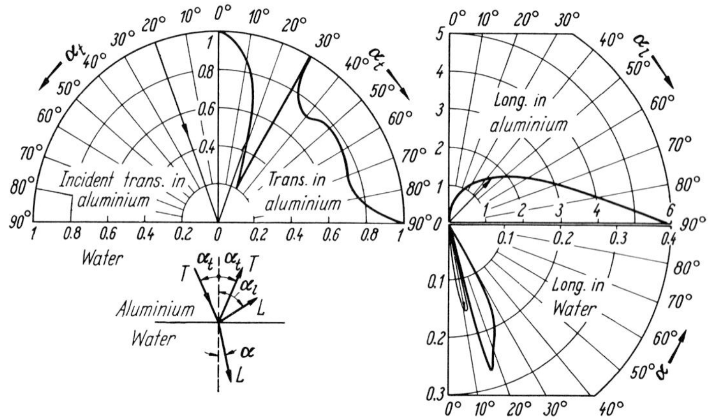

Fig. 1.24 Interface aluminium/water with incident transverse wave.

at 10°) a longitudinal wave enters the aluminium whose acoustic pressure and angle increase rapidly with increasing angle of incidence. Simultaneously, a weak transverse wave (quadrant right bottom) is formed with a maximum at 20° in aluminium. The angle of incidence of 13.56° is the so-called critical angle of the longitudinal wave because it disappears at this point from the aluminium. Immediately, however, a stronger transverse wave occurs and then remains with increasing acoustic pressure in the aluminium from approx. 30 to 90°, while the angle of incidence increases up to 29.2°. This is the second critical angle, viz. the critical angle for the transverse wave.

Above this range no wave whatsoever can be found in the aluminium and this range is of no interest for the testing of materials. The incident longitudinal wave is totally reflected in it. Of importance is the range between the two critical angles because only one single kind of wave, viz. the transverse wave, is available there when testing solid materials.

Since the acoustic pressures differ greatly, it was necessary to increase or decrease the scale of the presentation in some quadrants in Figs. 1.20 to 1.24 for the sake of clarity.

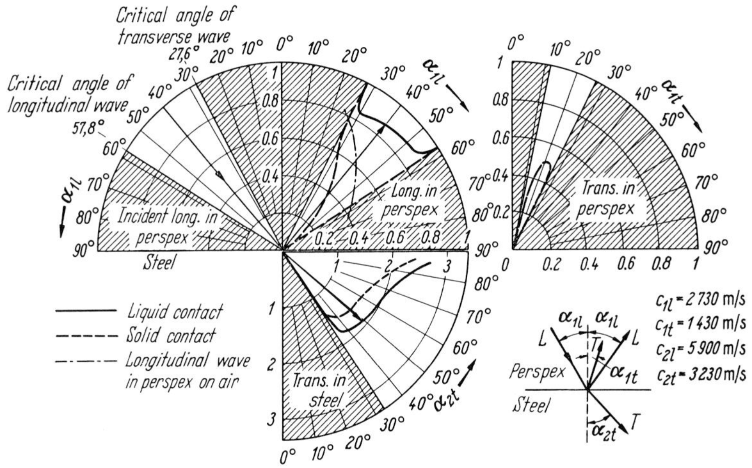

Fig. 1.25 Interface perspex/steel. Incident longitudinal wave in perspex.

Figs. 1.23 and 1.24 show the reverse wave path, viz. from aluminium into water, which is of importance for the echo method in the testing of materials, in order to find an answer to the question how much of the wave beamed into the test specimen returns from it as an echo.

Case d) solid/solid. In this most general case both longitudinal and transverse waves occur in the two contiguous materials. Consequently, the reflection formulas and the presentations become more complex. Thus far only a few individual cases have therefore been calculated.

As far as the acoustic contact between the two materials is concerned, two cases can again be distinguished:

d 1) Solid contact, i.e. the two materials are connected to each other by welding, soldering or by a thin, solid cementing layer.

d 2) Liquid contact, i.e. the two materials are in contact with a thin layer of liquid, resulting in the covering layer being able to transmit compressional forces but not, as in the case of d 1), shear forces as well. In practical testing of materials this case is by far the most important one. However, attention is drawn to the fact that if high compressional forces are applied (e.g. shrink fit) the two surfaces, owing to their roughness, may interlock to such an extent that shear forces also can be transmitted, thus representing physically case d 1 (see KÜHN and LUTSCH [211]).

In practice the refraction at the interface solid/solid with liquid contact finds wide application when beaming transverse waves obliquely into the material. Fig. 1.25 shows the acoustic pressure amplitudes of the refracted transverse wave and the reflected longitudinal and transverse wave for the transition of a longitudinal wave from perspex into steel, as calculated by KÜHN and LUTSCH [211]. Only the range between total reflection of the longitudinal and transverse wave, which is of main interest in practice, is shown. At the transition to solid contact (case d 1) the dotted line shows that both the acoustic pressure values of the refacted transverse wave and the reflected longitudinal wave decrease in favour of the reflected transverse wave. The pronounced dependence of the coefficient of reflection on the coupling conditions in the case of the longitudinal wave in perspex permit a practical coupling check [238]. For comparison the reflection of the longitudinal wave at the free perspex interface is therefore likewise shown (dash-dot-dash line).

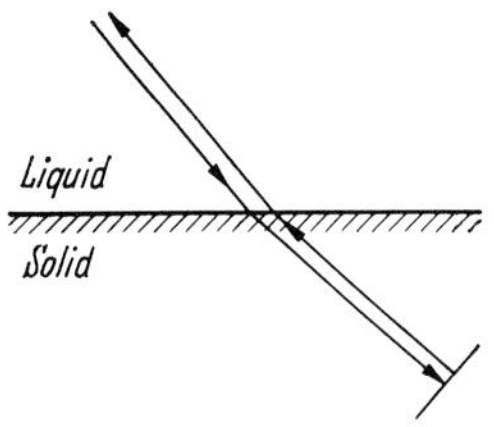

Fig. 1.25a Explanation of echo transmittance at an interface.

When using the echo method for testing purposes it stands to reason that it is desirable to transmit as much as possible of the sound wave into the test specimen and to receive a maximum echo. According to Fig. 1.22 approx. 80% of the acoustic pressure of the incident wave is lost in the reflected wave. Also in the reverse process as shown in Figs. 1.23 and 1.24, large portions of the two kinds of waves are lost again through reflection when leaving the solid body. Fig. 1.26 answers the question how much of the acoustic pressure is still returned at the different angles in the case of the two kinds of waves along the outgoing and return path when penetrating the interface twice. Let us for this purpose imagine, as shown in Fig. 1.25a, that the sound beam is thrown back completely along its own path in the solid material, e.g. from a large smooth crack surface. The calculation requires only multiplication of the transmittance in the one direction with the transmittance in the other to obtain the *echo transmittance*. In solid materials one can operate either with the longitudinal or with the transverse wave, furnishing the echo transmittances E_{ll} or E_{lt}. Since these quantities are very important when testing at oblique angles, both are shown in Fig. 1.26 for different liquid and

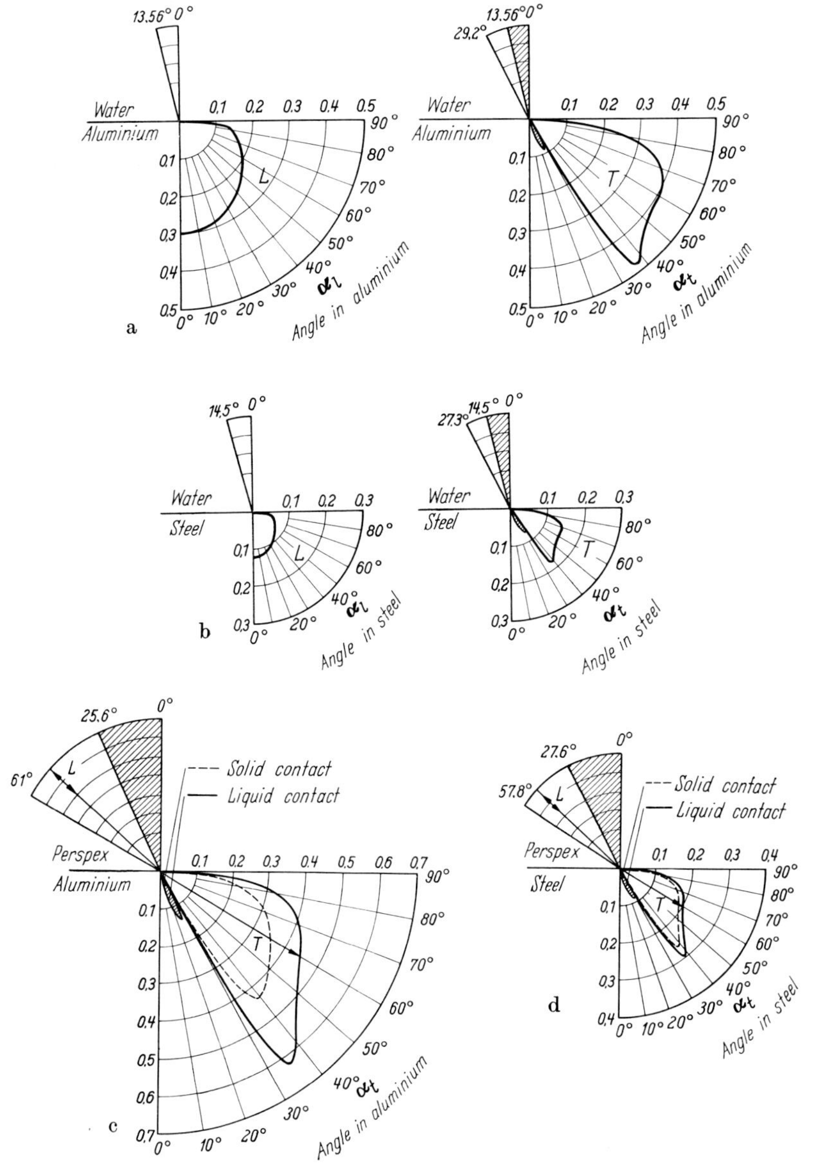

Fig. 1.26 Echo transmittance at various interfaces. a) Water/aluminium, b) water/steel, c) perspex/aluminium, d) perspex/steel.

solid materials. As in the previous case, it is furthermore assumed that the acoustic pressure of the incident wave is 1. The length of the vector then indicates the acoustic pressure of the returning wave.

For water/aluminium (Fig. 1.26a) an echo is obtained via the longitudinal wave from the aluminium at small angles of incidence below 13.56°, containing up to 30% of the incident acoustic pressure. At the same time the transverse wave furnishes only a weak echo of less than 10% (shaded sector). At greater angles of incidence up to 29.2° an echo is obtained only via the transverse wave, with good efficiency of up to nearly 50%. Fig. 1.26b shows the corresponding values for water/steel. Because of the greater difference in sonic hardness, the efficiency is in this case smaller. As far as the combinations liquid/metal are concerned, it can be stated quite generally that at angles of up to approx. 30° in metal it is best to operate with longitudinal waves. Above approx. 35° the transverse wave becomes more favourable, a fact widely exploited in the testing of materials. Above 80° the conditions are bad for both kinds of waves. The corresponding curves for the case perspex/metal are shown in Figs. 1.26c and d, but only for the transverse wave in metal, for which thus far the two different conditions, viz. solid and liquid contact, have been calculated (Kühn and Lutsch [211]). In the same way as in Fig. 1.25, the efficiency becomes surprisingly better for liquid contact than for solid contact. Owing to the improved matching of the acoustic impedances, it is of course also better than in the case liquid/solid. The combination perspex/aluminium returns more than 60% of the acoustic pressure at the most favourable angle with liquid contact.

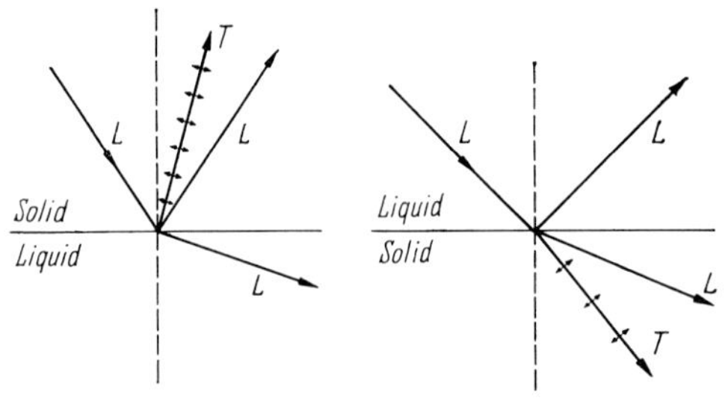

Fig. 1.27 The oscillation plane of a split off transverse wave is always parallel to the plane of incidence (= plane of the paper).

Regarding quantitative evaluation see formulas and tables in the Appendix.

Where transverse waves have been discussed in this Section, this concerns those whose plane of oscillation is in the plane of incidence (plane of drawing in the Figure). As shown in Fig. 1.27, only this kind of transverse wave is produced if a longitudinal wave is split at an interface. For vertical incidence the position of the plane of oscillation is of course unimportant; both the reflection and the transmission always obey the law (1.11). This is not the case at oblique incidence; a transverse wave having a plane of oscillation at right angles to the plane of incidence is reflected totally at all angles if the contiguous material is liquid or gaseous. It never splits off another kind of wave.

Transverse waves with arbitrary direction of oscillation can be resolved into two components, viz. one parallel and one perpendicular to the plane of incidence, which must then be treated separately.

As agreed, we have so far neglected the phase change during reflection at the sonically softer material (see 1.5). In Figs. 1.20, 1.23 and 1.24 the reflected wave should receive a negative sign because its phase is reversed, i.e. shifted one half wave length. This applies both to the longitudinal and the transverse wave with polarization parallel to the plane of incidence. However, the wave polarized at right angles is an exception: as long as the absorption in the contiguous material is low, its phase is preserved at each reflection. This is important when considering a wave incident at a very large (glancing) angle: since the value of the coefficient of reflection approaches 100%, both the longitudinal and parallel transverse waves cancel themselves near the interface because the direct wave interferes at every point with the reflected wave thus cancelling it. This is not the case with a transverse wave oscillating perpendicularly to the plane of incidence. At grazing incidence the amplitude of such a wave is doubled.

1.63 Reflection in a Right-angled Edge and in a Corner

In the testing of materials, reflections within an angle formed by the two planes of a test object are frequently encountered (Fig. 1.28). If a ray strikes such a right-angled edge perpendicularly, it is reflected parallel to itself, whatever angle it makes with one of the two faces, after a double reflection. In the case of a beam (Fig. 1.28b) in addition an interchange of its two sides occurs. If its axis does not strike the edge, it is furthermore transposed parallel to itself.

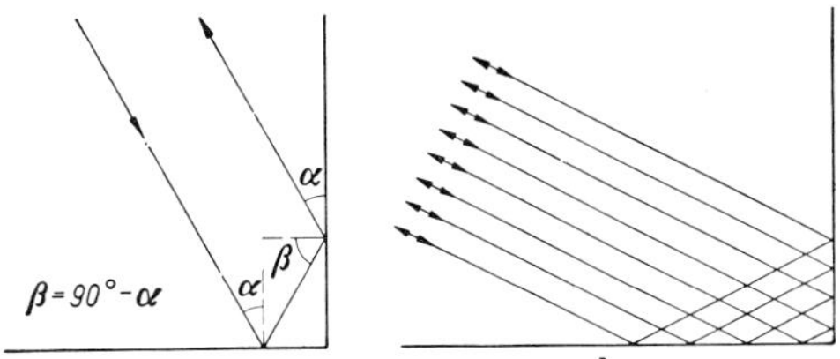

a b

Fig. 1.28 Reflection of an angle mirror. a) Single ray, b) beam.

A third plane face perpendicular to the other two faces forms with them a corner which reflects a beam, coming from any angle in space, parallel to itself. This effect is exploited optically in the "cat's eye" reflector.

A similar effect is obtained for a plane ultrasonic wave. Allowance must, however, be made for the results of the reflection: solid/gaseous, case a). At each of the two reflections a wave of the other type can be split off so that the total coefficient of reflection largely depends on the angle of incidence. Fig. 1.29 shows the angle reflection for a longitudinal wave (a) and a transverse wave (b) in steel. It is calculated as the product of the coefficients of reflection from Figs. 1.20 and 1.21 for the angles α_l and $90 - a$, and α_t and $90 - \alpha_t$, respectively.

Except for very flat angles to one of the faces, the longitudinal wave shows very bad angle reflection. The reason is that at one of the two reflections a strong transverse wave which does not return in the direction of the incident wave is always split off.

Because it is twice totally reflected the transverse wave is reflected completely in the medium range. On either side, however, there are *holes* in which practically no reflection occurs. At flat angles the transverse wave is theoretically again reflected more strongly. Here, however, the supplementary limitation must be made concerning both kinds of waves, that

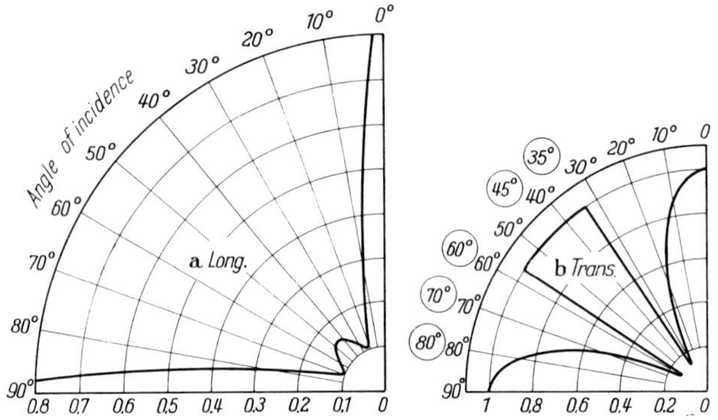

Fig. 1.29 Coefficient of reflection of an angle in steel for incident longitudinal wave (a) and transverse wave (b).

at flat angles an actual sound beam, in contrast to a fictitious plane wave, has lost its sensitivity. Cancellation by interference between the direct and the reflected beam occurs along the wall so that both curves in Figs. 1.29a and b again drop practically to zero at 0 and 90°.

Fig. 1.29b also shows the angles frequently used in the testing of materials. It can be seen that for an angle reflection as used for instance for the detection of an incipient crack starting at right angles to the surface, the angles 35° and 45° are favourable. The 60° angle is particularly unfavourable because it lies within a reflection trough.

At a corner it is possible to calculate certain *surfaces* of which those for the longitudinal waves likewise furnish only small reflection factors for the greater portion of the steric angle range. For transverse waves a total reflection range is obtained around the steric angle bisector of the corner, surrounded by a deep trench.

For aluminium the corresponding curves are all very similar, but the troughs are still more pronounced.

1.64 Splitting of Surface and Boundary Waves

The relatively simple theory described above according to which the reflection and refraction on interfaces has been calculated, covers only longitudinal and transverse waves. In reality, however, so-called boundary layer waves also occur, viz. near the critical angle of total reflection. One type of boundary layer wave has already been encountered in the surface wave occurring at the interface solid/gas. On other interfaces, viz. solid/liquid and solid/solid one speaks of boundary layer waves.

If a longitudinal wave strikes the interface liquid/solid at approximately the critical angle for total reflection of the transverse wave (in the case of perspex/steel, 57.8° in perspex according to Fig. 1.26), such a wave is produced along the interface, which is, however, strongly attenuated as far as the liquid (or perspex) reaches (Fig. 1.30). If immediately behind the point of incidence the interface is free, a surface wave travels unattenuated and with considerable amplitude from that point along the surface of the solid material. In practice this effect is exploited for producing surface waves. The strongest surface wave is obtained at an angle of incidence slightly greater than the critical angle where, according to the elementary theory, the incident wave should already be totally reflected.

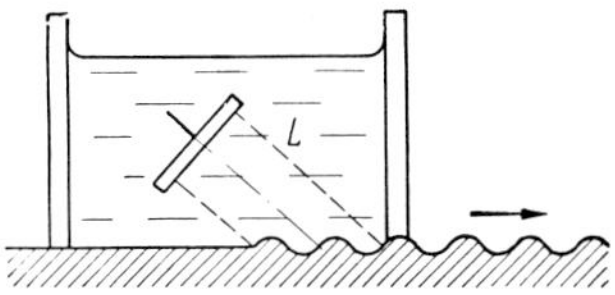

Fig. 1.30 Excitation of surface waves on a solid body. In practice the liquid space is usually replaced by a plastic wedge with a thin liquid film.

1.65 Acoustic Propagation in Plates, Plate Waves

In Fig. 1.6a it was shown that transverse waves, whose direction of oscillation is parallel to the surface of the plate concerned, can be propagated in plates. Possible means of excitation for such waves are shown in Fig. 1.31.

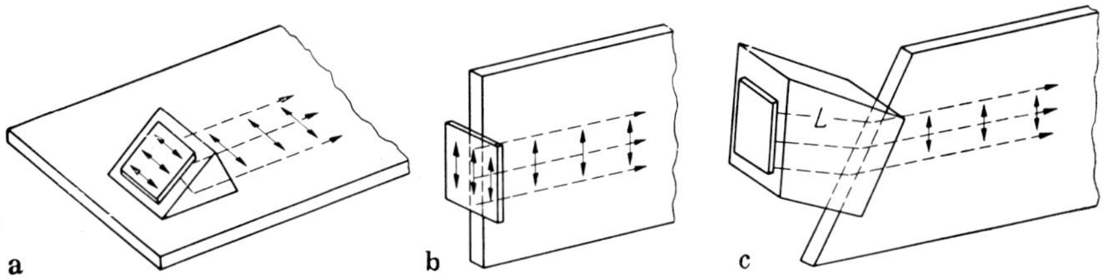

Fig. 1.31 Possible means for exciting transverse waves in plates; a) and b) with transverse wave generator (e.g. Y-cut crystal, see 1.10) in solid contact, through a wedge or at an edge; c) by conversion of longitudinal waves through a wedge in liquid contact along an edge.

Transverse waves whose direction of oscillation is perpendicular to the surface of the plate or longitudinal waves can, however, not be propagated in this way, i.e. in a direction parallel to the surfaces. In the case of glancing incidence of the sound such waves are reflected at the surfaces of the plates with a phase skip of 180°, so that incident and reflected waves cancel each other. These waves can, however, travel unimpeded through the plate at an angle α to the surface, i.e. along a zig-zag path as shown in Fig. 1.32a.

If, however, wider sound beams are used as shown in Figs. 1.32b and c, or if the thickness of the plate is very much smaller than the width of the beam B as shown in Fig. 1.32a, beam I partly covers beam II after a double reflection. As shown in Fig. 1.32b, the acoustic pressure peak may then coincide with the acoustic pressure minimum so that the beams partly cancel each other resulting in unfavourable sound propagation in the plate. At changed angle of incidence α the beams cover each other in proper phase relationship as shown in Fig. 1.32c. The pattern arising in this way and composed of mutually superimposed zig-zag reflected longitudinal and transverse waves is known as a Lamb wave [213, 20, 276, 19, 306]. For steel the most favourable angle for different plate thicknesses can be found in the diagram of Table 9 in the Appendix.

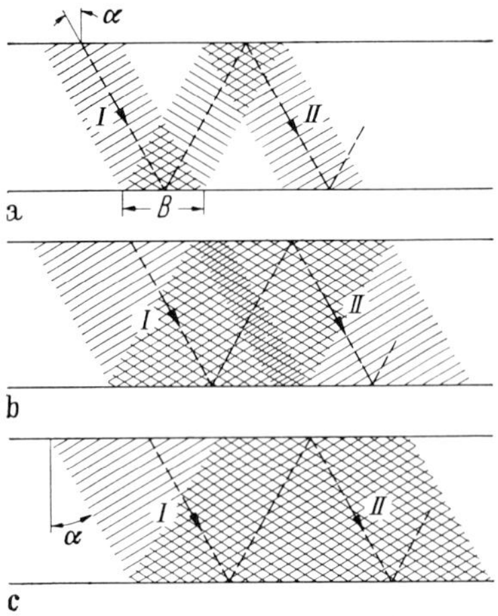

Fig. 1.32 Generation of the Lamb wave. a) Narrow, obliquely reflected beam; b) wide beam at unfavourable phase position, the edges of the beam cancel each other by interference; c) favourable phase position through adaptation of the angle α. Beams I and II cover each other in proper phase relationship.

At first glance it seems strange that such a simple geometrical requirement – that the reflected beams should not cancel each other – demands such a complicated relationship between plate thickness and most favourable angle as shown in Table 9. This complication results from the fact that in the case of the oblique reflection of sound on surfaces of solid bodies phase shifts occur which in turn depend on the angle (see [276]).

The relationships become even more complicated when one examines the velocity of these Lamb waves in a direction parallel to the surface. The phase shift during reflection results in the reflected beam being transposed relative to the incident beam so that the path of propagation is not zig-zag like but trapezoidal [277], [20, para. 19]. The extent of this transposition of the beam depends on the angle α and the frequency. It may amount to several wave lengths, particularly near the glancing incidence of the longitudinal wave (33.2° in steel), with the result that in the case of plates with a thickness of only a few wave lengths, the velocity differs greatly from the simple geometrical relation $c_t \sin\alpha$ and $c_l \sin\beta$ (β = angle between longitudinal wave and normal to plate) which could be expected to follow from the elementary presentation in Fig. 1.32. Only at $\alpha = 45°$ does the phase shift, and thus also the transposition of the beam become zero; in this case the simple geometrical sine relation is valid by way of exception.

In addition to these wave types which manifest themselves as longitudinal and transverse waves propagated along a zig-zag path, thick plates also have surface waves. If the thickness of the plate becomes less than the penetration depth of the surface wave, the latter degenerates and is split into two branches with different propagation velocities, viz. the branches marked a_0 and s_0 in Table 9. The correlated mode of oscillation has already been shown in Fig. 1.6. In a certain sense these waves a_0 and s_0, and the surface wave are also degenerated zig-zag propagations. The wave surfaces are almost perpendicular to the surface of the plate or are even inclined backward against the direction of propagation. Consequently, the wave beams no longer detach themselves from the surface, the oblique paths through the plate (I and II in Fig. 1.32) are suppressed, and the wave motion now consists only of the reflection at the plate surface and the continuous conversion of longitudinal waves into transverse waves resulting from this process. Mathematically this degeneration corresponds to the change of α from a real to an imaginary quantity, viz. $\sin\alpha$ becomes greater than 1. As far as the excitation of these wave types is concerned, it should be mentioned that like the true waves reflected along a zig-zag path they can be excited by exploiting the law of refraction [Eq. (1.13) and Fig. 1.19], in which the sine of the angle of refraction is made, purely formally, greater than 1 (values of $\sin\alpha$ in Table 9). This results in an entrance angle in the water or plastic wedge used for excitation, which is greater than the total reflection angle, as already mentioned in Sec. 1.64.

1.7 Geometric Ultrasonic Optics

1.71 Limits of Validity

Geometric optics uses light rays which can be drawn as straight lines. Applying the simple law of refraction and reflection at interfaces, it permits very clear presentation, e.g. of the effect of mirrors and lenses with curved surfaces. Also we have already used this convenient method, e.g. when discussing reflection and refraction in 1.5 and 1.6. In this connection it should, however, not be overlooked that this method fails to take into account a very important property, both of light waves and ultrasonic waves, viz. the wave structure. Already in optics this produces a number of departures from a geometric-optical construction: *diffraction phenomena* occur at gaps and small openings as well as at focal points, i.e. whenever the dimensions considered become small, or more precisely when they are no longer large compared with the wave length.

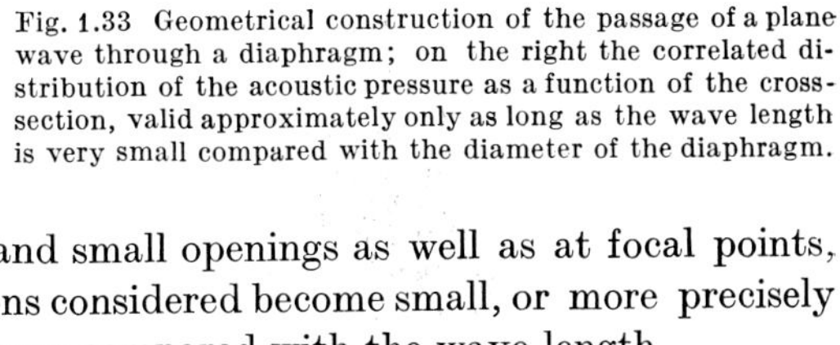

Fig. 1.33 Geometrical construction of the passage of a plane wave through a diaphragm; on the right the correlated distribution of the acoustic pressure as a function of the cross-section, valid approximately only as long as the wave length is very small compared with the diameter of the diaphragm.

The length of light waves is of the order of less than a thousandth of a millimetre whereas that of ultrasonic waves is of the order of millimetres. For the latter, diffraction phenomena therefore occur far more frequently, already at dimensions below 100 mm, i.e. in the range most commonly used in practice. The simple geometrical construction of an ultrasonic field behind a diaphragm as shown in Fig. 1.33, will therefore in reality be slightly changed for diaphragm dimensions around 100 mm, and in the case of still smaller dimensions, diffraction phenomena will change it completely (see 1.8).

In the following a few feasible applications of geometric ultrasonic optics will be discussed remembering, however, that where this concerns cases in which the wave length is *no longer* very small compared with the dimensions concerned, the results obtained are only more or less rough approximations.

1.72 Acoustic Pressure Distance Law for Spherical and Cylindrical Waves

Let us investigate how in the case of simple wave forms the acoustic pressure changes with the distance from the source. In a plane wave the pressure of course remains constant in each plane of the wave. In the case of waves which are not plane, energy considerations lead to a distance law. Fig. 1.34 shows 4 rays coming from the origin of a spherical wave, which determine a small square on the surface of a sphere with the radius a. On a further spherical surface with the radius 2a the 4 rays determine a square which is evidently four times greater. According to the law of conservation of energy, the ultrasonic energy passing through both squares per unit time must be identical. The energy density per unit surface, i.e. the intensity on the sphere with the double radius is thus only one quarter. Generally: the intensities at two different distances are, in the case of spherical waves, inversely proportional to the square of the distances from the source.

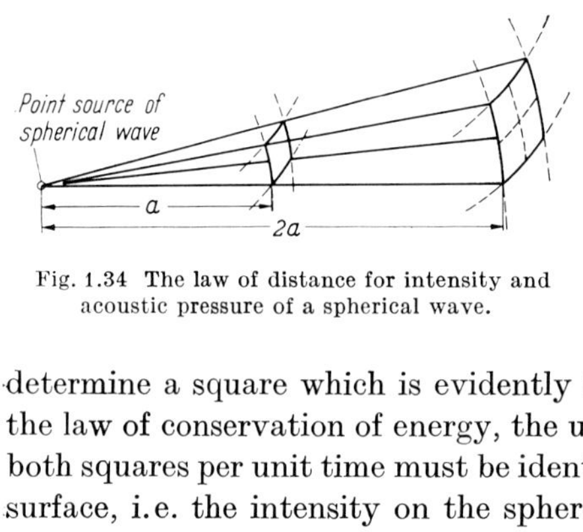

Fig. 1.34 The law of distance for intensity and acoustic pressure of a spherical wave.

Since according to Eq. (1.4) the acoustic pressure is proportional to the square root of the intensity, the acoustic pressures are inversely proportional to the distances:

$$\frac{P_2}{P_1} = \frac{a_1}{a_2}.$$

If $a_1 = 1$ and the acoustic pressure at this point is P_1, the law of distance for the acoustic pressure of the spherical wave furnishes

$$P = P_1 \frac{1}{a}. \tag{1.14}$$

According to this relation the acoustic pressure in the source itself would become infinite, which is just as unreal as a point source. Real sources always have finite dimensions and in close proximity to them the acoustic wave is usually not strictly spherical. The law (1.14) therefore applies only to distances very large compared with the dimensions of the source. If this condition is not yet fulfilled at a distance 1, P_1 refers merely to a quantity specified purely for determining the strength of the source.

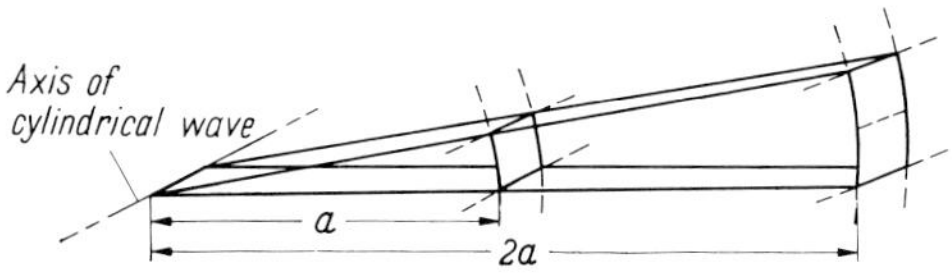

Fig. 1.35 The law of distance for intensity and acoustic pressure of a cylindrical wave.

In the case of a cylindrical wave the source is not a point, but a line, viz. the axis of the cylindrical wave. According to Fig. 1.35 the area determined by 4 rays on a cylindrical surface therefore changes only as a linear function of the distance. A square on the inner cylindrical face becomes a rectangle of twice the area on the cylindrical surface with double the radius. The intensity therefore changes only inversely with the distance i.e. it decreases at a slower rate than in the case of a spherical wave. Consequently, the acoustic pressure decreases only inversely with the square of the distance:

$$P = P_1 \sqrt{\frac{1}{a}}\,. \tag{1.15}$$

In the testing of materials the spherical wave, particularly where large test objects are concerned, is the most important wave form because the wave generated by a conventional ultrasonic resonator can be regarded at greater distances as a spherical wave. In practical testing this spherical wave frequently strikes flat, cylindrical, and more rarely also spherical surfaces, whereby it is subjected to changes by reflection and refraction, which will be discussed in the following Sections.

1.73* Reflection and Refraction of Spherical Waves on Plane Surfaces

The reflection of a spherical wave on a plane surface is shown geometrically in Fig. 1.36 where each ray is reflected at its own angle of incidence. The shape of the spherical wave is preserved but the reflected spherical wave seems to come from a point 0′ which is the mirror image of the real centre 0. A beam retains its angle of aperture δ, as can be seen from the two rays drawn in the Figure and which form the angle δ.

If one observes the acoustic pressure along a given ray, it is found that before being reflected it follows the law (1.14). After reflection, the coefficient of reflection for the angle of incidence and the type of interface concerned has to be taken into account, as described in 1.6:

$$P = P_1 \frac{1}{a} R .$$

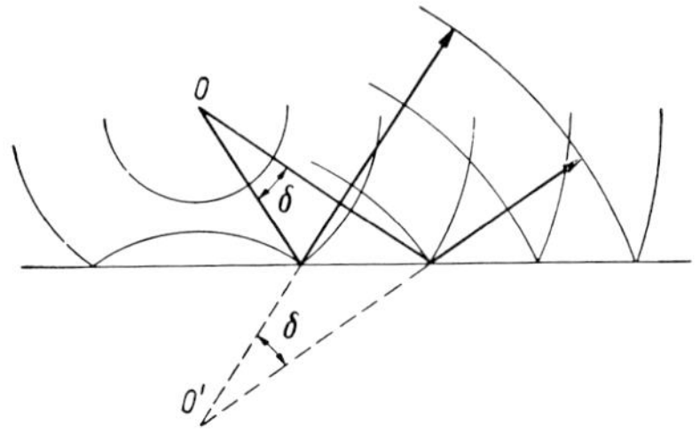

Fig. 1.36 Reflection of a spherical wave on a plane interface (wave surfaces only shown partially).

Since according to Fig. 1.20 and following diagrams, this coefficient R depends strongly on the angle, the distribution of the acoustic pressure on one of the spherical wave surfaces may be greatly changed by reflection. The spherical character of the wave is nevertheless preserved.

A simple example is the multiple reflection between two walls (Fig. 1.37). The axis of the beam of spherical waves (sound beam of a probe) is incident at right angles. If the walls border on air, the axial ray is reflected completely, viz. $R = 1$, and practically also rays at small angles as shown in Fig. 1.20 for steel in air. The path of the ray is then obtained by simple reversal of the free beam path around the corresponding mirror plane. The acoustic pressure distribution along the axis of the beam plotted above is obtained similarly. P has the following values

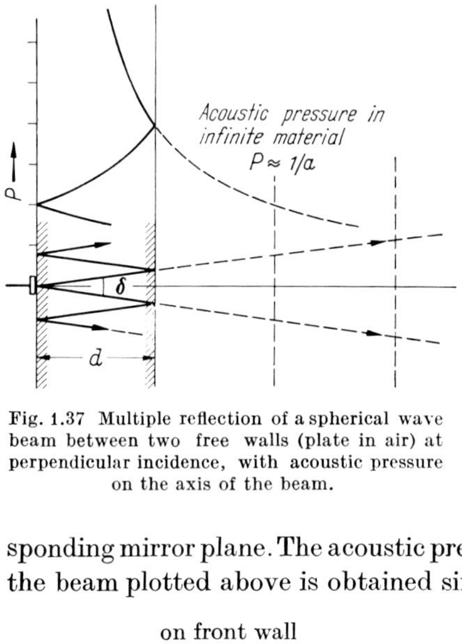

Fig. 1.37 Multiple reflection of a spherical wave beam between two free walls (plate in air) at perpendicular incidence, with acoustic pressure on the axis of the beam.

on front wall	on back wall
	$P_1 \frac{1}{d}$,
$P_1 \frac{1}{2d}$,	
	$P_1 \frac{1}{3d}$,
$P_1 \frac{1}{4d}$, etc.	

On the probe side the acoustic pressures of the wave are thus in the ratio $1 : 1/2 : 1/3 : 1/4$, etc. This presupposes that no disturbance is caused by interference, i.e. that pulses are used.

In the case of reflection of the spherical wave with wave mode conversion and refraction of the spherical wave, the wave no longer remains spherical, in contrast to the simple reflection. As an example, Fig. 1.38

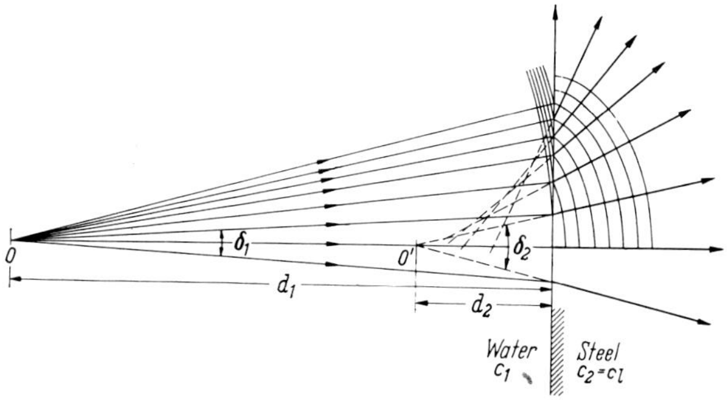

Fig. 1.38 Refraction of a spherical wave at the interface water/steel.

shows the refraction at an interface water/steel, in which only the longitudinal wave in steel is considered. Only rays which are almost perpendicular still intersect each other after refraction at a virtual centre 0′. The refracted wave can therefore be regarded as a spherical wave only in this particular zone. Geometry furnishes

$$d_2 : d_1 = \delta_1 : \delta_2 = c_1 : c_2, \quad \text{here } 1:4.$$

The angles of divergence of narrow beams incident at right angles are in the rate of the acoustic velocities, i.e. for longitudinal waves in steel they are four times greater than in water. The pattern of the acoustic pressure in the second material is determined by the virtual centre 0′ from which the distance a in equation (1.14) must be calculated. In the case of obliquely incident beams with both refraction and reflection with mode conversion, the angle of divergence is dependent on the angle of incidence, and therefore also the pattern of the acoustic pressure.

1.74* Curved Interfaces as Concave Mirrors and Lenses

If a plane wave strikes the curved interface between two materials 1 and 2, e.g. on a spherical surface (of which Fig. 1.39 shows a section), only the ray incident at right angles can pass through or be reflected without angular change. The formulas (1.11) for the coef-

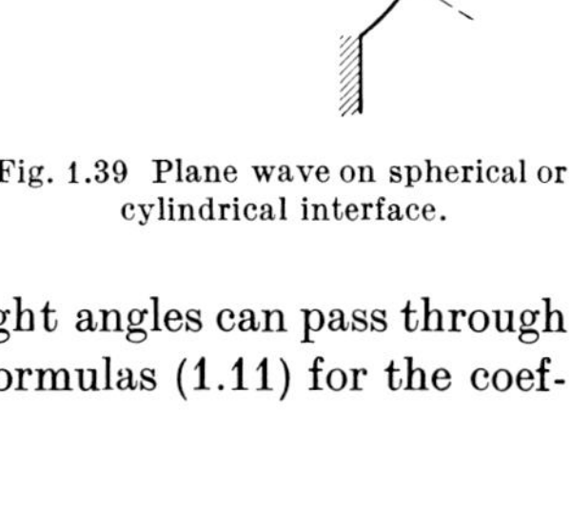

Fig. 1.39 Plane wave on spherical or cylindrical interface.

ficients of reflection and transmission apply only to this particular ray. Since the lateral rays are refracted or reflected at an angle, which is greater the further they are from the axial ray, concentration or dispersion occurs, viz. the acoustic pressure increases or decreases, as in the case of the similar optical phenomena produced by mirrors and lenses.

Fig. 1.40 shows the two possibilities of the concave concentrating mirror and the convex dispersing mirror. Let us assume an incident plane wave with the acoustic pressure P_0. If rays at small distance from the axial beam only are considered, a simple geometric construction shows that they meet at a *focal point* with the *focal distance*

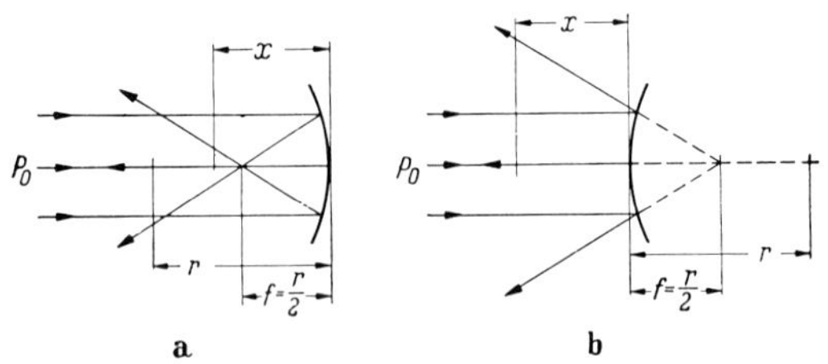

Fig. 1.40 Plane wave on a) concave mirror, b) convex mirror.

$$f = \frac{r}{2}, \tag{1.16}$$

measured from the point of symmetry on the mirror surface. Only in the case of the concave mirror is this focal point real, whereas in the case of the convex mirror a virtual focal point occurs behind the mirror, from which the rays extended backward seem to come.

This applies both to a spherical and to a cylindrical mirror. The spherical mirror has a focal *point* and the cylindrical mirror a focal *axis*. Fig. 1.40 shows both types of mirror, according to the manner in which their spatial completion is visualized. If the incident wave is a plane wave, a spherical mirror produces a spherical wave and a cylindrical mirror a cylindrical wave.

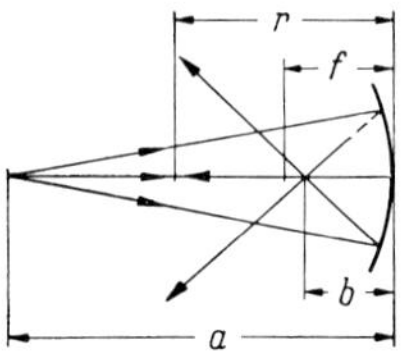

Fig. 1.41 Sperical wave on concave mirror.

If, as shown in Fig. 1.41, a spherical wave meets a concave mirror with the centre of the spherical wave at distance a from the point of symmetry on the mirror surface, a focal point is produced. This is called the image point with the image distance b. The relationship between the distances a and b and the focal distance f is given by the formula

$$\frac{1}{b} \pm \frac{1}{a} = \frac{1}{f} = \frac{1}{r/2}. \tag{1.17}$$

The plus sign applies to the concave mirror and the minus sign to the convex mirror. The focal distance should always be taken as positive.

If in the case of a concave mirror a negative image distance is obtained, this means a virtual image point behind the mirror. Conversely, if the direction of the rays is taken to be reversed (incident, convergent spherical wave) with apparent centre behind the concave mirror, the distance a should be taken with the negative sign.

In the case of the dispersing mirror all quantities should be taken with the positive sign. Either the image point or the centre of the spherical wave will always appear to be behind the mirror.

In order to calculate the acoustic pressure of the reflected wave, Eqs. (1.14) and (1.15) are used in which the distance from the correlated image point must now be taken. This image point, or *image line* in the case of a cylindrical wave, is the source from which the further propagation process can be recalculated, independently of the generation of the image point.

Let a plane and a spherical wave strike a spherical mirror or a cylindrical mirror; the acoustic pressures as a function of the distance from the apex x for the reflected waves are then:

	Plane wave on spherical mirror	Cylindrical mirror	
	$P_0 \dfrac{f}{x \mp f}$,	$P_0 \sqrt{\dfrac{f}{x \mp f}}$,	(1.18)
Spherical wave	$\dfrac{P_1}{a} \dfrac{f}{x \mp f(1 + x/a)}$	$\dfrac{P_1}{a} \sqrt{\dfrac{f}{(1 + x/a)(x \mp f(1 + x/a))}}$.	(1.19)

The upper sign applies to concave mirrors, and the lower sign to convex mirrors. P_0 is the acoustic pressure of the incident, plane wave, P_1 that of the spherical wave at distance 1 from the centre, so that P_1/a is its acoustic pressure at the apex of the mirror. In the latter case, viz. that of the spherical wave on the cylindrical mirror, which is the more important one in practice, neither a purely spherical wave nor a cylindrical wave is produced but a combination of two different spherical waves which, in accordance with the two terms below the root sign, have also two different image points.

For quantities under the root signs only absolute values will be calculated. In the case of the concentrating mirror the nominator can disappear in all terms, viz. at the real image points, where theoretically the acoustic pressure would become infinite. In reality the geometric construction fails here because of diffraction phenomena. The true concentration and increase of the acoustic pressure depends on the wave length.

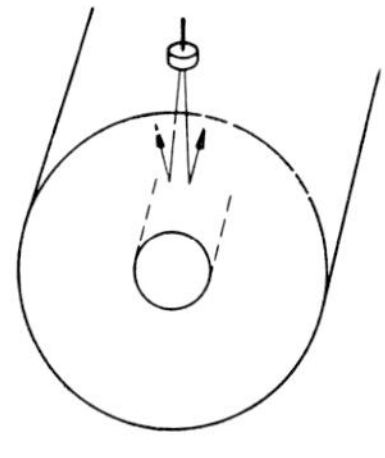

Fig. 1.42 Cylindrical mirror on a forging.

Fig. 1.42 shows a practical test in which the sound beam of spherical waves from the probe meets a cylindrical hole in a forging. The calculation will be made in 1.75.

In this case the surfaces of the object border on air and the rays incident at right angles are totally reflected, as also assumed in Eqs. (1.18) and (1.19). According to Fig. 1.20, the rays not strictly normally incident, are no longer totally reflected. The deviations are, however, only very slight, viz. for longitudinal waves at 16° only approx. 10%. Since Eqs. (1.16) and (1.17) are being used, the observation should in any case be limited to narrow beams about the normally incident ray.

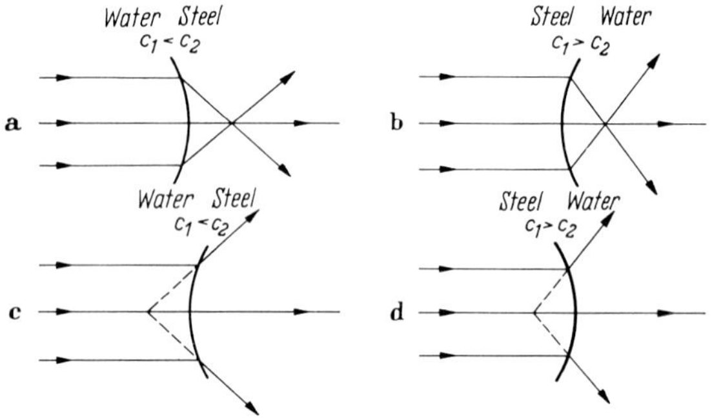

Fig. 1.43 Lens effect of a curved interface water/steel.

If the reflected surface does not border on air but e.g. on water, the reflection will be reduced. Formulas (1.18) and (1.19) must then be supplemented by the coefficients of reflection R according to Eq. (1.11). Naturally, this does not change the shape of the reflected wave, e.g. the position of the image point.

The curved interface acts on the transmitted waves in the contiguous material like a lens on light (Fig. 1.43). This may involve either a condensing lens or a dispersing lens, depending both on the orientation of the curvature and on the ratio of the acoustic velocities c_2/c_1.

In contrast to the concave mirror, where no differences exist compared with the optical mirror, there are two basic differences in the case of lenses compared with the customary treatment of optical lenses: since optical lenses are usually considered in air, the index of refraction $n = c_1/c_2$ is in this case always greater than unity. This is not the case in our example and we shall therefore avoid the expression index of refraction. Furthermore, optical lenses are always used with two boundaries on air. In our case it is preferable to consider the effect of a single interface.

Fig. 1.43 shows the four possibilities of a lens illustrated by the example water and steel:

	Fig. 1.43	Curvature	c_2/c_1
Condensing lens	a	concave	>1
Condensing lens	b	convex	<1
Dispersing lens	c	conacve	>1
Dispersing lens	d	convex	<1

In cases a and b a spherical wave (Fig. 1.44) also has a real image point, in the other case only a virtual one. Here also, in the case of an incident plane wave, the focal distance f is again determined by the distance of the axis intersection of the curved surface from the real or imaginary focal point. For a narrow beam this leads to

$$f = \frac{r}{1 - (c_2/c_1)}\,. \tag{1.20}$$

The focal distance shall here always be regarded as being positive, as well as the axial distances a and b of the centre of the spherical waves and their image points from the convex surface. The lens formula

$$\frac{1}{b} - \frac{c_2/c_1}{a} = \frac{1}{f} \tag{1.21}$$

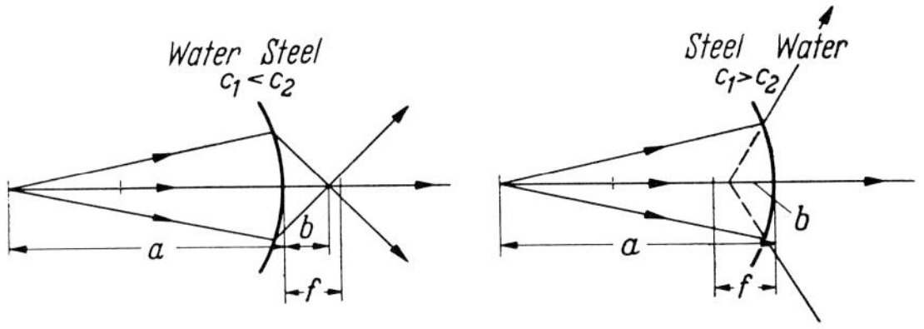

Fig. 1.44 Spherical waves in cases a) and d) of Fig. 1.43.

links all three quantities. Anything said above concerning lenses, including Figs. 1.43 and 1.44, also applies to cylindrical lenses. If again a plane and a spherical wave is to pass through a spherical lens or a cylindrical lens, the resultant acoustic pressures are

Plane wave through spherical lens	Cylindrical lens	
$D P_0 \dfrac{f}{x \mp f}$,	$D P_0 \sqrt{\dfrac{f}{x \mp f}}$,	(1.22)
Spherical wave		
$D \dfrac{P_1}{a} \dfrac{f}{x \mp f\left(1 + \dfrac{x c_2}{a c_1}\right)}$,	$D \dfrac{P_1}{a} \sqrt{\dfrac{f}{\left(1 + \dfrac{x c_2}{a c_1}\right)\left(x \mp f\left(1 + \dfrac{x c_2}{a c_1}\right)\right)}}$.	(1.23)

(The upper, negative sign applies to condensing lenses, case a and b in Fig. 1.43, and the lower, positive sign to dispersing lenses; under the root sign only absolute values shall apply.) D is the transmission coefficient according to Eq. (1.11).

As far as the focal points are concerned the same reservations as above apply. Figs. 1.43 and 1.44 clearly indicate the strong refracting effect of a water/steel lens. In optics the greatest index of refraction is only 2.4 (diamond), compared with the value of $c_2/c_1 = 4$ in our case. This is the reason for one of the difficulties encountered when testing objects with curved surfaces in liquids ultrasonically.

For the sake of clarity excessively wide beams are used in the illustrations, for which in reality the boundary rays would no longer intersect each other at the focal point.

When testing materials, the mirror and lens effects are produced unintentionally by the given surfaces of the test objects; sometimes, however, also intentionally in order to change the direction, shape or intensity of a wave. The plane mirrors used for this purpose consist of a metal or plastic membrane stretched over a flat surface leaving a thin layer of air. The layer of air can of course be very thin without becoming transmissive. As a precaution a dry sheet of paper is inserted. This foil should be thin compared with the wave length. Convex mirrors are best made of solid material, e.g. steel or lead, with losses of 10 to 20%. An absorbing material such as lead can be used to prevent the return of transmitted waves from other interfaces. Superior to a spherical mirror is a parabolic mirror in which also the boundary rays converge at the focal point.

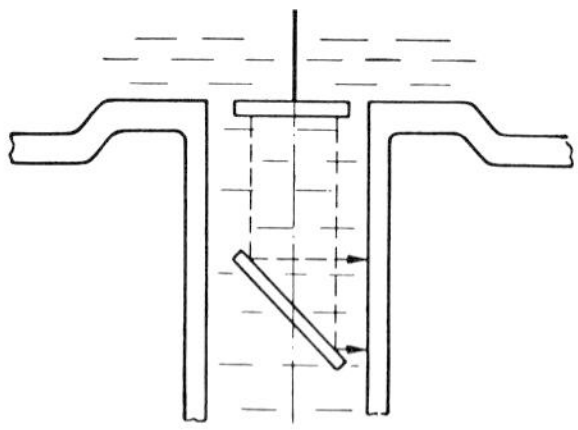

Fig. 1.45 Exploitation of mirror effect for measuring the cylinder wall thickness of an engine block under water.

Occasionally, when testing a complex specimen, the reflection by means of mirrors can be exploited to reach points difficult of access (Fig. 1.45). Other examples are shown in Figs. 3.84a and 3.164; in the latter case the work piece has intentionally been given a special form to be able to carry out the test by means of the mirror effect.

To obtain high efficiency in the case of ultrasonic lenses, it is important to keep the reflection losses small. According to Eq. (1.11) this means that the acoustic impedances of lens and contiguous material should be as nearly equal as possible. On the other hand Eq. (1.21) indicates that in order to produce satisfactory refraction, the acoustic velocities should differ as much as possible. The first requirement rules out lenses made of metal and immersed in liquid, whereas those made of plastics, e.g. perspex or polystyrene are superior, at least for lower frequencies at which their absorption is not excessive. Liquid lenses consisting of containers made of thin, spun metal sheets, have also been successfully used. (For details see Bergmann [1]).

Finally, one has taken from optics, and applied successfully to ultrasonic testing, the principle of Fresnel and zone lenses [362].

1.75* Spherical Waves in Hollow and Solid Cylinders

The application of the results of the last section will now be illustrated by the practical cases in which a sound wave passes through a hollow or solid cylinder, either through direct contact (e.g. entrance point of spherical wave on surface) or while immersed in a liquid (at a given distance from the centre of the spherical wave).

For a cylinder with co-axial hole as shown in Fig. 1.42, e.g. a generator rotor with hollow shaft, the result of the calculation of the acoustic pressure according to Eq. (1.19) is plotted in Fig. 1.46 for different ratios of internal and external radii. On the surface of the hole the acoustic pressure of the incident spherical wave has been given the value which corresponds to the arbitrarily assumed value 1 on the axis. After reflection this value decreases rapidly and remains appreciably smaller than in the case of a reflection from a flat back wall at the same distance.

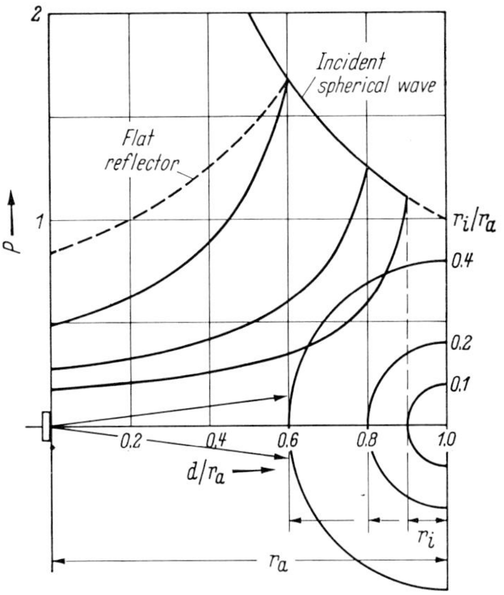

Fig. 1.46 Relative acoustic pressure P of an incident spherical wave after reflection on a cylindrical hole (acoustic pressure of spherical wave at distance $d/r_a = 1$, arbitrarily set equal to one).

Of particular interest is the magnitude of the reflection from the hole, measured at the entrance point of the beam, as compared with the reflection on a flat back wall.

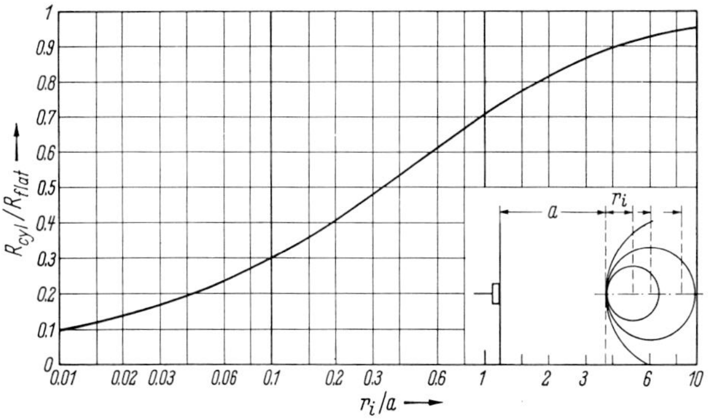

Fig. 1.47 Ratio of reflected acoustic pressures at cylindrical hole and flat backwall, measured for incident spherical wave at entrance point of beam.

This law is shown in Fig. 1.47. This diagram shows for instance that a hole of 100 mm radius produces at a distance of 500 mm only 40% of the reflection from a flat backwall ($r_i/a = 0.2$). The function is derived from

Eq. (1.19) for the cylindrical mirror as convex mirror (therefore lower sign), if $x = a$ and if divided by the acoustic pressure $P_1/2a$ which the flat backwall would produce:

$$\frac{P_{\text{cyl}}}{P_{\text{flat}}} = \sqrt{\frac{r_i}{a + r_i}}. \tag{1.24}$$

In the case of reflection in the solid cylinder, the beam entrance point is usually located directly on the surface of the cylinder as shown in Fig. 1.48. In this case the backwall concentrates the wave along a focal line F between axis and backwall, viz. at 1/3 radius from the axis. The corresponding law is again derived from (1.19) for the concave mirror with $a = 2r = 4f$. The presentation in Fig. 1.49 uses the distance d instead of x, measured from the beam entrance point.

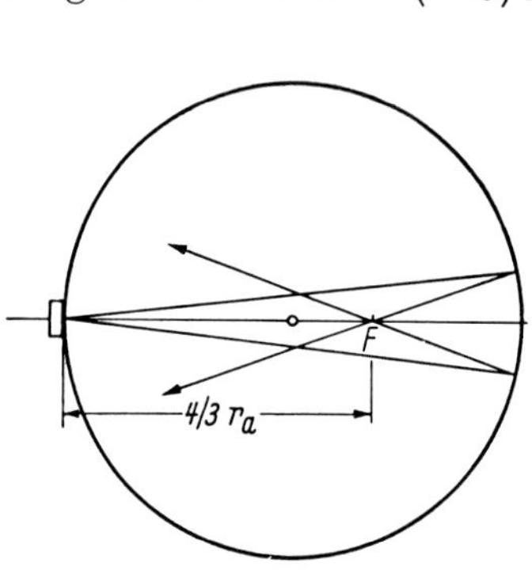

Fig. 1.48 Reflection of a spherical wave in a solid clyinder.

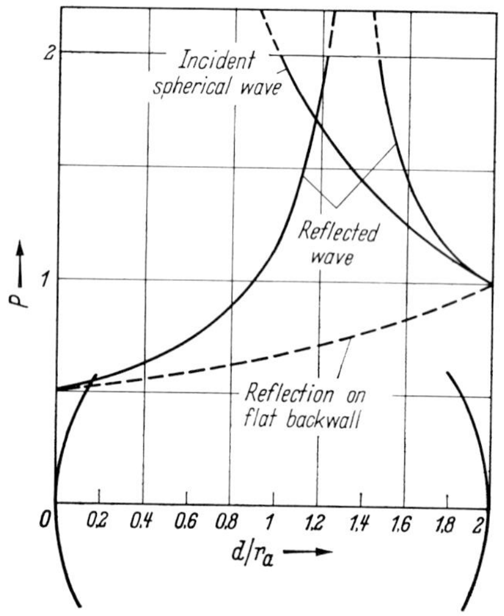

Fig. 1.49 Relative acoustic pressure P of an incident spherical wave and reflection in solid cylinder (see Fig. 1.48) (acoustic pressure of spherical wave at distance $d/r_a = 2$ arbitrarily set equal to one).

Also in this case the simple formula fails to give the true value of the acoustic pressure along the focal line, but in practice considerably higher acoustic pressures are reached than produced by the incident wave at that point. For practical echo sounding this focussing method may result in a small, reflecting flaw producing at this point a much stronger echo wave over the longer path via the backwall (W-reflection, Fig. 1.50), than along the direct path to the beam entrance point.

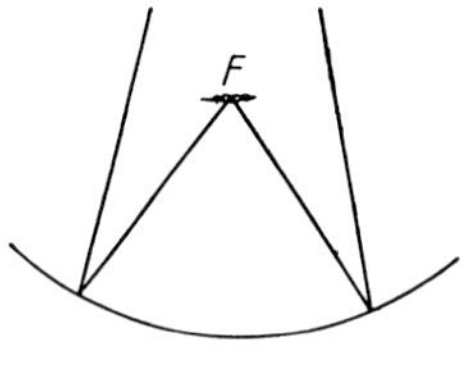

Fig. 1.50 W-reflection from flaw F.

The acoustic pressure of the reflected wave is also greater along its entire path through the cylinder than in the case of a flat backwall, plotted for comparison in Fig. 1.49. They become equal only immediately at the beam entrance point, i.e. when comparing a solid cylinder and an

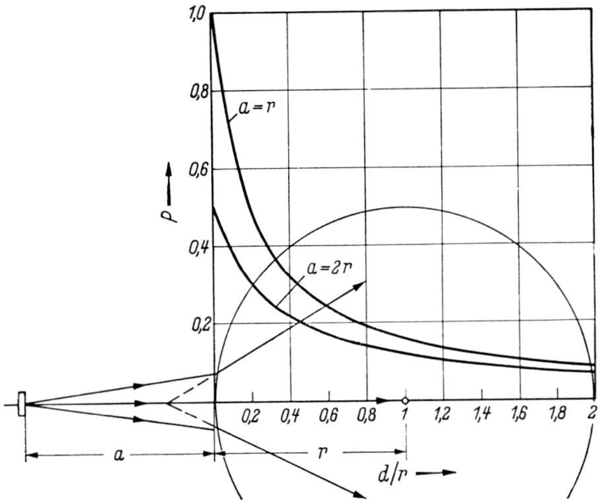

Fig. 1.51 Relative acoustic pressure in solid steel cylinder for an incident spherical wave from distance a in water.

equally thick flat plate the *backwall echoes* are equally strong for equally strong entering waves, which also applies to the multiple echoes as confirmed by a simple calculation.

Often cylindrical test objects are immersed in a liquid, the sound generator being at a distance a from the test object. Fig. 1.51 shows that the acoustic pressure in the steel cylinder immersed in water decreases rapidly with the distance from the surface. With the probe at a distance of 1 radius, viz. $a = r$, the side facing away from the probe receives less than 1/10th of the initial acoustic pressure. At a greater distance ($a = 2r$) the initial value decreases but the pattern becomes generally more uniform.

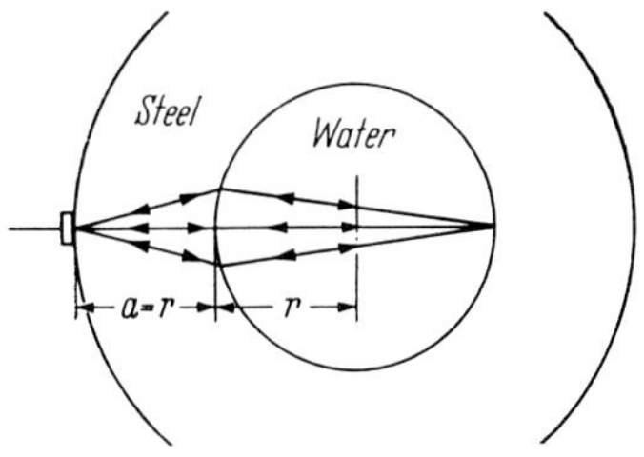

Fig. 1.52 Path of rays in a water cylinder inside steel.

Conversely, in the case of a liquid cylinder inside a solid material, for instance a thick pipe filled with water or a hole in a machine component filled with oil, a focusing effect is produced: Fig. 1.52 shows the case for water in steel. The spherical wave coming from distance $a = r$ then has its image point exactly at the backwall of the cylinder, i.e. it is thrown back along its own path with the coefficient of reflection R, and concentrated again in the sound generator.

Along its path the spherical wave has passed the interface twice in opposite directions with the transmission factor D according to Eq. (1.11), i.e. compared with the incident wave it has only been attenuated by $D_{1/2}D_{2/1}R$. The geometric construction does not supply the true acoustic pressure at the beam entrance point because this is the location of the image point. Compared with an equally thick layer of water with flat walls it can, however be said in a general way that the backwall, owing to focusing in the case of the cylinder, produces a much stronger echo. For this reason the backwall echo of an oil-filled hole in a given machine component is always indicated very strongly. It is located behind the echo of the front wall of the hole at a distance which, due to the ratio of the acoustic velocities, corresponds approximately to the four-fold diameter of the hole. Although the focusing effect depends on the distance of the sound generator it is still pronounced at distances greater than the radius.

1.8 Wave Physics of Sound Field, Sound Diffraction

1.81 Elementary Description

Before becoming acquainted in Sec. 1.10 with the structure and mode of operation of ultrasonic generators, let us visualize an *oscillator* in the form of a plate which transmits to the particles of the contiguous material its own longitudinal or transverse motion, viz. over its entire surface with the same phase and amplitude. If such an oscillator is mounted in an extended, rigid wall whence it radiates into a liquid, a sound field is obtained similar to that behind a diaphragm of the same diameter as the oscillator in the wall if struck by a plane wave (Fig. 1.53). The particle motion in the diaphragm is then the same as that immediately in front of the oscillator.

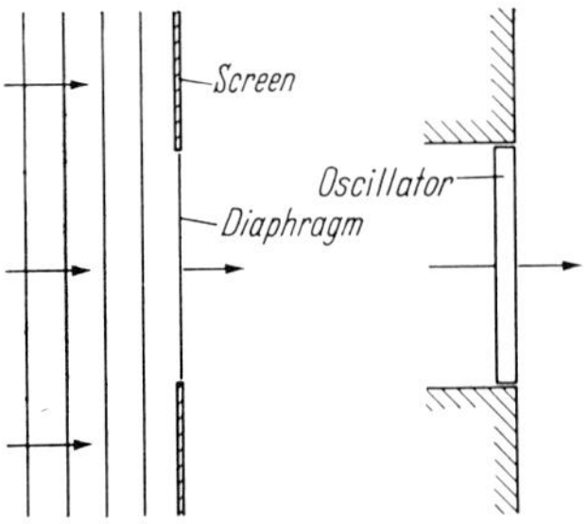

Fig. 1.53 Oscillator in rigid wall produces same effect as a diaphragm in a flat wave with rigid screen.

According to geometric principles the plane wave would beam through the diaphragm a sharply defined cylinder surrounded by a *shadow field*. In reality the sound field, owing to diffraction phenomena, is changed considerably in both regions. This can be illustrated qualitatively by applying Huygens' principle mentioned in 1.3. As in Fig. 1.10, the spherical elementary waves again form plane wave surfaces in the centre zone of the diaphragm. To this is added the edge effect. In the case of a straight edge the elementary waves of the edge form a cylindrical wave whose axis is the edge, while in the case of a circle an annular wave is produced. Superposition upon the plane wave produces a field of maxima and minima of the acoustic pressure, of which some are indicated in Fig. 1.54. This is clearly demonstrated in Fig. 1.55 where the actual sound field in front of an oscillator has been made visible (OSTERHAMMEL method [280]).

Both pictures are instantaneous exposures of the sound field. The maxima in Fig. 1.54 travel with the wave along the dotted curves towards the axis.

The ratio of oscillator diameter D to wave length λ determines the spread of the interference field and the number of maxima and minima, In Fig. 1.54 $D/\lambda = 6$, and in Fig. 1.55 6.7.

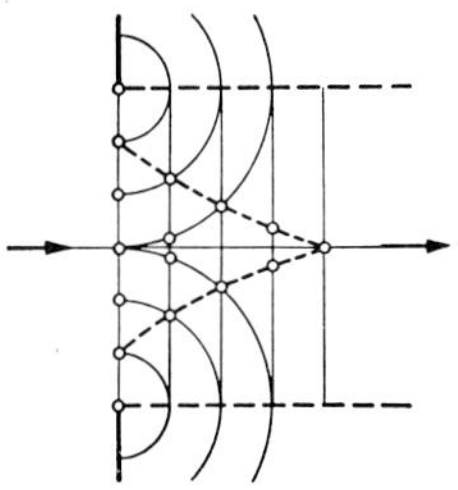

Fig. 1.54 Interference structure of sound field behind diaphragm according to Huygens' principle.

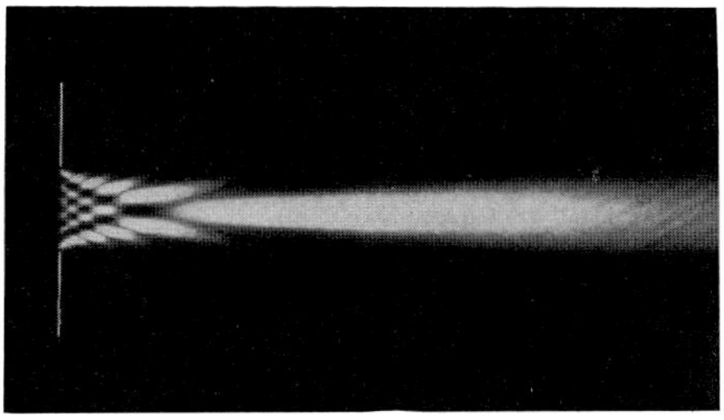

Fig. 1.55 Sound field in front of an oscillator with $d/\lambda = 6.7$ (photograph by LINHARDT and RIECKMANN [228]).

The graphic construction according to Fig. 1.54 gives the correct position of the maxima and minima only in the case of a narrow long gap perpendicular to the plane of the drawing, but not in the case of a circular diaphragm. A more accurate method for constructing the interference field will be discussed in Sec. 1.82.

Behind the diaphragm in the direction of the sound is a last maximum located on the axis, viz. the main maximum, whose distance from the diaphragm is given according to an accurate calculation by

$$N = \frac{D^2 - \lambda^2}{4\lambda}. \tag{1.25}$$

Since the interference field is also called the near field in contrast to the continuous, interference-free, far field, the last maximum determines the end of the near field. N is therefore the length of the near field. For wave lengths which are short compared with the diameter of the diaphragm or the oscillator, λ^2 can be neglected in the numerator so that in most practical applications the approximation

$$N = \frac{D^2}{4\lambda} = \frac{R^2}{\lambda} = \frac{F}{\pi\lambda} \tag{1.25a}$$

(with the radius R or the area F of the oscillator) suffices, particularly because this value serves not as a sharply defined boundary but only for orientation in the sound field.

Fig. 1.56 shows the sound field of an oscillator with 24 mm dia. and a wave length of 1.5 mm, corresponding to a frequency of 4 MHz in steel. This presupposes continuous excitation of the oscillator, or at least very long pulses. The influence of short pulses is discussed in 1.83.

Immediately at the oscillator the mean acoustic pressure equals approximately that which would occur in a plane wave, i.e. far to the left of the diaphragm in Fig. 1.53. The actual local pressure fluctuates, how-

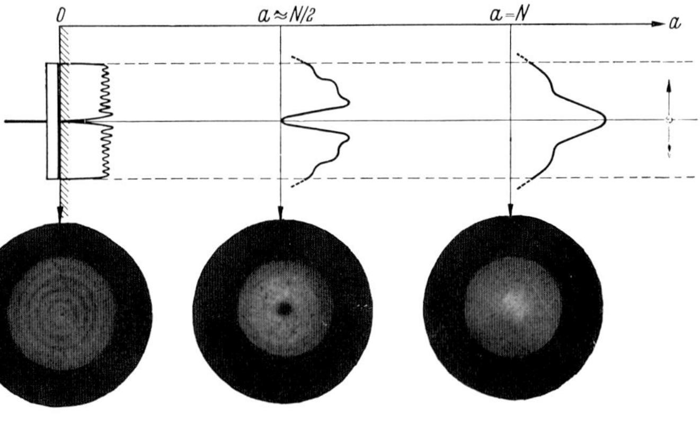

Fig. 1.56 Near field in front of an ideal piston oscillator or behind a circular diaphragm in a plane wave with distributions of the acoustic pressure along sections spaced $a = 0$, $N/2$ and N, for $d/\lambda = 16$, with correlated photographed simulated images of the beam cross-section.

ever, around the mean pressure from point to point in accordance with the many maxima and minima of which only the middle one becomes large. The number of maxima is D/λ, i.e. in our case $24/1.5 = 16$. In the case of an odd number a maximum is obtained in the centre with double the mean acoustic pressure. The acoustic pressure along the axis of the oscillator fluctuates between zero and double the mean value (Fig. 1.57). Simultaneously the maximum or minimum in the centre becomes broader and shifts the many smaller fluctuations around it laterally into the shadow zone, where immediately behind the diaphragm the acoustic pressure is still zero. Approximately at the position $N/2$, only a low minimum remains on the axis, surrounded by a maximum. A further cross-section at the end of the near field shows only one remaining maximum with double the initial mean value. None of the acoustic pressure curves of the cross-sections are smooth like sinusoidal curves; even the last maximum has a broader base which slowly decreases towards the outside.

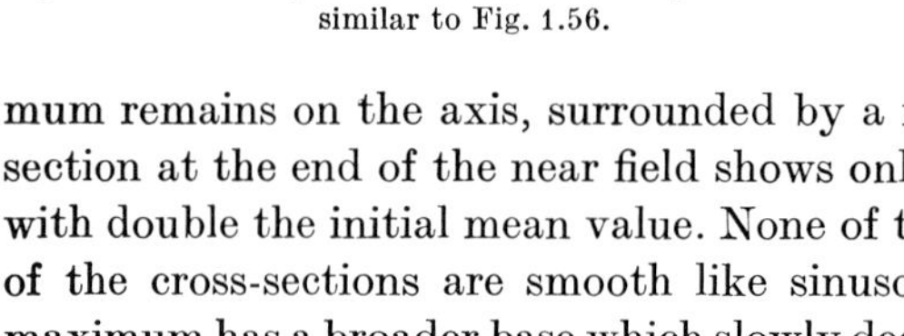

Fig. 1.57 Acoustic pressure on the axis of a piston oscillator similar to Fig. 1.56.

Since it is very difficult to obtain distinct pictures of such acoustic beam cross-sections, the images in Fig. 1.56 were produced artificially by photography on the basis of the calculated cross-section curves. Intense brightness means high acoustic pressure.

In contrast to the complex pattern of the acoustic pressure, both along and transverse to the axis in the near field, the far field is simpler

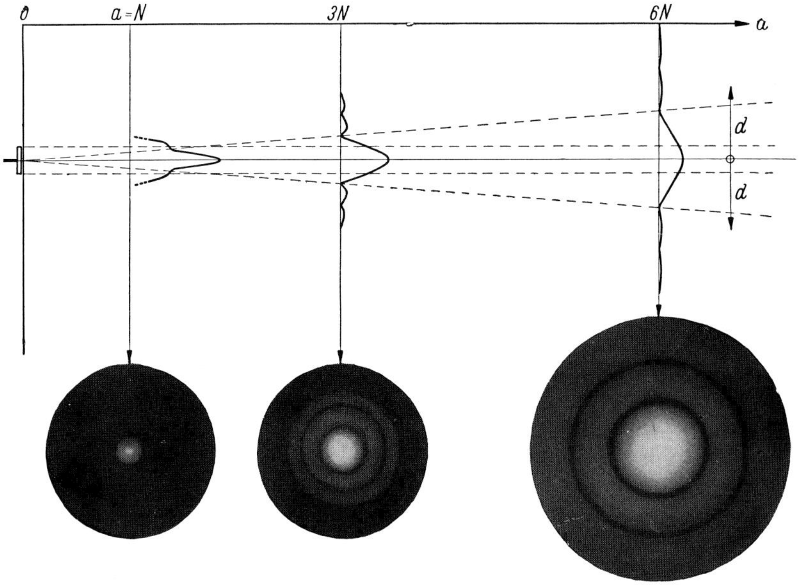

Fig. 1.58 Transition from near field to far field with acoustic pressure distributions in cross-section as shown in Fig. 1.56, but reduced 1 : 4.

(Fig. 1.58). The steep maximum at the end of the near field widens with increasing distance and at $3N$ already shows a nearly smooth curve with zero points and secondary maxima whose peaks decrease rapidly towards the outside. On doubling the distance, the width of the curve in cross-section doubles while the height is halved. This shows that it opens at a definite angle, which is obtained for instance for the first zero point by connecting it to the centre of the radiator along the broken lines shown. The angle of one of these lines with the axis of the radiator is the angle of divergence γ_0. This angle is calculated according to the theory of diffraction

$$\sin\gamma_0 = 1.2\frac{\lambda}{D}\,. \tag{1.26}$$

In our example with $D/\lambda = 16$ we obtain $\sin\gamma_0 = 0.075$, i.e. $\gamma_0 = 4.3°$ Since in the case of such small angles the sine can be replaced with sufficient accuracy by the arc, one obtains approximately

$$\gamma_0 = 1.2 \frac{\lambda}{D} 57.3 \quad \text{in degrees.}$$

Formula (1.26) is valid only for small values of λ/D, i.e. only small values of the angle of divergence are obtained correctly. If λ/D approaches 1, the stricter theory gives an angle of divergence of 90° const., i.e. directional characteristics

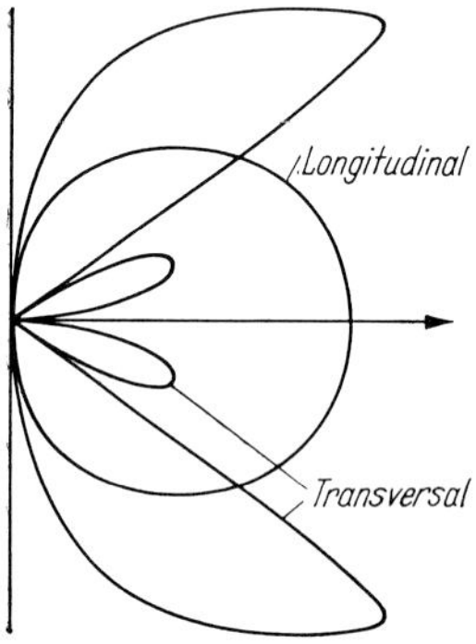

Fig. 1.59 Directional characteristics of a very small radiator (large λ/D ratio) in a solid body, calculated by RODERICK for Poisson's ratio $\sigma = 0.25$).

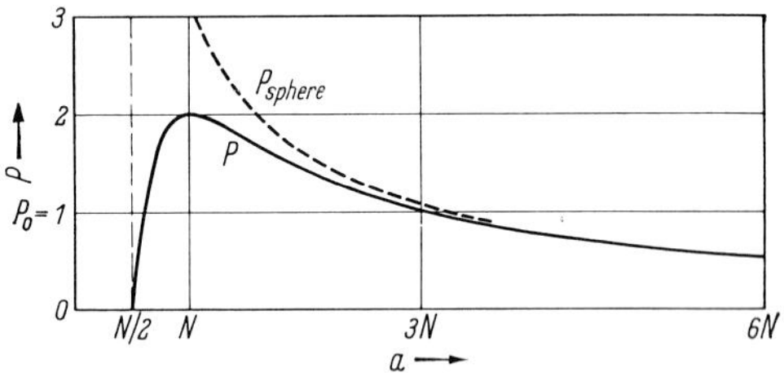

Fig. 1.60 Acoustic pressure P on the axis of the radiator as shown in Fig. 1.57; dotted line acoustic pressure of spherical wave.

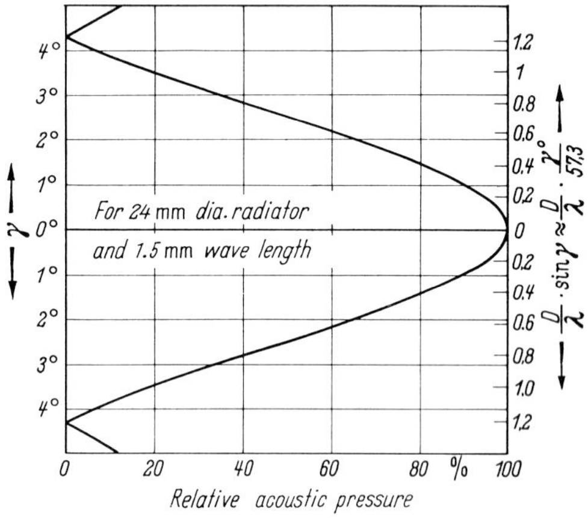

Fig. 1.61 Relative acoustic pressure in the far field plotted against angle γ for $D/\lambda = 16$.

which more closely resemble the spherical form and not, as frequently but erroneously assumed, the hemispherical form. This is shown in Fig. 1.59 according to a calculation by RODERICK [312]. At the same time an oscillator of this type shows strongly pronounced lateral sensitivity for transverse waves, as both transmitter and receiver, particularly at angles greater than 33° in steel. Furthermore, with increasing λ/D ratio, such an oscillator always radiates more energy in the form of surface waves as compared with the radiated longitudinal waves. The characteristics of the longitudinal and transverse waves were confirmed experimentally by FILIPCZYNSKI [97].

According to Fig. 1.60 the acoustic pressure decreases continuously along the axis in the far field, as will be discussed in greater detail below. Fig. 1.61 shows the centre position of the cross-sectional distribution, enlarged and plotted above the angle to the oscillator centre. In this way the curve can be evaluated for arbitrary distances from the radiator.

Example: At what distance d from the axis does the acoustic pressure become zero at a distance $a = 500$ mm from the radiator?

$$d = a \sin \gamma_0 = 500 \sin 4.3° = 37.5 \text{ mm}.$$

With these data of the radiator the acoustic beam thus "illuminates" at a distance of 500 mm a circular disc of 75 mm diameter in such a way that the shadow field starts just at its edge.

For other values of D and λ the scale on the right-hand side in Fig. 1.61 is used.

Example: At what angle is the acoustic pressure still 50% of the maximum pressure on the axis for a radiator with $D/\lambda = 4$ (say $D = 24$ mm and $\lambda = 6$ mm, i.e. at 1 MHz in steel)? The scale on the right-hand scale reads at 50% acoustic pressure:

$$\frac{D}{\lambda} \sin \gamma = 0.7 \,,$$

therefore $\gamma \sim 10°$.

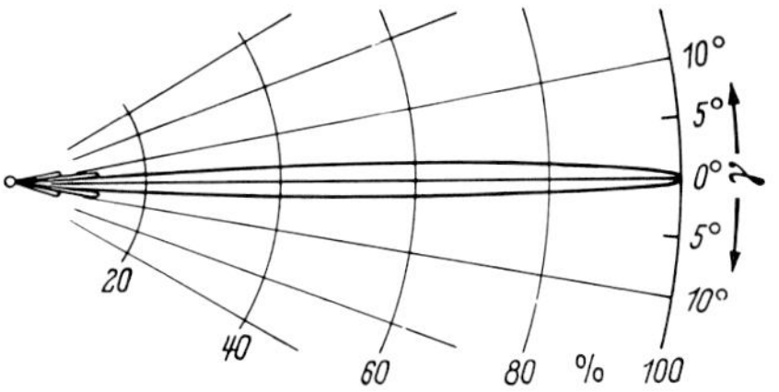

Fig. 1.62 Same directional characteristic as in Fig. 1.61 ($D/\lambda = 16$), but in polar diagram.

Angles of divergence at which the acoustic pressure has decreased to a definite fraction of the maximum pressure, e.g. 50% or 70%, are also written γ_{50} or γ_{70}, respectively.

When applying the echo method the directional characteristic of the radiated sound field is of less importance than the sensitivity for indicating a small flaw off the axis. It is important to know at what percentage, referred to the maximum indication on the axis, a given flaw is still indicated at a definite angle. Since the directional characteristic for a given radiator acting as a transmitter is the same as when it is operated as a receiver, the sensitivity characteritic in the echo method is equal to the square of the directional characteristic of the sound field. This should be noted wherever angles of divergence are given: γ_0 is identical for both, but not γ_{70}. Since $0.7^2 = 0.49 \sim 0.5$, we have

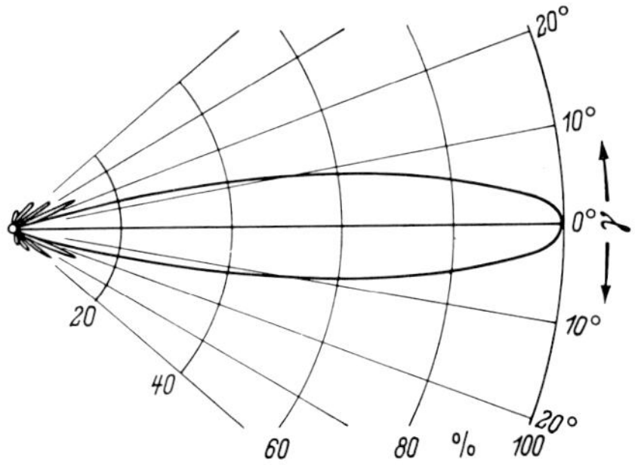

Fig 1.63. Directional characteristic for $D/\lambda = 4$.

$$\gamma_{70 \text{ (sound field)}} = \gamma_{50 \text{ (echo)}} \,.$$

Instead of plotting the angle γ linearly as in Fig. 1.61, the relative acoustic pressure can also be presented in a polar diagram as in Fig. 1.62. At low acoustic pressures in the zone of the secondary maxima this *directional characteristic* of the radiator is, however, difficult to evaluate. Fig. 1.63 shows it for a value of $D/\lambda = 4$, as compared with Fig. 1.62, i.e. when the radiator diameter is reduced from 24 to 6 mm, or the wave length increased from 1.5 to 6 mm. The angle of divergence then becomes approx. 10°. Of course the directional characteristic provides no information on the change of the actual acoustic pressure with D and λ.

Let us investigate the pattern of the acoustic pressure along the axis more closely. Fig. 1.57 shows this in the near field, while Fig. 1.60 shows it in the far field (reduced to 1/4 scale and omitting the many maxima and minima of the near field). In both diagrams the acoustic pressure is given by the function

$$P = P_0 2 \sin\left(\frac{\pi}{\lambda}\left(\sqrt{\frac{D^2}{4} + a^2} - a\right)\right) \tag{1.27}$$

with the initial acoustic pressure $P_0 = 1$. However, only positive values are plotted. At large distance a the curve can be approximated by

$$P = P_0 2 \sin\left(\frac{\pi D^2}{8\lambda}\frac{1}{a}\right) \approx P_0 \frac{\pi D^2}{4\lambda}\frac{1}{a}; \qquad \left(a \gg \frac{D^2}{4\lambda}\right). \tag{1.28}$$

Finally, if we insert in Eq. (1.25a) the length N of the near field or the area F of the radiator, the acoustic pressure along the axis of the far field becomes:

$$P = P_0 \pi \frac{N}{a} = P_0 \frac{F}{\lambda a}. \tag{1.29}$$

This curve is indicated in Fig. 1.60 by a dotted line as P_{sphere} because, in view of the dependence on $1/a$, this is the acoustic pressure of a spherical wave: in the far field our sound beam follows the law of distance of a spherical wave, as already used in 1.7.

To simplify the calculation the actual pattern of the acoustic pressure in the far field is often replaced by that of the spherical wave; in this connection it should be noted that at $a = 2N$ the error according to Fig. 1.60 is approx. 10% along the axis. At $a = N$ the ratio becomes $\pi/2 = 1.6$.

Furthermore, Fig. 1.60 indicates that at distance $3N$ the mean acoustic pressure is again reached immediately in front of the radiator, or in the example quoted at approx. 300 mm from the radiator: this shows that the radiator produces an intrinsic focusing effect on the radiation with a *focal point* at the end of the near zone, at double the mean acoustic pressure at the radiator. From thereon the acoustic pressure decreases slowly and regains the mean value only at 3 times the distance.

The results concerning the sound field can be summarized as follows:

1. The character of the acoustic beam is determined by the ratio of *diameter to wave length* of the radiator. If this value is large we get a sharply defined and far extending beam, with a long near zone.

2. The magnitude of the acoustic pressure at a given distance is determined by the ratio of *area to wave length* of the radiator.

3. At a sufficiently great distance the sound field follows the distance law of a spherical wave, i.e. the acoustic pressure decreases inversely with the distance.

So far sound fields produced by uniform excitation in a diaphragm or at the circular contact face of a radiator have been discussed. Departures from this excitation greatly change both the near field and the far field. The influence of a non-uniform excitation on the near field will be treated separately in 1.83. Two examples for other excitation surfaces follow.

If a conventional circular radiator makes only partial contact with a workpiece, its angle characteristic always becomes broader, possibly asymmetrical, with more radiation in secondary lobes. As an example let us consider an oscillator placed on a test object with an indented or conical hole as shown in Fig. 1.64, which makes contact only along an annular boundary zone. Its radiation, compared with the undisturbed radiation (Fig. 1.62), shows a broader main maximum and pronounced secondary lobes. In addition the acoustic pressure in the far field along the axis, according to Eq. (1.29), is reduced in proportion to the radiating area.

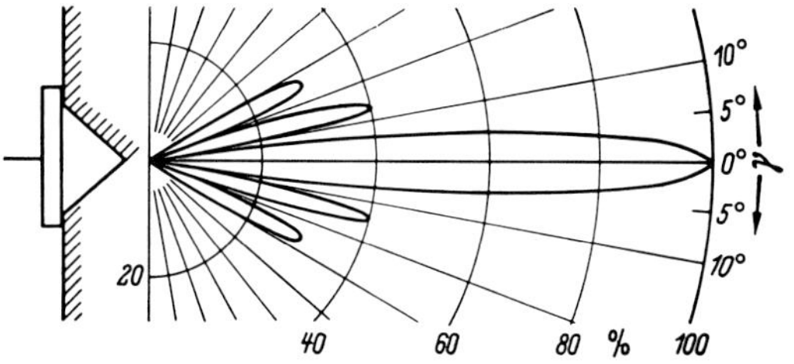

Fig. 1.64 Directional characteristic for $D/\lambda = 16$ in the case of an annular radiation area (see also Fig. 1.62).

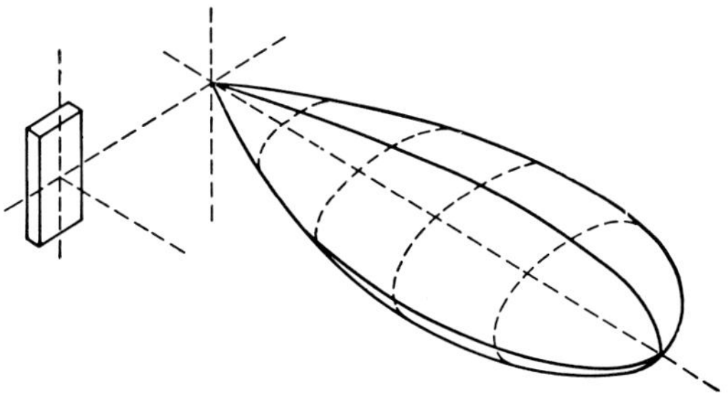
Fig. 1.65 3-dimensional view of directional characteristic of a rectangular radiator (without secondary lobes), ratio of sides 2 : 1, $D_1/\lambda \sim 4$, $D_2/\lambda \sim 2$.

The characteristic of a rectangular radiator (Fig. 1.65) is no longer axially symmetrical. It has become broader in the plane which contains the axis and the narrow side of the radiating rectangle, and vice versa. Spatially it represents a flattened lobe. The angle of divergence of this lobe in one of the two sectional planes may be calculated from Eq. (1.26), as for the circular disc, by inserting the factor 1.0 instead of 1.2, and the corresponding side D_1 or D_2 of the rectangle instead of the diameter D of the circular disc. A square radiator with the sides D thus has a slightly more pointed characteristic than a circular disc of the same diameter. A narrow and long rectangular radiator produces a beam in the form of a runded broad and flat paint brush.

Mathematically the directional characteristic shown in Fig. 1.61 is expressed by the function

$$\Re(\gamma) = 2\,\frac{J_1(x)}{x} \quad \text{where} \quad x = \pi\,\frac{D}{\lambda}\sin\gamma\,.$$

J_1 is a Bessel function whose value can be taken from Tables, e.g. in [14].

The function for the rectangular radiator is

$$\Re(\gamma_1, \gamma_2) = \frac{\sin x_1}{x_1}\,\frac{\sin x_2}{x_2} \quad \text{for} \quad \begin{aligned} x_1 &= \pi\,\frac{D_1}{\lambda}\sin\gamma_1, \\ x_2 &= \pi\,\frac{D_2}{\lambda}\sin\gamma_2. \end{aligned}$$

See also [9] for further functions.

Unless very small microphones are used for precise measurements in a given sound field, they easily disturb the sound field proper and indicate instead of the true, local acoustic pressure, merely a mean value according to their size. However, in materials testing comparatively large microphones are used for detection, viz. probes of the same shape as the transmitting radiator, or frequently the latter itself. As a result of this averaging effect, the sound field is sometimes presented greatly simplified as shown in Fig. 1.66: in a cylinder having the same length as the near field in front of the radiator and having the same diameter, the acoustic pressure is constant at all points but zero outside this zone. To it the far field is connected in the form of a cone in which the acoustic pressure decreases from the axis towards the shell surface. Such a simplification may only be used with reservations.

Compared with the above simplified description, actual sound fields show certain differences as confirmed by measurements. In liquids these are unimportant from the point of view of materials testing as long as one does not operate in the near field close to the radiator, or in the far field in the range of large angles to the axis. These differences are explained by the deviations from the condition of an ideal radiator in a rigid wall. In solid materials it is found, however, that this simple description overlooks the coupling of the various wave types: a sound field of longitudinal waves also contains portions of transverse waves and surface waves which in certain circumstances may cause disturbances (Roderick [312], see also Sec. 1.59).

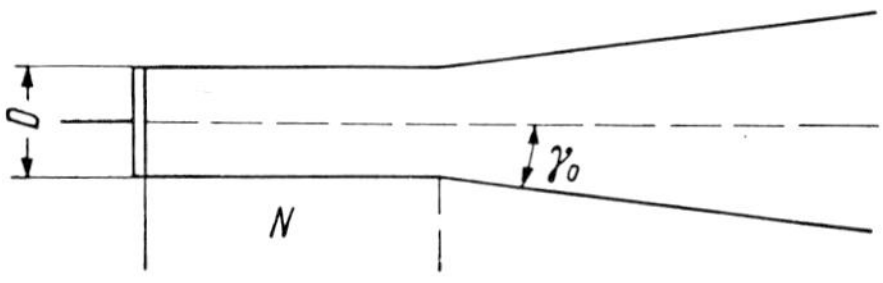

Fig. 1,66 Simplified presentation of the sound field.

It is often of interest to know how a sound field behaves in its near and far zone when passing through the interface of two different materials. In the testing of materials for instance, when applying the immersion method, the ultrasonic beam first passes through a liquid before it enters the test object. In the case of a flat interface at right angles to the beam the following simplified presentation can be used: irrespective of the location of the interface in the sound field, whether in the near zone or the far zone, the field in the solid test object appears shortened in the sound direction, in the ratio of the acoustic velocities. In the case of water/steel the value is approx. 1/4. Consequently the rest of the near zone in the test object is shrunk to 1/4 and the angle of divergence of the far field has increased 4-fold, as long as small angles are involved. In addition, the acoustic pressure values in the test object have been reduced by the transmittance factor of the interface for vertical incidence. This neglects the transverse and boundary layer waves separated at the interface. However, a rigorous treatment of the phenomena involved falls outside the scope of this presentation.

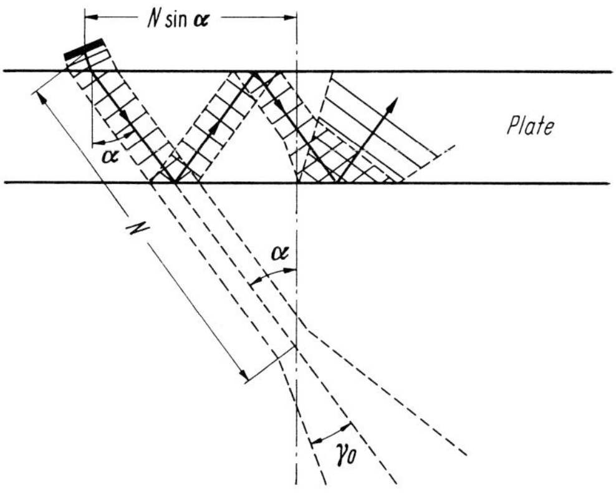

Fig. 1.67 Shortening of near field in the case of a plate wave. For the sake of clarity the beams are drawn so narrow that they do not cover each other after reflection.

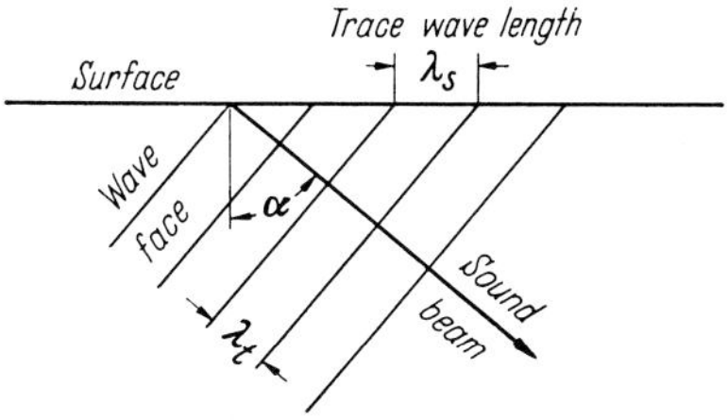

Fig. 1.68 Trace wave length $\lambda_s = \lambda_t/\sin\alpha$ of plate wave.

More complex is the sound field of wave types in finite bodies, such as plate or surface waves. In the case of plate waves it is necessary first to consider the length of the near field of the sound beam along the zig-zag propagation path of the longitudinal and transverse wave components. As indicated in Fig. 1.67 the near field at the surface of the plate appears to be shortened by the factor $\sin\alpha$, while the divergence of the beam appears increased by the factor $1/\sin\alpha$ because the process is viewed from a direction perpendicular to the surface and towards a beam directed obliquely downward or upward. The propagation angles α of the transverse components for the plate and surface waves are shown in Table 9.

Basically the formulas (1.25) to (1.37) can, however, also be applied to these wave types if the "trace wave length" is inserted as wave length λ_s of the plate wave, which is defined as the distance between two co-phasal wave planes along the surface. It is calculated from the wave length of the transverse wave λ_t in the contiguous medium as shown in Fig. 1.68, by using the relation

$$\lambda_s = \frac{\lambda_t}{\sin\alpha}.$$

The trace wave length must *not* be determined from the basic relation (1.1), viz. wave length = velocity of propagation : frequency. To be able to use this relation purely formally, the "phase velocity" has been defined for plate waves as the velocity of propagation of a wave crest along the surface of the plate. It is calculated from:

$$c_{\text{phase}} = c_{\text{trans}}/\sin\alpha\,.$$

The surface wave is one of the few types of waves in finite bodies for which the velocity of propagation is equal to the phase velocity.

Since, in casual observation, plate and surface waves seem to be purely areal wave fields, the opinion is occasionally expressed in literature that these wave types show a divergence only in the plane of the surface but not normal to it. Consequently the amplitude in the distant field would decrease inversely with the distance a as $1/\sqrt{a}$, and not as in the case of spatial propagation of waves as $1/a$. This assumption of a purely two-dimensional wave propagation is, however, not tenable. Experiment also gives a distance law of $1/a$, which corresponds to a normal, spatial wave propagation, as can be expected in accordance with the model of wave propagation along a zig-zag path [276, 336)].

1.82* Zone Construction of Sound Fields

For a better understanding of the properties of the sound field described in the previous Section, a method for its construction will be dis-

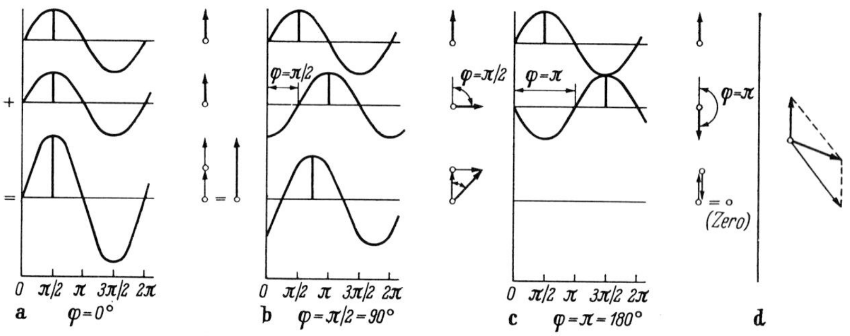

Fig. 1.69 Vector addition, a), b) and c) with identical amplitude and different phase, d) with different amplitudes. a) $\varphi = 0$, b) $\varphi = \pi/2 = 90°$, c) $\varphi = \pi = 180°$, d) intermediate value.

cussed which is a further development of Huygens' principle, viz. the zone construction according to FRESNEL. In simple cases this also permits practical, graphic determination of the acoustic pressure at any arbitrary point of the sound field, without mathematical effort.

Differences of the acoustic pressure at different points of the sound field result from the fact that Huygens' elementary waves have not travelled along the same paths from all points of the radiating surface. In addition their acoustic pressure decreases inversely with the distance. The individual acoustic pressure values of the elementary waves can therefore not simply be added but their path differences must be taken into account: two equally strong waves with a path difference of exactly one half wave length cance. each other completely. Path differences between zero and 1/2 wave length thus result in acoustic pressure values between double the value and zero. This can be presented very conveniently by *vector addition* as shown for a few cases in Fig. 1.69. This no longer determines the path difference of two elementary waves by a linear measurement but by an angle measurement in which one full wave length corresponds to an angle φ of 360° or 2π. Generally, the path difference l corresponds to the phase angle

$$\varphi = 2\pi \frac{l}{\lambda}. \tag{1.30}$$

In Fig. 1.69 the sinusoidal patterns of the acoustic pressures of two elementary waves superimposed at a point, are added for given moments and for different path differences and phase angles. In each case the corresponding vectors are added on the right hand side. The result is identical but much simpler and clearer. At arbitrary acoustic pressures and phase angles therefore the correlated vectors form a parallelogram, the diagonal indicating the acoustic pressure of the resultant wave in both magnitude and phase.

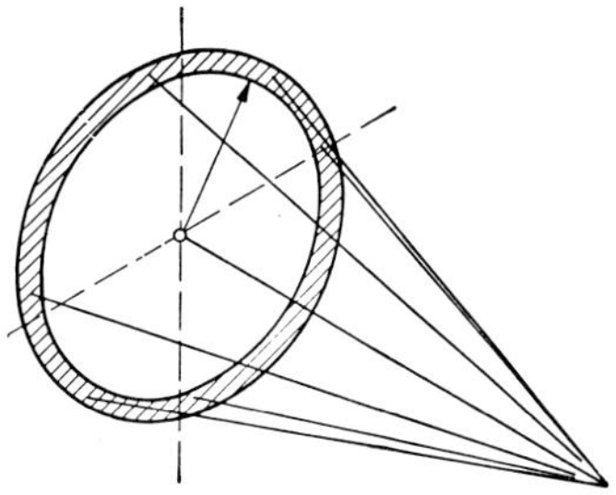

Fig. 1.70 Elementary waves radiated from the face of a circular ring.

In the Fresnel method of presentation, all elementary waves radiated from a given surface and producing at a point of the sound field a resultant acoustic pressure by adding their individual vectors, are first sorted into groups. Such a group should have approximately the same phase angle, i.e. the same path length from the area concerned to the point of summation. For a flat radiating surface this is true for instance for all waves radiated from an annular zone whose centre lies at the foot of the vertical (Fig. 1.70). If the radiator oscillates uniformly inside such a zone all its waves can be added up to a single acoustic pressure which is proportional to the area of the zone, and inversely proportional to its distance from the point of observation (since they are spherical waves). In the case of a flat area the suitable zones are concentric, circular rings of which the n-th ring produces the acoustic pressure

$$P_n = C \frac{F_n}{a_n}. \tag{1.31}$$

C is a proportionality factor which is the same for all zones if the radiation is uniform every where (if this is not the case C_n is different for each zone). It is convenient to choose rings of equal area. This area is

$$F_n = \pi\,(r_n^2 - r_{n-1}^2).$$

If we choose

$$r_n = r_1\sqrt{n}$$

all areas will be equal, i.e. equal to the central circular area

$$F_n = \pi\,r_1^2 = F_1.$$

Such a system of zones is shown in Fig. 1.71. For addition of vectors we furthermore require the path a_n which is calculated for the n-th zone according to Fig. 1.72 as:

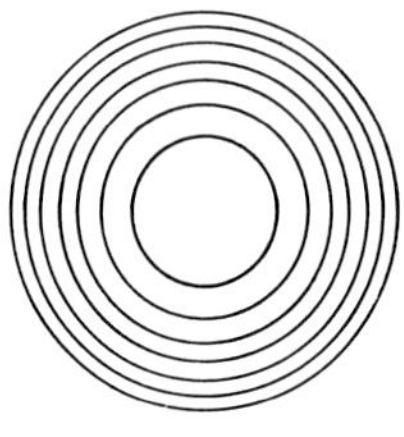

Fig. 1.71 Fresnel zones of equal area. (The radii are in the ratio of the roots of integers.)

$$a_n = \sqrt{r_{n-1}^2 + a^2} \quad (\text{for } n = 2, 3 \text{ etc.}, a_1 = a). \quad (1.32)$$

This also gives the phase angle with the vector of the 1st zone:

$$\varphi_n = \frac{2\pi}{\lambda} a_n \quad (\text{for } n = 2, 3 \text{ etc.}, \varphi_1 = 0). \quad (1.33)$$

If the point of observation is located on the axis of a circular disc radiator with radius R, one can choose $r_n = R$, with the result that the entire surface of the radiator is divided into n equal zones. The construction for this case is shown in Fig. 1.73 for a radiator with $D/\lambda = 16$, at two different points on the axis. The dimensions are chosen so that in the first case a is equal to the length N of the near field, and in the second to half the length of the near field:

$$a = \frac{D^2}{4\lambda} = \frac{R^2}{\lambda} \quad \text{or} \quad = \frac{1}{2}\frac{R^2}{\lambda}.$$

The surface of the radiator has been divided into 12 zones with vectors Nos. 1 to 12 whose lengths are given by Eqs. (1.31) and (1.32) and the angles by (1.33). In the case of distances a which are long compared with the diameter of the radiator, the values of a_n change so little compared with a that the difference is hardly discernible in the drawing. Similarly, the differences from one angle φ_n to the next become practically identical, viz. for $a = N$, $\varphi_1 = (\varphi_n - \varphi_{n-1}) = 15°$, for $a = N/2$ 30°, as readily confirmed by calculation.

In the first case the chain of the P_n vectors forms a curve closely approximating a semi-circle whose diameter gives the wanted acoustic pressure P at $a = N$. In the second case the vector chain forms a complete circle and the result is zero. This may now be compared with Fig. 1.57

whose pattern now becomes understandable. As the point on the axis approaches the radiator, the links of the chain become inversely longer with the distance while the angle increases proportionally, resulting in

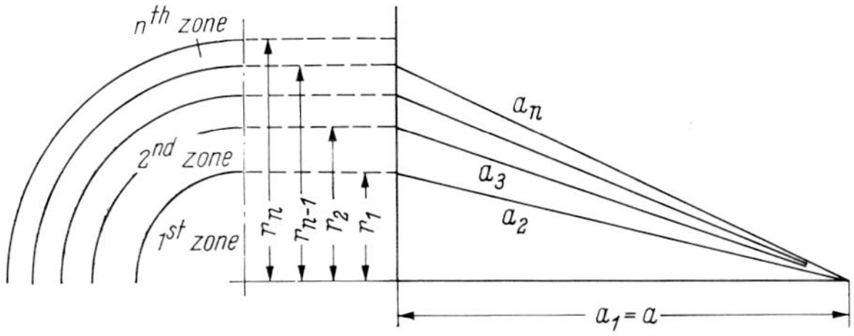

Fig. 1.72 Construction of zones, path $a_n = \sqrt{{}^{2}_{n-1} + a^2}$.

the chain being wound up. At every minimum in Fig. 1.57, beginning and end have just met, P becomes zero. Between is always a maximum in which P equals the diameter. The more subdivisions are made, the more closely will be the result in agreement with that of Fig. 1.57. It can be seen that for practical purposes 12 zones are already sufficient.

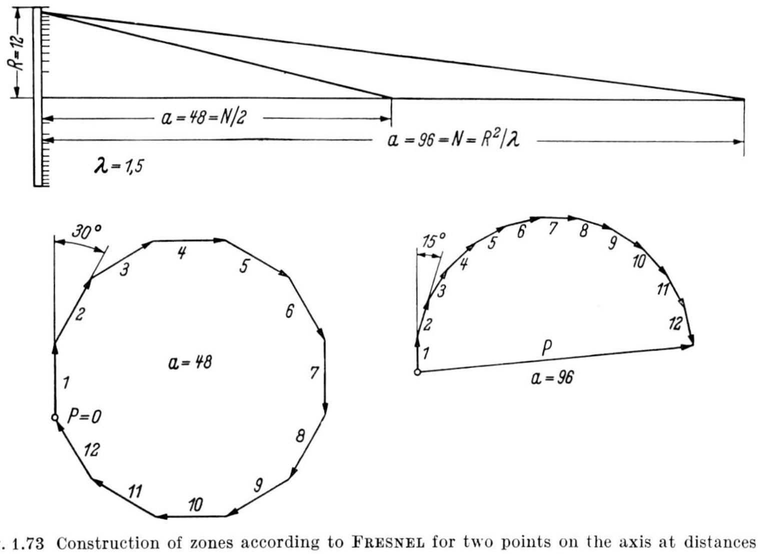

Fig. 1.73 Construction of zones according to **Fresnel** for two points on the axis at distances $a = R^2/\lambda = 96$ mm and $1/2\,R^2/\lambda = 48$ mm, at $R = 12$ mm, $\lambda = 1.5$ mm ($D/\lambda = 16$, as in Figs. 1.56 to 1.58).

In this simple case the mathematical solution is not difficult and on the basis of the above discussion, leads directly to formula (1.27).

In Fig. 1.73, P_{12} is at $a = N/2$, approx. 3% shorter than P_1, i.e. the configurations are, at moderate distances, no longer regular polygons and the zero points in Fig. 1.57 are therefore not located exactly at $N/2$, $N/3$, $N/4$, etc. In the case of irregular polygons the graphical solution also furnishes correct results and is suitable for any distances a. For large distances of course it becomes particularly simple.

For distances a greater than N the chain of the P_n vectors gradually approaches a straight line and becomes correspondingly shorter. In this case these P_n vectors can simply be added without taking the angles into account and without any great error; the radiator behaves like a spherical wave radiator with 12 times the strength of a single zone. If with $a = N$ the addition in Fig. 1.73 were made *without* regard to the angles, the result would be a straight line and thus too long by a factor equal to the ratio of the circumference of the semi-circle to the diameter, i.e. $\pi/2$ times as long. This has already been shown in Fig. 1.60; the acoustic pressure of the spherical wave (broken line) at distance N is exactly $\pi/2$ times as great as the actual pressure.

It is furthermore interesting to investigate, with the aid of the zone construction in Fig. 1.73, the influence of the individual zones on the result obtained. At $a = N$ the outer zones contribute little to the magnitude of the acoustic pressure. One or two of the zones can readily be neglected or the radiation reduced (the vectors shortened), with the result that the acoustic pressure changes essentially only its phase, its magnitude hardly at all. This, however, is different at $N/2$: any masking or attenuation of the outer zones immediately increases the acoustic pressure from zero to high values, i.e. the zero points are sensitive to uneven radiation.

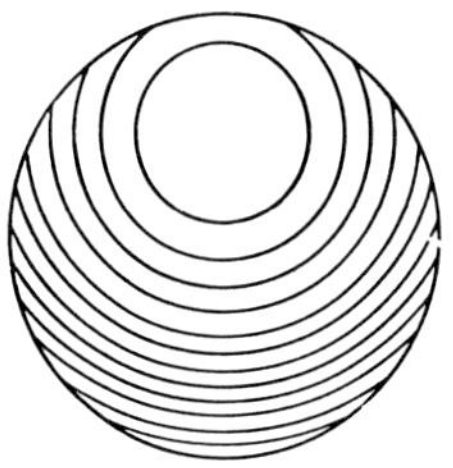

Fig. 1.74 Fresnel zones for a point not on the axis.

If half of the zones are screened out at $N/2$, viz. numbers 7 to 12, the acoustic pressure again reaches the same value as for the unchanged radiator at distance N: this would correspond exactly to the near field distance of a radiator with radius $R' = \sqrt{6/12}\ R = R/\sqrt{2}$, whose near field is $N' = R'^2/\lambda = 1/2N$. These experiments, which can readily be carried out with ultrasonic radiators in water, demonstrate particularly clearly that, owing to the wave structure of the sound field, the results can sometimes be *stepped up* by cutting down (masking) the radiator area – which would be unthinkable from the point of view of geometric ultrasonic optics.

For points not on the axis, all circular ring zones are no longer located entirely on the surface of the radiator (Fig. 1.74). The areas F_n are no longer identical and the lengths of the P_n vectors become different. But even in this case the construction by the graphical method is simple. The areas are determined by counting the squares in a drawing of the system on millimeter graph paper. This method is then not limited to circular radiator surfaces.

If the point of observation not on the axis moves very far away, the phase difference for two points of the radiator surface depends only on the angle γ at which this point appears relative to the axis (Fig. 1.75).

The ring system with far distant centre then appears as a system of parallel strips which for a given path difference Δl have the distance $b = \frac{\Delta l}{\sin\gamma}$. If a path difference of half a wave length is chosen, two adjacent strips will cancel each other at the point of observation if their areas are equal. Such a system is shown in Fig. 1.76 for the radiator conditions: $D/\lambda = 16$, angle $\gamma = 20°$. It can be seen that the black strips are practically completely counterbalanced by the white strips, so that

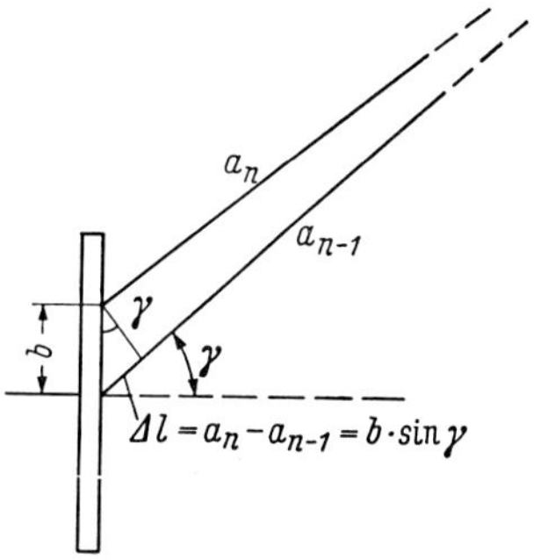

Fig. 1.75 Path difference between two elementary waves for the case of a distant point of observation.

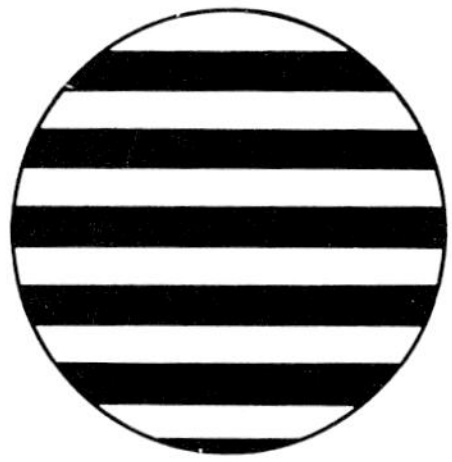

Fig. 1.76 Zonal strip with path differences of $\lambda/2$ at $D/\lambda = 16$ and with $\gamma = 20°$ (see also Fig. 1.62).

nothing, or almost nothing, is left in this direction. This explains the angle characteristic of the radiator in the far field. At small angles the strips become wider and the total area of the white strips may then greatly exceed that of the black strips, – the condition corresponding to the main maximum of the radiation.

In this discussion and in the previous section, a radiator has been assumed which oscillates continuously and sinusoidally at a given frequency. The directional characteristic and the pattern of the near field are valid only for a definite frequency. A composite oscillation must be resolved into its component oscillations and the complete sound field determined for each separately. The individual fields are superimposed. The acoustic pressure which is then measured in the total field has in general a chronological pattern different from that of the oscillation of the radiator itself. For instance, the high frequencies are radiated preferentially in the direction of the axis of the radiator. The share of the various frequencies changes with the radiation angle. The total acoustic pressure is defined by the mean value

$$P = \sqrt{P_1^2 + P_2^2 + P_3^2 + \cdots},$$

where in this case the P_n values are the acoustic pressure of the partial frequencies at the point of observation.

1.83 Sound Field at Non-uniform Excitation of the Radiator, for the Case of Pulse Excitation and Focusing Radiators

The complex structure of the sound field which, particularly in the case of radiators with large D/λ ratio, manifests itself in the numerous maxima and minima of the near field and the secondary lobes of the directional characteristic, results from the elementary waves with large path differences, i.e. by the zone near the rim. If the excitation of the radiator is permitted to decrease towards the rim the field becomes more uniform.

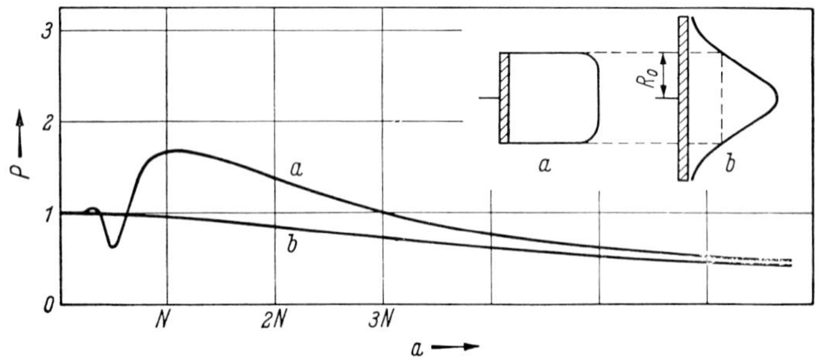

Fig. 1.77 Unevenly excited radiators, distribution of excitation over the cross-section and acoustic pressure on the axis, calculated *a* schematically for ordinary oscillators, *b* for Gauss oscillators.

In contrast to the theoretical piston oscillator, the rim of the piezoelectric disc in the case of the ordinary probe in fact is already less strongly excited than the centre. Fig. 1.77 (*a*) shows schematically the excitation curve and the corresponding, flattened-out acoustic pressure curve. The exact pattern depends on the type and shape of the radiator and its mounting.

If an excitation in the form of a bell-shaped curve is purposely chosen, the irregularities disappear almost completely, which is very desirable in non-destructive testing. For it should be born in mind that the multiple maxima in the near field transverse to the axis make the exact location of a flaw more difficult, and fluctuations of the acoustic pressure along the axis make any estimation of the size of the flaw on the basis of the height of its echo rather uncertain, a point which will be discussed again in 1.84 ([206, 133, 228]).

The distribution function which gives optimum smoothing is the Gauss function

$$e^{-\varrho^2/R_0^2}$$

with the radius co-ordinate ϱ and a constant R_0. This distribution and the co-ordinated acoustic pressure curve are shown in Fig. 1.77*b*. R_0 refers to a given radius. The greater the radius of the radiator compared with this value, the better is the constancy in the near field. The extent of the near field of the Gauss oscillator is calculated from R_0:

$$N_0 = \frac{R_0^2}{\lambda}.$$

In the distant field the Gauss oscillator in any case behaves completely like a piston oscillator with the diameter $2R_0$. However, the angle of divergence can no longer be defined by a zero point of the directional characteristic because no such zero point exists, but if it is referred to a definite decrease in acoustic pressure, e.g. 70%, it is greater than in the case of a piston oscillator of equal size, i.e. equal to the angle of divergence of a piston oscillator with the diameter $2R_0$. Quite generally the angle of divergence in the case of a given diameter of the oscillator can never be made smaller by changing the excitation, only greater. The maximum beaming accuracy is always obtained with a uniformly excited oscillator.

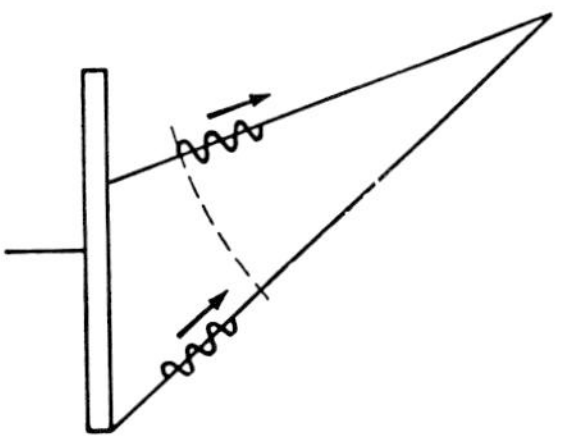

Fig. 1.78 Interference is no longer possible in the case of pulses with greater path differences.

If in the case of a continuously excited radiator only the mean value in time is of interest, e.g. when measuring the acoustic pressure or the intensity with a measuring instrument of sufficient inertia, the irregularities of the sound field can also be equalized by *wobbling*, i.e. by rapid fluctuations of the excitation frequency over a given range. Since the length of the near field changes with the frequency, the scale in Fig. 1.77 would be lengthened and shortened periodically by frequency sweeping, and at a given point in the measured field the minimum of the acoustic pressure curve, for instance, would rapidly travel back and forth so that a higher mean acoustic pressure would be indicated. It can be seen, however, that only a considerable frequency change, of at least 30%, could flatten out the minimum effectively. Naturally, simultaneously the amplitude should be kept as constant as possible, which technically is by no means simple.

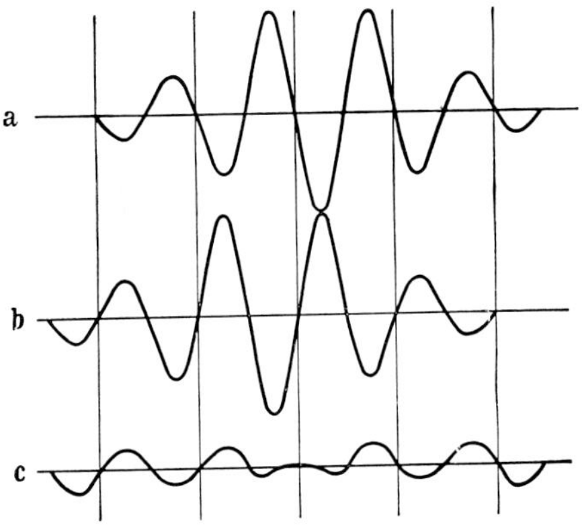

Fig. 1.79 Short pulses no longer cancel each other completely, even in the case of 1/2 wave length path difference (a + b = c).

Excitation in the form of short wave trains, i.e. pulses, can greatly influence the sound field. As shown in Fig. 1.78, pulses coming from different points of the radiator may be unable to produce interference because they do not arrive simultaneously at the point of observation. Where they are still superimposed partially (Fig. 1.79), the cancellation will always be incomplete, even in the case of a phase difference of 1/2 wave length or odd multiples of it, particularly at the head and the tail. In a sound field excited by pulses there are therefore no longer total minima. This

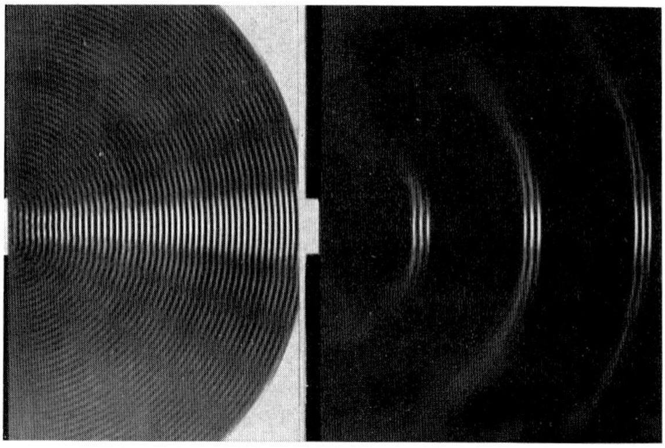

Fig. 1.80 Simulated picture of a sound field with $D/\lambda = 6$ at continuous excitation (a) and pulse excitation (b). The secondary maxima become faded in the case of pulse excitation.

is shown by the simulated picture in Fig. 1.80. It can be seen that for pulse radiation the minima and maxima of the lateral radiation are *smudged*. Although this makes the sound field of a piston radiator more uniform, as desired the pulses will be distorted at the points of the previous minima (Fig. 1.79). The original shape of the pulses can hardly still be distinguished from the complex superposition curve, and in particular the height of the pulse, which must be measured as echo height when testing materials, is no longer clearly defined and measurable.

Such pulse distortions, therefore, must be expected in the case of a piston radiator operated with short pulses of only a few oscillations, both in the far field at larger angles to the axis as well as in the near field on the axis. Only in the far field on the axis are short pulses radiated, in shape and duration, as they would be measured immediately in front of the radiator.

Strictly speaking, the pulse is still distorted on the axis even in the far field. It must not be overlooked that it represents a mixture of frequencies in which, in addition to the fundamental frequency, a portion of higher frequencies is present, which is the greater the shorter the pulse. According to Eq. (1.29) the acoustic pressure on the axis in the far field is inversely proportional to the wave length for a given radiator area. Therefore in the far field, the higher frequency components represent a larger proportion as compared with their proportion close to the radiator and therefore they distort the pulse.

The above-mentioned Gauss oscillator whose sound field is independent of the length of the pulse, essentially avoids the disadvantages of pulse distortion and is therefore more suitable for a method in which the height of the echoes is measured (see also 1.84).

The effect on the sound field of curved radiator surfaces remains to be discussed. In 1.7 the sound fields of curved mirrors and lenses were investigated with the aid of geometrical constructions. This method always results in the acoustic pressure at a focal point becoming infinite. On the basis of the correct treatment of wave physics it is now, however, possible to determine the true acoustic pressure at the focal point. For this purpose a radiator in the form of a spherical cup will first be assumed (Fig. 1.81). Evidently this radiator has a focal point at the centre of the correlated sphere.

For the acoustic pressure on the axis of a flat radiator the pattern in the far field has been found according to Eq. (1.29), as indicated in Fig. 1.60 by a dotted line. In the derivation the path differences between the individual elementary waves were not taken into account, which in the case of the far field makes little difference in contrast with the transition to the near field. In the case of the concave radiator all elementary waves converging at the focal point have the same path length, and the approximation formula for the flat radiator therefore gives the correct value for the concave radiator in the centre of the sphere.

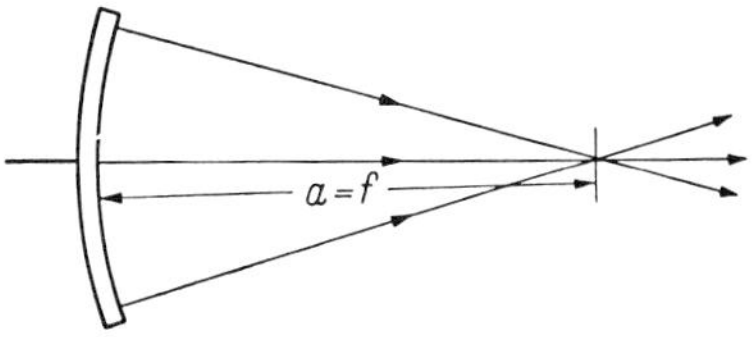

Fig. 1.81 Concave radiator.

The difference arising from the addition of elementary waves with and without making allowance for the path differences (phase angles) is demonstrated clearly by a zone construction according to Fresnel (Sec. 1.82).

If the flat radiator with the area F is visualized to be curved into a spherical surface, the acoustic pressure at the focal point with the distance f (= radius of sphere) according to Eq. (1.29) becomes

$$P_{\text{foc}} = P_0 \frac{F}{f\lambda}. \tag{1.34}$$

Thus, the acoustic pressure increases if the wave length decreases. If the wave length is further decreased, this is equivalent to a transition to geometric acoustic optics with infinite acoustic pressure at the focal point.

The above formula is valid only for the focal point. About the focal point, path differences again make themselves felt; an interference field forms both along the axis and transverse to it. This is demonstrated by the simulated picture in Fig. 1.82 which according to POHL [17] is best viewed at a small angle to the direction of the axis. This clearly reveals the interference rings around the axis. Figs. 1.83 and 1.84 show the sound fields of a concave radiator which have been made visible (according to WILLARD [388]) and a plastic condenser lens (according to SETTE [331]) with an incident, plane wave packet. Because the wave lengths used are small compared with the dimensions of the radiator and the lens, the form of the sound field largely corresponds to the geometrically constructed form. Particularly in Fig. 1.83, however, one can recognize also the interference structure of the field near the focal point.

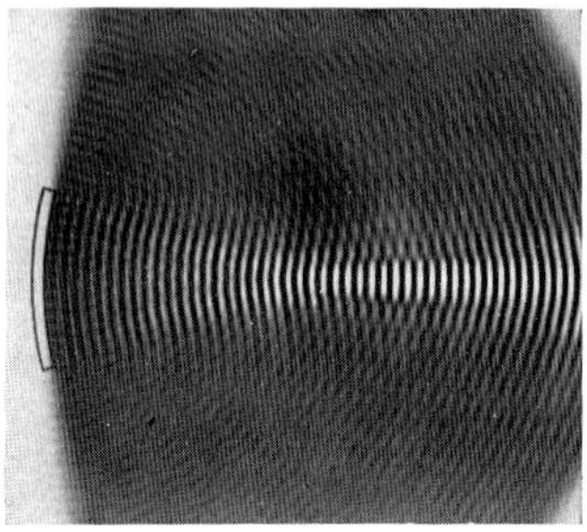

Fig. 1.82 Picture of a simulated sound field in front of a concave radiator.

Finally, we shall briefly discuss the cylindrically curved radiator, e. g. a rectangle with the sides a and b, of which a shall have a radius of curvature equal to the focal distance f. In this case the acoustic pressure at the focal point cannot be calculated as simply as in the case of a spherical radiator because the maxima and minima of the interference field correlated to the straight side b, play their part on the axis in quite the same way as in the case of the circular disc radiator in Fig. 1.57. In the case of an unfavourable ratio of the radius of curvature f to the side b, it can happen that a minimum coincides with the focal point, resulting in the acoustic pressure there becoming zero, at least theoretically for long pulses and continuous excitation.

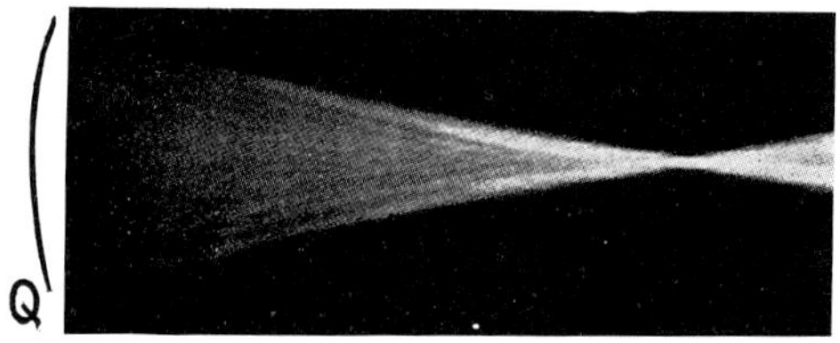

Fig. 1.83 Sound field in liquid in front of a concave radiator (according to WILLARD).

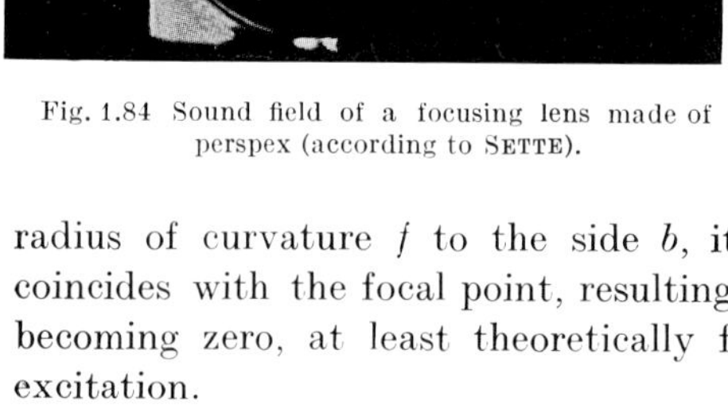

Fig. 1.84 Sound field of a focusing lens made of perspex (according to SETTE).

Therefore, the side b would have to be chosen so that its near field length $b^2/4\lambda$ is approximately equal to the focal distance, so that the last maximum occurs at the focal point. However, also in this case the calculation gives an acoustic pressure which is insignificantly higher than is much more simply obtained with a flat circular disc radiator of equal area, viz.

$$P_{\text{foc}} = P_0 \frac{F}{f\lambda} 0.64, \tag{1.35}$$

whereas the factor for the circular disc radiator according to 1.81 was $2/\pi = 0{,}637$ at the end of the near field.

Only for focal distances considerably shorter than the length of the near field in respect of side b, can a cylindrical radiator offer greater advantages than a circular disc radiator; in this case the interferences are somewhat smudged and the acoustic pressure of the radiator, because of the focusing effect of side a, becomes greater than that of a circular disc radiator, although always considerably smaller than in the case of a spherical radiator.

When using the pulse technique only the spherical radiator has the advantage that at its focal point the form of the pulses has no influence on the focusing because phase differences play no part.

1.84 Echo and Shadow of an Obstacle in the Sound Field

A given flaw in a test object, e.g. a cavity in a casting, represents an obstacle to the sound wave. Information on this flaw can only be obtained either via the reflected wave, i.e. its *echo* when using the echo method, or by its shadow when applying the method of sound intensity measurement. Information obtained from the echo and the shadow on the basis of purely geometric-optical concepts can be obtained only in the case of very large and regularly shaped flaws: in the case of a flat, smooth transverse crack in a roll the incident wave is reflected as on a mirror, resultin g in a total shadow zone behind the crack. In most instances however natural defects are so small, that diffraction phenomena determine both the echo and the shadow. Therefore defects are classified according to their dimensions transverse to the beam, as large or small defects. The designation *small* of course constitutes no evaluation of the seriousness of the defect in respect of the usefulness of the test object concerned.

Natural defects may be very irregular and of complex shape, permitting no simple evaluation by calculation. Therefore, as a first step, simple forms shall be substituted for them, of which separations in the material in the fo m of circular discs at right angles to the sound beam are particularly easy to calculate; for various purposes these can also be realized approximately and easily in the form of flat-bottomed holes. Since, however, natural defects with their uneven and rough surfaces and with their main dimension not always at right angles to the sound beam, in practice usually produce smaller echoes than circular disc defects of equal cross-section, the size of a circular disc defect is equal only to the minimum size of a natural defect producing an echo of equal amplitude.

The effect on the sound field of a flaw is shown in the simulated picture in Fig. 1.85. Fig. 1.85a shows only the wave reflected by the front of the flaw, i.e. without the incident wave. Of course, with a continuous, incident wave no separate echo wave could be observed because it would be superimposed on the former thus producing a standing wave field. Whereas according to geometrical concepts the shadow behind the flaw disc should be absolute, the sound is in fact also diffracted around the edge into the shadow space, where a field consisting of maxima and minima of the sound pressure is formed.

a 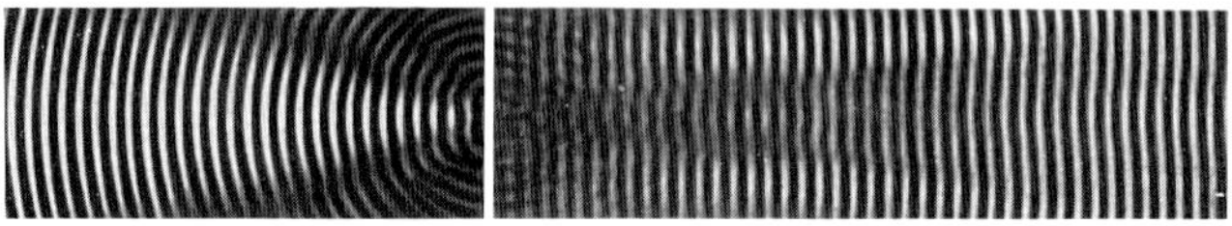 b

Fig. 1.85 Simulated picture of echo and shadow produced by a small flaw in the case of a plane wave. a) Wave reflected on the flaw alone, i.e. without incident plane wave; b) shadow of flaw. When viewing the picture at a glancing angle to its surface the interference structure of the shadow with alternating maxima and minima on the axis, becomes clearly visible.

In Fig. 1.85 a plane wave is assumed to be incident on the flaw, whereas in practice this would be a sound beam. The echo method requires that the wave reflected by a defect in such a sound beam be known, both for different distances and sizes of the defect.

Later we shall also analyse the shadow, but for the sake of simplicity for a plane wave only. Finally, the investigation will cover an oblique position of the flaw and the influence of rough surfaces.

The *echo wave* produced by a *circular disc flaw* can be analysed most conveniently if we first consider a small circular disc placed on the axis at a great distance from the radiator. This circular disc will then be *illuminated* almost uniformly because it is much smaller than the diameter of the beam. Every point of the disc becomes the origin of elementary waves as discussed in the case of the diaphragm in a plane wave. The form of the reflected wave is thus identical with that of the wave transmitted by a diaphragm: the area of the flaw in the beam becomes a new radiator whose sound beam can be calculated from the formulas given in 1.81 on the assumption that the wave length is still appreciably smaller than the diameter. Thus, the flaw has its own near zone according to Eq. (1.25a), a sound beam with an angle of divergence according to

Eq. (1.26), and a sound pressure along the axis calculated according to Eq. (1.28). P_0 is then the sound pressure over the area of the flaw. Fig. 1.86 shows clearly that the sound pressure of the incident wave at the flaw equals the initial sound pressure of the reflected wave, because it has been assumed that the flaw causes complete reflection (air gap of sufficient width).

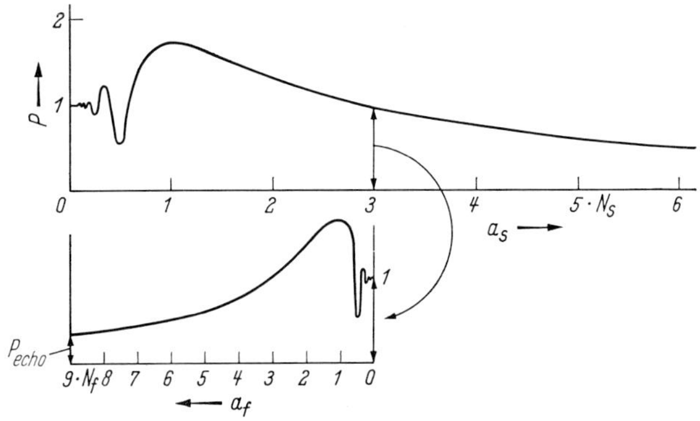

Fig. 1.86 Sound pressure on axis (schematic) for the incident wave (top) and the wave reflected from a defect corresponding to a circular disc (bottom).

The sound pressure of the reflected wave on the axis may thus be calculated from Eq. (1.29) as

$$P = P_0 \frac{F_s}{a_s \lambda} \frac{F_f}{a_f \lambda}, \tag{1.36}$$

where the suffixes s and f refer to the radiator and the flaw, respectively. If in turn the radiator is also the receiver of the echo, we have $a_s = a_f$. At a sufficiently great distance from the defect the radiator will likewise be uniformly illuminated by the reflected sound beam and is thus a measure of the sound pressure of the echo. The latter is called *echo height* H because, as will be described below, it can be read directly on the luminescent screen of a pulse echo instrument by measuring the height of a peak above the zero line. Referred to the initial sound pressure $P_0 = 1$, the height of the echo is thus given by

$$H_f = \frac{F_s F_f}{a^2 \lambda^2} \tag{1.37}$$

for a small flaw in the form of a circular disc on the axis in the far field. With a given radiator (F_s and λ) this height is therefore directly proportional to the area of the flaw and inversely proportional to the square of the distance.

Similarly, it is also possible to derive the echo height of a very large flaw which is much greater than the cross-section of the sound beam, e.g. the flat backwall of a test object at distance a. In this case the sound beam is reflected straight back along its own path and the radiator acting as receiver measures the sound pressure in its own sound beam apparently at distance $2a$. At a sufficiently great distance of the backwall its echo height can therefore be written

$$H_r = \frac{F_s}{2a\lambda}. \tag{1.38}$$

Following Ref. [206], a simplified presentation of Eqs. (1.37) and (1.38), which also lends itself to a graphic presentation of general validity, may be derived if, using the length of the near field N of the radiator, one introduces the reduced distance of the flaw

$$A = \frac{a}{N}$$

and the ratio of flaw diameter to radiator diameter as reduced size of the flaw:

$$G = \frac{D_f}{D_s}.$$

As already done in Figs. 1.57, 1.60 and 1.86, the distance of the flaw is measured in lengths of the near field. In the latter diagram for instance the flaw has the reduced flaw distance $A = 3$. A and G are dimensionless quantities which reduce the Eqs. (1.37) and (1.38) to the simple form

$$H_f = \pi^2 \cdot \frac{G^2}{A^2}, \tag{1.39}$$

$$H_r = \frac{\pi}{2} \cdot \frac{1}{A}. \tag{1.40}$$

The advantage of writing the formulas in this form is that they no longer contain directly the characteristics of the probe which change from one case to another, its near-field length which in turn contains the wave length, and its radiator diameter. Both relationships, as shown in Fig. 1.87, can be presented in a form of general validity, which if logarithmic co-ordinates are used appear as straight lines. The straight line of smaller slope, top right, represents Eq. (1.40), viz. the backwall echo, and the family of steeper straighter lines with the parameter G, the echo of the flaw according to Eq. (1.39). Both equations apply only to the far field, and are only subject to the condition that the wave length remains smaller than the diameter of the flaw.

The extension of the diagram in the direction of the near field has as yet been carried out theoretically only for the backwall echo of a piston radiator [329]. Additional information can therefore be gained only on the basis of measurements, as made for instance in Fig. 1.88 for a radia-

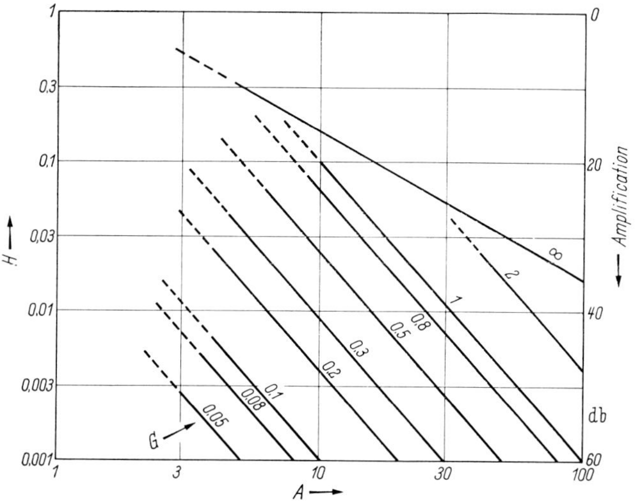

Fig. 1.87 Relation between distance of flaw A, height of echo H or amplitication V and size G of a flaw having the form of a circular disc in the far field (AVG diagramm or DGS diagramm from Distance, Gain and Size).

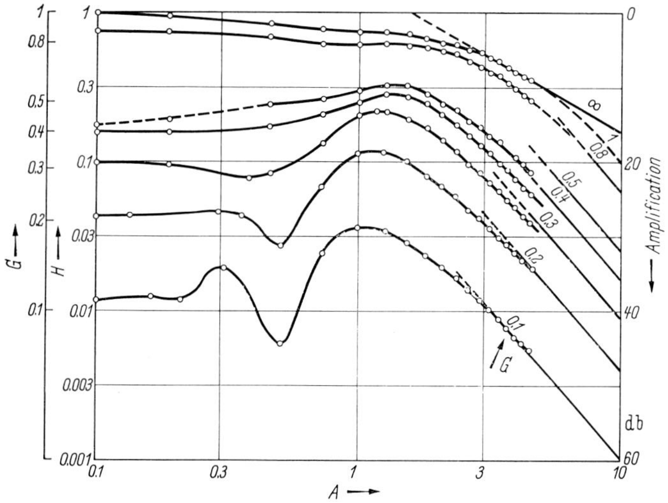

Fig. 1.88 AVG or DGS diagramm in the near field, mearsured in water with a 2 MHz radiator of 24 mm diameter.

tor in water (according to [206]). Whereas the far field is generally valid both for short and long pulses and for any type of radiator, the near-field contains interferences which depend on the pulse form and the excitation of the radiator. In this zone the diagram therefore loses its general validity; at shorter pulses the fluctuations of the curves are less pronounced particularly for small flaws. They would disappear completely for radiators excited according to the Gaussian curve.

For flaws in the form of circular discs located immediately in front of the radiator ($A \approx 0.1$) a theoretical approximate solution for the echo height can be found by assuming a plane wave, a portion of which is likewise reflected by the flaw as plane wave. In the case of a uniformly excited radiator the echo height is therefore proportional to the square of the reduced size of the flaw, as long as the flaw is smaller than the radiator:

$$H_f = G^2 \quad (\text{for } G < 1)$$

and

$$H_f = 1 \quad (\text{for } G \geqq 1).$$

As indicated in Fig. 1.88, the measurements essentially confirm this law. In the case of a Gauss rad.ator, however, the law changes due to the uneven distribution of the sound pressure immediately in front of the radiator. In this connection it should also be borne in mind that the size of the flaw should be referred to the effective diameter $2R_0$ (Fig. 1.77). The actual diameter is no longer of consequence.

The arbitrary assumption that the initial sound pressure $P_0 = 1$, made above means that the echo of the defect is given the value 1 for $G \geqq 1$ immediately in front of the radiator. The backwall echo of a thin plate with a diameter greater than that of the radiator thus becomes the reference echo with the value 1. Therefore, if the ratio of a flaw echo to this plate echo is measured, the size of the flaw of an equivalent defect in the form of a circular disc can be determined by calculation from Eqs. (1.37) or (1.39), or more simply from the diagram, provided the length of the near field and the diameter of the radiator of the probe used are known. A complete diagram, as obtainable by combination of the calculated and measured curves in Fig. 1.87 and 1.88, either for a given type of probe or preferably for Gauss radiators makes it possible to apply this method also to the near field. Similar diagrams have been determined by Zottmann [398] for cylindrical holes at right angles to the sound beam, on the basis of measurements.

From the group of *small* flaws considered above, one can still separate a sub-group of *smallest* flaws for which the wave length is no longer small compared with the diameter of the flaw concerned. Fig. 1.89 shows the cross-section of the distribution of the sound pressure of the scattered wave, on a flaw in the form of a circular disc in a solid body, according to Filipczynski [96]. For flaws which are very small compared with the wave length, the longitudinal wave reflected in a scattered form shows a spherical characteristic and is practically independent of the form of the flaw and its orientation relative to the incident wave. At right angles to the direction of incidence a transverse wave is scattered which shows an annular characteristic. With increasing size of the flaw the longitudinal wave reflected at the glancing angle is given preference, and the transverse wave diffracted transversely to the direction of the incidence becomes weaker.

The sound pressure of the reflected wave is proportional to the third power of the diameter of the flaw, and inversely proportional to the

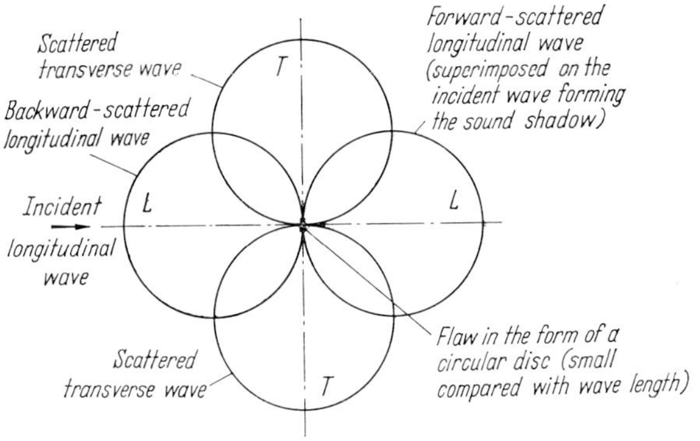

Fig. 1.89 Sound reflection and scatter from a flaw having the form of a circular disc, in a solid body. The flaw in the form of a circular disc is small compared with the wave length.

square of the wave length. The rapid decrease of the echo inversely as the third power of the diameter means in practice that the smallest flaws soon defy detection because of the limited sensitivity of the instrument.

Let us now discuss the *shadow of a flaw* in the form of a *circular disc.* For this purpose a plane incident wave shall be assumed in which therefore the sound pressure P_0 is uniform at all points in the absence of a flaw. To facilitate the analysis we understand the sound field behind the flaw as the superposition of two waves, viz. the original, undisturbed wave, and an interfering wave emanating from the back of the flaw. As far as the reverse side of the flaw is concerned the following statement on the interfering wave applies: Since on the basis of geometrical concepts the shadow on the reverse side of large flaws must be total, i.e. zero sound pressure, the interfering wave has at these points a sound pressure opposite to that of the incident wave because these waves must cancel each other completely. Therefore, the interfering wave has at every point on the circular disc the sound pressure P_0, with a phase shift of half a wave length relative to the incident wave. This, however, is exactly the same distribution of sound pressure as produced by the reflected wave on the front of the disc. This then also completely determines the whole sound field of the interfering wave. In contrast to the reflected wave, which, provided pulses are used, can be observed separately from the incident wave, the interfering wave cannot be observed alone but only in its superposition with the undisturbed wave. The result is the shadow.

The assumption of an interfering wave, which at first may seem to be merely a device for calculation purposes like saying 1 – 1 instead of 0, thus provides the entire field behind the flaw. If P_s is the sound pressure of the interfering wave, the sound pressure at any given point in the shadow zone is

$$P = P_0 - P_s.$$

The result, however, cannot be stated quite so simply because this addition must be carried out with due consideration of the phase, which has so far been disregarded in the sound field of the circular disc radiator. Let us state the result for the axis of the flaw. In this connection it should be recalled that the phase in the far field of the circular disc radiator coincides with that of a plane wave radiated from the face of the circular disc. However, nearer to the radiator the phase rotates relative to the former so that at the end of the near field the phase difference is $\pi/2$, which is equivalent to a path difference of $\lambda/4$. At the first minimum the difference is π, or $\lambda/2$.

In the far field of the flaw, i.e. at a distance a very much greater than the length of the near field of the flaw,

$$N_f = \frac{D_f^2}{4\lambda},$$

simple subtraction thus gives

$$P = P_0 - P_s.$$

and therefore according to Eq. (1.29)

$$= P_0\left(1 - \pi\frac{N_f}{a}\right).$$

At a very great distance a the disturbance, as could be expected, becomes negligible. At short distances, e.g. $a = 6N_f$, the sound pressure in the shadow zone is smaller than in the undisturbed wave, but only along the axis. Fig. 1.90 shows the calculated pattern transverse to the axis. Thus, the darker centre is surrounded by several bright rings. This diagram is based on the beam cross-section of Fig. 1.58, at $a = 6N$, making allowance, however, for the fact that the phase position in the secondary crests opposes that of the main maximum.

At distances along the axis shorter than $6N_f$, the change of phase of the interfering wave must be taken into consideration. The result is shown in Fig. 1.91, obtained by the addition of vectors (see also 1.82). The shadow along the axis is darkest at approximately $4N_f$ but it never becomes completely black. Towards the flaw it becomes gradually lighter. Near $a = N_f$, the acoustic sound pressure reaches values as much as 2.4 times the height of the undisturbed wave. Here it is lighter in the shadow than outside – another of the paradoxes resulting from the wave nature of the sound field. In the near field the values of the sound pressure fluc-

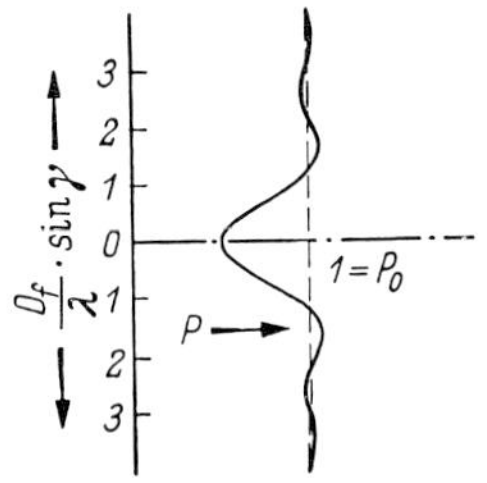

Fig. 1.90 Distribution of sound pressure in the shadow zone of a circular disc flaw, calculated for a section transverse to the axis at distance $a = 6N_f$.

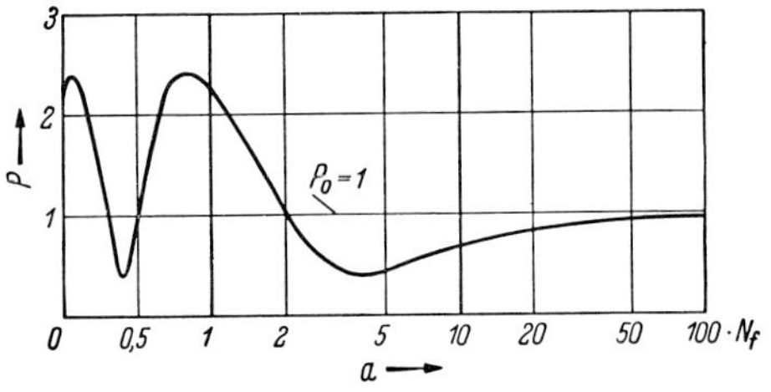

Fig. 1.91 Sound pressure in the shadow zone of a circular disc flaw, calculated for points along the axis.

tuate in quick succession, but only for a strictly circular flaw. These theoretical values are therefore of minor interest in practice where in this zone the sound pressure decreases more or less rapidly towards zero, in the shadow zone proper, as is to be expected in view of the geometric sound optics applied here.

However, only a very small receiver would measure the sound pressure as shown in Fig. 1.91, while a larger receiver would smooth out the difference by its averaging effect. The testing of materials requires that the flaw should be indicated as clearly as possible, i.e. the receiver should indicate a maximum difference between the non-disturbed wave and the shadow. This means that the receiver should not be too large. It can therefore roughly be stated: If it is required that a given flaw should still produce a 10% reduction of the indication, then immediately behind the flaw the receiver should have maximally an area ten times greater, i.e. a diameter approximately three times greater. In the far field the receiver should not cover more than the main maximum in Fig. 1.90 whose angle of divergence is determined by the relation

$$\sin \gamma_0 = 1.2 \frac{\lambda}{D_f},$$

i.e. the receiver should not be larger than

$$2a\gamma_0 \approx 2.4a \cdot \lambda / D_f.$$

Let us now determine the smallest possible flaw which can still be detected by a 10% reduction of the indication if the receiver complies with the above conditions. Fig. 1.91 shows that at $a = 30 N_f$ the sound pressure along the axis is still approximately 10% lower than the undisturbed sound pressure. However, in the zone from 2 to $0.5 N_f$ the sound pressure becomes greater and this zone is therefore unsuitable and must be excluded. The limits are drawn in Fig. 1.92 for a smallest flaw diameter of 1/3 wave length, because in the case of still smaller flaws the above calculation of the sound field is certainly invalid and because the sound pressure decreases rapidly to zero. These evaluations should be regarded as a rule of thumb.

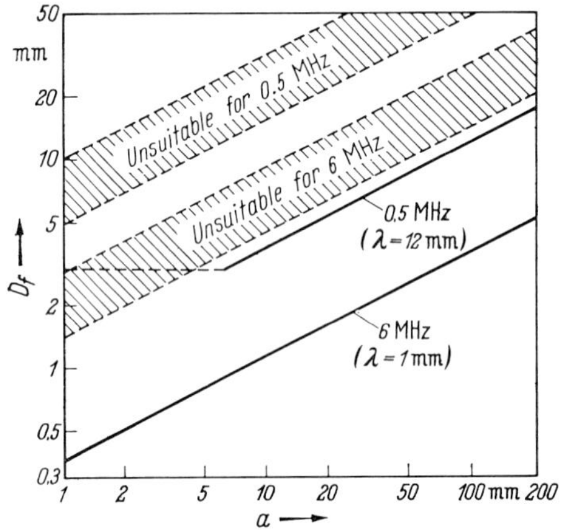

Fig. 1.92 Minimum diameter of circular disc flaws, which can still be detected by a 10% reduction in sound pressure in their shadow zone at a distance a calculated for an incident, plane wave in steel or aluminium at 0.5 and 6 MHz, respectively. Condition for receiver diameter: below unsuitable zone: $D_e < 2.4 a\lambda / D_f$, above unsuitable zone: $< 3 D_f$.

Above the two bold lines in Fig. 1.92, flaws in the form of circular discs can be detected by their shadows at a reduction of the undisturbed sound pressure of at least 10%. However, in the shaded zones the sound pressure caused by the flaw becomes greater and detection in this zone is therefore doubtful.

Example: Let it be assumed that a sheet 10 mm thick contains in its centre plane disc-shaped laminations of various diameters. It is further assumed that a plane wave strikes the sheet at right angles and that the receiver touches the back surface, thus placing it at a distance a of 5 mm from the flaw. According to Fig. 1.92 flaws with a diameter between 0.8 and 3 mm, and again above 7 mm, could be detected at a frequency of 6 MHz, but not flaws between 3 and 7 mm. Furthermore, the receiver should have a diameter of less than 4 mm. Laminations of 3 to 10 and above 25 mm diameter could be detected at a frequency of 0.5 MHz.

In practice the condition of a plane, incident wave can usually not be fulfilled, e.g. if the transmitting radiator is of small diameter and is placed close to the flaw. In this case the detection limits shown in Fig. 1.92 can be reduced and the chances for detecting small flaws increase. RIECKMANN *[310]* has carried out tests on the possibility of exploiting the shadow for the detection of flaws.

Let us now investigate *obliquely orientated flaws* in the form of *circular discs*. According to Fig. 1.93 the directions of both the echo and the shadow wave are determined by a simple application of Huygens' principle: this shows a wave surface of the incident, plane wave which has just reached the more distant edge of the circular disc. Elementary spherical waves have radiated from both the front and the back of the disc; they form the echo wave and the shadow wave, respectively. It is clear that the shadow wave must have the same direction as the incident wave, while in the case of the echo wave, as in geometric sound optics, the angle of reflection equals the angle of incidence.

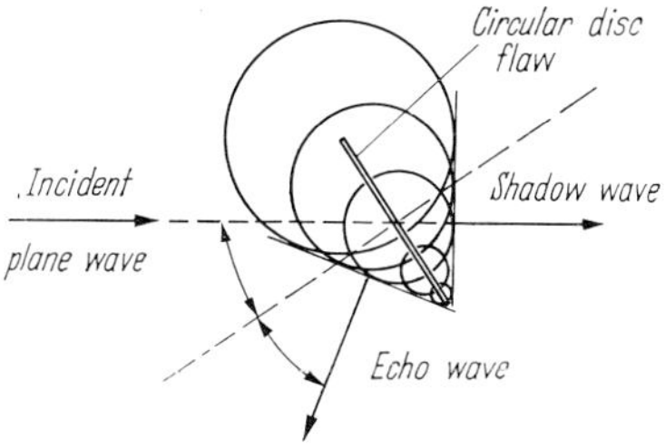

Fig. 1.93 Directions of echo wave and shadow wave of an obliquely orientated flaw plotted according to Huygens' principle.

At moderate oblique orientation of the flaw the form of both waves does not differ greatly from that produced by a flaw orientated at right angles. In Fig. 1.94 both waves were calculated with their angular distribution for a flaw with a diameter of 4 wave lengths. Only the weak sound pressure which fluctuates rapidly with the angle and which comes from the side lobe region returns to the probe. Consequently, when applying this method and using *the same* probe as both transmitter and receiver, *detection* of an obliquely orientated flaw is perhaps still possible, but any estimation of its size on the basis of the sound pressure of the echo is questionable. Therefore, provided the form of the test object permits it, one would take into account also the shadow of the flaw because it is less influenced by the oblique position than the echo wave.

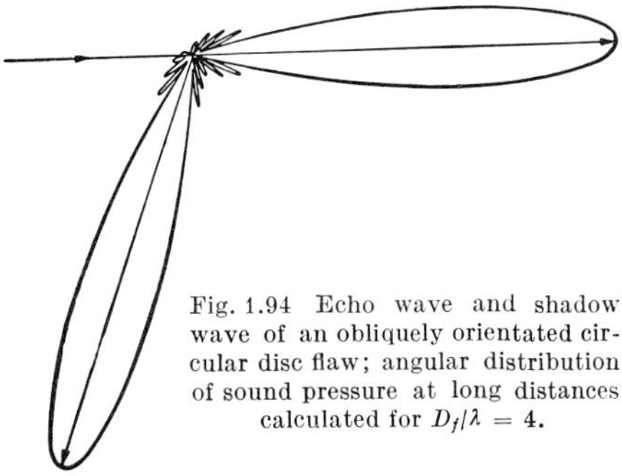

Fig. 1.94 Echo wave and shadow wave of an obliquely orientated circular disc flaw; angular distribution of sound pressure at long distances calculated for $D_f/\lambda = 4$.

Only in rare cases will it be possible to detect the main lobe of the echo wave by means of a separate receiver, to assess the size of the flaw in this way, as in the case of perpendicular incidence. In practice, this would require that the position of the flaw already be known approximately and that the test object has a suitable form.

In practice, the oblique position of a flaw does not affect the echo wave as adversely as it may seem.

Firstly, in the case of short pulses, the secondary lobe region has already been deformed, giving a more or less uniform decrease of the sound pressure.

Secondly, in the case of flaws which are no longer large compared with the wave length, the angle distributions of the echo wave and the shadow wave can no longer be given separately as in Fig. 1.94, viz. they merge to form a connected, scattered wave. With decreasing ratio of diameter to wave length this scattered wave becomes more nearly spherical in form (see Fig. 1.89) so that finally the influence of the oblique position disappears altogether for very small flaws; it should, however, be remembered that the sound pressure also becomes very small. By choosing a lower frequency (longer wave length) it is therefore possible within certain practical limits to change the reflection characteristic of obliquely orientated small flaws so that they become more favourable for the detection and estimation of their size when applying the echo method (see also measurements by KLEINT [177]).

Natural flaws in work pieces differ from the artificial, *substitute flaws* in the form of circular discs, also in several other respects. In general their boundary is not circular, their surface not flat, nor smooth, even if it could be regarded as approximately flat.

The last-mentioned point will be discussed first: How does a rough, flat surface differ from a smooth surface when struck by an ultrasonic beam? The measure of the qualities rough and smooth is again the wave length. If the differences in height of the surface irregularities are less than approximately 1/3 of the wave length, this surface can be regarded as smooth, as measurements by KLOTH [181] have shown. The surface reflects the sound beam in the same way as an optical mirror reflects the beam of a search light in the dark. For an observer outside the reflected beam the mirror is practically invisible; at the most its edge only. With increasing roughness the surface exposed to the sound beam behaves like a dust-covered mirror in a searchlight beam. In addition to the reflected beam the light is also scattered in all directions. In the case of the echo method such a rough surface therefore returns an echo to the transmitting radiator also if the beam is not incident at right angles. On the other hand, the reflected beam, compared with that returned by a smooth surface, becomes weaker. This roughness may be either regular and uniform, e.g. like machine-turned grooves, or irregular, producing quite different results as confirmed by measurements by KLOTH in the arrangement shown in Fig. 1.95. For the case of an irregular, artificially produced roughness of approx. 0.8λ, Fig. 1.96a shows that a residual, mirror-like reflection remains at perpendicular incidence which is accompanied by a relatively uniform scatter at greater angles. However, the

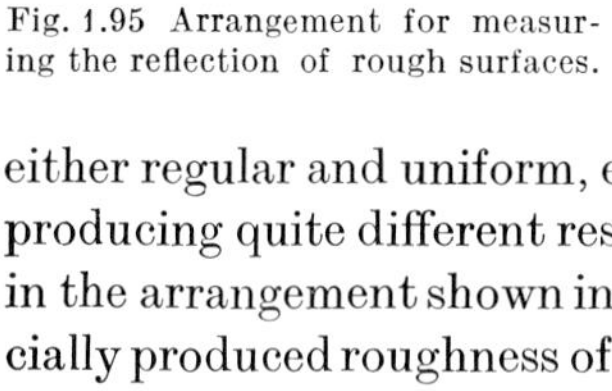

Fig. 1.95 Arrangement for measuring the reflection of rough surfaces.

effect of regular roughness of uniform height is shown in Fig. 1.96b; it produces pronounced maxima at definite angles, which can be explained and calculated like the diffraction from an optical grating. In this experiment long pulses with many oscillations were used. In the case of short pulses this phenomenon, like all interference phenomena, is less pronounced, but in practice it may still lead to wrong interpretation if not taken into account.

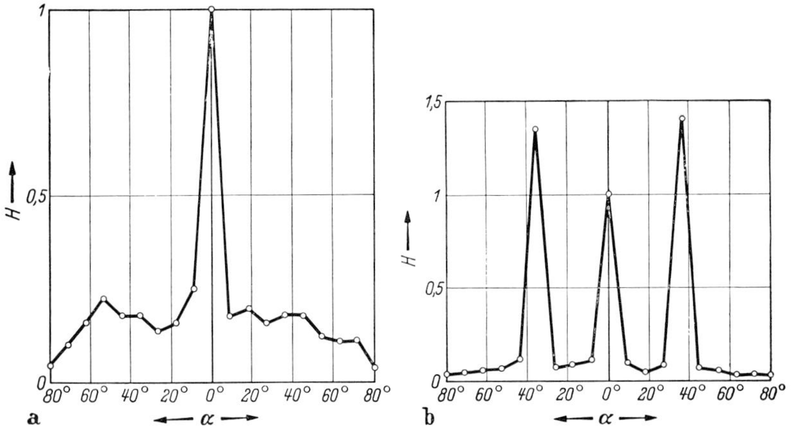

Fig. 1.96 Reflection on rough surfaces. Relative echo height *H* versus incident angle according to measurements by KLOTH. a) Irregular roughness in the form of centre-punch indentations of approximately 2 mm depth and at 2.4 mm wave length; b) regular roughness in the form of milling grooves of approximately 2 mm depth and spacing, at right angles to the sound beam.

If the roughness is equivalent to one wave length and more, the mirror-like reflection gradually disappears completely, e.g. on badly corroded surfaces and on certain natural flaws, e.g. cavities in castings. The echo produced by such surfaces is weak and spread out compared with a mirror-like reflection, and its shape and amplitude change rapidly with every change of the incident sound beam, for it is the result of superposition of and interference between numerous elementary waves of different intensity and transit times. The echo may in some cases disappear altogether, e.g. in the case of a sponge-like structure in castings, or clusters of pores.

The reflection produced by rough surfaces can be improved to some extent by a suitable choice of the frequency or wave length; a surface of given roughness appears in the case of a longer wave length smoother and thus produces a more mirror-like reflection and less scatter, and vice versa; a shorter wave length produces more scatter reflection in the case of oblique incidence. If the wave length and the length of the pulses are greatly reduced, the pulse length will finally be shorter than the difference in transit times from points of different depths, e.g. on a corroded wall, and not all elementary waves will produce interference, resulting in separate echoes received from such points.

In the case of flaw surfaces which are very rough it is of course no longer possible to deduce the size of the flaw from the height of the echo. Natural flaws can, however, frequently be regarded as smooth, at least for the usual wave lengths of 1 to 12 mm, e.g. crack surfaces, cavities, blisters and inclusions which are forged or rolled flat, etc. If they are not flat, a mirror-like reflection will nevertheless be obtained from individual points from which, however, no deductions can be made regarding the size of the flaw. Defects of this nature then show up like a piece of corrugated or crumpled silver paper in a search-light beam: the reflections returned from various points of the paper change with its orientation. If however such flaws can still be regarded as sufficiently flat, e.g. small flakes, and if the sound beam can be directed at right angles to their surface, their size can be estimated by comparing them with artificial defects in the form of circular discs. Such an estimate gives a minium size because all deviations from the flat and circular form which occur in practice reduce the echo. (This disregards the improbable case where the surface of the flaw forms a concave mirror which returns the sound beam focused, thus possibly producing a stronger echo than an equivalent flaw in the form of a circular disc.)

According to Ref. [181] spherical reflectors with a diameter of more than 3 wave lengths produce approximately only 1/50th to 1/60th of the echo of a circular disc flaw of equal diameter. It will thus readily be seen that in the case of greater deviations from the form of a circular disc the estimate may give a value which is smaller than the actual cross-section of the flaw by more than 1 order of magnitude.

Deviations from the shape, as well as slight deviations from the perpendicular orientation produce a smaller influence, the greater the wave length compared with the dimensions of the flaw. It is therefore recommended that for such comparative measurements the wave length be chosen as large as possible provided that a sufficiently clear echo of the flaw can still be obtained.

When trying to estimate very long, cylindrical flaw shapes it may be preferable to compare them with artificial flaws in the form of holes drilled at right angles to the beam. According to Ref. [181] their distance law differs from that of a flaw in the form of a circular disc: the echo is not proportional to $1/r^2$ but to $(1/r)^{3/2}$, so that at greater distance their reflection is stronger than that of flaws in the form of circular discs. At a distance of only a few near field lengths, however, their reflection is weaker, i.e. approximately only 1/10th of the echo of a circular disc flaw.

Natural flaws may also differ from circular disc flaws in that they are not filled with air or gas, as has been assumed, but that they contain non-metallic inclusions, oxides, slags or liquids. In the case of materials of high acoustic impedance, e.g. steel, the influence on the height of the echo is usually not very pronounced. In light metals, however, it seems that any cavities filled with oxides accompanied by strong compression can greatly reduce the flaw echo.

Another cause of echoes which are smaller than would be expected from the size of the actual flaw can be the fact that the transition from the flawless section of the work piece to the flawed section is not well defined, covering a zone in which the elastic properties change more or less continuously.

Example: Cavity in a casting surrounded by fine pores (sponge), in which the porosity decreases gradually from the outside towards the inside. This zone dissipates the wave more or less completely. In this case the actual flaw is shielded by an absorbing or scattering layer. The effect of such a transition zone is minor if its thickness is small compared with the wave length. It is therefore sometimes possible to improve the reflection of an indistinct boundary by using longer waves.

1.9 Attenuation of Ultrasonic Waves in Solids

1.91 Absorption and Scattering

So far ideal materials have been assumed in which the sound pressure is attenuated only by virtue of the spreading of the wave. A plane wave would thus show no attenuation whatsoever of the sound pressure along its path, and a spherical wave, or the sound beam of a probe in the far field, would merely decrease inversely with the distance from the source. Natural materials, however, all produce a more or less pronounced effect which further weakens the sound. This results from two causes, viz. scattering and (true) absorption which can both be combined by the concept of attenuation (sometimes also extinction).

The scattering results from the fact that the material is not strictly homogeneous. It contains boundaries on which the acoustic impedance changes abruptly because two materials of different density or sound velocity meet at these interfaces. Such inhomogeneities may either be inclusions, e.g. non-metallic inclusions in a forging, or pores. They may be genuine flaws of the material concerned, or also natural or intentional flaws such as porosity in sintered materials. There are, however, also materials which by their nature are inhomogeneous, e.g. cast iron, in which an agglomeration of elastically completely different ferrite and graphite grains occurs. In other materials crystallites of different structure and composition are mixed, as in brass and steel. Even when only a single type of crystal is present, the material may still be inhomogeneous for ultrasonic waves if the grains are orientated at random, viz. if the crystal concerned has different elastic properties, i.e. different sound velocities in different directions. In this case it is called *anisotropic*. In the case of metals, however, elastic anisotropy is the rule, but in different metals it manifests itself to a varying degree.

In a material with very coarse grain compared with the wave length the scatter can be visualised geometrically: on an oblique boundary the wave is split into various reflected and transmitted wave types. This process repeats itself for each wave at the next grain boundary. Thus, the original sound beam is constantly divided into partial waves which along their long and complex paths are gradually converted into heat because of the always present true absorption (see below).

In the frequency range used in testing materials the grain size is usually smaller than the wave length. Under these conditions scatter occurs instead of geometric division, as when the light of a headlamp is scattered by the small water droplets in fog. In the case of grain sizes of 1/1000th to 1/100th of the wave length, scatter is for all practical purposes negligible. It increases very rapidly however, approximately as the 3rd power of the grain size, to make itself felt at sizes from 1/10th to the full value of the wave length, to such an extent that testing may become impossible if the material concerned is anisotropic.

The second cause of the attenuation, viz. absorption, is a direct conversion of sound energy into heat, for which several processes can be responsible [12] discussion of which here would fall outside thes cope of this book. Absorption can roughly be visualized as a sort of braking effect of the oscillations of the particles, which also makes it clear why a rapid oscillation loses more energy than a slow oscillation; the absorption usually increases as the frequency, i.e. at a rate much slower than the scattering.

Both losses set limitations to the testing of materials, but in slightly different ways. Pure absorption weakens the transmitted energy or the echo from both the flaw and the backwall. To counteract this effect the transmitter voltage and the amplification can be increased, or the lower absorption at lower frequencies can be exploited for this purpose. Much more awkward, however, is the scattering because in the echo method it not only reduces the height of the echo from both the flaw and the backwall but in addition produces numerous echoes with different transit times, the so-called *grass* in which the true echoes may get lost. The scattering can be compared with the effect of fog in which the driver of an automobile is blinded by his own headlights and is unable to see clearly. Apparently this disturbance cannot be counteracted by stepping up the transmitter voltage or the amplification because the "grass" effect increases simultaneously. The only remedy is to use lower frequencies, which sets a natural and insuperable limit to the detectability of small flaws.

The sound pressure of a plane wave, which decreases only as a result of attenuation, can for the purpose of calculation be written in the form of an exponential function

$$P = P_0 e^{-\alpha d}. \tag{1.41}$$

P_0 and P are the sound pressures at the beginning and the end, respectively, of a section of length d and with the attenuation coefficient α.

In common with many other natural phenomena of growth and disappearance, the process of attenuation has the property that the amount of the increase or decrease over a given interval, of time or space, is proportional to the momentarily existing quantity. For instance, the increment in timber of a forest is proportional to the momentarily existing quantity of timber. The latter therefore changes according to an exponential function with a positive exponent. In the case of a decrease the exponent is negative.

In literature the attenuation coefficient α is sometimes referred not to the sound pressure but to the intensity. If the latter is called α_I the attenuation law of intensity can be written

$$I = I_0 e^{-\alpha_I d}.$$

Since the intensity is proportional to the square of the sound pressure one obtains

$$e^{-\alpha_I d} = e^{-2\alpha d},$$

therefore

$$\alpha_I = 2\alpha.$$

The natural logarithm of Eq. (1.41) gives

$$\alpha d = \ln \frac{P_0}{P} \text{ Np}. \tag{1.42}$$

This is the *attenuation* proper, or the total attenuation over the distance d, a dimensionless number which is expressed in *nepers*. The attenuation coefficient can therefore be given in neper/cm. Following the practice in electrical measurement, however, another unit is being given preference, viz. the decibel/mm or abbreviated dB/mm. The decibel measure is obtained if in Eq. (1.42) instead of the natural logarithm, Brigg's logarithm with base 10 is used and multiplied by 20:

$$\alpha d = 20 \log \frac{P_0}{P} \text{ dB}. \tag{1.42 a}$$

Since $\log x = 0.434 \ln x$ the one unit can be converted into the other as follows:

numerical value in decibel = 8.68 · numerical value in neper.

If the coefficient is referred to the millimetre unit of length, the numerical values of dB/mm and Np/cm become almost identical, which is then easier to remember:

numerical value in dB/mm = 0.87 · numerical value in Np/cm.

In what follows α will always be given in the unit 10^{-3} dB/mm (= dB/m) because in the frequency range of interest and the materials in question the numerical values, which lie approximately between 1 and a few hundreds, can be memorised more easily. For instance, water as well as other materials with low attenuation have values from 1 to $4 \cdot 10^{-3}$ dB/mm.

The decibel unit can be memorised more easily than the neper unit because the transition to powers of ten is more simple. 20 dB is a power of ten, and an attenuation of 20 dB is equivalent to a reduction to 1/10th; 40 dB 1/100, 60 dB 1/1000, and conversely an increase by 20 dB means a ten-fold increase, and so forth. Further, 1 dB means a change by approx. 10%, 0.1 dB approx. 1%. If the attenuation coefficient of a given material is 1 dB/mm, the wave is attenuated by a 1 mm layer approx. 10%, by a 20 mm layer approx. 90 %; at 100 mm the attenuation is the 5th power of 10 and the sound pressure is 10^{-5}. This would already be a very severe attenuation.

Table 1.2 facilitates the conversion of dB values to ordinary figures. The second column applies to negative dB values and gives the attenuated amplitude in %; the third column applies to positive values and gives the amplification factor.

Intermediate values are obtained by adding the dB values and multiplying the ordinary numerical values. Example: A decrease of the amplitude by 23 dB = 20 + + 3 dB, corresponds to 10% · 71% = 7.1% amplitude, requiring an amplification factor of 10.0 · 1.41 = 14.1.

Table 1.2

dB	Attenuated amplitude in %	Gain	dB	Attenuated amplitude in %	Gain
0.0	100	1.00	10.0	32	3.16
0.5	94.5	1.06	12.0	25	3.98
1.0	89	1.12	14.0	20	5.01
1.5	84	1.19	16.0	15.8	6.31
2.0	79	1.26	18.0	12.6	7.94
2.5	75	1.33	20.0	10.0	10.00
3.0	71	1.41	30.0	3.2	31.62
3.5	67	1.50	40.0	1.0	100.00
4.0	63	1.59	50.0	0.32	316.23
4.5	60	1.68	60.0	0.10	1,000.00
5.0	56	1.78	70.0	0.032	3,162.30
6.0	50	2.00	80.0	0.010	10,000.00
7.0	45	2.24	90.0	0.003	31,623.00
8.0	40	2.51	100.0	0.001	100,000.00
9.0	35	2.82			

A table of attenuation coefficients for various materials would be of doubtful value. Where values have already been reliably measured, which is very difficult below $10 \cdot 10^{-3}$ dB/mm (see 3.63), such values, in the case of metals, depend very much on the state (see 1.92). Table 1.3 therefore provides only general information.

Table 1.3 *Attenuation of longitudinal waves at 2 MHz and room temperature in various materials*

<table>
<tr><th>Attenuation coefficient α in 10^{-3} dB/mm</th><th>Low
1 to 10</th><th>Medium
10 to 100</th><th>High
above 100</th></tr>
<tr><td rowspan="6">Material</td><td rowspan="6">Cast: aluminium, magnesium, pure and slightly alloyed
Worked: steel, aluminium, magnesium, nickel, silver, titanium, tungsten (all pure and alloyed)

Non-metals: glass, porcelain</td><td colspan="2">Predominantly absorption</td></tr>
<tr><td colspan="2">Plastics
(polystyrene, perspex, rubber, PVC, synthetic resins)</td></tr>
<tr><td></td><td>Plastics with fillers, and rubber, vulcanized rubber, wood</td></tr>
<tr><td colspan="2">Predominantly sacttering</td></tr>
<tr><td colspan="2">Cast aluminium and magnesium, alloyed</td></tr>
<tr><td>Cast steel, slightly alloyed, high-quality cast iron
Worked: copper, zinc, brass, bronze, lead, hard and sintered metals</td><td>Cast steel, highly alloyed, lowstrength cast iron, cast copper, zinc, brass, bronze
Non-metals: porous ceramics, rocks</td></tr>
<tr><td>Max. thickness that can be tested</td><td>1 to 10 m</td><td>0.1 to 1 m</td><td>0 to 0.1 m, can frequently no longer be tested</td></tr>
</table>

For a few values of α from 1 to $300 \cdot 10^{-3}$ dB/mm, Table 10 in the Appendix shows the decrease of the sound pressure of a plane wave as a function of the distance in the form of a graph. It shows the attenuation in dB or that of the amplitude in per cent if the pulse echo method is used, i.e. the height of the echo. If the decrease of the amplitude to 0.1 % is defined arbitrarily as the range, Table 10 indicates for light metals and fine-grained steel ($\alpha = 1$ to $3 \cdot 10^{-3}$ dB/mm) transmission ranges above 5 m when using the echo method, but for grey cast iron (order of magnitude of α approx. 300) only 100 mm. This presentation draws attention to the fact – which in practice is frequently overlooked – that the attenuation can increase very rapidly with the thickness of the layer concerned. While for instance 20 mm grey cast iron can still be measured with 25 % of the echo height of a good quality steel when applying the echo method, which can easily be compensated on the gain control, the echo in the same material but 100 mm thick has dropped to 0.1 %, i.e. to a value which most likely can no longer be measured, which of course depends on the transmitter voltage, design of the probe and the gain. If with increased gain it is nevertheless possible to increase this backwall echo from a thickness of 100 mm to the same value as obtained from a thickness of 20 mm, the material at the distance of 20 mm is subjected to a sound pressure 250 times greater than previously, resulting in grain boundaries and small flaws in the near range now being indicated excessively large. This is erroneously referred to as increased scattering, although compared with the test at 20 mm thickness nothing has changed. Where there is high attenuation in a given test piece, a comparison of flaw echo and backwall echo may therefore lead to completely wrong conclusions (see Fig. 3.158).

In view of the fact that at greater layer thicknesses one is no longer working with plane waves but must regard them as spherical waves, additional allowance has to be made for the decrease of the amplitude due to the divergence of the beam. According to Eq. (1.29) the sound pressure at distance a from the probe can therefore be written

$$P = P_0 \pi \frac{N}{a} e^{-\alpha a} . \tag{1.43}$$

A numerical example will make it clear that both causes of the decrease follow essentially different distance laws, so that the range will in the one case be determined more by the divergence of the beam and in the other by the attenuation.

Let the sound pressure at a distance of 100 mm be set arbitrarily at 100%. The sound pressure then is in per cent

at a distance of:	100 mm	1 m	10 m
due to the divergence of the beam alone:	100	10	1
due to the attenuation alone at			
$\alpha = 1 \cdot 10^{-3}$ dB/mm:	100	90	32
$10 \cdot 10^{-3}$ dB/mm:	100	35	0.001
$100 \cdot 10^{-3}$ dB/mm:	100	0.003	–

Since the two contributing factors have to be multiplied by each other, the divergence of the beam determines the range in the case of materials which can readily be penetrated (fine-grained steel and aluminium at 2 MHz), whereas in the case of greater attenuation the proportion of the latter predominates.

With few exceptions (e.g. magnesium) transverse waves are attenuated more strongly than longitudinal waves, particularly in plastics. This is readily understandable in view of the fact that in the case of transverse waves, because of the shorter path length, approximately twice as many wave lengths are apportioned to the same layer thickness.

The attenuation usually increases with the temperature, particularly in plastics.

In the case of surface waves, plate waves and rod waves the weakening influence of the roughness of the guiding surfaces is added; this can be nominally taken into account by adding a certain quantity to α. In this case also the decrease of the amplitude follows an exponential law.

If an attempt is made to avoid the attenuation of the material by using lower frequencies when trying to detect small flaws, a compromise has to be made: there is an optimal frequency, because the effect of the flaw on the sound field decreases simultaneously. For instance, in the case of a spherical flaw whose diameter is much smaller than the wave length, the echo amplitude is determined according to RAYLEIGH [18] by the ratio

$$\frac{D^3}{\lambda^2}.$$

If the dependence of the attenuation coefficient on the frequency is known from measurements and can be expressed say by the formula

$$\alpha = p + q f^m$$

where p, q and m are constants, one obtains according to MALECKI [185] for a given flaw distance a the optimal frequency

$$f_{\text{opt}} = \frac{1}{\sqrt[m]{m q a}}.$$

1.92* Attenuation in Metals, Anisotropy and Cast Structure

In view of the fact that the attenuation, particularly the scattering in the material, is one of the main difficulties encountered in ultrasonic testing, and often is the only factor limiting its application, it is of great practical importance to be able to estimate the influence of the crystal structure on the attenuation. So far no general solution has yet been found because both theoretical and measuring difficulties are encountered, and because indubitably, in addition to the directly measurable quantities such as grain size and anisotropy, many other parameters which are difficult to determine intervene. There are for instance the nature of the grain boundaries and the internal stresses. Frequently, however, not even the grain size can be clearly defined, as demonstrated by polished microsections of steels with their complex structures.

A clear and logical law of behaviour can therefore be expected only in the case of simple structures with only one type and form of crystal and a minimum of impurities. This need not necessarily apply to pure metals since alloys with mixed crystals are no exceptions in this respect. In such cases the influences of anisotropy and grain size which can readily be interpreted are observed. If for instance two samples of cast aluminium and cast brass of identical grain size are compared the attenuation in brass is much greater than in aluminium. Further, if two samples of the same material but of different grain size are tested it is found that the change of the attenuation due to grain size is much more pronounced in brass than in aluminium. This last-mentioned comparison can also be made with shorter wave lengths instead of larger grain size. A greater ratio of grain diameter to wave length is thus accompanied by an attenuation which is the greater the anisotropy.

According to Roth [317] a number of important materials can be classified according to increasing anisotropy:

W	Mg	Al-Cu	Al	Fe	Ag	Cu	Pb	α-brass	β-brass
		(95 + 5%)						(72 Cu + 28 Zn)	(58 Cu + 42 Zn)

The coarser grain produces a disturbance which is the greater, the further to the right the material appears in the above series.

According to Roth, and also Mason and McSkimin [251, 252], the anisotropy can also be specified numerically, which will not be discussed here, especially since the sequences are not identical for different concepts. In the case of transverse waves permutations in the series may result.

Tungsten should be completely isotropic like non-crystallized materials, e.g. glass. Tests on samples, however, are usually hampered by porosity introduced during manufacture.

A case in point is the low attenuation of the pure light metals and aluminium copper alloys with only a few per cent copper. As far as the testing of materials is concerned the grain size is immaterial.

After iron come the strongly anisotropic materials of which the copper alloys metals in particular cause many difficulties. As far as is known β-brass is the most strongly anisotropic material.

Iron is considered here only alloyed with carbon and with other metals in the form of steel. The influence of the grain size is considerable, which is the main reason why when testing steel, essentially only frequencies below 5 MHz should be used. Reliable measurements on a number of carbon steels and low-alloyed steels [165] (see below) in this range have only recently become known.

In the case of steel the structure is usually not a simple one with only *one* approximately uniform grain size and *one* type of crystal. It is therefore not surprising that the results are as yet unclear. As a first approach the grain size should be replaced by the maximally occurring structural dimension.

Example: If a forging of nickel-chrome-molybdenum steel (C = 0.25, Ni = 2.5, Cr = 0.6, Mo = 0.25%) is cooled slowly, a structure forms in which the large γ-grains originally present, remain clearly outlined by ferrite segregation on their boundaries, resembling a bird's eye view of fields framed by hedges. However, inside the frames the original γ-grain has decomposed into several, smaller α-grains. The strong scattering in such a material is then determined by the relatively large dimensions of this cellular structure and not by the much smaller α-grain or the still smaller ferrite grain in the boundaries. If the ferritic cell structure is eliminated by further heat treatment, a process called homogenisation, the remaining determining structural dimension is a smaller grain and the material can now be penetrated more easily (Bastien, Bleton and Kerversau [33]). The structural dimension responsible can be recognized also in this case, and quite generally, most simply by the structure of a fracture face.

Segregations at the grain boundaries, e.g. impurities, are much thinner than the ferrite boundaries of the above example. Their detection and investigation is also more difficult. Nevertheless, they too may greatly influence the scattering because the penetration of the sound at the interface between two grains is no longer determined by the elastic properties of the contiguous grains alone but is also affected by this intermediate layer. Thus, two samples of a given material of identical grain size may in certain circumstances show different scattering because of different conditions of the grain boundaries.

Most materials show a particularly pronounced reduction of the attenuation of sound if their cast structure is destroyed by working, cold or hot, e.g. during forging, rolling, extruding, etc. To a small extent this effect may be the result of true compaction of the structure by a reduction of the pore volume. In the main, however, the deformation process leads to a destruction of the larger grains of the cast structure, resulting in reduced scattering.

The reduction of the pore volume is usually indicated directly by an increase of the specific gravity, e.g. cast copper has a specific gravity of 8.3 to 8.9 but this changes to 8.9 to 9.0 if hammered. Since porosity reduces the velocity of sound the densification should manifest itself by an increase of the acoustic velocity.

However, if the large grains of the cast structure are crushed this certainly does not result in newly created grain boundaries, which have the same properties as the original grain boundaries, and differ only in their dimensions. This would hardly explain the sometimes very considerable changes in transmittance. Their very character must have changed, which seems plausible because, if produced at low temperatures, they show no grain boundary segregations. The fact is that a cast structure almost invariably has a lower tensile strength and ultimate elongation than a worked structure. This is a result of the weaker mechanical bond at the grain boundaries which also reduces the transmittance of the sound oscillations at the grain boundaries of the cast structure. Basically the transmission of sound also involves only a mechanical stress of the material by tension and compression or shear, although it is non-destructive.

The effect of the working on the attenuation of the sound is particularly pronounced in the case of non-ferrous metals as well as high-alloyed steels. While in the structure as cast even small thicknesses can frequently not be penetrated, they can readily be penetrated even after the first pass during rolling. Particularly disturbing in such materials therefore is a zone in the finished piece in which the cast structure has not yet been sufficiently crushed because of insufficient deformation. A special condition of crystallization, e.g. an austenitic structure, has apparently no great significance in itself, but it is important to know whether this condition is present in the cast structure or the deformed structure. For instance the material of austenitic pipes can readily be penetrated, while an austenitic weld in it usually shows bad transmission because of its cast structure.

It may be mentioned briefly that the improved mechanical properties of centrifugal casting as compared with chill castings, sand castings or continuous castings, immediately manifest themselves in their ultrasonic behaviour: the centrifugal casting shows better ultrasonic transmittance and is therefore easier to test. It is debatable whether this is merely an effect of the finer grain or of a simultaneously changed condition of the grain boundaries. This has been observed not only in cast iron but also in non-ferrous metals [347].

According to Mason and McSkimin [251] the *theoretical interpretation* of the correlation between attenuation coefficient, frequency and wave length, grain size D_k and anisotropy can be based firstly on the assumption of a true absorption which is proportional to frequency, which also seems plausible on the basis of measurements at frequencies lower than customarily used in the testing of materials. If the attenuation frequency is then subdivided into an absorption coefficient and a scatter coefficient,

$$\alpha = \alpha_a + \alpha_s \tag{1.44}$$

we have

$$\alpha_a = C_1 f \tag{1.45}$$

where C_1 is a constant unaffected by grain size and anisotropy. Depending on the ratio of grain size to wave length there are two possibilities for formulating the scattering: for small D_k/λ Mason and McSkimin apply the concept of Rayleigh [18] concerning the scattering of a single, small flaw, to the agglomeration of crystals with anisotropy, and obtain

$$\alpha_s = C_2 F_A D_k^3 f^4 \quad \text{(as long as } D_k \ll \lambda) . \tag{1.46}$$

thus indicating a dependence on the third power of the grain diameter, the fourth power of the frequency, as well as on the anisotropy by a factor F_A. Thus, in the case of tungsten and light metals the factor F_A would be almost zero. On the other hand, if the grain diameter becomes much greater than the wave length, the scatter coefficient should be independent of the frequency and inversely proportional to the grain size:

$$\alpha_s = C_3 F_A \frac{1}{D_k} \quad \text{(as long as } D_k \gg \lambda) . \tag{1.47}$$

Measurements seem to limit the first range approximately to $D_k < \lambda/3$, and the second to $D_k < 3\lambda$. Since D_k^3 is proportional to the grain volume V, the formula can also be written (with λ instead of the frequency f)

$$\alpha = C_1' \frac{1}{\lambda} + \begin{cases} C_2' F_A V \frac{1}{\lambda^4} & \text{for} \quad D_k < \lambda/3\,, \\ C_3' F_A \frac{1}{D_k} & \text{for} \quad D_k > 3\lambda\,. \end{cases} \tag{1.48}$$

For very small and very large grain diameters at least, the formula seems plausible; the scatter portion disappears if D_k/λ becomes very small, even in the presence of anisotropy. On the other hand, the scatter portion should likewise disappear for very large grain diameters, which is equivalent to a transition to the single crystal.

Measurements made on aluminium and magnesium [317, 251, 252], i.e. materials with simple structure and definite grain size, qualitatively confirm the formula with calculated constants and anisotropy factor. The dependence according to the third and fourth power of grain size and frequency, respectively, is not reliably confirmed. Measurements on steels [313] are not in agreement with this formula. Numerous, more qualitative measurements of the attenuation in steels, and their discussion [33, 11] still require confirmation by a reliable measuring procedure first developed by Ivens [167] for frequencies below 10 MHz and for longitudinal waves. In the frequency range limited to 2 to 5.5 MHz Ivens finds in the average for various steels with perlitic and intermediate structure for each group, a dependence of the attenuation coefficient on the third power of the grain diameter as required by Eq. (1.46), but only on the third instead of the fourth power of the wave length and frequency, respectively. His results can be summarized empirically in the form

$$\begin{aligned} \alpha &= 100 \cdot (D_k/\lambda)^3 \cdot 10^{-3}\,\text{dB/mm} \quad \text{for perlitic structure,} \\ &= 35 \cdot (D_k/\lambda)^3 \cdot 10^{-3}\,\text{dB/mm} \quad \text{for intermediate structure.} \end{aligned}$$

In addition to the difficulties in the measuring methods involved (see also 3.63) it is very difficult in such a series of measurements to keep all but one of the many variables constant in a given series of tests.

For the practical purpose of non-destructive testing the result can be summarized by rule of thumb as follows:

1. The scattering produced by a given material increases rapidly with increasing grain size or decreasing wave length if the grain size is about 1/10th of the wave length or greater. However, the effect becomes disturbing only if the material appears far to the right in the anisotropies series.

2. In complex structures the grain size should then be defined as the maximum structural dimension which occurs.

3. A cast structure produces stronger attenuation than a deformed structure, even in the case of identical grain size.

4. By taking recourse to lower frequencies the attenuation can be reduced considerably, but this step is promising only if the smallest flaws to be detected are still large compared with the grain size.

According to newer concepts true absorption in crystals is explained by energy-consuming oscillations of dislocations in the lattice (Reid [304], see also Mason's book [12] with further bibliographic references). This theory also explains the increase in attenuation if the material is stressed by tension or compression, as well as the fatigue behaviour of materials (see 3.63, reports by Truell et al. [144, 127, 368, 369]).

1.10 Generation and Reception of Ultrasonic Waves

1.101 The Piezoelectric Effect

So far we have discussed the propagation and behaviour of ultrasonic waves in various materials without presupposing anything regarding their generation except that they are excited in the material concerned by the contact face of a *radiator* which oscillates with the desired wave-form and frequency. For detection a *microphone* has been assumed which likewise has a contact face and which is capable of measuring the sound pressure of an incident wave. Both devices are referred to in materials testing as a *probe*, or search unit, and where applicable as a transmitting probe or a receiving probe. We shall now discuss its mode of operation, which is based almost exclusively on the piezoelectric effect. Other methods for generating ultrasonics are therefore discussed only briefly in 1.105.

A piezoelectric material has the property that if deformed by external mechanical pressure electric charges are produced on its surface. This effect was discovered in 1880 by the brothers Curie. The reverse phenomenon, according to which such a material, if placed between two electrodes, changes its form if an electric potential is applied, was discovered soon afterwards (1881). The first is called the direct piezoelectric effect, and the second the inverse piezoelectric effect. The first is now used for measuring, the second for producing mechanical pressures, deformations and oscillations.

Since then a great number of materials have been found to be piezoelectric, of which however, only a few are suitable for our purposes. They will be described in greater detail in 1.104. The effect will be explained briefly for the most important piezoelectric crystal, viz. the quartz. More detailed data are found in the books by BERGMANN [1], HÜTER and BOLT [9], MASON [11] and CADY [4].

The piezoelectric effect is a property of the crystal structure and is linked to an asymmetry in it which can be characterized by the appearance of one or several *polar* axes. These are crystal axes in which one direction differs from the opposite direction so that any rotation of the crystal in which the front and back ends of such an axis are interchanged never gives the same position of the crystal. It is impossible to make it coincide with itself in this way. In the case of quartz which occurs in the form of hexagonal prisms in nature (Fig. 1.97) there are three such polar axes, viz. X_1, X_2, and X_3 each of which passes through two opposite edges. The Z-axis of the crystal is parallel to the axis of the prism and is also called optical axis. In addition there are three Y-axes normal to the Z-axis and the X-axes, i.e. they pass through the centres of two opposite sides of the hexagon.

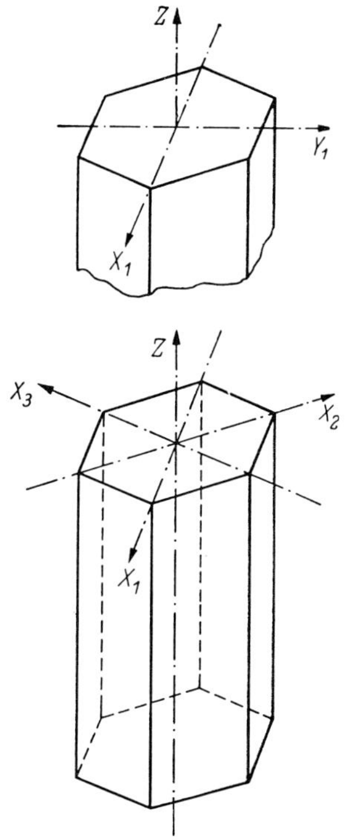

Fig. 1.97 Position of crystal axes in quartz (idealized crystal).

The piezoelectric effect is best analysed by using plates cut from the crystal at right angles to an X-axis, as shown in Fig. 1.98. In this socalled X-cut the Z-axis and one Y-axis are located in the plane of the plate.

Any pressure on this plate slightly reduces its thickness because it is elastic. This shifts the electrically charged elements of the crystal lattice, i.e. in the case of quartz the silicon and oxygen ions, in a way relative to each other such that the plate becomes polarized. As a result free positive charges appear on one side of the plate, and negative charges on the other. This can readily be demonstrated by an experiment. For convenient discharge of the electric charge, metal electrodes, e.g. silver layers are used, which are firmly attached to both sides of the plate. These layers form an electric capacitor with the crystal as dielectric. In the presence of polarization, resulting from pressure exerted on the plate, the capacitor is charged to a voltage measurable on a voltmeter. However, one must provide for perfect insulation and loss-free measurement. Otherwise only a voltage surge is recorded when pressure is applied, the charge being removed by a flow of current. Changing the thickness of the crystal by dilatation poses a more difficult problem. In this case it is found that the charges reverse their sign.

If therefore the pressure changes its sign and becomes tension, the potential on the plate likewise changes its sign. If a sound wave with its alternating tension and compression impinges on the plate, the latter

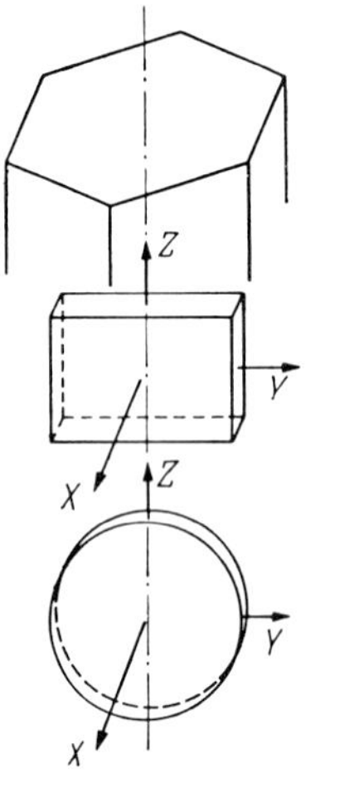

Fig. 1.98 Orientation of sections for rectangular and round X-cut quartz plates.

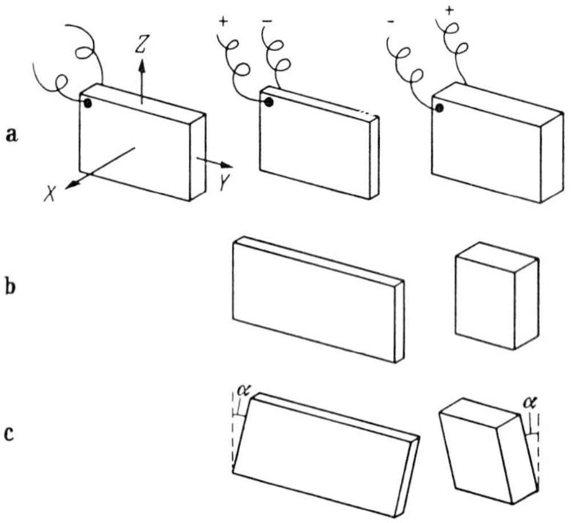

Fig. 1.99 Deformation of an X-cut quartz plate with dimensions $x \cdot y \cdot z = 5 \cdot 30 \cdot 20$ mm, at a voltage of 1000 V, drawn on an exaggerated scale of 1,000,000 : 1. a) Change of thickness alone, b) with additional change of width (Y-direction, c) with additional shear (in the YZ plane).

produces an alternating voltage with the frequency of the wave. The generated voltage is proportional to the sound pressure: the plate becomes a microphone. One of its sides serves as receiving surface which is not adversely affected by a sufficiently thin metallized layer.

The direct piezoelectric effect thus provides a receiver for ultrasound. The reciprocal effect can be used for generating ultrasound: If a voltage were placed on an X-cut plate as shown in Fig. 1.99, the thickness of the plate would change as shown in Fig. 1.99a. If the plate were prevented from expanding it would produce compressive forces on the neighbouring material, which are proportional to the voltage applied. If an alternating voltage is applied it produces an alternating pressure and radiates a longitudinal wave. As already shown in 1.8, the form of the wave depends on the frequency and on the dimensions of the plate, and also on the properties of the ambient medium.

However, the quartz plate does not comply strictly with the behaviour of such an ideal radiator because it experiences other changes of form as shown in Figs. 1.99b and c.

Even in the case of an ordinary, solid and elastic material, a form change alone as shown in Fig. 1.99a is not possible because it always produces a change of the transverse dimensions. In the case of quartz, as for all piezoelectric materials, the conditions are much more complex and, depending on the crystal structure, differ from one material to the other. They can only be described by means of mathematical analysis. The additional deformations for quartz are indicated in Figs. 1.99b and c. The Y-direction is greatly elongated or shortened. This is accompanied by shear which distorts an original rectangle on the surface of the plate into a rhomb. These are merely the primary deformations caused by the action of the electric potential. To this must be added other deformations resulting purely from mechanical coupling, e.g. compression in the Z-direction, which we shall neglect here.

As a result of the Y-elongation an X-cut plate always radiates some transverse waves in addition to the longitudinal waves, if the plate is cemented firmly to a solid material. On the other hand, the shear action interferes less in practice.

Occasionally the Y-elongation is also used for radiating longitudinal waves from the narrow $X \cdot Z$-face, particularly for exciting low frequencies, because the correlated natural frequency (see 1.102) is very much lower than that of the thickness oscillation. Other piezoelectric materials, besides quartz, in which the change in thickness is linked to a strong change in the transverse direction, e.g. barium titanate in particular (see 1.104), are sometimes used in this way. An advantage in this connection is that the radiating and contact faces of the oscillator carry no metal electrodes.

In the case of an X-cut quartz crystal the transverse waves are not transmitted in the X-direction in liquids, nor in solid bodies if coupled to them by a liquid layer. In this case the crystal radiates only longitudinal waves. It nevertheless does not behave strictly like a piston oscillator, because of the *fringe effect*: strictly speaking, the change in thickness of the plate is not determined by the electric potential placed on it but by the electric field strength produced. Because the field lines bulge near the edge, the field strength there is lower than in the centre. The effect of the reduced fringe radiation on the shape of the sound field has been discussed in 1.83.

Fig. 1.99 shows the deformations of the quartz plate in the correct relative ratio, although enlarged 1 million to 1 in relation to the actual changes in length and shear angle. The calculation was based on the dimensions $x = 5$ mm, $y = 30$ mm and $z = 20$ mm, at a potential of 1000 V, i.e. values used in practice. This shows that the actual deformations are extremely small. The elastic limit of the quartz alone sets a limit so that these deformations can never approach the dimensions shown, even for much higher potentials. They are linearly proportional to the potential only up to a few thousand volts.

Besides the X-cut quartz plate discussed above, which in non-destructive testing is used extensively for generating and receiving longitudinal waves, the Y-cut is occasionally also encountered, viz. for generating transverse and surface waves in solids. Fig. 1.100 shows the position of the crystal axes and the deformation of the plate by shear. Compared with the deformation in the case of the X-cut quartz plate, this is very considerable and is therefore shown in the drawing on an enlarged scale of only 200.000 : 1, the dimensions of the plate and the potential applied being otherwise identical with the above.

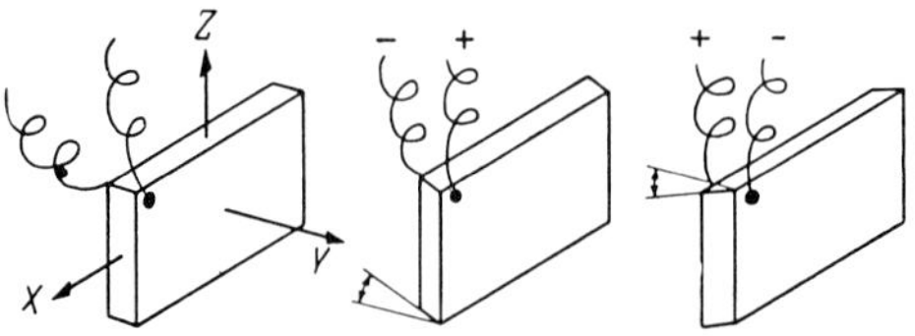

Fig. 1.100 Deformation of a Y-cut quartz plate, dimensions and potential as above, angle of shear exaggerated on a scale 200,000 : 1. To this must be added the shear in the ZX-plane, as in the case of the X-cut.

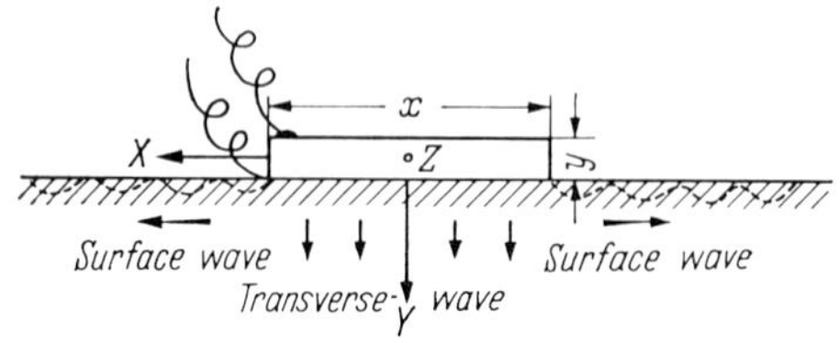

Fig. 1.101 In the solid material the Y-cut quartz plate generates a transverse wave normal to the surface, and a surface wave in the X-direction. The latter is particularly strong in the case of steel if $x : y \sim 7 : 1$.

Superimposed on this main shear is an additional shear action which deforms the rectangular surface of the plate as shown in Fig. 1.99c for the X-cut quartz plate. This secondary shear action is, however, moderate and in practice can be neglected.

A Y-cut quartz plate generates in a solid a transverse wave if a solid, or sufficiently tough, cement is used as couplant. In the case of smooth, flat surfaces transverse waves can, however, also be transmitted if the crystal is pressed on dry. Liquid coupling transmits from a Y-cut quartz plate only strong surface waves radiated from both sides in the X-direction (Fig. 1.101). According to Firestone [107, 104], a Y-cut quartz plate is particularly suitable for this purpose in the case of steel and aluminium if the plate in the X-direction is approximately 6 to 8 times thicker than the thickness Y. The length in the Z-direction is arbitrary because it only influences the angle of divergence of the flat beam.

1.102 The Piezoelectric Plate as Transmitter and Receiver of Ultrasonic Waves

Let us assume in the following an ideal X-cut quartz plate, i.e. a pure thickness oscillator with no other deformations. The static case of the two piezoelectric effects can then be written in an elementary way as follows:

1. Let the applied potential U_s (transmitting voltage) be given. Find the change in thickness Δx_s:

$$\Delta x_s = d_{11} U_s \,\mathrm{m} \tag{1.49}$$

with the constant

$$d_{11} = 2.3 \cdot 10^{-12}\,\mathrm{m/V} \quad \text{or} \quad \mathrm{As/N},$$

where d_{11} is the *piezoelectric modulus*[1].

2. Let an externally produced change in thickness Δx_e (reception) be given. Find the corresponding open-circuit voltage, i.e. the voltage on the quartz without any load being applied by measuring instruments or through insufficient insulation:

$$U_e = h_{11} \Delta x_e \,\mathrm{V} \tag{1.50}$$

with the *piezoelectric deformation constant*

$$h_{11} = 4.9 \cdot 10^{9}\,\mathrm{V/m} \quad \text{or} \quad \mathrm{N/As}.$$

In the case of other crystals, naturally other axes and numerical values apply.

In the latter case one can also start from the pressure P_x which produces the change in thickness. The receiving voltage then depends additionally on the thickness d:

$$U_e = g_{11} d P_x \,\mathrm{V} \tag{1.50 a}$$

with the *piezoelectric constant*

$$g_{11} = 0.057 \frac{\mathrm{V/m}}{\mathrm{N/m^2}} \quad \text{or} \quad \mathrm{m^2/As}.$$

Assuming that the entire change in thickness of the transmitting quartz is transferred to the receiving quartz, i.e. $\Delta x_e = \Delta x_s$, the ratio of receiving voltage to transmitting voltage according to Eqs. (1.49) and (1.50) becomes

$$\frac{U_e}{U_s} = d_{11} h_{11} = k^2 = 1.1 \cdot 10^{-2} \quad \text{(for quartz)}. \tag{1.51}$$

The quantity k defined by this equation is the electromechanical coupling factor which for a piezoelectric material is a reference for the efficiency of the conversion of electric potential into mechanical displacement and vice versa. Under the above assumption approximately 1/100 of the transmitting voltage reappears as receiving voltage in the case of quartz,

[1] Units in MKS system, in agreement with common practice. For conversion see [1, p. 96 et seq.]. Ampere-second can also be replaced by Coulomb.

but in reality this is considerably less, usually less than 1/1000. The value of k is usually given in per cent. According to Eq. (1.51) k is approx. $0.1 = 10\%$, but there are considerably better piezoelectric materials with a coupling factor exceeding 60% (see also 1.104).

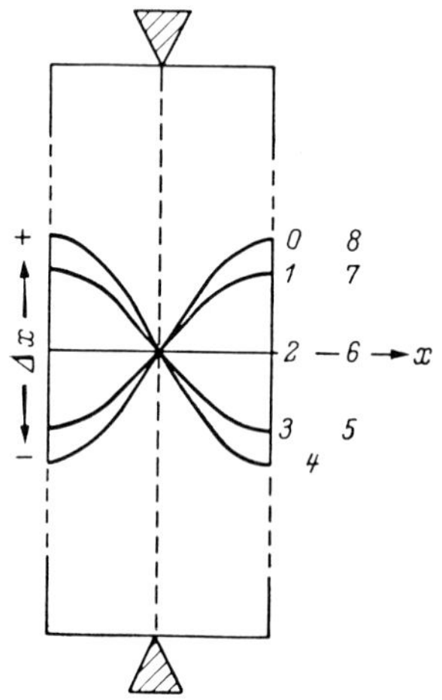

Fig. 1.102. Fundamental oscillation of a plate. Displacement of particles plotted at successive moments 0 to 8 as a function of the plate thickness.

The above discussions only apply to the static case, i.e. all changes must be so slow that the mass effect or the forces of inertia of the quartz plate do not come into play. A plate, apart from its piezoelectric properties, can however also oscillate mechanically, like a system consisting of a mass suspended from a spring. In the case of a plate, however, both the mass and the force of the spring are distributed evenly, so that in contrast to a mass suspended from a spring it can produce in addition to a fundamental wave also harmonics, like a taut string.

Let us now consider the fundamental or first characteristic oscillation of a plate held firmly along its edge as indicated in Fig. 1.102. The particles of both surfaces swing simultaneously outward and at a later moment inward, while the central plate remains constantly at rest. If the displacement of the particles for different moments 0 to 8 is plotted at right angles to the axis of the plate as shown in Fig. 1.102, the result is a bunch of sinusoidal curves with different amplitudes. This is a well-known phenomenon: we have here a standing wave which as explained in Fig. 1.7 is composed of two waves travelling in opposite directions. The thickness oscillation of the plate can therefore also be described as follows: a plane wave travels at right angles through the plate, is reflected at one of the surfaces, returns in the opposite direction and after a further reflection on the other surface meets itself in phase because the displacement amounts to a full wave length. Thus two opposing waves travel constantly through the plate.

If the wave is reflected on the free surface or at the interface of a contiguous and sonically soft material it is, however, necessary to add a phase shift of half a wave length each time which together just form a full wave length and thus do not interfere.

Taking c as the velocity of sound for longitudinal waves in quartz, we have

$$\text{Plate thickness } d = \frac{\lambda}{2} = \frac{c}{2 f_e}. \tag{1.52}$$

The characteristic frequency f_e of the plate is therefore

$$f_e = \frac{c}{2d}. \tag{1.53}$$

Consequently a thickness oscillation can also have transverse waves, which are of interest for the Y-cut plate. For both cases one obtains experimentally for a plate thickness d, calculated in mm:

$$\begin{aligned} f_{el} &= 2.88 \frac{1}{d} \text{ MHz} \quad (X\text{-cut quartz, thickness oscillation}), \\ f_{et} &= 1.92 \frac{1}{d} \text{ MHz} \quad (Y\text{-cut quartz, thickness oscillation}). \end{aligned} \tag{1.54}$$

For the thickness oscillation of a quartz plate to fall just within the audible range, it would therefore have to be approximately at least 20 cm thick. For thicknesses of the order of millimetres we approach the range of ultrasonic frequencies as required for non-destructive testing.

Fig. 1.103 shows the higher characteristic oscillations of the plate. Standing waves can also occur if the wave length is shorter, viz. if it is exactly one, half or one third, etc., of the original wave length, so that exactly 2 or 3, etc., half-wave lengths are apportioned to the plate thickness. This results in several node planes where the particles are constantly at rest. The higher characteristic frequencies f_n are the n-fold multiples of the characteristic frequency f_e.

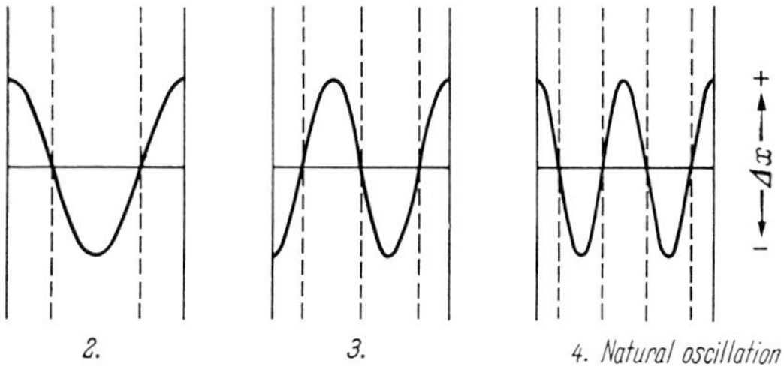

Fig. 1.103 Higher harmonics of a plate. Particle displacement for points taken across the plate thickness at time 0 corresponding to Fig. 1.102.

For the odd characteristic frequencies $f_n = f_1, f_3, f_5$ etc., the particles of the surfaces are subjected to opposing oscillations, simultaneously inward or outward, i.e. the thickness of the plate changes in the ryhthm of the oscillations. In the case of even characteristic frequencies, f_2, f_4, etc., the particles oscillate simultaneously in the same direction; the thickness of the plate remains unchanged and the plate, viewed from a point outside, merely oscillates back and forth as a whole.

Mechanical excitation, e.g. a shock, can produce in a plate, in addition to the fundamental, also higher characteristic oscillations as well as bending oscillations, resulting in a rather complex situation. Thanks to the piezoelectric effect quartz plates can, however, be excited electrically in the fundamental characteristic oscillation by applying to the metallized surfaces an alternating voltage corresponding to the characteristic frequency.

If a briefly excited plate is left to itself so that it oscillates freely, its sinusoidal oscillation does not remain constant because the plate constantly looses energy for two reasons, viz. internal friction and energy convection in the form of ultrasonic waves transmitted to the mounting and the ambient material. The first cause is usually rather insignificant compared with the second which is the real purpose of the oscillator. Due to the loss of energy the oscillation is damped and the amplitude

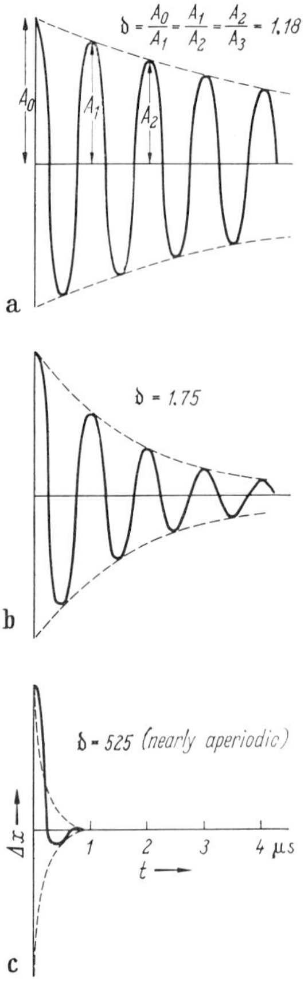

Fig. 1.104 Decay of oscillation of a thickness oscillator at different damping coefficients ծ (oscillator as in Fig. 1.105).

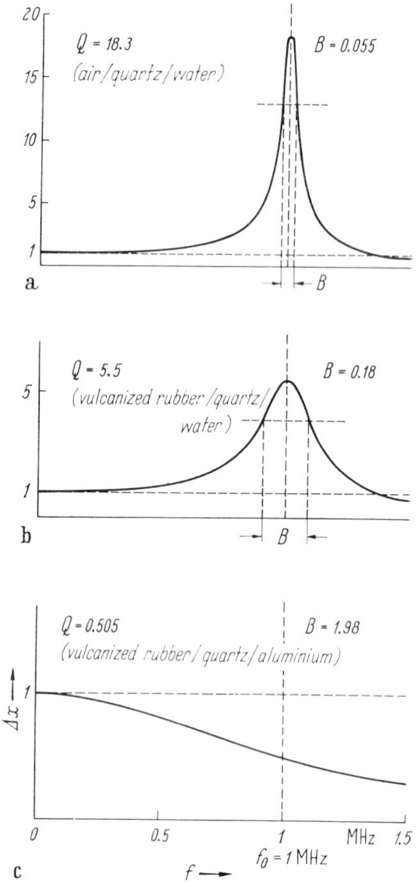

Fig. 1.105 Resonance curves of forced oscillations of a thickness oscillator as in Fig. 1.104. [Quality: a) 18.3, b) 5.5, c) 0.505].

decreases from one oscillation to the next by the factor ծ, known as the damping coefficient (Fig. 1.104). As will be explained later, this quantity depends essentially on the coupled material. In the case of the damped oscillation the frequency is likewise practically that of the characteristic frequency of the oscillation without damping; only for very high values of damping are the frequency deviations considerable.

If the piezoelectric plate is excited by an alternating voltage of different frequency, it oscillates at this frequency after buildup as a forced oscillation with constant amplitude. This amplitude, however, depends on the frequency (Fig. 1.105): for very small frequencies it is practically identical with the static thickness change Eq. (1.49) which is arbitrarily taken to be 1 in Fig. 1.105. Up to the resonance frequency f_0 it increases to a maximum whose value depends on the coefficient of damping, whereupon it drops again.

This increase at resonance, also called *quality* or quality factor which is designated by the letter Q, is defined as the ratio of the amplitude at the resonance frequency to the static thickness change:

$$Q = \frac{\Delta x_{f_0}}{\Delta x_{stat.}}. \tag{1.55}$$

The quality is linked to the damping coefficient $\mathfrak{d}$:

$$Q = \frac{\pi}{\ln \mathfrak{d}} \quad (\ln \mathfrak{d} = 2.303 \log \mathfrak{d}). \tag{1.56}$$

The quality is linked also to the band width of the resonance curve. If the band width B of the resonance maximum is defined according to Fig. 1.105, measured at 70% (more accurately at $1/\sqrt{2} = 0.707$) of the maximum value, the following equation applies if the damping is not excessive, i.e. for Q-values above say 10:

$$B = \frac{f_e}{Q}\,\text{MHz} \quad (f_e \text{ in MHz}). \tag{1.57}$$

Formulas (1.56) and (1.57) should be regarded only as approximations because their derivation presupposes that the oscillating piezoelectric plate behaves like a mass suspended from a spring. However, this is only approximately so, because, particularly in the case of high damping, the deviations are considerable. In the testing of materials by means of sound pulses damping coefficients of this order are necessary, so that when calculating the resonance advantage and the band width, considerably more complex, exact calculations should be used [94, 318].

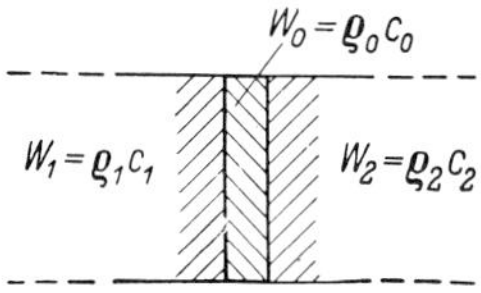

Fig. 1.106 Radiator between two materials 1 and 2.

When using a piezoelectric plate as an ultrasonic generator, the correlation between the damping coefficient and the constants of the contiguous materials is of interest. Let it be assumed that the plate is located between two materials 1 and 2 with the acoustic impedances W_1 and W_2 ($W = \varrho c$) (Fig. 1.106). As long as W_1 and W_2 are both smaller than W_0, the acoustic impedance of the piezoelectric material, i.e. for sonically soft coupling on both sides, the following applies:

$$\mathfrak{d} = \frac{(W_0 + W_1)\,(W_0 + W_2)}{(W_0 - W_1)\,(W_0 - W_2)}\,. \tag{1.58}$$

(Evaluation of equations in [318].)

Eq. (1.58) is also valid if both contiguous materials are sonically harder than the piezoelectric material. If, however, one of the two materials is sonically softer while the other is sonically harder, the piezoelectric plate oscillates only at $\lambda/4$ resonance, i.e. the characteristic frequency of the plate damped in this way is only half as high as given by Eq. (1.53), and the damping coefficient in this case is:

$$\mathfrak{d} = \frac{(W_0 + W_1)^2\,(W_0 + W_2)^2}{(W_0 - W_1)^2\,(W_0 - W_2)^2}\,. \tag{1.59}$$

Example: Let it be assumed that a quartz plate is mounted so that one side borders on air and the other on water. From the values $W_1 = 0.4 \cdot 10^3$, $W_2 = 1.5 \cdot 10^6$, and $W_0 = 14.5 \cdot 10^6$ kg/m²s it follows that $\mathfrak{d} = 1.18$ (Fig. 1.104a). This quartz is now cemented at the back to vulcanized rubber. From $W_1 = 2.8 \cdot 10^6$ we get $\mathfrak{d} = 1.75$ (Fig. 1.105b). This applieds not only to a plate of 1 MHz, but according to Eq.(1.58) the damping coefficient is independent of the resonance frequency. If, however, we now let the quartz cemented to vulcanized rubber radiate into aluminium instead of water, so that $W_2 = 16.4 \cdot 10^6$, the natural frequency of the plate is now only half as high. To facilitate the comparison Figs. 1.104 and 1.105 have, however, been drawn as if a plate of half the thickness were used for this test. In this case the damping coefficient should be caluculated according to Eq. (1.59); this gives $\mathfrak{d} = 525$, i.e. in this case the plate is already damped almost aperiodically because the amplitude of the second oscillation is now only 1/525 of that of the first and the third only $1/525^2 = 1/275{,}000$. For practical applications it must, however, be taken into consideration that a thin layer of cement between crystal and aluminium reduces the effective acoustic impedance of the material so that invariably smaller damping values will be obtained in tests.

In practice, the coupling conditions of a probe may fluctuate considerably with the surface quality, surface shape and material of the test piece, and therefore also the damping. In order to reduce excessively large fluctuations the unchanged acoustic impedance W_1 of the damping body cemented to the back can be chosen high. However, this can be done only at the expense of sensitivity because the amplitude of the oscillator, and therefore also the amplitude of the radiated sound, decrease with increasing damping factor.

So far the fundamental oscillation of a piezoelectrically excited plate has been discussed. The harmonics will now be analysed; for this purpose we assume that also in this case the plate is on both sides in contact with sonically soft materials. It is found that only the odd harmonics can be excited piezoelectrically, i.e. after the fundamental f_e, further resonances occur at $3f_e$, $5f_e$, etc. Fig. 1.105 should be supplemented on the right towards the region of higher frequencies by these additional resonance peaks. The correlated attenuation values increase with the order of the harmonics, i.e. they are proportional to 3, 5, etc. Therefore, at constant exciting voltage, the amplitude of the radiated sound wave decreases at the same rate.

The even harmonics of the plate may be present to the same extent as in the case of a taut string. That they cannot be excited piezoelectrically results from the fact that the piezoelectric effect produces a thickness change of the plate. In the case of the even harmonics the thickness of the plate, however, remains unchanged. In practice they can nevertheless be excited, even if only very weakly, by certain devices or as a result of irregularities in the crystal structure.

In spite of their lower amplitude, use is made of excitation by harmonics for the purpose of generating ultrasonic waves of high frequencies advantageously. For instance, instead of using an X-cut quartz crystal of approx. 0.1 mm thickness for 30 MHz, it is preferable to excite a crystal of 0.3 mm in its third harmonic because this quartz crystal is much less fragile and has a higher dielectric strength.

Even if the resonance curve shown in Fig. 1.105 is supplemented by the resonance peaks of the harmonics, it still differs from any measured curves because every quartz plate always has additional resonance points produced by additional deformations, linked to the thickness oscillation, which have been neglected here.

As far as the testing of materials is concerned, the oscillation amplitude of the piezoelectric plate is less important than the sound pressure of the radiated sound wave. The sound pressure is proportional to the oscillation amplitude and the frequency, so that at frequency 0 the resonance curve starts at zero and not with a finite value as shown in Fig. 1.105. Further, the resonance peak is symmetrical about its resonance frequency. Only in the case where the piezoelectric plate borders on the one side on a sonically hard material and on the other on a sonically soft material, is the resonance peak shifted from the above-mentioned $\lambda/4$ point towards higher frequencies and becomes asymmetrical.

Inversely, if a similar plate is used as receiver, the no-load voltage produced at the plate (i.e. without the load of measuring instruments) is proportional to the amplitude of the oscillation. Therefore, this receiving voltage of the piezoelectric plate again has an asymmetrical form as shown in Fig. 1.105.

If similar plates are used as transmitter and receiver (or, as in the echo method, the same plate is used first as transmitter and then as receiver) and if we consider the ratio of receiving voltage (no-load voltage) to transmitting voltage, the frequency curve with its resonance advantage appears as a factor twice. Fig. 1.107 shows curves of this type calculated according to [318]. It should be mentioned here that electrical matching of the receiver plate to an amplifier can deform the curves considerably. In calculating the curves shown in Fig. 1.107 it was assumed that no loss of sound pressure occurs between transmitter and receiver as a result of the conditions of propagation. The magnitude of these sound losses is shown in Fig. 1.88.

It should be pointed out that the ratio receiving no-load voltage to transmitting voltage is independent of the size and thickness of the piezoelectric plate. Fig. 1.107 is therefore valid for all quartz plates. The size of the plate influences only the conditions of sound propagation (divergence, length of near field).

The sound field of a piezoelect ic plate used as transmitter has been discussed in 1.81 and 1.83. It should be added that if the piezoelectric plate is used as receiver it has a similar field of sensitivity. According to a general principle, viz. the reciprocity theorem, the transmitter characteristic equals the receiver characteristic. As far as the far field is concerned this means for instance that an incident wave of constant sound pressure but variable angle of incidence produces in the receiving oscillator a voltage which reaches a maximum at perpendicular incidence, and which decreases in the case of oblique incidence according to a characteristic as shown in Figs. 1.62 et seq.

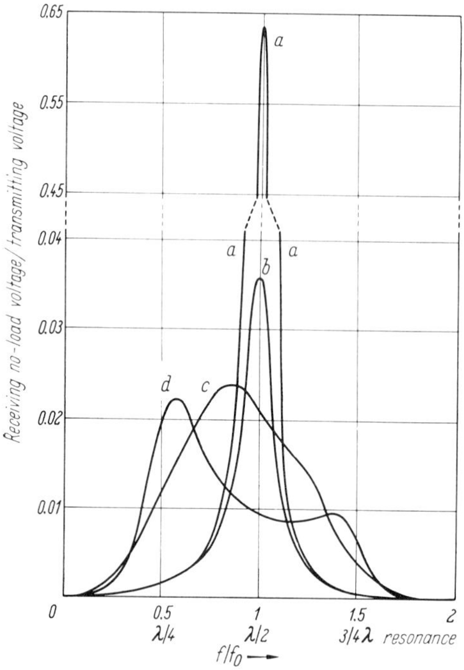

Fig. 1.107 Quartz plate operated simultaneously as transmitter and receiver. The ratio, receiver no-load voltage to transmitting voltage, is plotted for the following damping conditions: Sound radiation in water (curves *a* and *b*), in aluminium (*c*), in steel (*d*). Damping at back: *a* air; *b*, *c*, *d* vulcanized rubber (as in Figs. 1.104 and 1.105) (piezo-electric constant $h = 4.9 \cdot 10^9$ V/m, see Table 1.4). Loss-free propagation of sound between transmitter and receiver has been assumed.

In the echo method where the radiator functions both as transmitter and receiver, the directional characteristic in the far field therefore enters twice as a factor. The same applies to the near field. The ratio of receiving to transmitting voltage is therefore determined in the case of a small reflector movable in the sound field, by the square of the functions described in 1.8 exclusively for the sound field of the transmitter. The characteristic consequently becomes more pointed.

1.103* Piezoelectric Plate with Pulse Excitation

Let us first answer the question as to why a low damping of a given piezoelectric plate is not always advantageous. In order to radiate a continuous sound wave at maximally possible sound pressure and a given frequency, it is logical to excite a suitable plate at its natural frequency and to keep its damping at a minimum. For this purpose it is advantageous to let it be damped only by the coupled material while it borders on air at the back. In non-destructive testing this is rarely the case, because even if continuous ultrasonic sound is used for the test it will usually be necessary to sweep the frequency to avoid the creation of standing waves in the test piece (see also 1.10 and 1.83). In this shifting of frequency the amplitude should remain as constant as possible which, however, a narrow resonance curve does not permit. Ideal would be a frequency curve with a partially flat region, which, however, is difficult to achieve if one does not want to operate with very small amplitudes at frequencies far from the resonance point. A compromise is then made and the resonance curve is broadened as required by introducing suitable damping, resulting in the *band* not being completely smooth but decreasing to only 70% of the maximum value at its limits.

An adequate band width is particularly important when transmitting short pulses. In the echo method the length of the pulse may prevent the detection of flaws near the surface and pulses of minimum duration are therefore desirable. At high frequencies these pulses may still consist of a large number of oscillations. This advantage is, however, offset by the fact that the damping of most materials increases with the frequency. It is therefore necessary to generate and transmit pulses at frequencies which are not excessively high and with a minimum number of oscillations; it may even be advisable to produce completely aperiodic, i.e. so-called shock pulses.

Every pulse can be presented in sinusoidal form by a Fourier series as the sum of a given number of partial oscillations unlimited in time and contained in a frequency band of given width. Before and behind the pulse these partial oscillations cancel each other exactly. The shorter the pulse, regardless of its shape, the broader is the frequency band of appreciable amplitude. If some of the frequencies are suppressed in the case of pulse transmission by a mechanical or electrical system, the transmission distorts the pulse, and in particular lengthens it. The rule applies that in order to transmit a pulse of duration T without considerable distortion, a frequency band of width $B = 1/T$ is sufficient even if the latter has already decreased to 70% at both ends, as in the case of the resonance curve shown in Fig. 1.105.

A band width of 0.18 MHz shown in Fig. 105b therefore could transmit, with practically no distortion, a pulse of $1/0.18 = 5.5$ μs duration, e.g. 5 oscillations of 1 MHz frequency, each lasting 1 μs. If one attempts, however, to place on such a piezoelectric plate a pulse of 1 μs duration, the corresponding frequency band of 1 MHz is not transmitted, and the transmitted pulse would not be shorter than 5 μs as already indicated by the decay process of the plate shown in Fig. 1.104b.

If a transmission circuit contains several series-connected elements, e.g. transmitting radiator, receiving radiator and amplifier, the above statement applies to the total transmission curve which is the product of the individual transmission curves. The various elements must therefore fit to one another and it is futile to connect a wide-band radiator to a narrow-band amplifier, and vice versa. Also, the material through which the pulse passes in the form of a sound wave may reduce the frequency band, because its damping increases rapidly at higher frequencies.

Let us consider various types of electrical pulses and investigate how the piezoelectric plate behaves in these cases. First, let us take an alternating voltage train with 10 oscillations at the characteristic frequency of the plate (Fig. 1.108a). At the beginning and end this train suddenly disappears. However, because of its inertia and the elastic forces, the plate tends to resist any sudden changes and smoothes them out at the beginning and at the end of the oscillation by build-up and decay processes. The actual oscillation of the plate is therefore composed of the motion of an inertialess plate subjected to the influence of the voltage, which the plate follows precisely, and the transient oscillations. In Fig. 1.108 the curves *a* and *b* should therefore be added, so that the actual oscillation of the plate is obtained in *c*. Here again a damping coefficient $\mathfrak{d} = 1.75$ was assumed, as in Fig. 1.104b. The transient oscillation is the free characteristic oscillation of the plate, and Fig. 1.108b is therefore identical with Fig. 1.104b; the latter oscillation, however, as a build-up process, should be taken to be negative because it opposes the electrical excitation. However, at the end of the pulse, it acts in the same sense, i.e. it tries to support the electrical excitation.

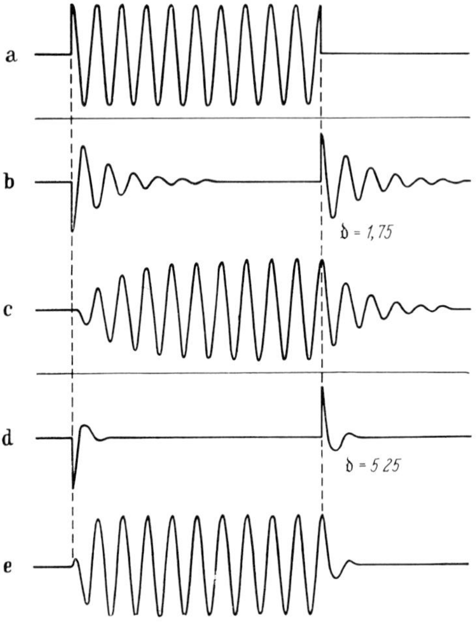

Fig. 1.108 Excitation of a piezoelectric plate by an alternating voltage train with damping coefficients 1.75 and 525, excitation frequency equals natural frequency. a) Alternating voltage train, identical with oscillation pattern of an inertialess plate; b) transient oscillation of actual plate for $\mathfrak{d} = 1.75$; c) oscillations occurring in the actual plate, i.e. the sum of a) and b); d) transient oscillations for $\mathfrak{d} = 525$; e) oscillation of plate, i.e. sum of a) and d).

With higher damping (Figs. 1.108d and e for $\mathfrak{d} = 525$) the effect of the transient oscillation is less important and the actual oscillation already resembles the exciting voltage much more closely. It should, however, not be overlooked that the amplitude decreases inversely with the damping coefficient; in the illustration this has not been taken into account

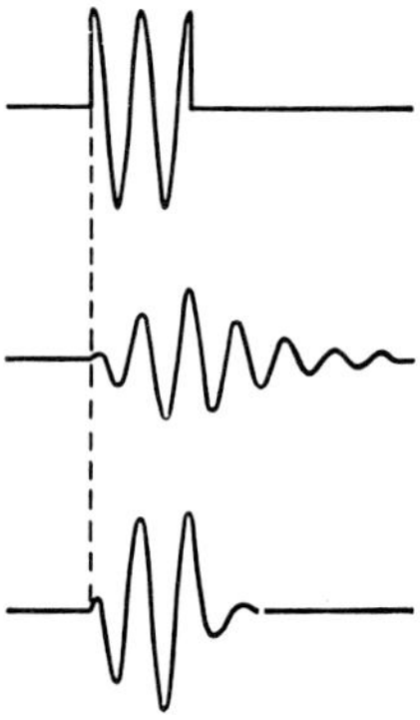

Fig. 1.109 As in Fig. 1.108, but with shorter pulse (see also Figs. 1.108a, c and e).

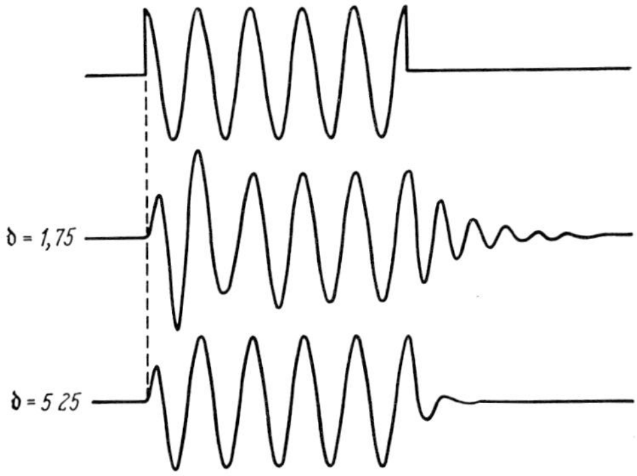

Fig. 1.110 As in Fig. 1.109, but with exciting frequency below characteristic frequency of plate (exciting frequency/characteristic frequency = 1 :1.6).

The build-up of the natural oscillation depends entirely on the impressed conditions, for which a particularly simple and clear case has been chosen here, viz. appearance and disappearance of the pulse voltage exactly at each maximum. Otherwise the correlated build-up process always develops in such a manner that it exactly cancels the motion of an intertialess plate at the beginning.

The greater the proportion of transient oscillations in the pulse, the shorter the duration of the excitation and the lower the damping of the plate. In Fig. 1.109 a pulse of only two oscillations of the characteristic frequency was used for excitation. With $\mathfrak{d} = 1.75$ the oscillation of the plate already fails to reach the maximum value, and build-up and decay already start to overlap. The plate with the greater damping still transmits the pulse almost undistorted, but with smaller amplitude. This disadvantage is partially offset by the fact that this plate reaches its oscillation peak earlier than the less damped plate.

As a last example of excitation by an alternating voltage let us consider a longer pulse but with a frequency lower than that of the characteristic frequency (Fig. 1.110). If the difference between the frequencies is not excessive the plate oscillation can still be synthesised approximately as in the previous example, so that the build-up frequency again equals the characteristic frequency of the plate. The result is a mixture of frequencies in which the exciting frequency can be recognized clearly only after the build-up.

In the latter case the plate is in reality excited not only in its fundamental but also its harmonics, which becomes more evident, the more the characteristic frequency differs from the fundamental frequency and the shorter the duration of the exciting pulse. Particularly in the case of aperiodic exciting voltages with very wide frequency bands, it is very difficult to obtain a satisfactory result in this simple way.

Since, however, short pulses are particularly important in non-destructive testing, the results of a more rigorous treatment of the piezoelectric plate, which makes it possible to construct correctly the pulse of the sound pressure of interest for arbitrary, exciting voltages by using a rather simple and fruitful method [66, 305], shall now be described.

Without presenting its derivation, it is recommended that the following basic rule concerning piezoelectric plates operated as transmitters be memorized (see Fig. 1.111):

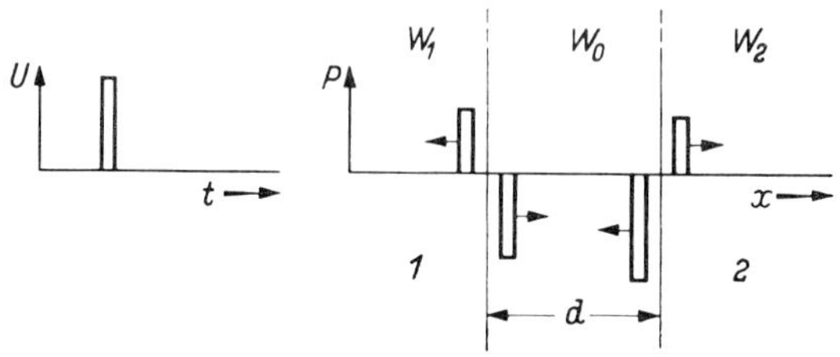

Fig. 1.111 Acoustic pressure waves, excited by the voltage U as a function of time, along the axis of a transducer plate sandwiched between two materials 1 and 2. For reasons of simplicity, the same acoustic velocity has been assumed in 1 and 2 and the scale chosen so that the pulse width is the same both in space and in time.

If an arbitrary voltage is applied to a piezoelectric plate, sonic pressure waves which show the same chronological pattern as the voltage radiate simultaneously from both surfaces. They travel into the plate as well as into the materials coupled to it externally, but inside the plate their phase is opposite to that outside. Their amplitudes depend on the acoustic impedances of the materials concerned as follows:

Material 1 (W_1)	Material 0 (W_0) (Piezoelectric plate)		Material 2 (W_2)
$\leftarrow \frac{W_1}{W_0 + W_1}$	$\frac{W_0}{W_0 + W_1} \rightarrow$	$\leftarrow \frac{W_0}{W_0 + W_2}$	$\frac{W_2}{W_0 + W_2} \rightarrow$

If the waves inside the piezoelectric plate strike the boundary, the well-known formulas given in Eq. (1.11) apply for their reflection and refraction, together with the rule: phase reversal at reflection on sonically softer material. Further, they are superimposed upon each other without distortion.

It is at this stage already no longer surprising that two waves travel in opposite direction in the plate, if it is realised that we have come to regard the oscillation of a plate in its fundamental and harmonic modes as a standing wave which may be composed of two waves travelling in opposite direction. This concerned the special case of sinusoidal waves, a limitation which is now discarded. Instead of the square waves in Fig. 1.111, any other arbitrary voltage and wave form may be used.

The above rules will now be applied to various boundary conditions and pulse forms. First, a short square wave pulse, as in Fig. 1.111 will be assumed in a thick plate so that the delay in the plate exceeds the duration of the pulse. Further, let us first take the simple case of a reflection-free boundary on both sides, viz. $W_1 = W_0 = W_2$, which can approximately be realised experimentally by a quartz plate sandwiched between aluminium, resulting in the four waves being identical.

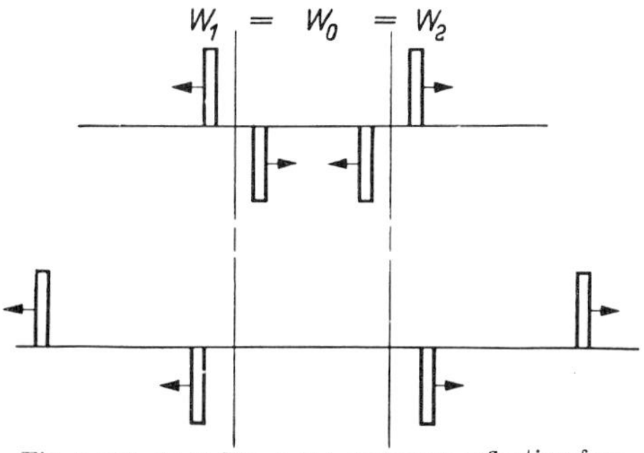

Fig. 1.112 As in Fig. 1.111, but with reflection-free matching on both sides.

The internal waves pass unimpeded through the opposite faces and completely leave the piezoelectric plate (Fig. 1.112). Thus, outside the plate, two identical, opposing pulses follow each other at an interval determined by the delay in the plate.

Fig. 1.113 shows the case where the plate on the left borders on air. The wave from the right is totally reflected with phase reversal. In Fig. 1.114, however, the matching on the right is no longer reflection-free, W_2/W_0 being chosen 0.25, which corresponds approximately to quartz/perspex. This results in a sequence of pulses which follow each other at the delay distance of the plate, Fig. 1.115 showing the first eight pulses on an enlarged scale. The second pulse is always twice as large as the first and the later pulses decrease in a constant ratio.

Other terminal conditions, e.g. the sonically hard termination, can be similarly treated. Here, however, only the length of the square wave voltage will be increased, again with reflection-free termination on both sides (Fig. 1.116). If the duration of the square wave voltage equals the transit time, the sound pressure has the form of a square wave oscillation, and if it becomes much longer (or if the piezoelectric plate is thin) only narrow pulses remain at the beginning and at the end. Between these pulses, the next wave (from the opposite plate surface) exactly cancels the first wave because of its reversed sound pressure. In the case of a thin plate, a step voltage therefore produces only one narrow pulse if the plate has reflection-free termination. If the square wave voltage is replaced by a sinusoidal voltage, only a very low sound pressure remains because two opposing half waves must be added at only a slight relative time lag.

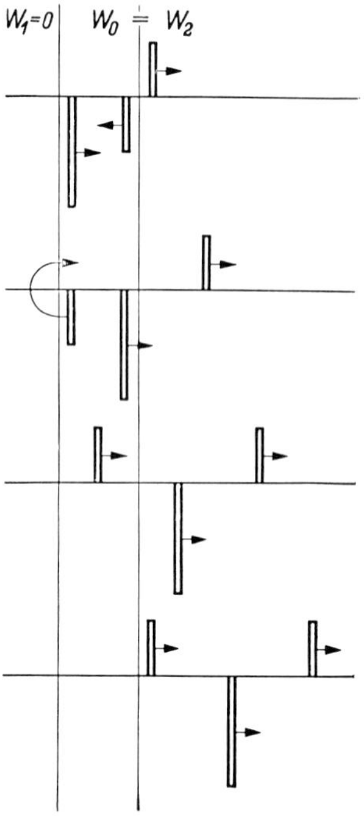

Fig. 1.113 As in Fig. 1.112, but with free boundary on the left and reflection-free matching on the right.

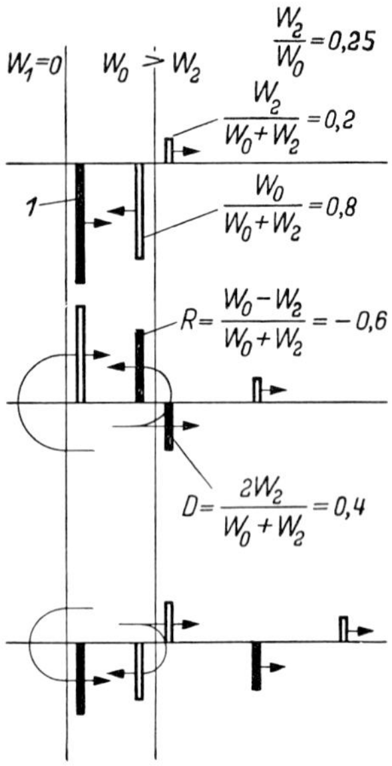

Fig. 1.114 As in Fig. 1.113, but with sonically soft matching on the right, $W_2/W_0 = 0.25$.
transmission;

$$D = \frac{2\,W_2}{W_2 + W_0} = 0.4;$$

reflection:

$$R = \frac{W_2 - W_0}{W_2 + W_0} = -0.6.$$

For clearer interpretation the waves coming from the left boundary are blackened.

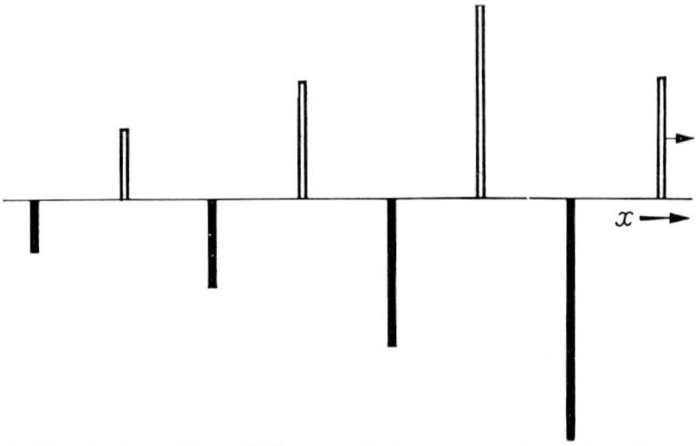

Fig. 1.115 The first 8 pulses of Fig. 1.114 shown on enlarged scale over path x.

In the case of excitation by several consecutive pulse voltages it is merely necessary to obtain the result for a single pulse and to add similar results, shifted according to the time lag of the pulses, respectively. In this way the sound wave corresponding to a given train of sinusoidal

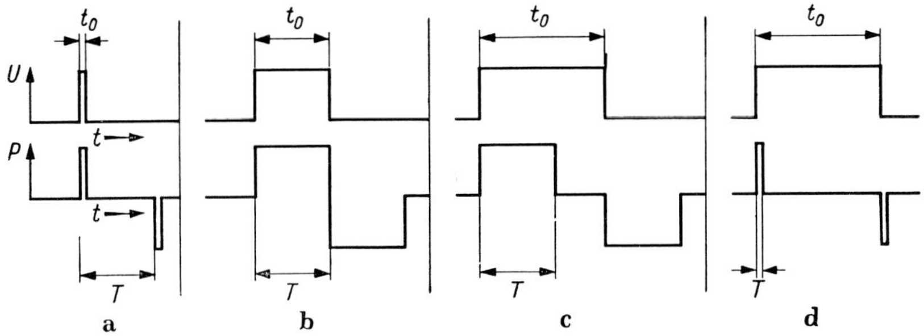

Fig. 1.116 Excitation of a reflection-free terminated oscillator by square wave voltages of different duration relative to the transit time in the oscillator. Pulse duration t_0, transit time T. a) $t_0 < T$, b) $t_0 = T$, c) $t_0 > T$, d) $t_0 \gg T$ (thin transducer plate).

waves can be plotted on the basis of the result of a sinusoidal half wave and one can thus determine the build-up and decay processes also in the absence of resonance. In practice this is done by calculation or graphically.

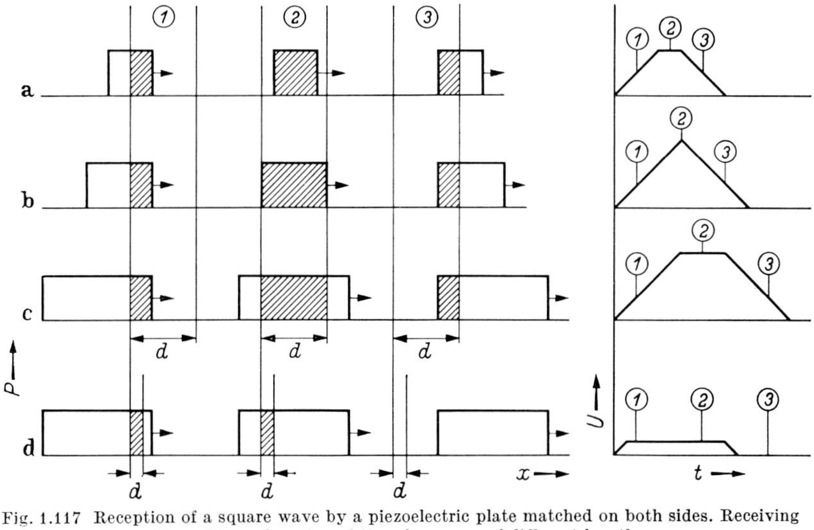

Fig. 1.117 Reception of a square wave by a piezoelectric plate matched on both sides. Receiving voltage U as a function of time for waves of different length. a) pulse duration t_0 < delay T, b) $t_0 = T$, c) $t_0 > T$, d) $t_0 \gg T$ (thin receiver).

As far as the receiver is concerned, the following rule applies (Fig. 1.117):

If an arbitrary sonic pressure wave enters a piezoelectric plate, an electric no-load voltage is produced at its electrodes which is proportional to the area of the sonic pressure curve of the wave which has already entered. If several waves are propagated in the plate simultaneously, e.g. by zig-zag reflection, their areas are added with due regard to sign.

The example in Fig. 1.117a shows a square wave which enters a thick plate (duration of wave shorter than transit time). The area inside the plate (shaded) increases linearly, and therefore also the voltage. It remains constant as long as the whole wave travels inside the plate. Since it has been assumed that the back of the plate is matched reflection-free, the wave leaves the plate unimpeded and the voltage therefore again drops to zero.

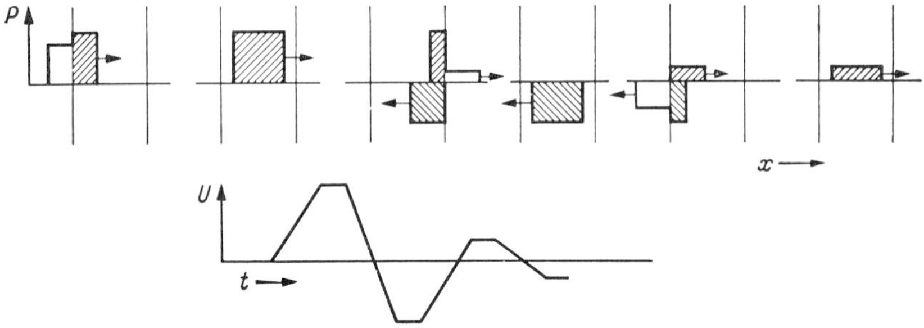

Fig. 1.118 Reception by a piezoelectric plate with sonically soft termination on both sides, left $W_0/W_1 = 2$, right $W_0/W_2 = 9$. Receiving voltage U as a function of time.

If the wave is longer, it can fill the plate completely and the voltage reaches a maximum which persists as long as the plate is filled. Finally, if the wave is very long compared with the transit time (Fig. 1.117d), it increasingly resembles the voltage curve. Thus, if the back of a piezoelectric plate is matched correctly, and the thinner the plate a sound wave can be transformed into a voltage with increasing faithfulness. In this case, however, the amplitude of the voltage decreases with the thickness of the plate because the area is reduced.

In practice it is not an easy matter to terminate a piezoelectric plate reflection-free. If the termination at the back is sonically soft, reflections at this point are produced with phase reversal. A single, short pulse therefore produces an alternating voltage of decreasing amplitude (Fig. 1.118).

Finally, Fig. 1.119 shows a case of practical interest calculated by the method described; this concerns the transmission from an X-cut quartz plate backed by vulcanized rubber through water, a similar oscillator acting as receiver. The exciting voltage, as is frequently done, is the damped oscillation of a resonating circuit with the characteristic frequency of the plate. Both the resonating circuit and the plate have the damping coefficient $\mathfrak{d} = 1.75$, wherein it is assumed that the plate produces no reaction on the resonating circuit and the rest of the generator circuit. This applies approximately to quartz with its loose electromechanical coupling.

The example shows how resonance of both the transmitter and the receiver changes the original pulse. The build-up is flattened and the decay

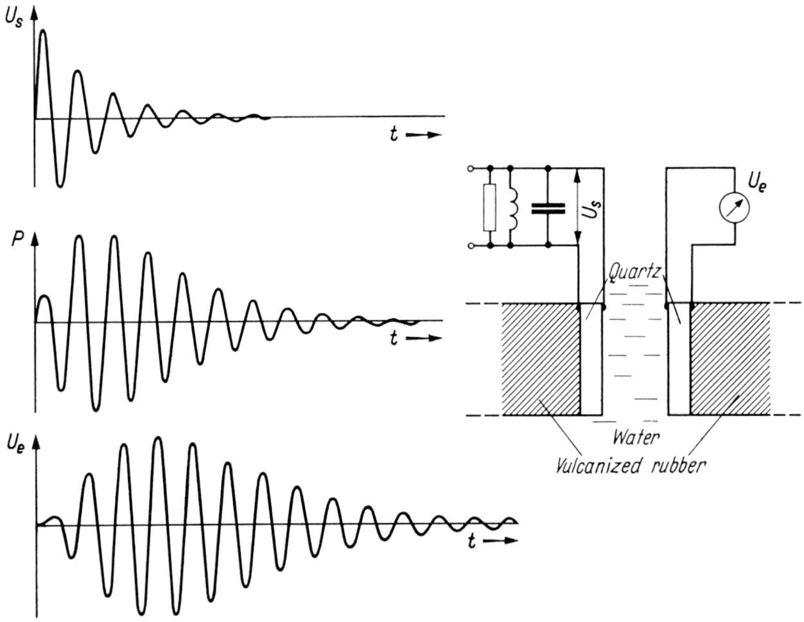

Fig. 1.119 Transmission of an electric pulse in the form of a damped oscillation with $\mathfrak{d} = 1.75$ from transmitter to receiver in resonance at $\mathfrak{d} = 1.75$. Transmitting voltage, sound pressure and receiving voltage as functions of time, maxima arbitrarily shown equally large.

increased considerably. Special attention is drawn to the build-up of the receiving voltage, which due to the formation of the area integral is always very flat. The considerable distortion of the pulse can be reduced by better damping as well as by off-resonance excitation.

When coupling an oscillator to a solid via a thin layer of liquid the problem becomes more complex due to the multiple reflections in this layer. Basically it can, however, also be solved by adding the individual waves according to amplitude and phase. It turns out that this considerably changes the resonance curve of the oscillator, particularly by the appearance of two peaks (Filipczynski [94]).

1.104 Piezoelectric Materials

Of the many materials with piezoelectric properties mainly quartz, barium titanate, lithium sulphate and lead meta-niobate are used for the non-destructive testing of materials; their constants are given in

Table 1.4. For use in special cases, seignette's salt or rochelle salt (sodium potassium tartrate, abbreviated KNT crystal), potassium dihydrogen phosphate (KDP), ammonium dihydrogen phosphate (ADP), dipotassium tartrate (DKT), ethylene diamine tartrate (EDT), as well as turmaline, may also be mentioned.

Quartz, the oldest piezoelectric material, is pellucid and very hard. It is attacked chemically by only a few substances. The plates which may be dull to clear, depending on the polishing, are cut from natural crystals, usually of Brazilian origin or nowadays also from artificially grown crystals. The electrodes can be deposited by evaporation in vacuum, but are superior and more durable if produced by burning in silvering liquids. The wires can be soldered on directly if solder compatible with the silver plating is used.

All the other piezoelectric materials are mechanically less resistant. Lithium sulphate, or more accurately lithium sulphate hydrate, is the most sensitive. At 75 °C it looses its water of crystallization and decomposes into powdery lithium sulphate and water. The crystals are grown artificially from the solution. Electrodes can be deposited by evaporation or by painting with a suspension of flaky silver powder and varnish. The connecting wires are attached by cementing them into the deposit or by dusting a non-conducting cemented joint with metal powder.

Barium titanate and lead meta-niobate, as well as a number of materials on lead-zirkonate-titanate base (PZT) which resemble barium titanate, are used as sintered, ceramic materials because it is not possible to produce larger single crystals from them. The ground, raw material mixed with binders is moulded as required by pressing and sintering above 1000 °C, and is then shaped accurately by grinding. All these are white to yellowish materials of lower hardness and resistance to wear than quartz; their dull surface can be silver-plated very durably by a baking process. In contrast to quartz, lithium sulphate and the other natural crystals, they are given their piezoelectric properties by *polarization*. For this purpose a direct voltage of a few thousand volts per centimetre thickness is applied to the substance while being heated to a temperature which is characteristic for each material, viz. the Curie temperature, given in Table 1.4 as critical temperature, whereupon the material is permitted to cool off while the voltage is still applied. This aligns one axis of the small crystals previously orientated at random, which is then *frozen*. Provided the material is not reheated close to the Curie temperature, it remains piezoelectric although its constants may decrease slightly due to ageing. The material can be repolarized as often as necessary. The PZT ceramics have still closer electromechanical coupling (up to 70%) and higher Curie temperatures than barium titanate (up to 350 °C).

Table 1.4 *Constants of some piezoelectric materials*[1]

	Quartz SiO_2	Lithium sulphate $LiSO_4$	Barium titanate $BaTiO_3$	Lead meta-niobate $PbNb_2O_6$	
Density ϱ	2.65	2.06	5.7	5.8	10^3 kg/m^3
Acoustic impedance W	15.3	11.2	35	16	10^6 kg/m^2
Velocity of sound c	5760	4720	4400	2800	m/s
Characteristic frequency f_c of a plate 1 mm thick	2.88	2.36	2.2	1.4	MHz
Critical temperature	576	75	115 to 150	550	°C
Dielectric constant ε	4.5	10.3	1,700	225	
Internal damping coefficient $\mathfrak{d}$	1.00003		1.008	1.3	
Electromechanical coefficient of coupling k for thickness oscillation	0.10	0.35	0.52	0.42	
Coefficient for coupling of thickness with radial or shear oscillation (interfering oscillation)	0.10	0	0.37	0.07	
Piezoelectric modulus d for thickness oscillation	2.3	15	190	80	10^{-12} m/V
Piezoelectric constant of deformation h	4.9	8.2	1.1	1.1	10^9 V/m
Piezoelectric pressure constant g	57	165	11	37	10^{-3} V/m

[1] According to Ref. [1, 167, 12]. The data for barium titanate and lead meta-niobate depend on the exact composition and are only reference values.

Instead of sintering the polarized material used in ceramic transducers, it can also be made into a paste by mixing it with an electrically non-conducting liquid, which at a constantly applied high bias likewise becomes piezoelectric (Lutsch [241], see also [61]). Such paste transducers can be applied directly to the test piece without the use of an intermediate coupling liquid, allowing more uniform coupling on rough surfaces, but their sensitivity is considerably lower than that of conventional transducers [241].

Furthermore, powdered materials of this type can be mixed with molten or curable binders, thus providing solid transducers which, although their sensitivity is likewise low, nevertheless have high internal damping.

If the constants of the four most important materials listed in Table 1.4 are compared, the piezoelectric modulus d shows that at the same transmitting voltage, considerably greater thickness changes can be obtained in the case of the last three materials than in the case of quartz. Barium titanate, coming before lead meta-niobate, is the best transmitter material in this respect. However, if used as sound pressure receiver, lithium sulphate comes first (compare constant g). Both for mechanical damping and for coupling a low acoustic impedance of the material is desirable, which is by far the highest for barium titanate. Since the effective acoustic impedance is only a few millions kg/m^2s in the case of radiation in liquids or liquid coupling to a solid, the matching of barium titanate is always unsatisfactory and its sensitivity cannot be fully exploited. Lead meta-niobate and lithium sulphate are far superior in this respect, particularly the former, because of its mechanical properties. This is also the case if the *same* crystal is used as transmitter and receiver, as is customary.

However, lead meta-niobate offers still other great advantages for non-destructive testing. In order to produce short pulses, allowance must be made for the mechanical characteristic oscillations of the plate by attaching a damping body to the back of the crystal. This should not only damp the crystal but in addition should completely absorb the wave radiated from the back in a layer of minimum thickness. In the case of crystals with high acoustic impedance it is therefore not so simple to produce satisfactory damping bodies because in practice the required properties usually conflict with each other. Here again, lithium sulphate and lead meta-niobate are the best. However, the intrinsic internal damping of the latter is high ($\mathfrak{d} = 1.3$) so that for many purposes it can be used without additional damping, which again benefits the sensitivity.

A further considerable advantage of lithium sulphate and lead meta-niobate is their low coupling factor for oscillations in the plane of the plate, compared with the thickness oscillation. The transverse deformation of a piezoelectric plate caused by the thickness change results in decay processes in the plane of the plate if excited by pulses, which, because of the much greater transverse dimensions, last much longer than the decay of the thickness oscillations. In the case of quartz this concerns the Y-direction of the plate, and in the case of ceramic materials similar deformations occur in all radial directions, giving rise to concentric radial oscillations. These oscillations can be damped only partially, by a damping body at the back, and it is preferable, but more difficult from the design point of view, to apply damping which circles the edge. Therefore in the case of quartz, and much more so in the case of barium titanate, it is impossible to generate very narrow pulses, in contrast to lithium sulphate and lead meta-niobate. Summarizing the various points of view, the last-mentioned material is therefore by far the most suitable for use in the pulse-echo method. Its sole disadvantage is the low characteristic frequency f_e of a plate if high frequencies are to be produced, which would require very thin, and therefore fragile, lead meta-niobate plates (see also [121]).

Lithium sulphate, if used under water, must be protected by waterproof layers, usually cold-setting polymerization cements, which at the same time can be used for matching the acoustic impedances, and if given a curved surface, also as sound lenses for focusing. Since these layers have low resistance to wear and because the crystal would immediately be destroyed at the slightest defect of the protective layer if immersed in water, it is necessary to protect these probes, should they ever be used while in direct contact, by additional protective layers.

When working in direct contact with electrically conducting surfaces, the metallization on the front face can be omitted in the case of quartz. Any ordinary silver plating would in any case wear off rapidly. A contact spring in the probe must then establish electric contact between the surface, the return circuit, and the chassis of the instrument, without which the sensitivity is greatly reduced because the crystal is excited less strongly if the circuit is closed capacitively only. In the case of materials with high dielectric constants, such as barium titanate and lead metaniobate, a contact spring would also be of little use. As shown in Fig. 1.120, the crystal and the oil film form a capacitor with two layers of which the oil film, in spite of its thinness, has a smaller capacitance than the crystal. Both together form a voltage divider in which the higher voltage is on the smaller capacitance, so that the crystal receives only a fraction of the total transmitting voltage. If water or paste is used instead of oil, the effect is slight. Otherwise barium titanate must always be fitted with an electrode making direct contact, which in the case of quartz is recommended only for non-conducting surfaces. The relatively soft silver layer can be strengthened for direct contact by copper and hard chromium or glued-on protective discs of quartz or sapphire.

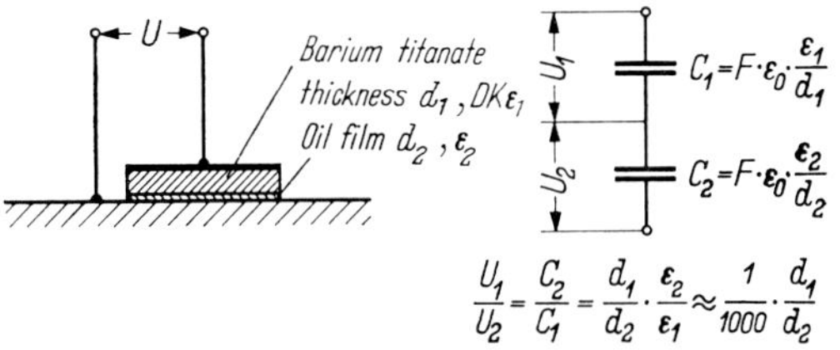

Fig. 1.120 Barium titanate transducer without metallised front, coupled through an oil layer to a metal base. Since the order of magnitude of the values of the dielectric constants of $BaTiO_3$ and oil are as 1000 to 1, in reality only a fraction of the applied total voltage is placed on the oscillator.

Ceramic piezoelectric materials can also be used for obtaining transducers with curved surfaces by sintering and grinding, in which the piezoelectric axis is orientated automatically at every point normal to the surface during polarization. In the case of a quartz plate ground with a curve this is of course no longer the case: the next Y-axis already lies at an angle of 30° to the X-axis in the XY-plane. Thus, if the transducer is ground excessively concave or convex, these faces no longer contribute to the radiation of longitudinal waves. In the case of ceramics, however, even greater angles of divergence, up to a closed cylinder, can be obtained so that considerable concentrations of the sound field along the axis of the cylinder can be achieved. To reduce costs, focusing transducers for non-destructive testing can be constructed also in the form of mosaics which must be laid out so that the piezoelectric axes are orientated uniformly in order to produce cophasal oscillations.

Reversing the polarity of a piezoelectric crystal also reverses the polarity of the radiated pulse, for instance, it then starts with a pressure minimum instead of a maximum. If the same crystal is also used as receiver, the form of the electrical pulse remains the same in both cases. Only when using separate transmitters and receivers, can the sign of the echo be reversed, depending on the polarity of the two transducers, i.e. for instance the echo can start with a negative instead of a positive voltage wave.

Finally, the matching of the piezoelectric plate to the electric transmitter will briefly be discussed. Greatly simplified, a piezoelectric plate of thickness $d = \lambda/2$ excited in the fundamental oscillation can be replaced by its static capacitance C_0 in parallel with an ohmic resistance R_s, as long as the plate is not excessively disturbed by contiguous materials (Fig. 1.121).

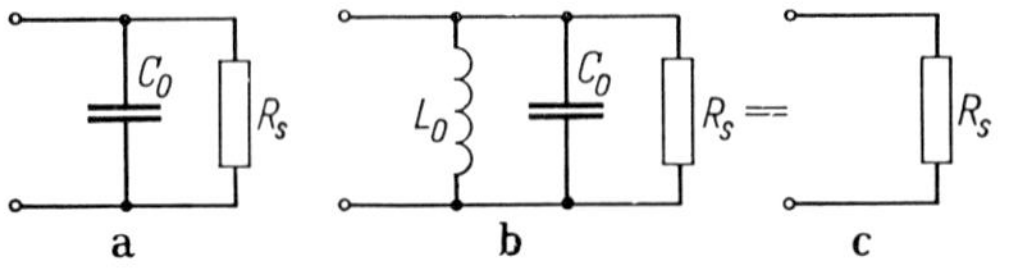

Fig. 1.121 Equivalent circuit diagram of a piezoelectric plate at fundamental resonance (a). If the static capacitance C_0 of the plate (including the capacitance of the circuit and the cable) is adjusted by means of coil L_0 to electric resonance at the fundamental frequency, only the effective radiation resistance R_s remains (b and c) if other losses are neglected.

This *radiation resistance* shown in the equivalent circuit, consumes the same energy as radiated by the plate into the contiguous materials. If the capacitance, as customary, is balanced by an inductance L_0 connected in parallel and tuned to resonance, only R_s remains. If W_1 and W_2 are the acoustic impedances of the materials adjacent to the piezoelectric plate, the acoustic impedance (converted according to [318], where a series circuit was assumed as equivalent circuit) is obtained from

$$R_s = \frac{1}{F f_e^2} \left(\frac{c^2 (W_1 + W_2)}{16 h^2 \varepsilon^2 \varepsilon_0^2} + \frac{h^2}{\pi^2 (W_1 + W_2)} \right) \Omega$$

where F (m²) is the area of the radiator, f_e (Hz) the fundamental frequency, and $\varepsilon_0 = 8.886 \cdot 10^{-12}$ As/Vm the universal constant. Typical constants c, h, ε of the piezoelectric material are given in Table 1.4.

Example: A quartz plate with the fundamental frequency $f_e = 10^6$ Hz (= 1 MHz) and the area $F = 0.001$ m² has the radiation resistance $R_s = 450$ kΩ if radiating in water ($W_2 = 1.5 \cdot 10^6$ kg/m²s) and damped at the back by vulcanized rubber ($W_1 = 2.8 \cdot 10^6$ kg/m²s), and $R_s = 2.1$ MΩ if radiating in aluminium ($W_2 = 16.9 \times \times 10^6$ kg/m²s). Under similar conditions, a barium titanate plate has a radiation resistance $R_s = 53$ and $R_s = 186$ Ω, respectively. In the case of quartz the radiation resistance is therefore approximately 1000 times greater than for barium titanate. In the case of radiation into aluminium it should be noted that the above calculation applies to the fundamental frequency ($\lambda/2$ plate). The resonance frequency, however, is lower, as shown in Fig. 1.106a, curve *c*. At this resonance point the radiation resistance is likewise lower than calculated above.

The equivalent circuit of a transmitter consists of the power supply U_s connected in series with the internal resistance R_i (Fig. 1.122). The transmitter reaches its maximum power if the connected load impedance, here the radiation resistance R_s, equals the internal resistance. Small

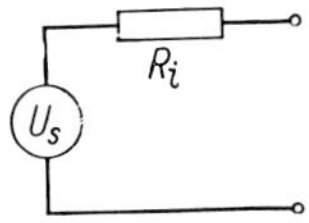

Fig. 1.122 Equivalent circuit diagram of a generator.

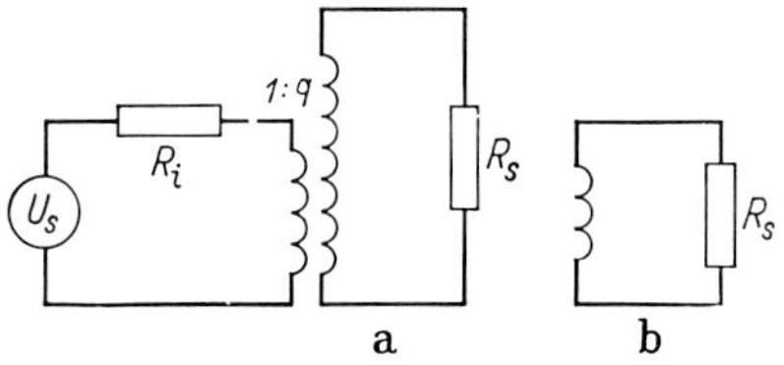

Fig. 1.123 Matching of transmitting radiator and generator. a) $R_s > R_i$, $q = \sqrt{R_s/R_i} > 1$ (quartz transducer at low frequencies); b) $R_s < R_i$, $q < 1$ (barium titanate transducer).

valve generators have an internal resistance of approx. 1000 Ω, indicating that the two radiators in the above example would be badly matched. They can, however, be matched correctly by interconnecting a transformer with the transformation ratio $1:q$, where $q = \sqrt{R_s/R_i}$. Thus, for quartz the voltage is stepped up and for barium titanate down (Fig. 1.123).

Since it is difficult to construct such transformers for transformation ratios above approximately 1: 10, and because it is furthermore undesirable to have high voltages on the quartz plate, it is much easier to match barium titanate at frequencies around 1 MHz and lower. For higher frequencies it is simpler to use quartz. Attention is drawn to the fact that the radiation resistance changes inversely with the square of the frequency.

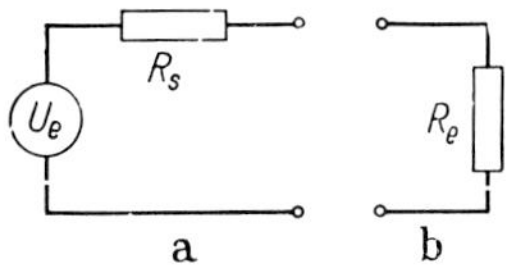

Fig. 1.124 Equivalent circuit of a piezoelectric plate as receiver at resonance, after the static capacitance has been balanced at resonance by a coil (a). Equivalent circuit of receiver with input resistance R_e (b).

Fig. 1.124 shows the equivalent circuit of a piezoelectric transducer used as receiver. It shows a voltage source equal to the no-load voltage in series with the radiation resistance R_s. As in the case of the transmitter, the internal losses of the piezoelectric plate have been neglected here. The static capacitance is balanced by an inductance. In this case the load is the input resistance R_e of the receiver, which in general far exceeds the internal resistance of the transmitter. Therefore, quartz is more suitable in this case and it usually requires no matching transformer, whereas in the case of barium titanate it would be necessary to step up the receiving voltage. Therefore, only if separate transmitters and receivers are used is optimal matching possible in both cases, while, if a single crystal is used for both purposes, a compromise has to be made.

1.105 Other Methods for Generating Ultrasound

The piezoelectric effect is particularly suitable for generating ultrasonic beams for testing materials because plates of only a few millimetres thickness produce suitable frequencies in conventional probes, which due to their high acoustic impedance, can radiate these frequencies from the crystal face directly into the test piece. Other methods are rarely used in practice.

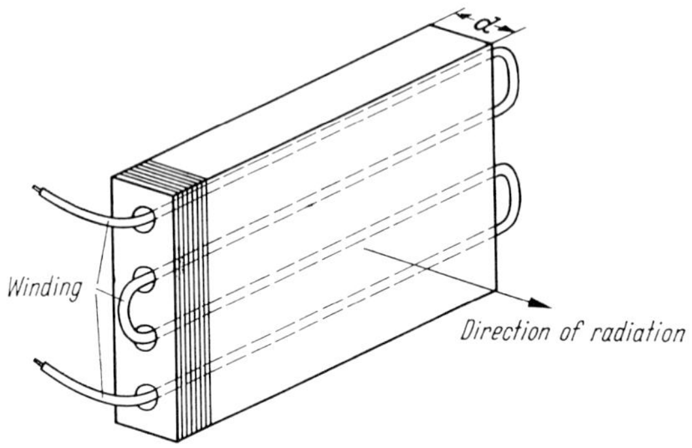

Fig. 1.125 Assembly of a magnetostrictive transducer.

Ultra-sound, as interfering sound, can, however, hamper the testing of materials if produced by mechanical working of the test piece during testing. Particularly in the case of highspeed grinding discs, milling cutters or steel brushes, ultrasonic waves of arbitrary direction and frequency are frequently generated at the machining points in addition to the audible noise. If these waves come into the probe in the axial direction, either directly or after multiple reflections in the test piece, their contribution in the frequency band of the instrument is amplified and indicated as noise level.

Amongst other generating methods the magnetostriction effect can be considered. It is similar to the piezoelectric effect: magnetostrictive materials change their form under the influence of a magnetic field. Magnetostrictive materials are in particular nickel and its alloys, and also steel and ferrites. A nickel rod placed in a coil experiences a change in length infunotion of the current which flows through the coil. If one wishes to exploit the mechanical length or thickness resonance as in the case of the piezoelectric plate, in order to produce greater amplitudes, one arrives at similar thicknesses of a few millimetres only, or even fractions of a millimetre, as above: however, while the generation of an electric field in the axial direction of such a plate is a rather simple matter – the plate serving as dielectric for a plate capacitor –, this is much more difficult in the case of a magnetic field because one face of the oscillator must remain accessible to transmit the radiation. To reduce the eddy current losses in such a plate to a minimum, it usually consists of a stack of laminations through which holes have been punched to accommodate the winding (Fig. 1.125). The thickness d of the stack determines the frequency of the fundamental resonance, which for values of 1 cm are of the order of 200 kHz. Transducers of this type can be used for generating low ultrasonic frequencies suitable for testing concrete and rock, as well as underwater sonic transmitters, because they are cheaper than the corresponding barium titanate transducers and because they have no low temperature limit. For higher frequencies, only generation in a harmonic could be considered. However, the probes then become too unwieldy. Furthermore, due to their high acoustic impedance, damping of these transducers causes difficulties.

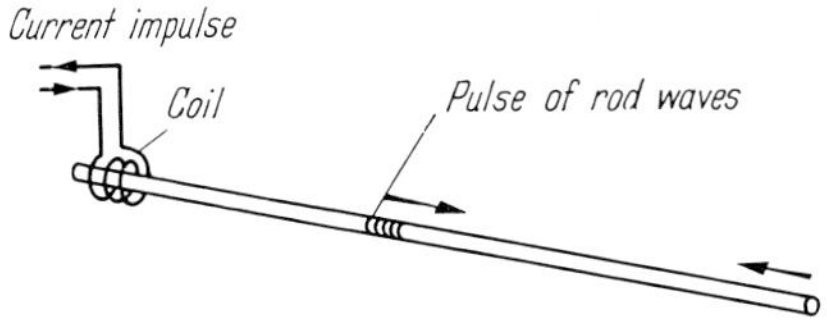

Fig. 1.126 Magnetostrictive testing of rod steel or steel wire.

The excitation of ultrasonic waves by the magnetostrictive effect, however, offers an interesting solution if they can be produced in the test piece itself and if its form and material permit it. As shown in Fig. 1.126, rod steel for instance can be tested in this way. A current impulse in the coil generates, at the end of the rod, an ultrasonic pulse in the form of a rod wave whose echo can be received by the generating coil, alternatively by a separate receiving coil. Flaws produce defect echoes or weaken the normal end echo of the rod if comparative tests are carried out. Naturally, only rods of identical cross-section and material can be compared with each other. This method has the very important advantage over the piezoelectric method, that no contact with the work piece is required. Furthermore, the influence of the condition of the surface is not very great. According to KAULE [173] coils placed on a flat or slightly

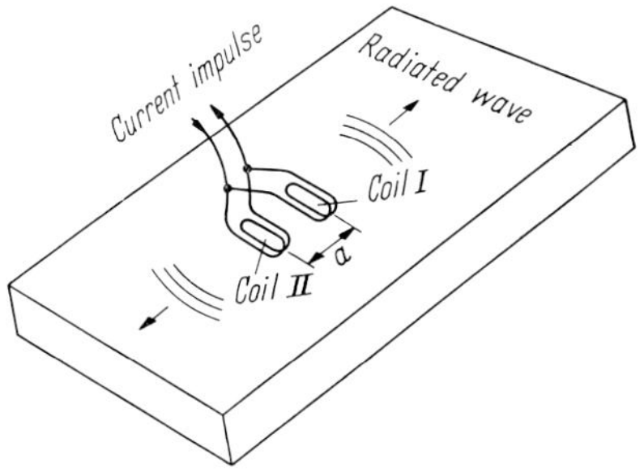

Fig. 1.127 Magnetostrictive excitation of plate or surface waves by staggered coils.

curved surface can produce also other wave types, such as surface waves or plate waves. If, as shown in Fig. 1.127, the coil is elongated, the radiated wave can be bundled as in the case of sound transmitters with piezoelectric plates with a diameter of several wave lengths. The laws determining the sound field, as discussed in Sec. 1.8, apply also in this case analogously. If two or more coils are operated in series or parallel, spaced at distance a, like coils I and II in Fig. 1.127, those wave forms are radiated preferentially whose "trace wave length" (see Fig. 1.68) equals the distance a, because in this case the waves radiated from the two coils are superimposed in phase. Since this phase relation no longer applies in the case of surface or plate waves radiated obliquely, this staggering of the coils produces an additional focusing effect.

For certain testing purposes it is undesirable that an arrangement as shown in Fig. 1.127 radiates sound equally in both directions. In such cases this can be remedied by exciting coil II with a high frequency voltage 90° out of phase with that of coil I and making the distance a 1/4 of the trace wave length. If the phase in coil II is leading, a wave excited by coil I reaches coil II in antiphase and is thus extinguished However, a wave coming from coil II arrives at coil I in phase and is thus amplified so that the sound is propagated only in the direction from coil II to coil I, and not in the opposite direction.

Curved coils, like curved piezoelectric plates, produce a focused sound field.

The same arrangement of coils can be used for receiving sound waves provided the work piece has been premagnetized near the coils by means of permanent magnets or electromagnets. Two effects determine the generation of receiving voltages in the coils:

1. The inverse magnetostrictive effect. The deformation of magnetostrictive materials produces a magnetic field which in turn by induction generates an electric voltage in the coil.

2. The magneto-elastic effect. The deformation of ferromagnetic materials changes the magnetic permeability and therefore also the magnetic flux through the receiving coil, with constant exciting field strength of the premagnetization circuit. This likewise induces a receiving voltage in the coil.

2 Methods and Instruments for the Ultrasonic Testing of Materials

2.0 Classification and Revue

It is useful to characterize all methods according to the *measured quantities* which they use, as in the general table below; this also gives the abbreviations and principal applications frequently referred to in what follows. As far as this classification is concerned the special *testing technique* discussed in detail in the various Sections, is of secondary importance. Methods which have not yet gained importance are marked "no", other ones "yes" and those which are particularly important are outlined in black. Among the latter the pulse transit time method with reflection has won most favour and is usually referred to as the pulse-echo method.

However, methods which have as yet remained unimportant may gain practical significance with the general advance in technology, at least for certain specific testing problems.

Measured variable	**Resonance frequency**	**Intensity alone**	**Intensity and transit time**		**Transit time only**
Name	Resonance method 2.1	Intensity method 2.2	Intensity transit time method 2.3		Transit time method 2.4
Abbreviation	R	I	Pulse transit time PT	Frequency modulation FM	T
Principal application	Wall thickness	Flaws in plates	General flaw location		Wall thickness
Testing technique	**Sound transmission**	Yes	Yes	No	No
	Reflection	No	**Pulse-echo method**	Yes	Yes
	Conduction	Yes	Yes	No	No
	Image projection	Sound-image method	No	No	No

2.1 Resonance Method

2.11 Principle and Revue of Applications

Acoustic resonances of objects are constantly encountered in daily life; every object has its own specific note. This results from the fact that sound waves of definite wave lengths, on being reflected back and forth or circling (rim of a cup) in the object concerned are superimposed exactly in phase, whereas other waves cancel each other. These preferred, so-called resonance frequencies are transmitted also into the air, thus reaching the ear. The accentuation of certain frequencies can readily be observed when singing in the bathroom. The enclosed air space with effectively reflecting walls starts to resonate at certain notes which are amplified.

The resonance method, using audible sound, is therefore probably the oldest of all non-destructive testing methods, being an old established practice, for instance, for detecting the presence of a crack in a ceramic vessel by its ring. For many other purposes this ringing test even today is still used as a non-destructive method. It can be very efficient if electronic methods are used both for excitation of the test piece and analysis of the resonance spectrum [326]. The resonance is influenced both by the material and the shape and dimensions of the test piece, furthermore also by the nature and the point of excitation and the unavoidable mounting of the specimen. All test conditions remaining constant, a change in the properties of the test piece can be detected by comparative measurements. However, a given flaw can produce an appreciable effect only if its dimensions are not too small compared with those of the test piece. For this reason, and also because the resonance pattern does not readily permit deductions concerning position and size of the flaw, this method is used less for flaw detection than thickness measurements or related test problems. Another field of application, viz. determination of the elastic properties of materials, which particularly in the case of transparent glasses and crystals also permit optical determination of the resonance, falls rather outside the actual scope of testing of materials (see also Bergmann [1]).

The basic principles of the resonance thickness measurement can be dealt with briefly because the thickness resonance of a plate has already been discussed repeatedly (1.5 and 1.102). If a thin plate (relative to its size) can oscillate freely on both faces, i.e. because it borders on an acoustically soft medium, it is possible to excite it to resonance in the direction of its thickness, as indicated in Figs. 1.102 and 1.103 by the corresponding particle displacement. Since resonance can also be described as a standing wave, the higher characteristic oscillations can best be indicated by the number of half wave lengths per plate. The fundamental or first characteristic oscillation thus has one half wave length per plate thickness and the n-th characteristic oscillation has n half wave lengths. Expressed as frequencies the n-th characteristic frequency of the plate is n times the fundamental frequency

$$f_n = n f_e \,. \tag{2.1}$$

If one tries to produce thickness oscillations of the plate, by, for instance, exposing it to the radiation of a plane wave in a liquid, resonance occurs only if the frequency of the wave equals one of the characteristic frequencies of the plate. For a given plate, the frequency of the exciting wave must therefore be changed continuously until resonance occurs. If it is certain that this has resulted in the excitation of the first characteristic frequency, i.e. that the frequency f measured is f_e, the thickness of the plate is determined by

$$d = \frac{\lambda}{2} = \frac{1}{2}\frac{c}{f_e} \tag{2.2}$$

where c is the known velocity of sound in the plate.

In general, however, it is by no means certain which of the characteristic oscillations has been excited and the number n is unknown. However, if one proceeds from one resonance point to the next by increasing the exciting frequency, e.g. from f_n to f_{n+1}, (2.1) states that the frequency difference Δf equals the fundamental frequency:

$$\Delta f = f_{n+1} - f_n = f_e \, .$$

The plate thickness is thus obtained by measuring the frequency difference between two successive resonance peaks:

$$d = \frac{c}{2\Delta f} \, . \tag{2.3}$$

This is the principle. Practical application, however, requires a simpler method of excitation than in a liquid bath, and in addition a method

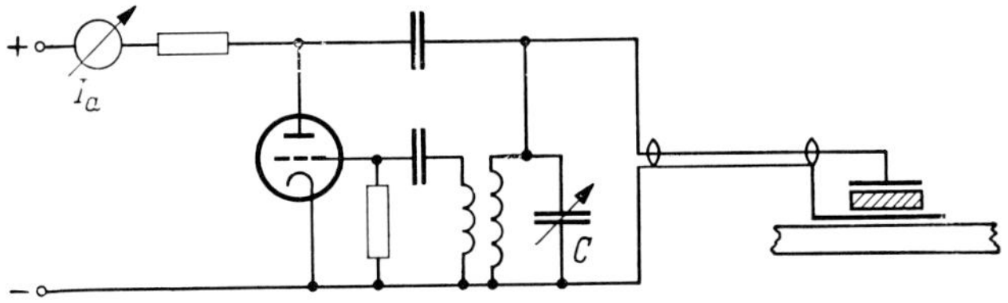

Fig. 2.1 Circuit diagram of a resonance thickness meter.

which indicates the resonance. Both are provided by a piezoelectric transducer fitted with electrodes and mounted in a holder with a damping body at its back, i.e. a *probe* which can be placed directly on the test piece. A shielded cable connects the probe to the instrument which consists essentially of a high-frequency generator with variable frequency. A simplified circuit diagram is shown in Fig. 2.1. The valve oscillates in a feedback circuit and generates a high-frequency voltage whose frequency is determined by the variable capacitor C. The plate current I_a can be read on a measuring instrument.

The piezoelectric transducer is excited below its own characteristic frequency so as to supply an acoustic pressure amplitude of maximum uniformity over the entire frequency range. The transducer should therefore be damped, which usually is achieved by cementing to its back a damping body with sufficiently high sound absorption, to avoid interfering resonance points. A small amount of liquid is used to couple the probe to the test piece.

Transducer and test piece form two coupled systems capable of oscillating, resulting in a resonance of the test plate reacting on the transducer which apparently reduces the load impedance of the resonant circuit. The oscillating test plate draws more energy from the transmitter when in resonance than outside resonance, which increases the plate current indicated by the instrument.

This simple arrangement, however, has the disadvantage that the test plate no longer oscillates unimpeded as assumed in the above derivation. Its resonance frequencies are shifted to higher values, this shift being the greater the closer the coupling, i.e. the smoother the surface and the greater the contact pressure of the probe. The error is the smaller, the higher the harmonic frequency of the test plate being excited; in all resonance methods it is therefore advisable to use the highest possible harmonic so as to be independent of the coupling conditions as much as possible.

For an exact calculation of the resonance frequencies it is no longer possible to consider the transducer and the test plate separately if they are coupled through a thin layer of oil, and the system must be considered as a whole. For this purpose the three elements, viz. transducer, oil film and test plate are represented in the electric equivalent circuit as electric *lines* forming part of the transmitter circuit [68, 152].

If the transducer is not coupled directly to the test plate to be measured but through an intermediate layer, one still obtains resonance peaks of the plate, but in addition resonances of the intermediate layer. With the aid of suitable electronic circuits the two resonances can be separated, as described below for the Vidigage instrument. This permits contactless thickness measurements through a liquid layer, which is important for continuous measurements.

Practical applications of the methods and of certain instruments are discussed in detail in Chapter 3 under Test Problems. Here it need merely be mentioned that this covers primarily wall-thickness measurements, particularly on containers and pipes where only one side of the wall is accessible. However, also flaws of a given test piece which result in the appearance or non-appearance of a thickness resonance or a shift of the resonance point can be detected by this method, e.g. laminations in sheets, corrosion, faulty adhesion in platings or at soldered joints of plates. The residual wall thickness which is of interest in the case of corrosion can, however, be detected by the resonance method only if the wear is uniform and if there is no pitting. In this case the pulse-echo method is more effective.

2.12 Instruments[1]

On the basis of patents granted to ERWIN and RASSWEILER [87], General Motors, USA, built the first resonanc thickness tester in 1947. The Sonigage instrument uses a mains-connected power supply and operates according to the basic diagram shown in Fig. 2.2. The high-

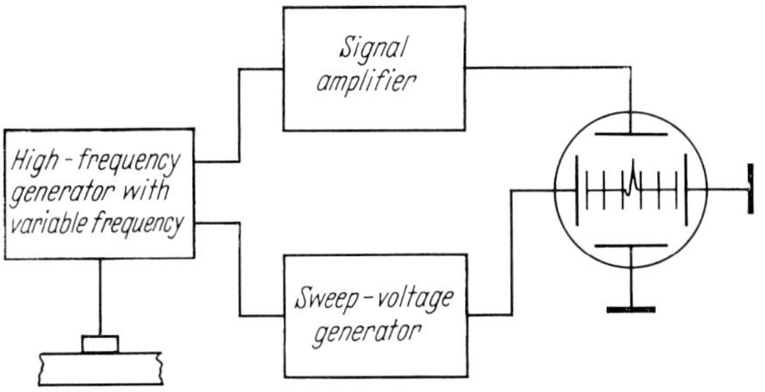

Fig. 2.2 Principle diagram of *Sonigage* resonance thickness tester.

frequency generator changes its frequency automatically over a range of approx. 1 : 2, e.g. from 0.75 to 1.5 MHz. This is achieved by the rotary capacitor shown in Fig. 2.1 being rotated by a motor at high speed. In order to cover also higher frequency ranges, viz. the contiguous octaves 1.5 to 3 and 3 to 6 MHz, the coil of the resonant circuit is changed by switching. This also makes it necessary to change the probe because every crystal has a natural frequency immediately above the frequency range concerned.

The plate current undergoes a rapid change when passing through a resonance point which via a signal amplifier appears as an indicating voltage on a CR tube. Simultaneously, a sweep-voltage generator generates a deflection voltage synchronously with the rotation of the motor. If this is a saw-tooth voltage, i.e. if it increases linearly and proportionally with the transmitter frequency, the horizontal deflection of the luminous spot on the screen of the CR tube is likewise proportional to the frequency. Instead of a frequency scale in front of the viewing screen, which starts on the right at 0.75 MHz and ends on the left at 1.5 MHz, a

[1] Specific instruments are mentioned only where this is of historic interest or if they have properties which are of considerable significance for the method and its application. This implies no specific appraisal of the instrument concerned. A general list of manufacturing firms is found at the end of this section. Any pertinent information is readily obtainable from the manufacturers.

scale calibrated directly in thickness values can be attached which has been calculated for a definite velocity. For steel with $c_l \sim 6 \cdot 10^3$ m/s the two scales are shown one above the other in Fig. 2.3. The measuring range thus covers the first resonance frequencies of plates 2 to 4 mm thick. If it is certain that a given peak shown on the screen indicates the position of the first characteristic oscillation, the thickness can be read directly. This is the case if for instance the approximate thickness is already known.

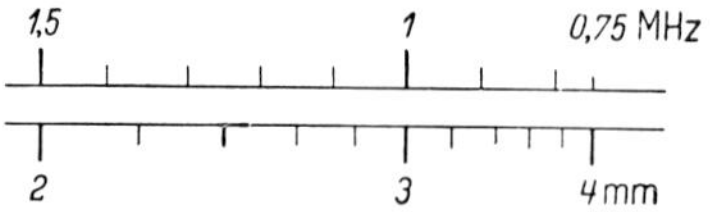

Fig. 2.3 Frequency scale and correlated thickness scale corresponding to an acoustic velocity of $6 \cdot 10^3$ m/s (e.g. steel or aluminium), calculated for the first characteristic oscillation according to Eq. (2.2).

If this is not the case additional resonance peaks are taken into consideration. Fig. 2.4 shows the screen traces at three different frequency ranges: 0.75 to 1.5 MHz, 1.5 to 3 MHz, and 3 to 6 MHz.

Since the ratios of the resonance frequencies are as 1 : 2 : 3, etc., the correlated resonance thicknesses are as 1 : 1/2 : 1/3, etc. In Fig. 24 peaks appear at

3.6; 1.8; 1.2; 0.9; 0.72; 0.6; 0.51 mm, etc., which corresponds to the 1st, 2nd, 3rd, 4th, 5th, 6th, 7th characteristic oscillation.

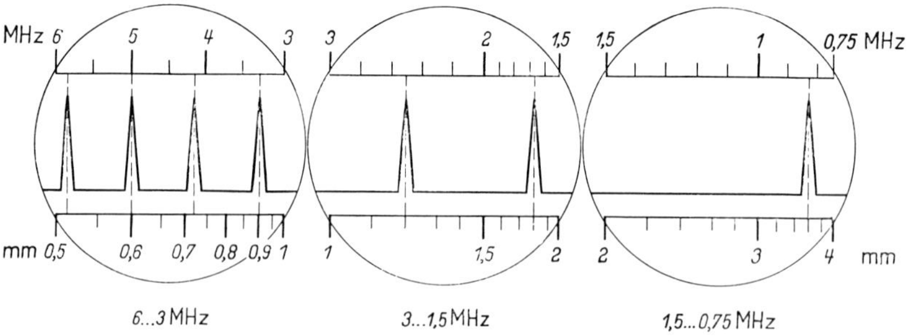

Fig. 2.4 Screen images at different frequency ranges with resonance readings of a steel plate 3.6 mm thick, at the 1st to 7th characteristic oscillation.

The true thickness is determined by the following simple rule: take two arbitrary peaks on the same or also on different ranges, with the thickness readings x and y. Between these readings let there be n gaps. The required thickness is then

$$d = \frac{n\,x\,y}{x - y} .$$

In the example shown two peaks appear on the centre measuring range with the thicknesses 1.8 and 1.2 mm. These are separated by one gap $n = 1$, therefore

$$d = \frac{1.8 \cdot 1.2}{1.8 - 1.2} = 3.6 \text{ mm} .$$

In general, these instruments therefore require the additional use of a slide rule which is unnecessary in the case of more modern instruments.

Messrs. Branson Instruments Inc., Stamford, Conn., USA, manufacture an instrument with visible indication, viz. the mains-operated *Vidigage,* and a portable instrument for battery operation with indicating instrument and headphones, viz. the *Audigage.*

The large scales of the Vidigage, 42 and 26 cm long, respectively, and the bright trace, facilitate reading even from some distance. Fig. 2.5 shows model 14 in operation while making a measurement of 4.2 mm steel.

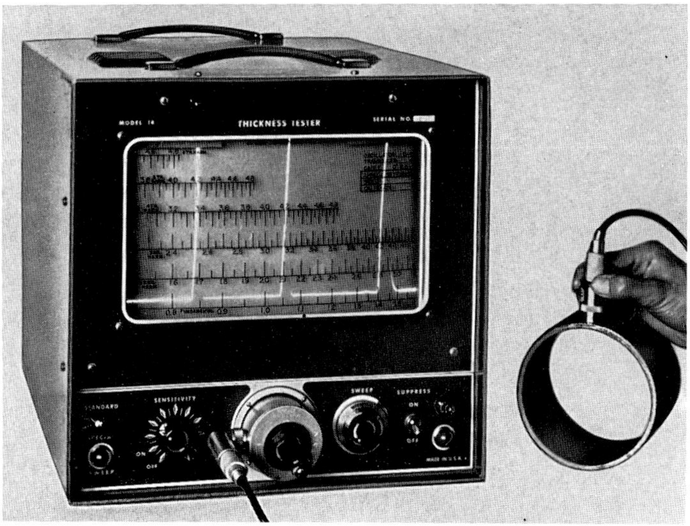

Fig. 2.5 *Vidigage,* model 14 (Branson), showing the wall thickness measurement of 4.2 mm steel.

The CR tube has a magnetic deflection system. The frequency change is no longer achieved mechanically by a motor but without mechanical motion by an electrically variable inductance of the resonant circuit. Depending on the model, the frequency band is swept 50 to 300 times per second, synchronously with the horizontal deflection of the luminous spot. The oscillator unit which determines the frequency range is exchanged whenever the range has to be changed; it is designed as a plug-in unit. It is connected to the probe by a high-frequency cable whose length at the same time determines the frequency, i.e. it cannot be chosen arbitrarily. To make it possible in spite of this to operate at very much greater distances from the instrument, the oscillator unit with the attached probe can be connected to the instrument by a long, multicore cable which carries no high frequency and whose length is therefore not critical. Such cables are available in lengths up to 300 m.

The peaks on the screen abscissa extend over the entire viewing screen, thus making it possible to read on several superimposed scales. To facilitate the reading, the rising edge is made particularly bright and is almost normal to the scales. At excessive gain interfering indications appear on the luminous screen in addition to the true resonance indications; the former can be suppressed in favour of the latter by using an amplifier with adjustable threshold.

Every oscillator unit is provided with certain probes which are readily distinguished by their colour code, and similarly distinguishable,

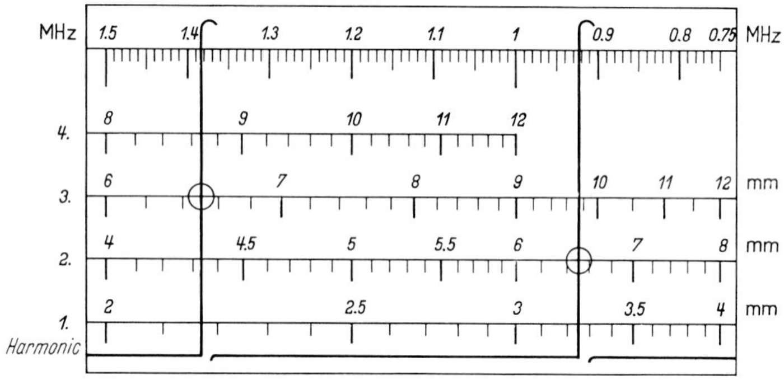

Fig. 2.6 Simplified scale of Vidigage for frequency range 0.75 to 1.5 MHz, with the 1st to 4th harmonic, resonance reading of a thickness of 6.5 mm at the 2nd and 3rd harmonic.

exchangeable scales. They comprise primarily a thickness scale for measurements with the first resonance (fundamental oscillation, Fig. 2.6). With the aid of calibration plates of known thickness the instrument is calibrated prior to the measurement at both ends of the scale by adjusting the single peak which should appear at the first resonance to the correct positions by expanding and shifting the entire screen picture. In subsequent measurements of unknown thicknesses by means of the first resonance only, the approximate thickness should, however, be known. A single peak may also indicate the second resonance point, a fact which is not readily recognizable because the thickness scale covers a ratio of only 1 : 2. Example (Fig. 2.6): A reading at 2.5 mm on the scale of the first resonance frequency may also be the second resonance of a thickness of 5 mm whose first resonance peak remains invisible on the 2 to 4 mm measuring scale because it falls outside of it on the right.

The universal scales of the Vidigage, which have several additional divisions for higher harmonics (Fig. 2.6), also permit the use of higher resonance peaks, without involving calculations. The thickness corresponding to the first peak from the left is read on the top scale (in Fig. 2.6, the division for the fourth harmonic) and one then checks whether the next peak gives the same value on the next lower scale. Should this be the case, the test confirms that the first peak in fact belongs to the top scale, i.e. in this case to the fourth harmonic, and that the reading gives the correct value.

Fig. 2.6 shows the position of two peaks. The one on the left indicates on the top scale (4th harmonic) a thickness of just under 8.7 mm, and the one on the right, on the next lower scale (3), 9.8 mm. The correlation is therefore wrong. Now the reading of the left indication on the third scale is taken which gives 6.5 mm; this is in agreement with the right indication on the second scale. The correlation is correct, the left indication belongs to the 3rd harmonic, the right to the 2nd. The correct reading points are marked in Fig. 2.6 by circles. With a little practice the correct value can therefore be determined reliably with several readings requiring no calculations. If there is only one peak, a different frequency range must be chosen if the thickness is completely unknown.

Since the scales must be calibrated for definite probes, one can also make approximate allowance for the frequency shift of the lower characteristic oscillations which results from the reaction of the probe. In contrast to Fig. 2.6 the multiples of a given thickness, e.g. on the righthand edge 12, 8 and 4 mm, are not aligned exactly one above the other, but the lower multiples are shifted towards the left, i.e. to higher frequencies. In the case of very close coupling, viz. on flat and very smooth surfaces, particularly in the case of materials with low acoustic impedance such as aluminium, the frequency shift may in reality become still greater than allowed for by the scale calibrated for average coupling conditions. In such cases the coupling should therefore be made less close by inserting spacer rings or thin plastic foils.

Both Vidigage models are supplied together with oscillator units of 0.75 to above 20 MHz and with separate scales according to range and material. Very high accuracy can be achieved if the instrument is calibrated immediately prior to use and if the reading is made at the calibrated points of the scale. Otherwise an error of 1 to 2% must be expected. This error may be greater near the ends of the scale.

For wall thickness measurements and coupling by means of an intermediate liquid layer, the instrument operates as follows. The transit time in the intermediate layer should be much longer than in the wall. The resonance points corresponding to the intermediate layer are then crowded together very closely on the viewing screen and would normally completely blot out the few simultaneously indicated resonance peaks resulting from the wall thickness. However, at these points energy is withdrawn over a small range by the resonance of the wall from the resonance of the intermediate layer, so that dents appear in the dense resonance spectrum. By exploiting the shortcoming of an amplifier, viz. jamming in the region of very densely packed resonance peaks, the indication is reversed; the dense resonance band becomes invisible but the dents in it appear as positive, sharp peaks, as in the old contact method [225, 132].

An auxiliary instrument, viz. the *automation converter*, is used for automating the operation which in a pre-selected range announces an indication by means of a signal and which in addition supplies a voltage for actuating a recorder. This voltage is proportional to the shift of the indication from the beginning of the selected range of the gate. This permits very accurate recording of thickness changes over a small range of the full scale.

The Vidigage model, with its relatively large size and weight, is intended primarily for stationary operation with mains connection; on the other hand the Audigage instrument with battery operation is a portable instrument for measurements on site. It has only a single frequency range, e.g. 0.65 to 2 MHz, for wall thicknesses above 1.5 mm.

The Audigage obtains its frequency changes by means of a rotary capacitor which is slowly turned by hand until a measuring instrument indicates resonance. Simultaneously with the resonance indication an audible signal can be placed on a headphone. This is achieved by an improvement of the simple circuit shown in Fig. 2.1 [53, 54]: An auxiliary audio oscillator modulates the frequency of the resonant circuit. The adjusted frequency therefore changes constantly around its mean value in the rhythm of the audio frequency. Thus, at a resonance point the plate current fluctuates likewise, and this is indicated both in the headphone and on a measuring instrument. If the resonance point is approached, the audible note first merely increases in intensity but then doubles its frequency if set exactly to the resonance frequency, and vice versa if the rotary capacitor is turned further.

Model 6 of the Audigage measures from 2.2 to 125 mm with an accuracy of 3 to 5%.

In the case of the "Sonizon" instrument of Magnaflux Corporation, Chicago, USA, a small glow lamp is connected firmly to the shaft of the motor-driven rotary capacitor, the lamp moving in a circle while the motor rotates. At the resonance points the change in plate current is used for passing a voltage pulse to the glow lamp. The latter therefore lights up periodically along its circular path at all clear resonance points, which can be observed on the dial of the instrument, resulting in the resonance frequencies being marked on a scale.

The accuracy is stated to be 1 to 2%. The measuring range extends from 0.6 to 150 mm and is subdivided into three switchable ranges with three different probes.

In addition to Messrs. Branson Instruments, Messrs. Dawe Instruments Ltd., London, also manufacture resonance wall thickness testers similar in design to the Branson instruments. Furthermore, SOKOLOV [22] mentions some instruments of Russian manufacture in his book without, however, giving details.

2.2 Intensity Method

2.21 Principle, Classification and Distinction from Transit Time Methods

The intensity method in which the intensity of the ultra-sound is measured after it has passed through the test piece, is the oldest application of ultrasonic waves for non-destructive testing. It dates back to 1930 and was originated by SOKOLOV and MÜHLHÄUSER [338, 270]. The

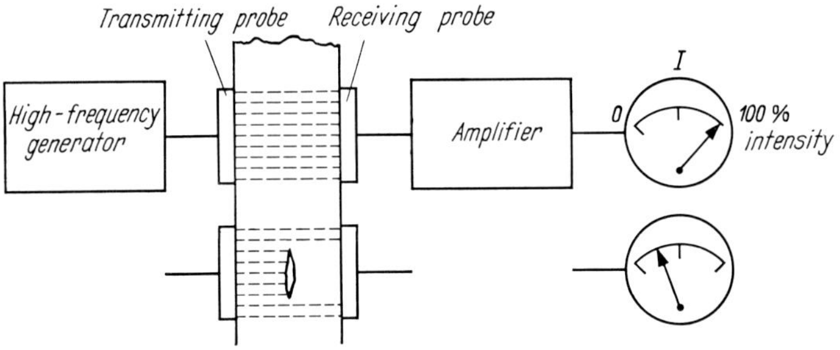

Fig. 2.7 Intensity method with sound transmission.

principle is shown in Fig. 2.7 in which the intensity method (abbreviated I-method) is portrayed schematically by passing sound through a test plate, at a flawless and alternately at a defective point.

The voltage produced by a high-frequency generator excites the transmitting probe to ultrasonic oscillations which are propagated in the coupled test piece. A second probe positioned coaxially on the opposite side receives a portion of the radiated wave and transmits to the input of an amplifier a high-frequency voltage which is proportional to the sound pressure at the contact point of the receiver. The amplified voltage is read on an indicating instrument. At the flawed point the propagation of the ultrasonic wave is impeded by the discontinuity in the material, resulting in reduced sound pressure at the receiver and thus a lower reading on the measuring instrument.

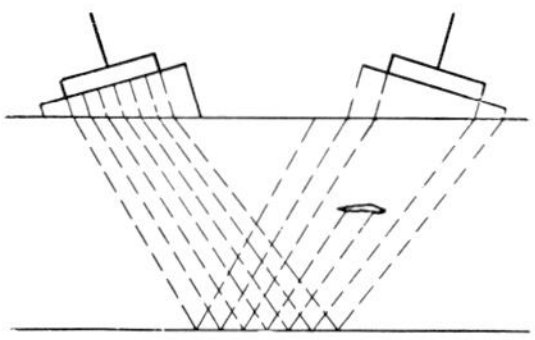

Fig. 2.8 I-reflection method.

Strictly speaking, therefore, this measures not the intensity but primarily the amplitude of the sound pressure if a piezoelectric receiver is used. Provided the characteristics of both the amplifier and the instruments are linear, the indication in this case is therefore proportional to the square root of the intensity. The designation *intensity method* will nevertheless be retained because it is not absolutely necessary to use piezoelectric receivers and because the indication is frequently squared electrically so that it is nevertheless proportional to the intensity, and because common usage has long established the designation "intensity" instead of "amplitude" in this connection. The real reason may be that the (genuine) intensity method using irradiation by X-rays or γ-rays and detection by means of films or counting tubes, has been applied to the ultrasonic method.

A warning is sounded here, particularly for the reader who is less familiar with physics, not to equate the schematic presentations of the ray paths indicated in Fig. 2.7 and many of the later diagrams, with the actual propagation of ultrasonic waves. As discussed in 1.7 and 1.8, this presentation of the rays based on geometric-optical concepts of *light* and *shadows* is only valid in the extreme case of wave lengths which are very short compared with the dimensions of the probes and the flaws, i.e. conditions which are usually not fulfilled in practice or if so, only with rough approximation. Unfortunately, wave physics does not lend itself readily to schematic presentation in the form of drawings.

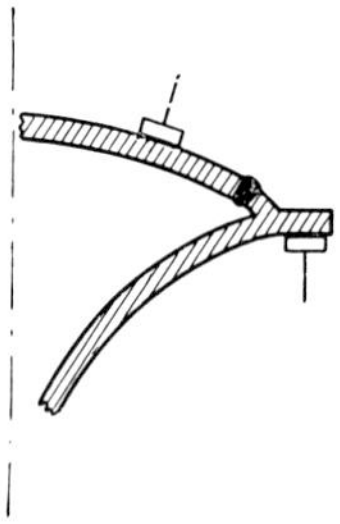

Fig. 2.9 I-conductance method.

The I-method can be applied in practice to four different testing techniques which are indicated schematically in Figs. 2.7 to 2.10, viz.: 1. sound transmission, 2. reflection, 3. conduction and 4. image projection (see 2.0).

Reflection occurs, if due to a directional radiation and receiving characteristic, a definite beam is reflected at the boundaries of the test piece. In the case of conduction, however, the ultrasonic energy fed at a given point is propagated in the test piece by arbitrary wave forms without it being possible to indicate a definite beam path preferred by the transmission. The two cases can also be referred to as quasi-optical and wave-physical propagation respectively. The criterion is the ratio of wave length to the smallest dimension of the test piece. As an example Fig. 2.9 shows schematically the testing of a welded seam in the cover of a conical valve, i.e. a complicated cross-section with thin walls. There is a gradual transition from one to the other of the three methods mentioned.

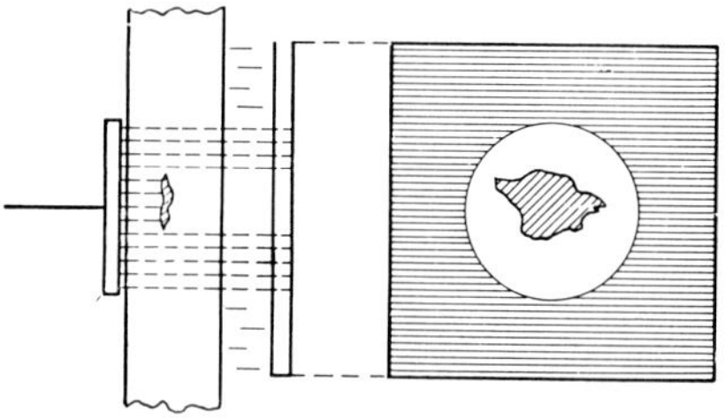

Fig. 2.10 I-projection method.

In the simplest case an image projection can be produced by the shadow of the flaw, whereby an *image converter* converts the intensity into visible light. An improved design uses acusto-optical image projection methods with lenses or mirrors. Because of the slight practical importance of the image projection methods they will be discussed only very briefly in the next Section when describing the instruments, and for further details the description by BERGMANN [1, pp. 325 and 754 et seq.] should be consulted.

As long as they use continuous ultra-sound of a given frequency, a considerable difficulty in all intensity methods arises from interference by standing waves: the sound pressure at a point of reception is not determined exclusively by the wave along the desired, usually shortest, path from transmitter to receiver and the effect of a flaw along this path; it also contains an interference factor which, depending on the phase, produces a higher or lower sound pressure due to interference. Usually only a very small portion of the direct wave is absorbed by the receiver while the rest is reflected back and forth repeatedly so that it fills the entire test piece and sets up a steric field of standing waves.

The standing wave in a plate as already discussed represents only the special case of a plane wave entering at right angles, which is realized approximately if the radiating face of a probe is much greater than the thickness of the plate.

The steric position of a given node or antinode depends on the difference in path length of the various transmitted waves, i.e. on the frequency of the wave and the dimensions of the test piece. If one of the two influencing factors changes, the interference field is shifted. When making comparative tests on different test pieces, great differences in intensity are therefore observed even if the form and dimension or the test frequency differ only slightly.

This is remedied by frequency wobbling, i.e. rapid periodic or aperiodic frequency modulation over a sufficiently wide range about the fundamental frequency. The required width of the range can be estimated as follows: Let the shortest possible path difference between two waves arriving at the test point be n wave lengths, e.g. double the plate thickness with perpendicular sound transmission through the plate. The interference maxima and minima can be averaged only if the path difference of the two waves for the lowest frequency differs by at least 1/2 wave length from that of the highest frequency, i.e. if the ratio of the two frequencies is n to $n + 1/2$. Therefore, the frequency must be changed by at least $1/2n$. For $n = 100$ wave lengths (e.g. for a 6 mm wave length, i.e. approx. 1 MHz in steel, plate thickness $6 \cdot 50 = 300$ mm), 0.5% frequency modulation is sufficient. For thin test pieces this value can become so great that it is practically not realisable especially also because the radiation of the transmitter and the frequency sensitivity of the receiver over the entire range should remain as constant as possible. Therefore, it appears to be preferable to use higher frequencies with thin test pieces.

Disturbances by interference can be avoided completely if the waves arriving at the receiver are separated according to their transit time, which is possible for instance if one uses pulse excitation of the transmitter instead of continuous excitation. These transit time methods will be discussed in the following Sections. In these methods the intensity is measured in addition to the transit time, e.g. on the screen of a CR tube as shown in Fig. 2.11, which anticipates the schematic presentation of the method as compared with Fig. 2.7. These methods are therefore

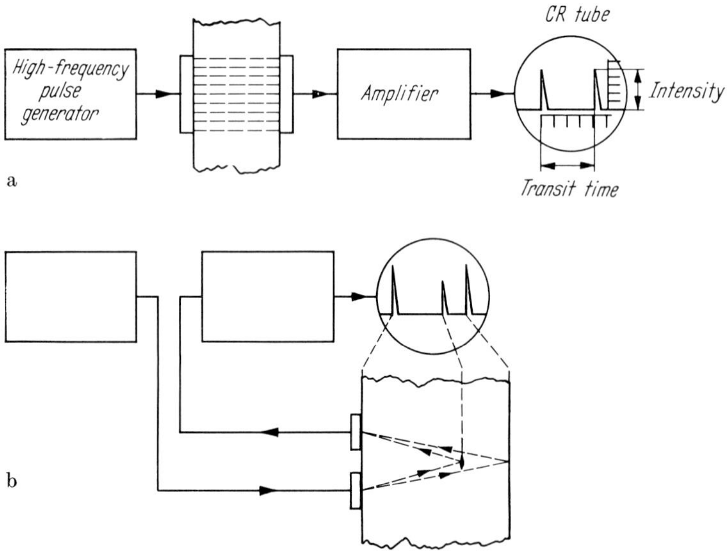

Fig. 2.11 IT-method (intensity transit time or pulse transit time). a) with sound transmission, b) with reflection.

called intensity transit time methods which, in contrast to many other presentations, thus do not differ basically from the simple I-method, but merely include and perfect it.

The frequently found subdivision into sound transmission and reflection, or echo methods, in no way characterizes the difference because these specific techniques, viz. sound transmission, reflection, conduction and image projection, are possible for each of these methods, for both the I-method and the IT-method (IT = intensity transit time method). To make this clear, Fig. 2.11 shows the first two techniques for the IT-method.

Even where the transit time as such is of no interest, as is for instance generally the case for pulse transmission according to Fig. 2.11a, the separation of the signals received according to transit times has the advantage over the simple I-method in that the disturbances through interference are eliminated completely.

Let us now return to the four testing techniques of the I-method. In the first three, viz. sound transmission, reflection and conduction, a measuring instrument is used for indication, which for a flawless test piece is adjusted to an initial value of, say, 100% by adjusting the transmitter voltage and the gain. In the image projection method the shadow, or an ultrasonic-optical image projection in the field of vision of an extended source of ultra-sound, is used for indication in the form of a visible image which may rely on differences in brightness or colour. The initial brightness or colour then corresponds to the undisturbed intensity. If then, according to the description in 1.8 and particularly the presentation of Fig. 1.92 for a given minimum flaw size and flaw position, a reduction of the measured value by a given amount, e.g. 10%, can be expected, the sum of all other influences on the measured value must be kept considerably below this reduction. Assuming satisfactory stability of tne electrical equipment, the relative position of the probes must be kept meticulously constant by a reliable mechanical mount. The only factor which may still vary then is the coupling between probes and test piece.

Coupling during testing is of maximum uniformity with an interconnected liquid layer (large compared with the wave length), e.g. immersed in a liquid (immersion technique). The image-projection methods therefore use exclusively the immersion technique. Direct contact through only a thin liquid layer between transducer and test piece is not recommended because, should their acoustic impedances be high, even slight thickness changes of the liquid layer result in large fluctuations of the transmittance (see also 1.5 and Fig. 1.7). The same difficulty arises when coupling through a sonically hard adaptor, e.g. to reduce wear. For this purpose a material whose acoustic impedance is as close as possible to that of the liquid, should be used, e.g. plastics (perspex or polystyrene) or rubber. The transducer is firmly coupled to the adaptor, e.g. by pressure or cementing.

Even with this type of coupling when using the measuring instrument method, a fluctuation of at least 10% from one test to the other in the measurement of amplitude must be expected, i.e. approx. 20% in intensity. Therefore, only considerably greater readings can be evaluated. These usable deflections can be intensified by means of a non-linear characteristic of the amplifier or of the instrument, and they can be *sifted out*, or evaluated directly by means of a relay in the form of a go/no-go indication.

The main application of the I-method, even after development of the more versatile IT-method, is the testing of plate-like or dished test pieces accessible from both sides and where the flaws are laminary and parallel to the surface. These are principally sheet metals of any given thickness containing laminations, short tubular bodies such as bearing boxes, laminated plastics and platings. In this case mainly straight transmission of sound is used, occasionally also reflection or conduction, where in the latter case the test piece need be accessible from one side only and the flaw does not necessarily have to be laminar and parallel to the surfaces in order to disturb the conduction. Example: thin sheets containing inclusions with banded structure, test by plate-wave conduction.

Of interest from the point of view of historic development is the fact that SOKOLOV, as well as CZERLINSKY had already tried to avoid the disadvantages of the simple I-method by using a transit time method: SOKOLOV used a frequency modulation method [342] and CZERLINSKY a pulse-transit time method with sound transmission [71].

2.22 Instruments for Intensity Measurements

In the experimental, non-destructive tests according to the intensity method carried out by SOKOLOV [340, 342], SCHRAIBER [333], KRUSE [209, 210], GÖTZ [118] on sheet metal, by MEYER and BOCK [259] on concrete beams, also by CZERLINSKY on bearings of metal and moulded laminates [70] and on sheets of plywood [71], measuring devices assembled in the laboratory were used. The high-frequency generators, in principle according to the circuit of Fig. 2.1 for voltages of up to a few 100 volts on

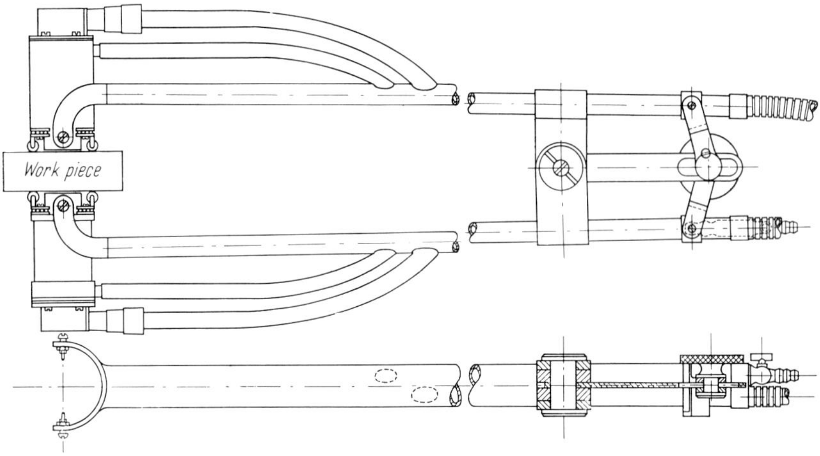

Fig. 2.12 Ultrasonic testing tongs according to TROST.

the quartz plate, were equipped in part with mechanical frequency modulation devices (rotating auxiliary variable capacitors) and in part also with electronic devices (e.g. noise modulation [70], i.e. completely aperiodic). Quartz plates were used in the probes. The multi-stage high-frequency amplifiers with subsequent rectification and measuring instrument showed no special features in their circuits compared with normal electronic circuits. To avoid direct transmission of high frequency from the transmitter to the amplifier by radiation or conduction, transmitter and amplifier were housed in separate cases effectively shielded from each other.

Laboratory-type measuring equipment was used also for the first practical tests on boiler plates to check for lamination, carried out by Messrs. AEG and Borsig, Berlin, during the first war years.

A useful advance in the mounting and control of the probe were the ultrasonic tongs (Fig. 2.12) suggested by Trost [367] and constructed by Messrs. Dr. Claren, Düsseldorf. It eliminates the water bath in the testing of sheet metal by using for coupling a flow of water which enters a cylindrical ante-chamber between sound transmitter (or receiver) and test sheet. On the side of the chamber open towards the sheet, the water flows through a relatively narrow gap kept constant by spacing rollers. The two probes are held in elongated mounts forming spring-loaded tongs which are slipped by hand over the test sheet. Once all air has escaped, one achieves very satisfactory and uniform coupling which, in a similar construction, is still used to-day for non-destructive testing, also with the pulse-echo method.

Instruments for the I-method were brought into mass production only after the war, first by Messrs. ACEC, Charleroi, Belgium, under the trade name *Ultrasonel.* The probes showed a marked improvement of the coupling on rough and curved surfaces when using a rubber cup filled with liquid and mounted in front of the transducer. When pressed on it adapts itself readily to the shape of the surface [150] (*palpeur turgescent*). A further interesting suggestion for improving the coupling, made by the same firm, is the *palpeur pneu* in which one or several fixed transmitters or receivers are mounted inside a closed rubber tyre which rolls over the test piece in a continuous test (Fig. 3.13). The probes are pressed against the walls by springs. Since the tyre is partially filled with liquid, acoustic contact is established through the filling liquid, the thin wall of the tyre, and a further liquid film between tyre and test piece.

At present the only instrument in production is the *Sonometer* of Messrs. Dr. Lehfeldt & Co., Heppenheim, Germany (Fig. 2.13). The high-frequency generator and amplifier are well-shielded from each other and are housed in one case. The instrument is available for one of the frequencies of approx. 0.1, 3 and 8 MHz, wobbled approximately 5% in the rhythm of the mains frequency. The probes are fitted with interchangeable contact tips shaped according to the specific purpose of the application. Instead of reading over the entire intensity range from 0 to 100%, the indications of the instrument can also be limited to a small zone of the total range by non-linear rectification. A relay is connected in parallel to it which displays a signal if less than one half the normal reading is obtained; thus it can be used as a convenient go/no-go gauge without the operator being distracted by minor coupling fluctuations.

The devices for testing thin sheet and heavy plate [46, 187] by means of an intensity method are described in Chapter 3 when the relevant test problems are discussed. This also applies to testing equipment for automobile tyres [268, 269, 220].

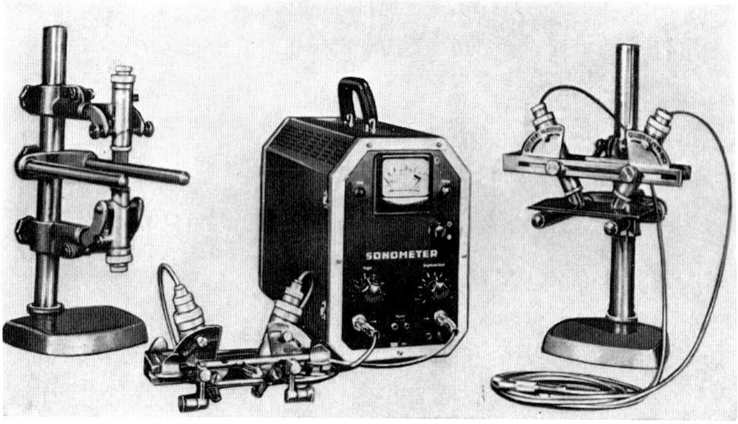

Fig. 2.13 *Sonometer* of Messrs. Dr. Lehfeldt & Co., Heppenheim, with three holding devices for probes.

2.23 Instruments for Sound Image Methods

In the instruments for ultrasonic-optical image projection the ray path of a projector is simulated for illuminating the test piece and producing an image. The source of light with condenser lens is, however, replaced by large, flat acoustic radiators, e.g. quartz plates of up to 60 mm in diameter, or quartz mosaics of up to 200 mm. The field of vision is partially enlarged still further by sound lenses so as to produce a complete picture also of large test pieces. From the test piece illuminated in this way a sound lens usually produces a reduced picture on the *image converter* which converts the intensity of the ultra-sound directly or indirectly into a visible image. Compared with the simple silhouette projection of Fig. 2.10 this image projection offers various advantages: the image is obtained at a readily accessible point at greater distance from the test piece; in the case of thick test pieces different planes can be focused on the image converter by shifting the lens, and the attainable resolution and detectability of small flaws is improved.

The first practical image converter was Pohlmann's cell [288, 289]. It consists of a chamber filled with liquid and placed in the beam path of the projector. Minute aluminium flakes small compared with the wave length are suspended in the liquid. If exposed to an ultrasonic wave, forces act on the flakes, and try to position them at right angles to the direction of sound propagation. Incidentally, the same effect is used for the absolute measurement of sound intensities in liquids and gases in the form of a *Rayleigh disc* suspended from a thread. The directive force of the sound wave is counteracted in the small discs suspended in the cell by the irregular Brownian molecular movement, so that within a range of the sound intensity of approximately 1 : 10 the minute discs are lined up more uniformly with greater intensity. If the cell is viewed from a direction opposite to that of the sound and if the suspension is illuminated by a beam of light, the points of greater intensity appear brighter because the lined-up small discs reflect more light.

An instrument equipped with this cell, viz. the *Schallsichtgerät*, had already been used earlier than 1945, for routine tests, e.g. in a special, large construction with a field of vision of 500 mm in diameter, for transmission testing of armour plate. After 1945, Messrs. Dr. Lehfeldt & Co., Heppenheim, constructed a smaller model with a diameter of 100 mm. Although in laboratory tests on plane-parallel aluminium plates, holes perpendicular to the direction of sound and with diameters smaller than the wave length could still be mapped at 4 MHz, the instrument found no further application in practice. Apparently the limited applicability to plate-shaped test pieces, a certain inertia of the cell, and the limited contrast are the reasons why the basically very promising method, in its present design, is not yet able to meet the requirements of practical non-destructive testing.

The same applies to the relief method used by Schuster [327] who designed an instrument at Messrs. VEB Jenoptik, Jena. The idea of the relief method was originated by Sokolov [339]. An ultrasonic image of the test piece immersed in a liquid is produced by a lens and is projected from the bottom by a plane mirror on to the surface of the liquid. At the points of high ultrasonic energy the surface of the liquid appears ruffled which, if kept free of external vibrations and illuminated correctly, makes it possible to recognise the image. The instrument has been constructed for testing large sheet panels but has not yet found practical application.

In the same year as Pohlmann's cell (1937) became known, Sokolov [341, 342] made the suggestion that the ultrasonic image of the test piece be scanned electronically and projected on the screen of a CR tube. The mechanical scanning of the test piece by means of a pencil-like ultrasonic beam, e.g. by moving the test piece back and forth horizontally with line-spacing between the fixed transmitter and receiver and subsequent modulation of a light source proportional to the measured intensity, is technically unsatisfactory because of the time required; except for a few instruments it has therefore found no wider use. On the other hand, electronic scanning involves practically no delay, as in the case of television scanning from which this principle has been borrowed. The image receiver is a quartz plate of the same diameter as the image (Fig. 2.14). In accordance with the intensity of the incident ultrasonic

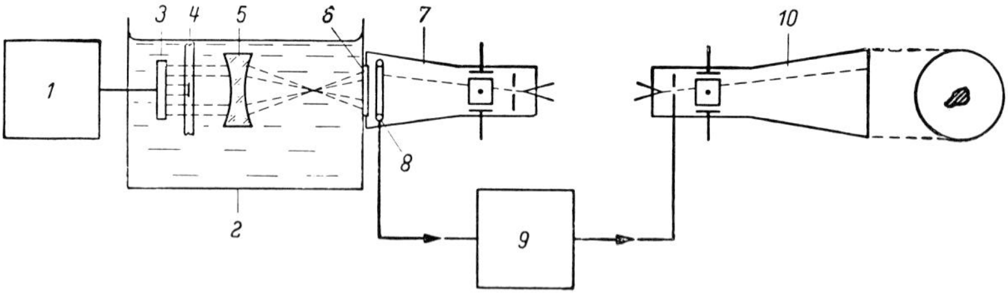

Fig. 2.14 Schematic diagram of an electronic image converter.
1 High-frequency generator, *2* water tank, *3* transmitting quartz plate, *4* test piece, *5* ultrasonic lens, *6* receiving quartz plate, *7* scanning tube, *8* collector, *9* amplifier, *10* picture tube.

wave which changes from point to point, piezoelectric charges appear on the quartz plate which cannot be discharged from the unmetallized surface. The plate forms the sealing window of an electronbeam scanning tube. The back of the plate is scanned line by line by means of a conventional scanning system and the resultant emission of secondary electrons is modulated by the charges of the plate. The electron current flowing to a collector is thus modulated by the image pattern. Amplification and transmission to a picture tube with synchronous deflection according to line change and image change correspond exactly to the methods used in television.

The first suggestion by Sokolov concerned a simple skiagraphic scanning device. Later publications of an instrument with ultrasonic optics called this device an *ultrasonic microscope* because it permits also enlarged reproduction. Instruments working on this principle have been constructed in the USSR and by VEB Jenoptik, Jena [109].

The Jena instrument uses a transmitting quartz of 60 mm dia. at 4 MHz, the picture frequency is 50, the number of lines 200 per second. It can therefore also be used for observing movements which can be filmed, e.g. for medical applications.

According to a further suggestion by Sokolov [343] the back of the receiving quartz plate is coated with a photoelectric cathode whose emission of photons on uniform illumination is influenced by the piezoelectric charges of the image produced under it. By means of post acceleration and electron-optical projection the electrons produce a visible image on the viewing screen in the same tube.

Compared with the scanning method, this method has the advantage that the image is produced strictly simultaneously at all points. In combination with a pulse-transit time method it is therefore possible to filter out a definite transit time in order to eliminate interfering reflections which otherwise would cause great difficulties (see also [22], and which also gives further data on image projection instruments manufactured in Russia). It is, however, not known whether an instrument has already been built according to this suggestion nor whether satisfactory results have been obtained.

There are a number of other possibilities for an image converter, viz. the chemical action on certain substances of ultra-sound which produces a colour change, the thermal action on heat-sensitive dyes, the blackening effect on photographic films, the extinction effect on excited phosphorescent screens, etc. All of them have the disadvantage of high inertia and high energy requirement. Their practical application to non-destructive testing at present appear to hold little promise. For further details see Bergmann [1] and Matauschek [13].

2.3 Pulse Transit Time Method

2.31 History and Principles

Of the methods which use both intensity and transit time, the pulse transit time method is the oldest. As an echo instrument it has been this since the first world war for locating objects under water. A suggestion by Richardson to locate icebergs at some distance by this method found practical realisation through Langevin in locating ships, particularly submarines. In peace time it was used in the form of Behm's depth sounder for measuring depths at sea, but only during the second world war was it applied to non-destructive testing.

In the meantime, however, the method had been applied to electromagnetic waves (short and ultra short waves) in air, first for sounding the ionosphere and later in radar technology for locating aeroplanes and ships.

Firestone [102, 105, 107] in 1940 was the first to recognise the importance of the pulse-echo method for non-destructive testing, particularly for the location of flaws. Earlier, Hiedemann et al. [142] had already used ultrasonic pulses for determining the velocity of sound on the basis of the transit time, but in a pure transit-time method, the so-called *sing-around* method described in 2.4. Sokolov [342] in 1941 was the first to publish another intensity-transit time method, the frequency modulation method, for non-destructive testing.

Although basically each of the four testing techniques can be applied to the pulse-transit time method, the second, viz. the reflection technique, was the only one to gain dominance in the form of the pulse-echo method. (The first two methods are shown schematically in Fig. 2.11.) In the other methods the transit time of the pulses provides no additional information on the flaw; however, by taking the transit time into account the disturbances caused by undesirable waves in the case of the simple I-method can be avoided. Instruments designed for an intensity-transit time method can of course always be used for separate application of either the intensity or the transit time method by disregarding the one or the other.

Fig. 2.11b shows the principle of the pulse-echo method: the sound pulse coming from the transmitter is radiated in a beam and encounters a flaw in its path. If this flaw is smaller than the cross-section of the sound beam, part of the beam by-passes the flaw and strikes the backwall. The flaw in turn transmits an echo wave which, depending on its form and size, is more or less specifically directed, of which a portion reaches the receiver. Receiver and transmitter need not necessarily be separate probes placed at different points on the test piece but can be combined in a single probe (Fig. 2.15). The echo wave coming from the flaw is indicated according to its transit time from the transmitter to the flaw and to the receiver. Later the wave reflected from the back, i.e. the back echo or bottom echo, arrives after a correspondingly longer delay. Both echoes are indicated according to their intensity, or rather amplitude, which is referred to as *echo height* because of their usual presentation as peaks above a horizontal zero line.

The transit time gives the distance to the flaw. Example: in steel with velocity of sound $c =$ approx. $6 \cdot 10^6$ mm/s, the pulse travels in a time $t = 1$ μs (microsecond) the distance $s = ct = 6$ mm. The flaw distance a is half of this, $a = 3$ mm. The delay scale can also be calibrated in flaw distances instead of μs, but this would apply only to a definite velocity of sound, i.e. for a definite material and definite wave mode.

According to Fig. 1.8 the height of the echo is determined by the size of the flaw but in addition is influenced by the position and form of the flaw and the instrument characteristics.

The advantage of this method as compared with the intensity-transmission method is made clear by the following example. If, in the latter method, a flaw within the sound beam reflects 5% of the total energy, the indication of the receiver decreases from 100% to 95% if it covers the entire sound beam. Usually, however, this decrease cannot be evaluated as flaw indication because the usual coupling variations and other disturbances by interference alone can produce much greater deviations if different test points are compared. 5% of the transmitted energy returned as echo can, however, readily be detected when compared with

0% from a flawless zone, and indeed a much lower energy because the echo can, within certain limits, be amplified considerably.

According to 1.8, such a simple division of reflected and transmitted energies is of course not permissible because size, shape and position of the flaw, as well as the characteristics of the probe, greatly affect the result.

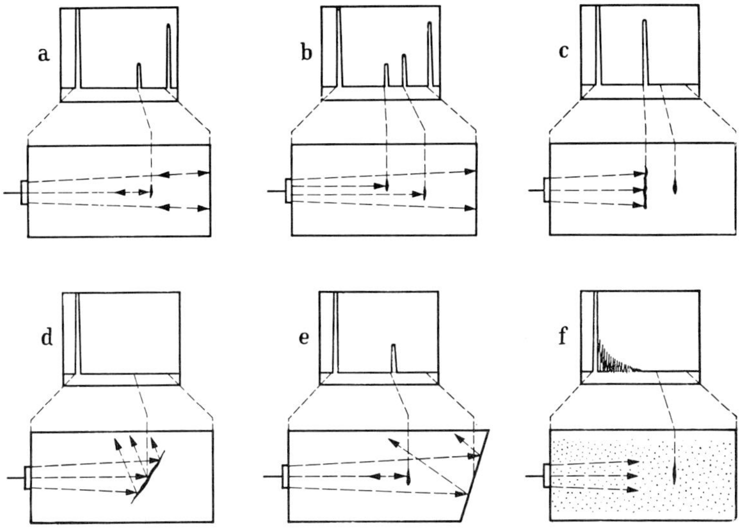

Fig. 2.15 Schematic screen pictures obtained by the pulse-echo method. a) Small flaw in sound beam; b) two small flaws in sound beam; c) large flaw in sound beam, smaller second flaw and backwall masked; d) large, obliquely orientated flaw, backwall masked; e) small flaw but no backwall echo because the axis of the beam is not incident at right angles on back wall; f) strong attenuation of sound beam due to scattering, no echo from flaw or backwall, only *grass*.

Fig. 2.15 shows schematically the traces on the viewing screen for various cases of flaw detection. It can be seen that in addition to the detectability of small flaws, the exact location of the flaw represents the decisive advance for most applications. If a backwall echo appears in addition to the echo from the flaw (provided the flaw is not too large and the beam is incident at right angles on the backwall), its transit time corresponds to the thickness of the specimen. The echo from the flaw divides the distance between the beginning of the time scale and the echo from the backwall, in the same ratio as the position of the flaw divides the distance between the front and the back of the specimen. If the time scale is linear, these three indications therefore provide an enlarged or reduced diagram of the location of the flaw. Even without measuring the transit time accurately, it is thus possible to state whether flaws are present and where they are located.

Several flaws in the sound beam can be indicated simultaneously (Fig. 2.15d) provided none of them are masked completely by another flaw. Sometimes, however, it is still possible to detect a small flaw behind a larger flaw, owing to sound diffraction around the edge of the masking flaw. Masking may also hide the backwall echo (Fig. 2.15c). A rough geometrical presentation indicates that this echo disappears if the flaw equals or exceeds the cross-section of the beam. This provides additional information concerning the minimum size of the flaw, which is particularly important if the latter is orientated obliquely (Fig. 2.15d). The backwall echo is also absent if the backwall is smooth and oblique relative to the axis of the beam, or if the attenuation of the sound in the specimen is too high because of scattering or absorption (Fig. 2.15e and f). Scattering is indicated by many irregular closely spaced echoes (*grass*) their height decreasing with the distance.

The height of the backwall echo in the IT-method thus gives the same information as the reading of a measuring instrument in the simple I-method, i.e. the transmitted intensity, with the difference however, that in the echo method the intensity is measured after a double transit. Provided the specimen is thick enough to be able to separate the backwall echo from the transmitting pulse, the IT-method can be used instead of the I-method, offering the advantage that only one side of the specimen need be accessible. If a flaw is located in the sound beam, it disturbs the wave twice, viz. along its outgoing and its return path.

A specimen with parallel boundaries yields not only one *single* backwall echo but a sequence of multiple echoes spaced evenly, provided the measuring range of the viewing screen is large enough (Fig. 2.16). These

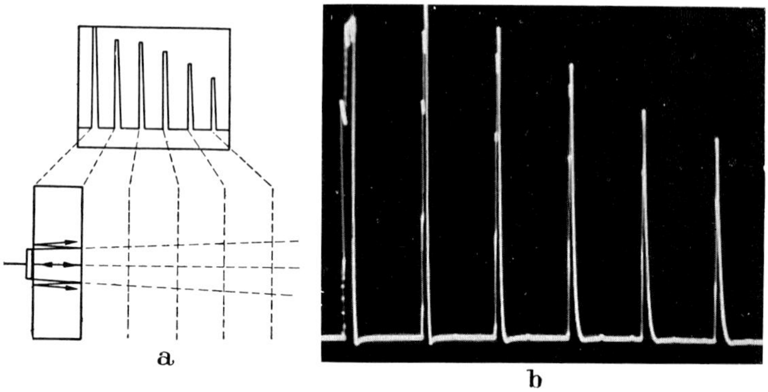

Fig. 2.16 Multiple echoes in a plate. a) Schematic; b) actual screen picture without time or thickness scale, steel plate 50 mm thick, frequency 4 MHz.

multiple echoes are obtained because the first wave reflected at the backwall transmits only a small portion of its energy to the probe when it arrives at the front wall. It is therefore attenuated only slightly when reflected from the front wall, and it passes through the specimen a second time, and so forth. The height of the multiple echoes decreases because, in addition to the slight energy loss in the probe, the wave is attenuated in the material, and because the propagation of the sound beam follows the laws laid down in Section 1.8.

The transit time spacings of the multiple echoes, i. e. with satisfactory linear time base also the spacing of the multiple echoes on the screen, are identical as long as the heights of the echoes do not differ greatly. This fact can be exploited for improved wall thickness measurement: the wall thickness can be read on a calibrated scale at the first backwall echo, but with increased accuracy at the n-th echo by dividing the result by n.

2.32 Construction and Mode of Operation of a Pulse-echo Instrument

A pulse-echo instrument consists essentially of an oscillograph with the correlated generators for the deflection voltages, the transmitter unit and the amplifier, as also the necessary mains-connected power supply or a battery. The mode of operation will be discussed with the aid of a block diagram, without going into the details of the various circuits. This information is given in the manufacturers' circuit diagrams or in text books on amplifiers and oscillographs.

The electric voltage pulse of the transmitter is supplied to the probe through a test cable. Along the same path the electric echo pulses reach the instrument where they are amplified and displayed on the screen of the CR tube (see also Fig. 2.17).

2.321 Sweep Section with CR Tube

The sweep section generates the deflection voltages for the CR tube, and simultaneously the control voltage for the high-frequency transmitter in the rhythm of the *repetition frequency* or *pulse repetition frequency* at which the transmitter transmits high-frequency pulses to the probe. The time sequence of all processes is shown on the right hand side in Fig. 2.17 where ① indicates the transmitter voltage; the example chosen is a highly damped, decaying high-frequency voltage.

The time deflection for the electrostatic CR tube is usually placed symmetrically on the two deflector plates for the horizontal time base, i. e. both receive the same voltage but with opposite sign. Only the small picture tubes in less sophisticated and small instruments use asymmetrical deflection which requires special design of the tube to avoid excessive distortion and lack of definition. ④ indicates the sequence of the sweep voltage: a period comprises the operating time t_a and the interval t_p. During the operating time the sweep voltage rises linearly and thus shifts the electron beam from left to right. During the return interval the voltage sweeps back in an arbitrary time pattern to its initial value and then rises again at the beginning of the next cycle. To prevent the return of the beam from producing a trace on the screen, the sweep section simultaneously controls the brightness of the beam by means of the square wave voltage (5) so that it remains bright only during the operating time.

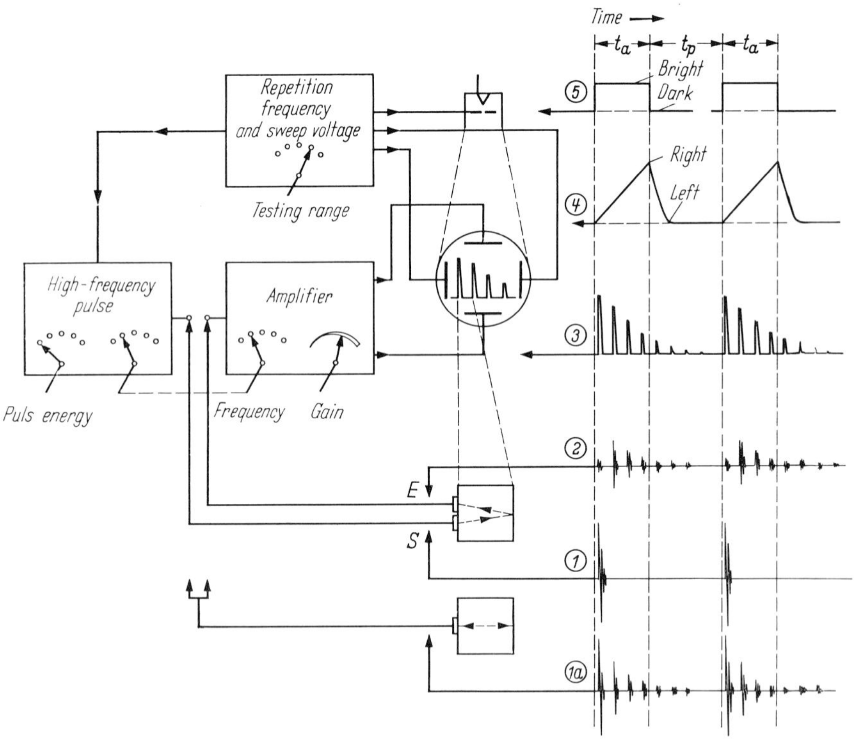

Fig. 2.17 Block diagram of a pulse-echo instrument, on the right hand side correlated voltage-time traces.

The image data (3) received from the amplifier are usually likewise symmetrically fed to the measuring plate for the vertical deflection. These data consist of the deflection which marks the moment of the transmitting pulse, and the subsequent echoes. Their transit time is determined by the thickness of the test specimen. The duration of the operating time t_a thus depends on the testing range and is adjusted on the sweep voltage unit either continuously or in steps, or by using both control methods. In the example shown of the multiple echoes returned from the specimen, only the first three fall into the display range, the remainder fall within the return interval and thus are invisible for the testing range chosen. They must have decreased to zero before the end of the return interval to prevent them from appearing during the next period. There they would simulate echoes from flaws, i.e. so-called *phantom echoes*. The interval must therefore be long enough – according to experience approximately 60 times as long as the operating time.

Sometimes, however, this is not yet sufficient, for instance if specimens of high acoustic transmittance, such as forgings of high-quality steel, particularly nickel steel, are tested at high sensitivity. It is then necessary either to reduce the repetition frequency, which at constant testing range amounts to an increase of the interval, or to learn to distinguish the phantom echoes from the true readings. The latter is possible because the repetition frequency of, for instance, 500 Hz is usually slightly modulated unintentionally with the mains frequency (hum). The time interval between two successive transmitting pulses therefore does not remain perfectly constant so that the delayed echoes likewise appear unsharp. Fig. 2.18 shows their cause and appareance on the viewing screen.

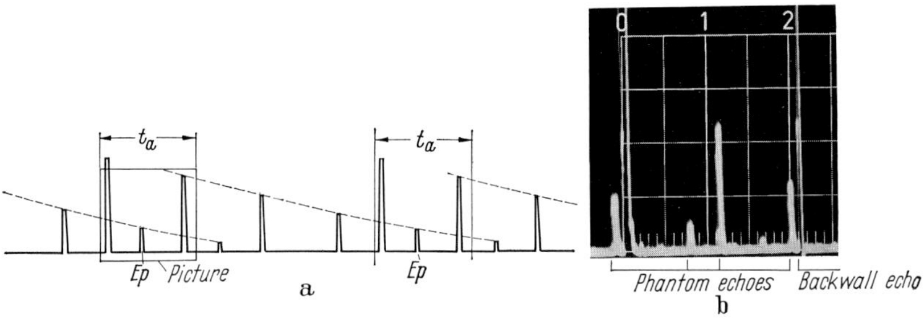

Fig. 2.18 Appearance of spurious flaw echoes (phantom echoes) if pulses are spaced too closely (repetition frequency too high) compared with the thickness of the specimen and its acoustic attenuation. a) Schematic; b) traces on screen showing indistinct phantom echoes, also to the left of the transmitting pulse.

Example:

Testing range in steel	Operating time t_a (time intervall for outgoing and return path for longitudinal waves)	Minimum pulse spacing $60t_a$	Max. pulse repetition frequency $1/60t_a$
100 mm	0.034 ms	2 ms	500 Hz
1000 mm	0.34 ms	20 ms	50 Hz

Satisfactory brightness of the picture requires a high repetition frequency (rate of successive pictures). The above values are therefore increased provided the form of the specimen remains constant and is unfavourable for the production of multiple echoes, e.g. when testing rails, and if experience shows that the frequency used is strongly attenuated by the material of the test piece. In the case of specimens thicker than 1 m the attenuation of the sound is usually so strong that the repetition frequency of 50 Hz can readily be maintained even for longer testing ranges.

In the case of simple instruments it remains constant, e.g. 50 Hz the mains frequency, but in most instruments it is changed with the testing range, while in others it can be adjusted independently of the testing range.

Fig. 2.19 shows the variation with time of the deflection voltage for the above numerical example with 1 m testing range in steel and 50 Hz repetition frequency. For continuous adjustment of the testing range between 0.5 and 2 m a pulse front of varying steepness is chosen at constant repetition frequency. This control is also necessary in order to calibrate a fixed scale placed in front of the screen, e.g. from 0 to 1000 mm, for a given acoustic velocity, if materials other than steel or waves other than longitudinal are used. For transverse waves in steel the operating time t_a should be chosen $1/0.55 = 1.8$ times longer for the same testing range because the velocity of the transverse wave is only 55% of that of the longitudinal wave.

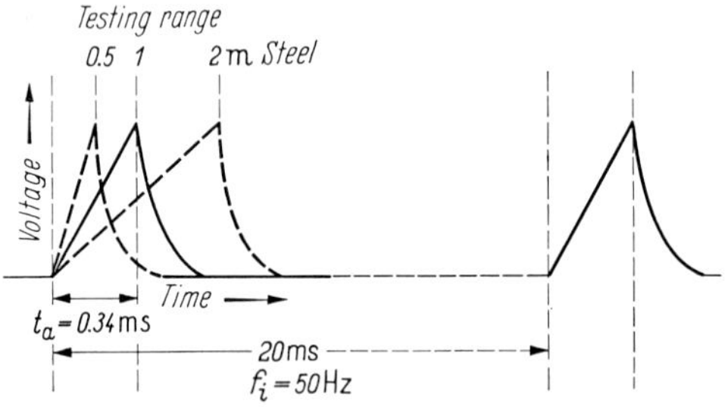

Fig. 2.19 Deflection voltage for a testing range of 0.5 to 2 m in steel and a repetition frequency of 50 Hz, voltage peaks up to a few hundred volts.

It is frequently desirable to be able to view a small section of the entire testing range with its echoes separately and magnified, the transmitting pulse being of no interest. For this purpose a section of the time base is expanded over the entire viewing screen by means of a steeper sweep voltage, as shown in Fig. 2.20. The position of this section can be shifted over the entire testing range, and in addition it is often possible to change the expansion arbitrarily. This device is called a *depth magnifier* or scale expansion. Fig. 2.20 shows the sweep voltage for a testing range of 1 m in steel together with its form with switched on scale expansion at a range of 250 mm. The effect is shown in Fig. 2.21.

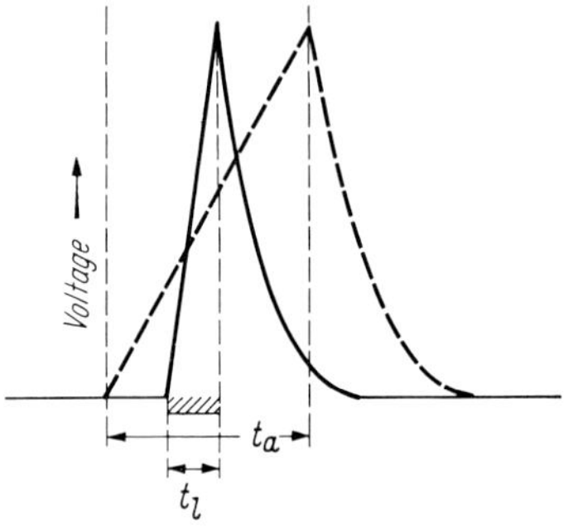

Fig. 2.20 Deflection voltage for time-base expansion of 250 mm range at 1 m testing range in steel.

Basically it is not difficult to expand the time base to a considerably greater extent. For instance, for wall thickness measurements (see Sec. 3.61) an expansion of 10 mm steel over the full screen width is desirable.

This, however, requires perfect stabilization of the operating voltages and high stability of the circuit elements to prevent trembling of the echoes.

According to Fig. 2.17 the sweep-voltage generator triggers the transmitting pulse, preferably with a delay such that it appears on the viewing screen slightly to the right of the beginning of the time base, so as to remain fully visible. Sometimes, however, the transmitting pulse is of no interest whatsoever, e.g. in the case of the so-called immersion tests where the sound is radiated into the specimen through a layer of water. In this case the range of the time base which is of interest, starts only with the entrance echo. For better utilization of the viewing screen the time base can then be triggered by the entrance echo (echo-start circuit of sweep-voltage generator). The entrance echo then replaces the transmitting pulse and thus appears on the viewing screen at the left end of the time base, irrespective of the length of the section in the water, even if the latter changes while scanning the test piece. The block diagram in Fig. 2.17 would then have to be changed so that the generator of the repetition frequency triggers the transmitting pulse only, while the generator of the sweep voltage is controlled by the amplifier.

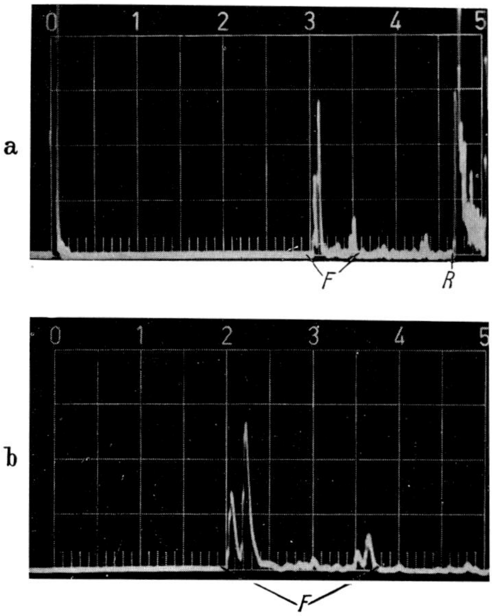

Fig. 2.21. a) Screen trace of a specimen with back-wall echo R and flaw echo group F in 1 m testing range in steel; b) group of flaws alone when viewed with scale expansion to 250 mm range.

In the usual echo-start circuit the entrance echo is no longer fully visible on the time base because it has to trigger the latter. If this shortcoming is to be avoided, the picture contents must pass through a delay line before they reach the picture tube.

The recording speed of the electron beam in the picture tube is very high, particularly for short testing ranges, e.g. the 100 mm range and display over 100 mm screen width (1 : 1 reproduction) for steel approx. 3 km/s on the zero line. At the flanks of the pulses the recording speed is still considerably higher, viz. up to 100 times higher. Since the traces should still be sufficiently bright to be observable also in the open, without cumbersome shielding devices, one should use tubes with high plate and post acceleration voltages, i.e. between 2 and 12 kV. Furthermore, for the same reasons, a reduced focusing sharpness of the trace due to higher electron beam intensity will usually have to be accepted.

Instead of electrostatic deflection systems which produce the best pictures with respect to image distortion, electromagnetic tubes have also occasionally been used. However, this makes it difficult to increase the upper cut-off frequency of the deflection system to an extent such that this does not involve a frequency limitation which would result in a broadening of narrow echoes.

2.322 Transmitter Unit

The transmitter unit receives the control pulse from the sweep voltage unit slightly later than the start of the rise of the deflecting voltage and the brightness control, so that the rise of the transmitting pulse appears on the viewing screen already slightly to the right from the beginning of the time base. The rise of the transmitting pulse serves as zero of the time delay or depth scale.

In unsophisticated instruments (Fig. 2.22a) a gas-filled valve, viz. a thyratron, generates a voltage surge by the sudden discharge of a capacitor charged to several hundred up to 1000 V. This surge excites a tuned circuit to its own, damped oscillation, viz. the electrical transmitting pulse. The damping can be increased by shunts parallel to the induction coil of the resonant circuit, which permits changing the oscillation amplitude, the *pulse strength* together with the pulse length.

The thyratron can also be replaced by controlled semi-conductor rectifiers, particularly in transistorized instruments.

If, as shown in Fig. 2.22b, the pulse of the thyratron is used first briefly to open a high-power output valve, similar shapes of the transmitting pulse are obtained. This, however, has the advantage that the valve again assumes a very high impedance parallel to the resonant circuit immediately after the transmitting pulse, whereas a thyratron, due to its de-ionizing time, may still have a very low impedance. This, however, is undesirable if the same probe used both for transmitting and receiving (single-probe operation), is required to indicate echoes of near flaws with a minimum delay after the transmitting pulse.

Certain applications require longer pulses which according to Figs. 2.22c or d can be produced either by means of an oscillator which builds up and decays again during a preset period (keyed transmitter), or by passing the voltage of a continuously oscillating transmitter through a final stage only during the pulse transmission time. This produces a pulse inside a square envelope whose sides, however, are rounded off by the build-up and decay phenomena of the resonant circuit (see also 1.103).

In order to produce pulses as short as possible so as to improve the resolving power for closely packed flaws or flaws near the surface, the first-mentioned circuits are preferred in practice, particularly because they are less complex. The continuously oscillating transmitting stage requires very careful shielding to avoid any direct electric transmission to the sensitive amplifier. In the case of pulse-keying this interferes less, par-

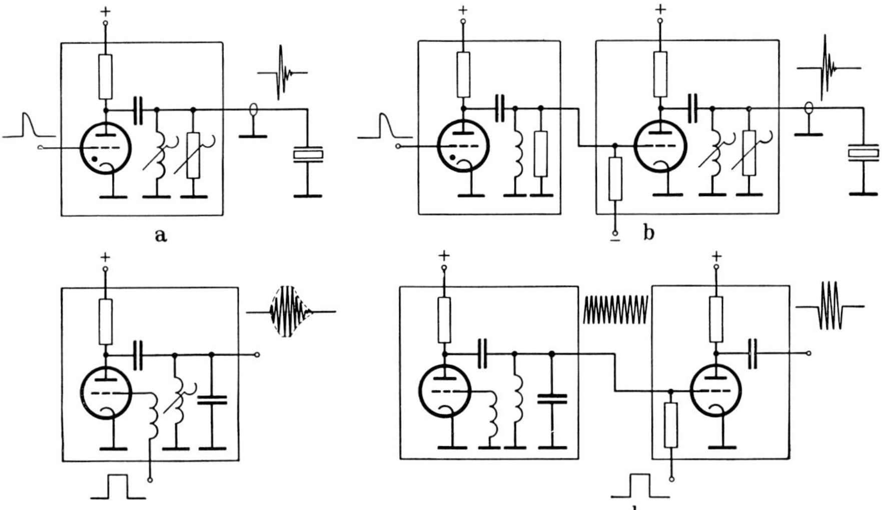

Fig. 2.22 Circuits for generating high-frequency pulses.

ticularly with single-probe operation, because the receiver must then in any case accept the full transmitting voltage as input voltage (see 2.323).

The shape of the transmitted electrical pulse is essentially predetermined by the connected probe and to some extent by its coupling conditions. In some instruments the frequency-determining circuit elements, particularly the coil, are not mounted in the instrument but in the probe so that the pulse oscillation can appear only after a probe has been connected. Without the probe the pulse is only a short, voltage surge, a so-called triangular pulse.

The shape of the electrical transmitting pulse as such is otherwise of no importance in the mode of operation of a given instrument; of importance is the pulse shape of an echo as it appears at the output end of the amplifier after it has passed through all elements of the whole transmission line. Influencing factors besides the amplifier are the double-conversion in the piezoelectric crystal, possibly also the frequency dependence of the acoustic damping in the test piece, and the reflection on a flaw. The two last mentioned factors are excluded when examining the sample pulse shape by using specimens with low acoustic damping, and the echo from the backwall reflection in a plate. Such pulse shapes are shown in Fig. 2.27.

The energy of the pulse (pulse voltage) can be regulated by adjusting the plate voltage of the transmitter stage. Frequently, however, this is achieved more simply by changing the load impedance of the output of the transmitter (Figs. 2.22a and b). This simultaneously influences the damping of the connected resonance circuit, which in turn changes the pulse length. In many cases of practical testing this additional effect is, however, of no consequence: if high pulse energy is used, longer pulses can usually be tolerated because this generally means great testing depth, and because resolution is not the main object. Conversely, in the case of small testing depth, particularly near the surface, a weaker but shorter pulse can be used.

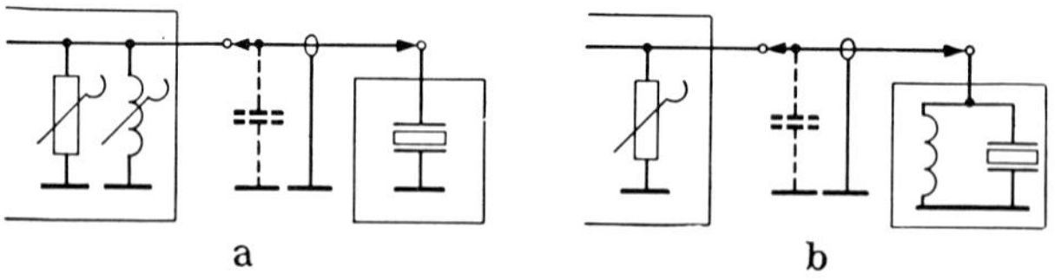

Fig. 2.23 The frequency of the transmitted pulse in cases a) to c) of Fig. 2.22 is influenced by the capacitance of the cable. The coil can be mounted in the transmitter unit of the instrument (a) or in the probe (b).

The frequency is usually selected by means of switchable coils unless the latter are already installed in the connected probe, making a separate frequency switch of the transmitter stage superfluous (Fig. 2.23). The effect, naturally, is the same. If the cable is not matched to its wave impedance (characteristic impedance) at both ends the frequency is influenced by the capacitance of the cable and the capacitance of the transducer and its holder. The cable therefore cannot be arbitrarily long. In the case of barium titanate probes its capacitance of approx. 30 to 60 pF per metre is not so important compared with the high capacitance of the radiator, and the cable can therefore be considerably longer than the usual 2 to 3 m. Very long cables, up to 100 m for instance, must be matched at both ends, i.e. the impedances of both the transmitter and the probe must be matched to the characteristic impedance of the cable (order of magnitude 100 Ω) by means of transformers.

To be able to draw maximum power from a given transmitter stage, the probe must also be matched correctly. However, the impedance of the probe depends very much on the piezoelectric plate used, barium titanate having a very low impedance, quartz a very high impedance. To be able to use different types of probes with a given instrument it should therefore also be possible to switch the matching on the transmitter. The simplest solution is to install in the probe, together with the coil determining the frequency, also the correct matching impedance in the form of an auto-transformer (Fig. 2.24).

If separate transmitting and receiving probes (Fig. 2.17) are used, in so-called TR-operation, the transmitter receives the pulses according to voltage pattern ①. Although the arriving echoes also produce echo voltages in the transmitting probe just as in the receiver, these are not further processed. The receiver receives a negligible transmitting pulse if shielded very carefully; some of it is received nevertheless, even if very much attenuated, ②. With single or multiple probe operation the transmitter and amplifier are connected to each other and simultaneously also to one or several probes (Fig. 2.25). Single-probe operation (Fig. 2.17 with ①) is most commonly used because of its simple maintenance and its sensitivity characteristics which can readily be checked. For flaws immediately below the surface a TR-probe is, however, more suitable because for single-probe operation the *dead zone* masked by the transmitting pulse may also mask such echoes. Finally, for special purposes which will be dealt with when discussing the various applications in detail, combinations of several parallel-connected probes in multi-probe operation offer certain advantages.

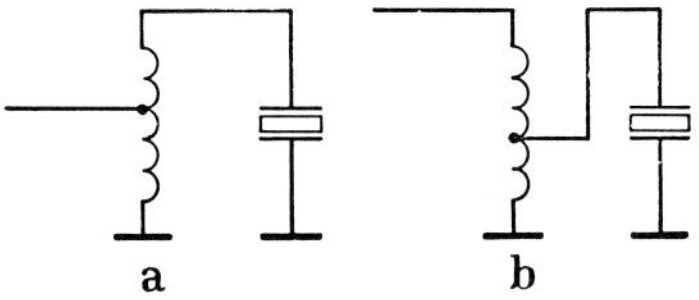

Fig. 2.24 Matching of probe and transmitter, a) in the case of high probe impedance (quartz), b) in case of low impedance (barium titanate).

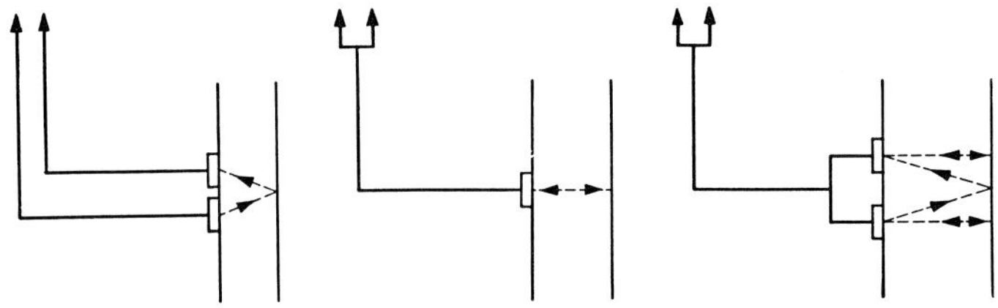

Fig. 2.25 TR, single-probe and multi-probe operation.

In this Section we have discussed only instruments for the generation of short pulses which are, however, still periodic. In 2.36 we shall investigate a pulse-echo method in which aperiodic, so-called shock pulses are used, which is therefore called the shockwave method and which in view of its special circuits and probe constructions will be discussed separately.

2.323 The Amplifier

The transmitting pulse at the output of the transmitter usually has a voltage of 100 to 1000 V, whereas the voltages of the echo at the input of the amplifier are much smaller, approx. 1/1000 to 1 V. Since the CR tube requires voltages of several 100 V for full modulation, the amplifier must have a gain of approx. 10^5 (100 dB).

On the viewing screen the pulses appear either in their high-frequency form, i.e. with deflection both above and below a central zero line [Fig. 2.17(1a)], or in rectified form, usually above a zero line (3). Most modern instruments use this last form.

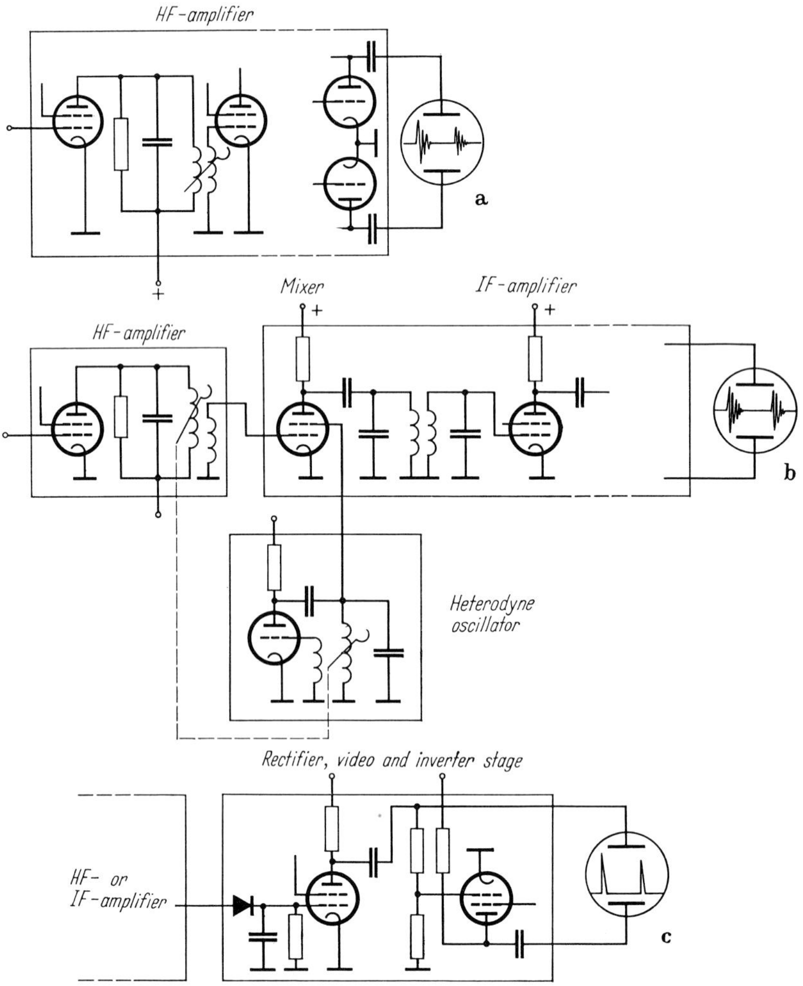

Fig. 2.26 Schematic amplifier circuits. a) High-frequency amplifier with push-pull output; b) heterodyne amplifier; c) high-frequency or intermediate frequency amplifier with rectifier, video and inverter stages.

The amplifier for the high-frequency display can be a straight high-frequency amplifier (Fig. 2.26a) with approximately four to six very similar stages and a push-pull output, to obtain symmetrical voltages for the plates of the CR tube. Alternatively, the heterodyne principle can be used to which after pre-amplification of the desired frequency a heterodyne frequency is added, whereupon the resultant differential or sum frequency is stepped up to the required voltage in a multi-stage IF-amplifier. The screen trace then no longer shows the frequency of the ultrasonic wave used, but an intermediate (usually higher) frequency (Fig. 2.26b). In the case of video display, a rectifier, usually with a video and inversion stage, is inserted between HF- or IF-amplifier and CR tube (Fig. 2.26c). Fig. 2.27 shows the relevant screen pictures.

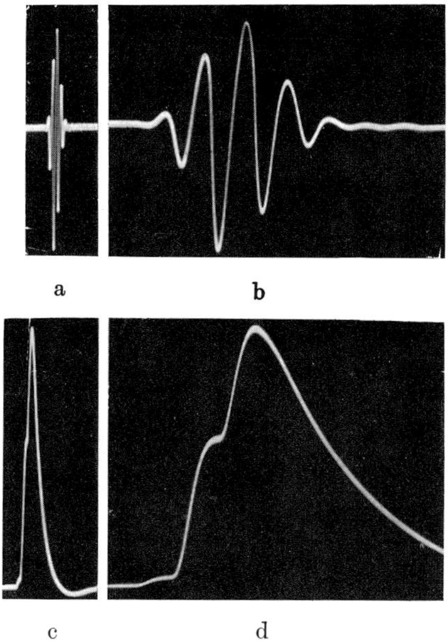

Fig. 2.27 Screen picture of 4 MHz echoes a) and b) with high-frequency modulation, c) and d) with rectified (video) traces.
Scale for a) and c): 21 mm = 10 μs, or 3.6 mm = 10 mm sound path in steel for longitudinal waves, i. e. 5 mm depth in steel on depth scale, scale for b) and d) expanded 10-fold.

Frequency response. The high-frequency amplifier can be of the pronounced broad-band type, i.e. covering all occurring ultrasonic frequencies, e. g. from 1 to 10 MHz. This makes switching over unnecessary if the frequency is changed. It has the advantage that short pulses with their wide frequency band pass through with little distortion or change, but there are also disadvantages: the amplifier noise (resistance and valve noise) limits the possible amplification. If the time base on the viewing screen clearly indicates noise, any further amplification is futile because the noise masks the small echoes (Fig. 2.28). The amplitude of the noise is proportional to the square root of the amplifier band-width; a narrow band amplifier therefore permits higher amplification. Furthermore, harmonics of the frequency of the probe frequently predominate in the frequency band of echoes as compared with the harmonics of the transmitted sound wave, particularly if they are caused by very small interference points which preferentially back-scatter the higher frequencies. This produces much undesirable background noise with which the larger flaws to be detected no longer contrast sufficiently. However, if the frequency band in the amplifier is clipped, e.g. already excluding the third harmonic (for 1 MHz below 3 MHz), the picture becomes clearer. An excessively narrow band width has the disadvantage that the pulses are broadened, resulting in reduced resolving power. The optimum will therefore have to be a compromise between opposing requirements, based on practical experience.

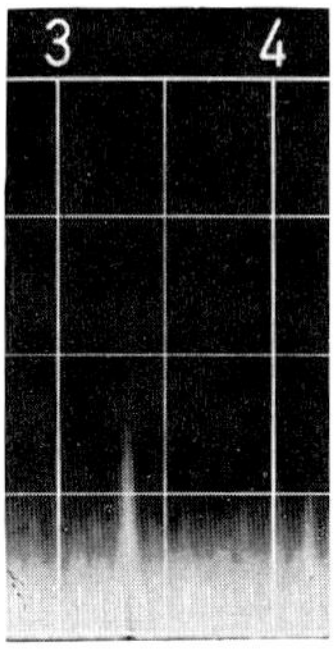

Fig. 2.28
Small echo masked by excessive amplifier noise.

In an instrument for scientific studies, which presupposes thoroughly trained operators, installation of a special bandwidth control would be justified; for practical applications one omits this in favour of fool-proof operation.

Theoretically and practically it can be shown that the slopes of the flanks of the amplification curve as a function of the frequency (frequency response of amplifier) should be as gentle as possible; in particular the upper frequency limit must not drop sharply to keep the distortion of the pulse to a minimum.

A similar compromise must also be made in respect of the upper frequency limit for the rectifier-video stage. If the frequency limit is high, the echoes are resolved into high-frequency oscillations cut in half (Fig. 2.29), when they have the minimum width and optimal resolving power. If the frequency limit is too low, the high-frequency peaks in the echo become very indistinct and at the same time the pulse is lengthened. Practical experience shows that the optimal solution resembles the form shown in Fig. 2.27 c. The actual choice, however, is largely a matter of taste. On some instruments the video frequency limit (high-frequency filter) can be changed so that it can be set to obtain the optimal form for the purpose in hand. Smoother echo forms are also obtained by full wave rectification before the video stage instead of the oneway circuit shown in Fig. 2.26 c. This obviously halves the spacing of the high-frequency peaks.

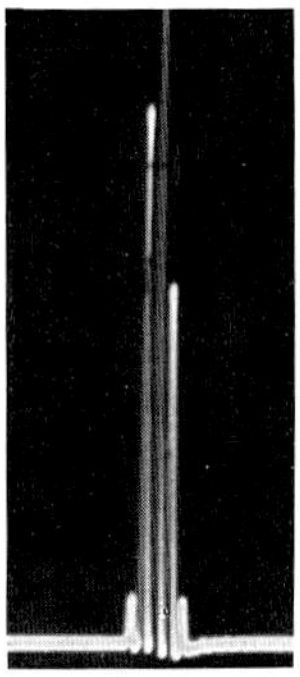

Fig. 2.29 4 MHz echo pulse as in Fig. 2.27 c but with higher upper frequency limit of video amplifier.

Amplification characteristic. The amplification characteristic shows the echo height of the trace as a function of the input voltage (Fig. 2.30). Usually a linear pattern as in Fig. 2.30 a is desirable because this makes it possible to compare the size of flaws of the same type and located at the same depth, on the basis of their echo heights. Double echo height would mean double flaw area.

With the conditions shown in Fig. 2.30 b the received echo voltages must exceed a certain threshold before they can be indicated at all. Smaller flaws might therefore be overlooked. This would be serious where the operator is unaware of this amplification characteristic. No threshold exists in the case of high-frequency display, but not always in the case of video display because at low voltages the rectifier has a more or less non-linear characteristic. However, the threshold can be limited to a tolerable value.

Since, however, a threshold is in many cases definitely desirable, e.g. in order to suppress amplifier noise as well as unimportant scatter echoes or even smaller flaw echoes which are of no consequence, some instruments permit adjustment of the threshold.

Curve *b* is linear along its rising section. To distinguish this clearly, curve *a* should therefore be called "linear proportional".

With rising input voltages, a point is reached in every amplifier where it is over-modulated and where the output voltage no longer increases proportionally. This saturation point may already be reached in the visible range on the viewing screen but, in the case of modern instruments, it may also start only at echo heights above the screen scale so that the latter is fully utilized.

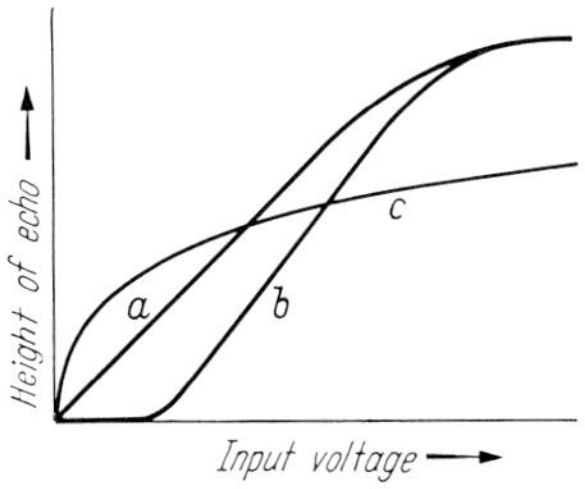

Fig. 2.30 Height of echo above input voltage, schematic. *a* Linear amplification; *b* threshold amplification; *c* logarithmic amplification.

When testing it is an advantage if all important echoes remain within the linearity range of the display so that it will be unnecessary to change the gain during testing. It is, however, hardly possible to detect echo ratios larger than 50:1 which corresponds to a 7 : 1 diameter ratio of circular-disc flaws. If in addition the height of the backwall echo and the great variation of the echo height with the distance of the flaw are taken into consideration, it is seen that a range of 50 : 1 will often be insufficient. Furthermore, any quantitative evaluation is no longer possible in the case of an echo of 1/50 scale height. In many cases it will therefore be absolutely necessary to change the gain even while testing. For this purpose less sophisticated and older instruments only have a continuously adjustable voltage divider at the input of the amplifier or between two of the earliest stages. This simple design, taken over from radio engineering, makes the gain control strongly frequency dependent. In addition the shape of the control curve shows considerable tolerances so that any adjustment on the arbitrary scale has no significance whatsoever in a comparison with a different instrument. Furthermore, the gain at for instance scale division 4 is not necessarily twice that at division 2, and finally the gain ratio for the two adjustments depends on the frequency used. Controls of this type are therefore unsuitable for any quantitative evaluation of echo heights.

It is therefore preferable to use common electronic measuring methods for this purpose in which the given maximum gain is reduced by means of a calibrated, frequency-independent attenuator. The unit generally used is the decibel (see page 91). Every echo is adjusted to an arbitrary, but in each case identical, height marked on the screen scale at approximately half level, and the dB value of the attenuator is read. A less experienced operator will, however, find it more logical if one speaks also in this case of gain and not of attenuation and if the control is therefore called a gain control which for maximum gain is turned to its end value, e.g. 80 dB, which in reality is equivalent to zero attenuation (see also Figs. 1.87 and 1.88, righthand ordinate scale). An indication of 50 dB, which therefore requires a gain of 50 dB to reach the reference level, is produced by a stronger echo than a reading of 70 dB. The former is 20 dB stronger than the latter, or in decadic measure exactly 10 times stronger. Controls of this type are available with continuous adjustment, but at large dB differences they are no longer reliable and in addition there is a reading inaccuracy at every point which exceeds 1 dB. A step-by-step control, e.g. with 40 steps of 2 dB each with a maximum error of 0.1 dB at any given point, meets all requirements.

With such an instrument it is therefore possible to compare echo heights in the ratio 1 : 10,000 (= 80 dB) with an accuracy of approx. 1% (= 0.1 dB).

Instruments with calibrated controls can of course also be used in the customary way. To be able to exploit the much wider and more accurate measuring possibilities fully, one must accept the disadvantage that the echoes to be compared can only be compared successively by adjusting the control by hand. In this connection it does not matter if the characteristic of the amplifier is unknown and non-linear because the amplifier is always used with the same setting.

In English the concept "dynamic range" has been coined for evaluating a given amplifier characteristic. A value of the "dynamic range" of e.g. 50 : 1 means that a given echo can just still be recognized as an indication on the zero line, while simultaneously another echo with a 50 times higher input voltage is also still visible on the same screen, viz. just below the saturation line. The calibrated gain control extends a value of 50 : 1 of the dynamic range practically to 10,000 : 1 or more, depending on the range of the attenuator.

If echo ratios greatly exceeding 50 : 1 are to be compared on the viewing screen and if no high accuracy is required, the amplifier can also be given a logarithmic characteristic over a range of approximately 40 to 60 dB, which is particularly important for recording purposes (curve *c* in Fig. 2.30).

In the USA, in addition to other measuring methods for other instrument characteristics, it has been suggested that the dynamic range be determined from the echo heights of artificial flaws [415]. This necessitates the use of aluminium test blocks with flat-bottomed holes of 1/64 to 8/64 inch spaced 3 inches from the surface. This method is not suitable for all frequencies and probes used in non-destructive testing, besides being very costly. If a calibrated gain control is used the amplification curve can be rechecked under any given conditions: an echo of arbitrary height is first brought to full scale height and then reduced step by step and its height measured. The general introduction of calibrated gain controls could thus in a simple way solve certain problems in the standardization of both instruments and test specifications.

The amplification curve, as shown for instance in Fig. 2.30, may differ intentionally or unintentionally at various points of the time base, which means that the characteristics of the amplifier can depend on the time interval behind the transmitting pulse. One form of intentionally time-controlled gain is "depth compensation" or "swept gain" intended for equalizing the drop in sensitivity with increasing distance of the flaw due to attenuation in the material and the beam spread. Since both influences differ from one case to another and since the actual pattern is rather complex, perfect compensation would be very costly. In most instances, however, it is sufficient if the gain increases more or less linearly over a given range. This makes it necessary in a given case to adjust it empirically, e.g. on the basis of artificial flaws at different depths in the material. The depth compensation is then, strictly speaking, valid only for the particular type of flaw concerned, and is not valid e.g. for backwall echoes which generally follow a different law. This device is therefore mainly used to facilitate evaluation by untrained operators and not so much for an accurate evaluation of the echo height.

For proportional (analog) recording of echo heights in continuous testing the great difference between height of backwall echo and flaw echo is a disadvantage. To remedy this the gain can be changed suddenly, e.g. reduced by 20 dB, beyond a certain adjustable depth.

Among the usually unintentional variations of the amplification curve as a function of the transit time, is the so-called dead zone behind the transmitting pulse. In single-probe operation the full transmitting voltage of the order of 1000 V is applied simultaneously to both the probe and the amplifier input, which latter immediately afterwards must be receptive for echo voltages of 1 millionth of this value. The amplifier is specially designed to produce this remarkable result. Nevertheless, a certain blocking effect behind the transmitting pulse cannot be avoided completely. Not only the gain may decrease considerably, but also the amplification curve may become pronouncedly non-linear and show a high threshold value. This effect can occur particularly easily in the video stage, not only behind the transmitting pulse, but also behind large echoes. It results in suppression of the trailing oscillations and the traces appear narrower and the resolving power seems improved. This effect, if intentional, and other electronic devices might be called "screen cosmetics" because it sometimes favours beauty at the expense of truth. The pulse trace on the fluorescent screen must not however produce the illusion, that both in the actual ultrasonic and in the high-frequency form of the pulse at the input of the amplifier, such residual oscillations have been suppressed by these measures.

A given amplifier can be checked for the presence of such effects by generating an artificial electronic pulse of variable delay and by shifting it continuously from the right towards the transmitting pulse or the echo concerned.

As shown in Fig. 2.31 this can readily be done by means of a variable reflection path in water with a second probe connected simultaneously. More versatile is the electronic generation of an artificial echo pulse in a so-called pulse-measuring instrument which in addition permits choosing any arbitrary frequency, pulse width and input voltage on the amplifier for the particular pulse selected.

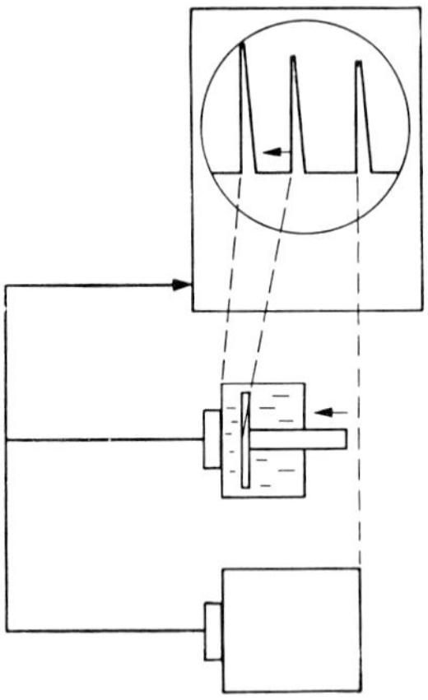

Fig. 2.31 Measurement of the *dead zone* with continuously adjustable measuring pulse produced by a liquid path.

A measuring pulse with adjustable and measurable input voltage is also the primary requirement for any exact determination of the amplification curve according to Fig. 2.30.

Because of interference with the trailing oscillations which are always present but merely suppressed on the screen, the measuring pulse during the approximation first shows maxima and minima and may finally disappear completely if the pulse has been trimmed too much. The point at which a reduction of about 1 dB (approx. 10%) is first obtained could thus be used for defining and measuring the dead zone behind the transmitter pulse as well as the amount of trimming of the echo. This requires in addition specification of the gain, e.g. in such a way that the echo of a smooth plate produces just full modulation on the viewing screen, or the ten or hundred times greater value. Fig. 2.32 shows the amplified echo curve measured in this way behind the transmitter pulse for 4 MHz. This parameter of the instrument, naturally, may be influenced by the probe and can also be used for testing the latter.

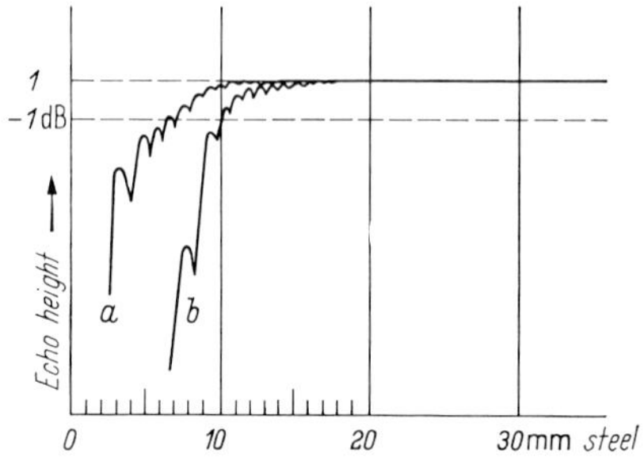

Fig. 2.32 Curve of echo height in dead zone, measured on a pulse-echo instrument by the method shown in Fig. 2.31; probe of medium damping at 4 MHz. *a* Normal gain (i.e. echo of plate full scale high); *b* 10-times normal gain. Reduction of echo height by 1 dB at 7 and 10 mm depth in steel, respectively.

Since good close-range resolution of a given instrument is important for many applications, many devices have been investigated which would shorten the dead zone of the amplifier and which would effect a genuine shortening of the overdriving time. This, of course, presupposes that both the transmitting pulse on the electrical side and the piezoelectric crystal on the mechanical side have already largely been freed of after-oscillations by correct damping and matching, which, converted into electrical receiving voltage, are comparable with the input voltage of the echoes.

When generating damped oscillation pulses according to Fig. 2.22a and b, the first half oscillation is negative and thus is not loaded and weakened by the connected grid cathode circuit of the first amplifier valve. The latter acts only on the positive, following half waves which produce a high grid current which damps them, and which in turn helps to shorten the transmitting pulse. The negative voltage surge on the first valve appears as positive surge on the second stage and overdrives it, and so forth. An attempt has therefore been made to cut off these overdriving peaks in the second and subsequent amplifier stages by means of diodes with small internal resistance; this can be done by connecting two diodes anti-parallel as leakage resistance of the grid in order to trim both voltage polarities. If necessary it is also possible to adjust the transmitted voltage range, for instance to 1 V max., by biasing the diodes.

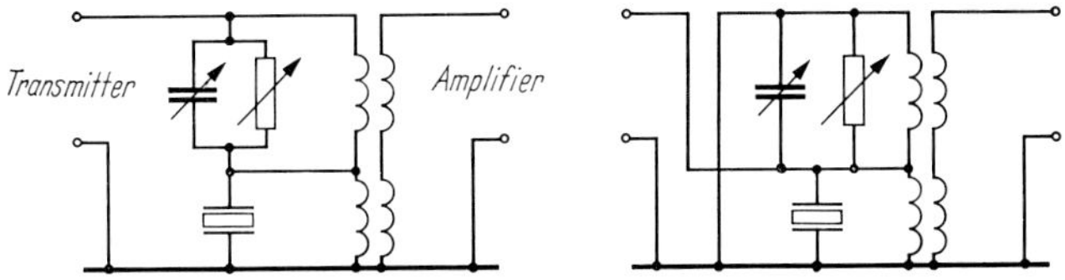

Fig. 2.33 Examples of circuits for suppressing the transmitting pulse at the amplifier input. In the circuit on the left-hand side the two transformers oppose each other.

Since positive overdriving is least desirable in view of the grid current, it has also been suggested that the amplifier be built using exclusively secondary emission valves which are not subject to phase reversal as in the case of conventional amplifier valves, and to operate only with negative voltage peaks.

Attempts have also been made to block the amplifier completely for the duration of the transmitting pulse by placing a specially produced negative blocking voltage on some of the grids of one or more stages. So far, however, none of these improvements seem to have found much favour.

This applies also to a suggestion to damp the transmitting pulse after a few oscillations by a parallel-connected gas discharge section, in which the length of the transmitting pulse can be varied by adjusting the delay of the ignition (FIRESTONE [102]), or in which an opposing pulse is placed on the piezoelectric crystal after a few oscillations in order to slow down the trailing oscillations (VAN VALKENBURG [371]). The bridge circuit of the probe proposed by BRADFIELD [51] and well known in telecommunication engineering (Fig. 2.33) makes it possible to ensure that, even in the case of single-probe operation, the transmitting pulse no longer reaches the amplifier input, but only the echoes. For this purpose the probe is simulated electrically in the simplest design by a capacitor and a resistor. The transmitting voltages then just cancel each other when they are received at the amplifier input whereas the echo voltages remain, because the latter occur only at the probe and not at its simulation.

Such measures can be quite effective but they require, for every probe and even for every coupling condition, fresh balancing of the simulation, which is undesirable in practice.

The simulation of the probe basically permits also measuring and checking the coupling conditions because the latter influence the radiation impedance of the crystal, which enters in the simulation.

Automatic gain control is sometimes desirable in order to equalize differences in the sensitivity of the method resulting from coupling variations [58, 440]. Circuits similar to the fading control in radio receivers can be used for this purpose. Any type of echo can be used for this control effectively, for instance the backwall echo. The gain control thus follows this echo and keeps it constant within the limits of the gain reserve.

The automatic gain control will achieve its purpose effectively only if the form of the sound field remains unchanged, and not for instance in the presence of non-uniform sound transmission through the coupling surface or if the backwall echo is masked by larger flaws in the path of the sound beam.

2.324 Distance Scale and Time Markers

The transit time of an echo, from which the flaw distance can be deduced, can be read on the viewing screen as distance of the flaw echo from the transmitting pulse if the zero line has a scale. The latter is linear, i.e. subdivided uniformly, if the deflection voltage rises linearly and if the CR tube introduces no distortions. Both requirements can be met in practice so accurately that once the beginning and end of the scale has been calibrated the measuring error is nowhere greater than approx. 2% of the total reading. This requires, however, that the measuring of the transit time of the echo peaks is defined more accurately. For most measurements it is sufficient to take as reading marks the flanks of transmitting pulse and echo which usually appear to rise very steeply from the zero line. As shown in Fig. 1.119 on a calculated example and in Fig. 2.27 on an actual echo pulse, the beginning of the pulse is not as sharply defined as may at first appear: if the gain is too small the first still small oscillations may not yet be measurable.

Still less clearly indicated is the zero point of the time scale, viz. the transmitting pulse. Here, the rise of the peak on the viewing screen merely corresponds to the beginning of the *electrical* transmitting pulse, i.e. the moment at which it arrives at the back of the piezoelectric crystal, because the electrical transit time in the leads can be practically neglected. Even if the transducer is in direct contact with the test piece, the transit time of the *ultra-sound* must be counted from a considerably later point of time. This difference is called the zero error. It is determined as follows (Fig. 2.34): In a sequence of multiple echoes of approximately equal height received from a test piece without sound attenuation, the echo spacings are very uniform and correspond to the true acoustic transit time. Therefore, if the multiple echoes with the rising front of their peaks are adjusted to the divisions of the time scale by successively expanding and shifting the echo pattern, the beginning of the transmitting pulse in steel is located a few millimetres to the left of the scale zero. This zero error is increased still further by every additional layer between transducer and test piece, as in the case of probes with protective layers or adaptors. It is always added to the transit time of the first echo, never to the spacing of the multiple echoes. Therefore, in order to determine the transit time accurately, only the spacing of the multiple echoes should be measured, particularly if the interference method is used (see also 3.62). In the case of the echo of an individual flaw without multiple echoes it is necessary instead to measure the transit time starting from the transmitting pulse and to deduce from it the separately determined zero error.

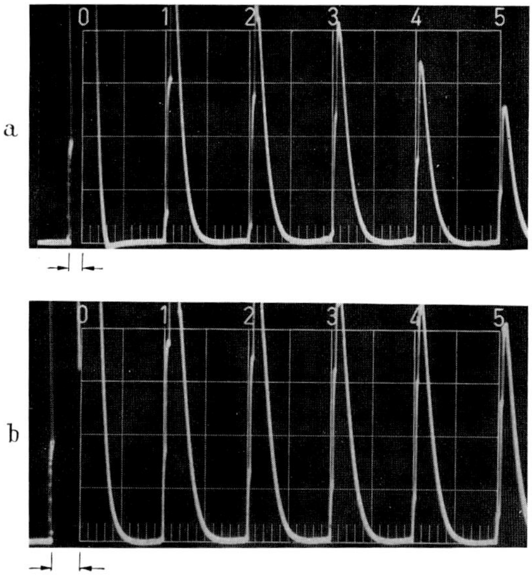

Fig. 2.34 Determination of zero error by means of multiple echoes from a plate (steel, 20 mm thick, a) probe unprotected (quartz plate in direct contact), b) probe protected by plastic layer approx. 1 mm thick.

The depth scale of the instrument should therefore permit determination of this correction value and its application. The simplest solution involves the use of a fixed scale which is placed in front of the viewing screen, and which can be calibrated by means of two controls of the screen picture, viz. by shifting the entire screen picture relative to the scale, and expanding it. By using test specimens, e.g. steel of known thickness, the scale can be calibrated directly in flaw distances in steel, the full scale corresponding to values from e.g. 50 mm to 10 m. If fluctuations of the mains voltage, which can cause fluctuations of the sweep voltages, are compensated by an effectively stabilized power unit, a single calibration will hold good a long time. Since the zero error depends on the probe used it must be determined separately for each probe for accurate measurements and short ranges; some instruments are supplied for this purpose with small calibration plates, e.g. corresponding to 10 mm of steel.

Such a scale can be subdivided very finely, thus permitting readings with an accuracy of 1 mm, i.e. approx. 1 % of the usual screen diameters of approx. 100 mm. A scale has, however, the disadvantage that the luminous trace on the inside surface of the tube is separated from it by the glass window which is several millimetres thick. This causes *parallax errors* when taking readings, which can only be avoided if the operator during calibration and subsequent readings does not shift his viewing position.

This shortcoming is avoided in CR tubes fitted with internal scales, which have recently become available. Another solution is offered by electronic time markers traced by the electron beam on the luminous screen. This requires that the electron beam for the time markers has the same plate and deflection voltages as used for the picture trace; this can best be achieved by using the same beam and the same deflection systems

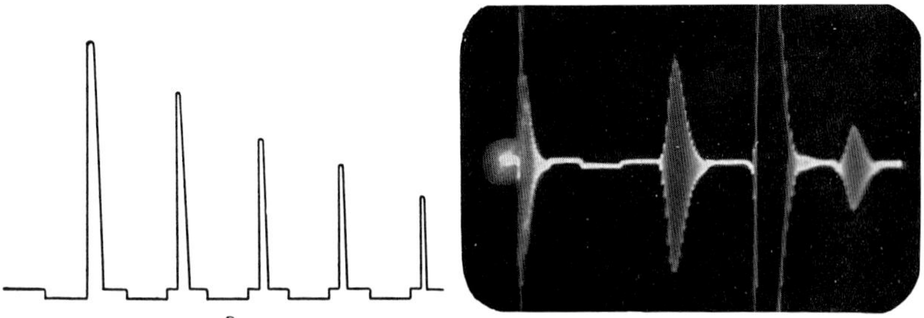

a b

Fig. 2.35 Electronic markers for depth or time with square voltages, traced simultaneously with the picture. a) Schematic with a few multiple echoes; b) screen trace (Sperry reflectoscope UR).

and voltages, both for the picture and the time markers. A periodical, e.g. a square voltage as shown in Fig. 2.35 is placed as time marker on the vertical deflection plates, together with the pulse voltages. In Fig. 2.17 an additional block for the time markers has to be added, which is triggered separately for each picture by the sweep voltage generator, and which produces such a voltage with variable periods, corresponding for instance to 10, 100 and 1000 mm steel. In addition to the zero shift, this should, however, also permit calibration for other velocities of sound (other materials and types of waves). The stability of the calibrations requires a rather complex electronic circuitry. Other disadvantages as compared with a scale on the front of the screen, result from the fact that it is very difficult to estimate even with moderate accuracy intermediate values of a few millimetres between the time markers, even if spaced as close as 10 mm, which can never be so sharply defined as a scale. Furthermore, reading takes slightly longer because the electronic scale cannot be fitted with numbers, thus making it necessary to count the scale divisions starting from zero. On the other hand, it is a great advantage that after calibration the time expansion of screen picture can be varied arbitrarily, whereby the time markers are shifted proportionally, also when expanding the time base (scale expansion).

A time marker as shown in Fig. 2.35 can no longer be read clearly if several echoes are present simultaneously. It is therefore preferable to trace the picture and the time marker alternately: The sweep voltage maintains its time rhythms, e.g. the frequency 500 Hz. This results in the repetition frequency of the transmitting pulse and the number of pictures of the echo trace being 250 Hz, which also happens to be the number of time marker pictures traced between them. The latter stand out clearly, even against a complex echo trace (Figs. 2.36 and 2.37).

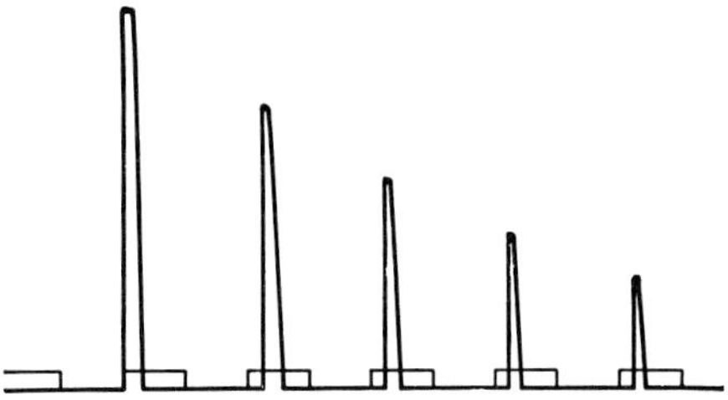

Fig. 2.36 Electronic time markers, traced alternately with the echo picture.

More accurate than on a scale, although also more time-consuming, is the determination of an unknown transit time of a given echo when comparing it with the known transit time of a variable delay line, e.g. in water. As in Fig. 2.31, both echoes are placed on the screen and shifted so that they produce interference by micrometric adjustment of the delay line. Coincidence can then be determined very accurately by the interference minima and maxima. Such a variable delay line is therefore also called an interferometer (see also 2.35 and 3.62).

The depth scale of pulse-echo instruments is usually calibrated for echo operation, i.e. for the go *and* return path. The echo of a plate 100 mm thick appears at scale division 100 mm, although the pulse has actually travelled 200 mm. If the same instrument is then used for straight sound transmission (Fig. 2.11a) the reading appears on the scale at 50 mm, but the multiple echoes are spaced 100 mm, i.e. at 150, 250 mm, etc.

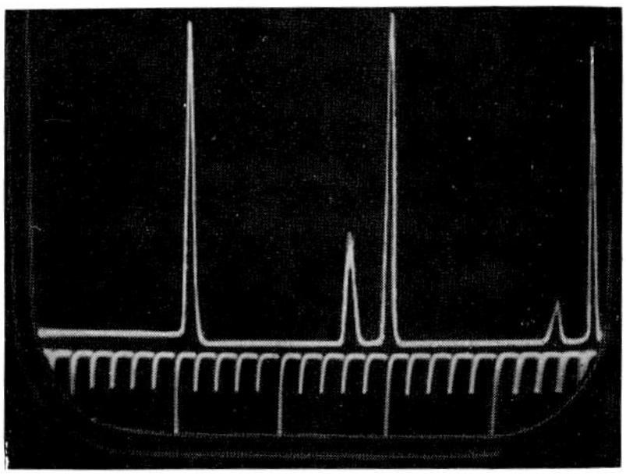

Fig. 2.37 Time markers in form of pips, traced alternately with the echo picture on a separate zero line (Lehfeldt Echoskop), spacing of the short time markers corresponds to 10 mm steel, test piece approx. 95 mm long with flaw at 80 mm.

2.325 Noise Suppression

In Germany, pulse-echo instruments are subject to the interference elimination regulations of the German Federal Post Office for high-frequency instruments. Other countries usually have similar regulations. The instruments must undergo a type-acceptance test and are given a test number. They may not produce any interference radiation, or transmit any interfering voltages into the mains exceeding a given, permitted value. The radiation from the probe is usually insignificant because frequencies of 0.5 to 10 MHz produce relatively long electromagnetic waves of which only very little is radiated from the small surface of a probe. If the probe has an earthed front electrode, this source of radiation is eliminated completely. More serious is transmission through the mains, which can only be suppressed by a multiple filter in the mains lead close to the mains plug. However, such a filter is also very important for the operation of the instrument in that it suppresses interferences from the mains, caused, e.g. by the sparking of rotating motors connected to the same mains (see also 3.16).

Because of the filters in the mains supply with their discharge capacitors connected to the chassis of the instrument, the latter always has a certain potential to earth unless it is earthed via a third conductor in the connecting cable (in Germany according to VDE regulations). Without this precaution the instrument can produce unpleasant, although quite harmless, electrical shocks between apparatus and earth.

2.33 The Probes

2.331 Normal Probes

The probe contains the piezoelectric transducer which converts high-frequency voltages into ultrasonic waves. In the normal probe these waves are normal to the radiating surface, i.e. in the case of contact with a given specimen they enter its surface at right angles. In the case of angle probe a wedge-shaped body is inserted between the radiating surface and the piezoelectric plate. When in contact with a test piece the waves are then refracted at the interface and penetrate the specimen obliquely.

In the most simple application the piezoelectric plate is wetted slightly with a liquid and pressed against the surface of the test piece, the electric pulse being placed on the metallized back of the plate. If the test piece is of metal and earthed, it forms the second plate of a capacitor whose field excites the crystal. In the case of a very smooth and flat surface, the damping of the plate by the coupling is sufficient where moderately short pulses are required. Adequate damping can be obtained also in the case of less satisfactory surfaces by firmly cementing the crystals to such surfaces by means of a cementing layer of minimum thickness. In practice this method can be applied only where the crystal can remain on the test specimen for subsequent repetitions of the test. If heat-resistent cements and plates with a high Curie point (see 1.104) are used, the test can also be carried out at higher temperatures.

If no particularly sharp pulses are required, the crystal plate wetted with oil can be pressed from the inside against the flat bottom of a metal cup so that it radiates through its bottom into the test piece. For most practical applications, particularly in the case of single-probe operation, the transducer plate should have good intrinsic damping, which is achieved by cementing a damping body to its back (Fig. 2.38). The front of the transducer plate can then be used directly or via an intermediate layer for making contact with the test piece.

The damping body has several functions. In order to damp the oscillation of the crystal sufficiently its acoustic impedance should be high; it could consist of solid and hard materials, e.g. metal or porcelain. It should, however, also absorb the waves which cannot be prevented from entering it, so as not to produce interfering echoes. This requirement is not so easily met, because the complete probe must remain small and handy. Finally, in the case of thin crystal plates, the damping body gives the necessary mechanical support and it should therefore not be deformed when pressed upon. Materials such as vulcanized rubber and moulded fibre plastics are satisfactory for moderate demands at higher frequencies. Preferable are composite materials based on curable synthetic resins or rubber in which other powdery admixtures have been incorporated. Natural and synthetic rubber have higher intrinsic absorption than moulded resins but their mixing and vulcanizing is cumbersome.

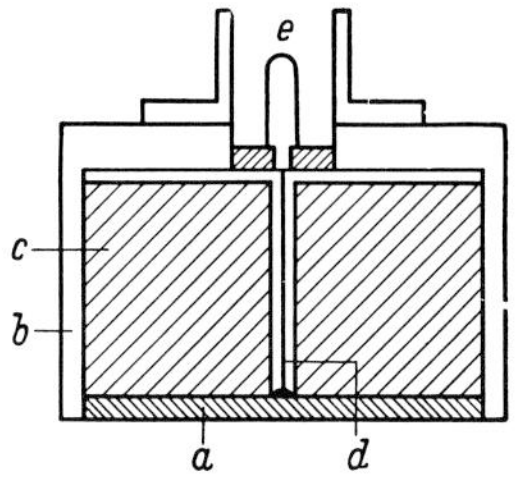

Fig. 2.38 Construction of a normal probe, schematic. *a* Piezoelectric plate; *b* metal case; *c* damping body; *d* lead; *e* plug.

The acoustic impedance can be increased by admixing metal powder or minium, and the absorption can be increased by adding finely ground materials, which combine high absorption with usually low mechanical strength. Attempts have also been made to scatter the waves by using sawdust or cellular structures. Such means, as well as disturbance of the plane reflection on the end of the damping body by oblique or sawtooth-shaped end faces, can be applied successfully only in combination with an already intrinsically effective absorption. Otherwise the various interfering echoes will be replaced by a background of *grass* behind the transmitting pulse.

If the content of admixed metal powder is high, the damping body can attain sufficiently high electrical conductivity for the high-frequency pulse. In the case of quartz the electrode can then be omitted but the damping body must be mounted insulated. However, barium titanate, with its high dielectric constant, definitely requires a metallic electrode directly on the piezoelectric plate.

The cementing layer between piezoelectric plate and damping body might again reduce the actual damping considerably, even in the case of a material of suitable properties. This layer should therefore be as thin as possible, or better still, eliminated completely by vulcanizing to the surfaces a rubber material or by applying to them pourable mixtures which are then cured.

A damping body attached to the back of the transducer damps mainly the thickness oscillation of the piezoelectric plate. However, interfering radial oscillations may also be present which are difficult to suppress, particularly in the case of barium titanate. They can be reduced by embedding the edge of the plate in the damping compound. In the case of thicker barium titanate plates, e.g. for 1 MHz and less, it is preferable to mill grooves into the plate from both sides to a depth of half its thickness which can then be filled with a damping compound (Fig. 2.39). Any radial oscillation can then be generated only in the smaller, interconnected sectional zones where they decay rapidly. The entire oscillator could of course also be constructed in the form of a mosaic with intermediate layers consisting of a damping compound.

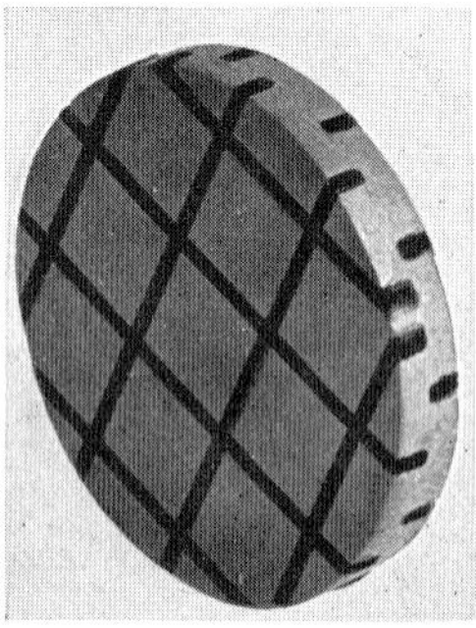

Fig. 2.39 Barium titanate plate with milled grooves for suppressing radial oscillations.

Good damping bodies can be characterized by the fact that they achieve attenuation of the backwall echo to 10^{-10} (200 dB) at a thickness of 4 mm for 4 MHz, and 9 mm for 1 MHz. In the case of quartz this damping gives mechanical Q-values of approx. 1 (see 1.102). Because of the loss in sensitivity which accompanies such strong damping, it is by no means always desirable. Therefore, usually less strongly damping materials are used, in which case a compromise has to be made between sensitivity and sharpness of pulse based on practical experience.

In the case of quartz and ceramic piezoelectric materials the most durable electrodes are obtained by spraying on liquid conducting silver, burned in at temperatures from 500 to 700 °C. The wires can then be soldered on with soft silver solder. In the case of barium titanate both the soldering on of wires and the milling in of grooves can be done after polarization if some care is taken. Lithium sulphate can be metallized by evaporating silver on the surface in vacuum or by painting the surface with cold-drying conducting silver. The wires should be glued on by means of a conducting cement.

If the front of the plate has to be used for direct contact, silver plating would not prove sufficiently resistant to the wear on surfaces to which the piezoelectric plate must be applied, which in practice are usually contaminated with very hard scale particles and impurities such as sand, resulting in excessive wear, particularly if the probe is applied by a sliding action, which can never be avoided completely. It is then preferable either to use a completely unprotected quartz plate whose gradual wearing off will have to be accepted, or the silver layer must be strengthened by applying a layer of copper and hard chrome with an overall thickness of a few tenths of a millimetre. This layer should be connected to the earth of the metal case via a metallized layer in an edgewise groove inside the

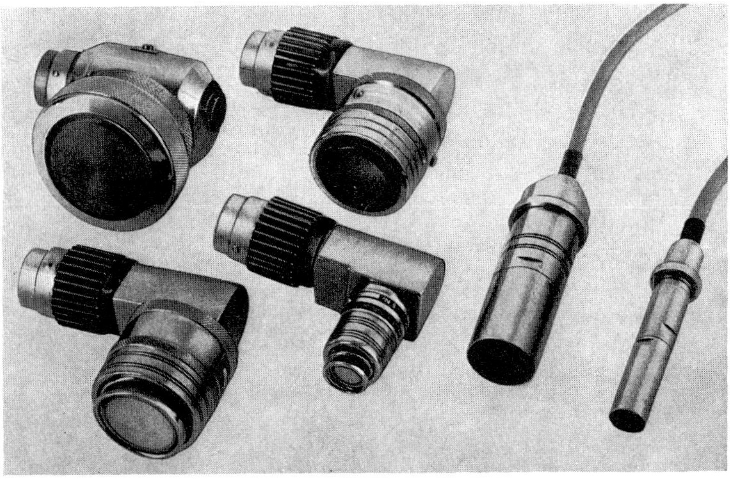

Fig. 2.40 Probes for pulse-echo method, top left for 1 and 2 MHz with metallised plate and plastic protective layer, bottom left for 4 and 6 MHz with non-metallised quartz plate and contact spring, right for 4 and 10 MHz with protective cover of epoxy resin for immersion testing.

probe because wires or strips soldered to the front may interfere. Such probes can also be used on non-metallic test pieces, e.g. porcelain, or test pieces with non-conducting coatings. In the case of unprotected probes it may be necessary to interpose thin metal foils or electrically conducting coupling liquids, e.g. water, to which if necessary additives have been added so as to increase both the viscosity and the conductivity.

A probe with non-metallized front requires an electric contact between its earth lead and the test piece. If this contact is unsatisfactory, the sensitivity becomes erratic and disturbances in the form of irregular pulse bursts, so-called *crackling*, appear on the viewing screen. A mount with metallic edge as shown in Fig. 2.38 no longer provides satisfactory contact once it has become worn. More satisfactory are spring-loaded projecting rings or simple spiral springs as in the case of some of the probes shown in Fig. 2.40.

Where maximum pulse sharpness and close-range resolution are not required, as is the case for most routine tests under rough operating conditions, it is preferable to prevent wear of the contact surface by means of a protective layer. Firmly attached protective layers of plastic material, whose wear can be reduced by admixing hard substances such as corundum powder, are being used. More durable are cemented-on thin discs of quartz or sapphire. However, where wear is excessive, the crystal will be destroyed and the probe can be repaired only by replacing the crystal. Thicker, metallic layers, such as steel foils firmly attached or cemented to the front have not proved successful. Usually readily exchangeable plastic foils are used; these are a few tenths of a millimetre thick and are stretched over the crystal by applying a little oil or grease (Fig. 2.40). Particularly suitable for this purpose are plastics with high resistance to wear and high absorption. Because of the thinness of the layer the high absorption has little influence on the sensitivity but it reduces multiple reflections in the layer, which could broaden the pulse [250].

Plastic intermediate layers as against direct contact have an additional advantage in that the coupling depends less on the pressing force and the roughness of the surface. This results from the fact that the acoustic impedance of the plastic material is much nearer to that of the coupling liquid than the acoustic impedance of the crystal; any change in thickness of the oil-filled gap therefore makes itself much less felt.

The problem of matching the transducer to the material of the test piece by means of intermediate layers of gradually changing acoustic impedance can be solved to some extent in the case of radiation in liquids with several layers in which the acoustic impedance decreases from layer to layer. Ideal matching would mean maximum sensitivity without lengthening the pulse by internal reflections. If only a single layer is used, its thickness should be a quarter wave length and its acoustic impedance the geometric mean of the acoustic impedance of the contiguous materials, viz. $\sqrt{W_1 W_2}$.

Most probes have circular radiating surfaces with diameters of approx. 5 to 40 mm. Diameters larger than 40 mm are unsuitable for most test problems because a corresponding flat contact surface is not available. The disadvantage of smaller diameters, particularly in the case of low frequencies, i.e. for large λ/D values, is the greater radiation of lateral transverse waves and surface waves as shown on page 58, Fig. 1.59. It should not be overlooked that the echoes of the various modes of waves cannot readily be distinguished. Another difficulty arising from the use of probes with small diameters is their greatly reduced sensitivity.

This results from the fact that the height of the backwall echo of a plate in the near field is proportional to the area of the transducer, but in the far field to the square of this area. Expressed differently, the sensitivity for backwall echoes in the far field decreases with the 4th power of the diameter. The first results from the fact that a piezoelectric receiver generates a receiving voltage which is proportional to its area if its terminating impedance is low (short-circuited), an assumption which will usually be a close approximation. The second then results from equation (1.38), where the initial sound pressure P_0 has to be proportional to the area of the transducer if transducers of different areas are compared. Where the transducer is operated as a transmitter, it is assumed that independently of its area it always receives the same transmitter voltage.

The corresponding length of the near field for the frequency range from 0.5 to 20 MHz can be read on the diagram, Fig. 2.41 top. The bottom diagram indicates the angle of divergence, on the left scale for γ_0 as calculated from Eq. (1.26) for the first zero of the directional characteristic, and on the right for γ_{70} for an echo height of 70% of the maximum height. While no real zero occurs in the sound beam of a pulse oscillator, α_{70} always furnishes valid data for the beaming accuracy of a given probe.

Example: An oscillator of 24 mm diameter has at 4 MHz a near field length of approx. 97 mm, $\gamma_0 = 4.3°$ and $\gamma_{70} = 1.3°$.

A good probe should have good sensitivity at long range and good resolution at close range. If, in order to meet the first requirement, the maximum diameter and the maximum frequency compatible with the attenuation in the given material, have already been chosen for a given piezoelectric transducer, the sensitivity can be still further increased only by reducing the damping. This, however, conflicts with the second requirement because it increases the length of the disturbed zone. With the piezoelectric material given, an optimal probe can be designed with regard to only one of the above two requirements.

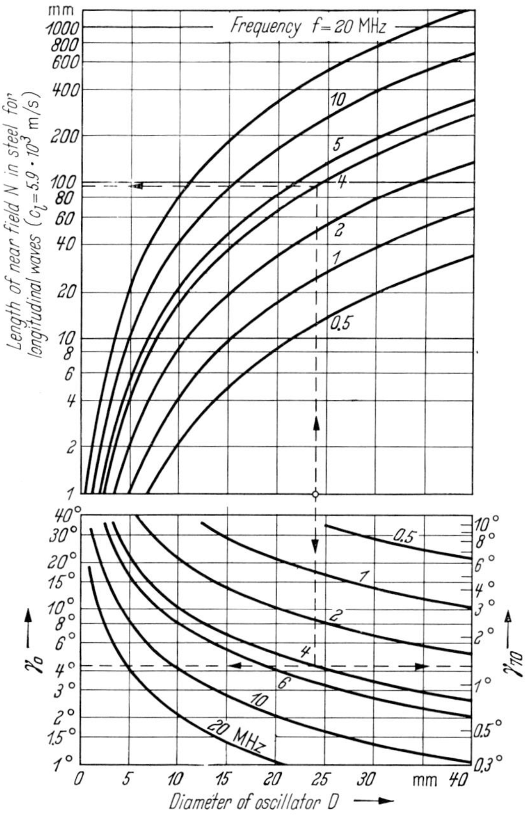

Fig. 2.41 Length of near field N, angles of divergence γ_0 and γ_{70} for probes with circular-disc oscillators of diameter D, calculated for steel and longitudinal waves (angle of divergence γ_{70} for echo height).

In the case of single-probe operation the close-range resolution is limited by the amplification characteristic of the dead zone as shown in Fig. 2.32. In this range TR (transmitting-receiving) operation is preferable if both the transmitter and the receiver are fitted with a "schnozzle" (coupling adaptor) and if the two probes are very carefully shielded from each other, both electrically and acoustically. Mechanically both probes can be combined in a single unit (Fig. 2.42) connected to the instrument by a twin cable to separate inputs for the transmitter and receiver.

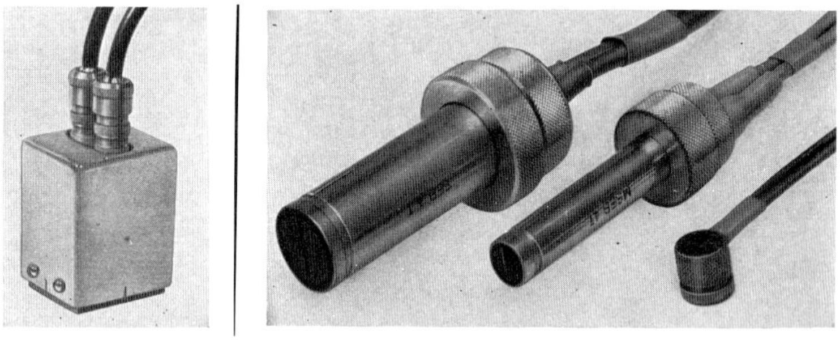

a b

Fig. 2.42 TR probes. a) Design Kelvin-Hughes, b) design Krautkrämer.

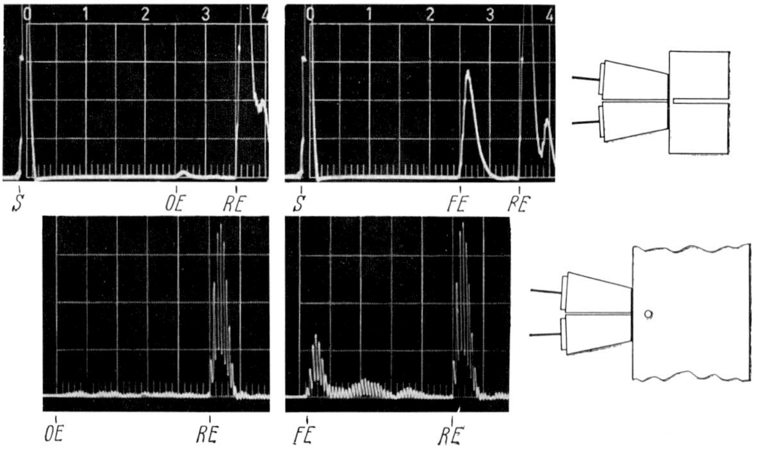

Fig. 2.43. Subsurface flaws as revealed by TR probe. Top: 4 MHz, flat-bottomed hole of 1.2 mm diameter, 2 mm below surface, aluminium 20 mm thick, *S* transmitting pulse, *OE* surface echo, *FE* flaw echo, *RE* backwall echo; bottom: 1 MHz, hole of 2 mm diameter parallel to surface and 5 mm below it, in grey cast iron (ASTM class 4) 100 mm thick, rough-cast surface, transmitting pulse shifted far to left, surface echo very weak. Screen traces on left side without, on right side with flaw indication.

As shown in Fig. 2.43 these probes can still detect flaws of a diameter and distance below the surface of the order of 1 wave length if the transducers are mounted at a flat angle relative to the surface. The transmitting pulse, which still "splashes over" electrically can also be shifted far to the left on the screen. The new zero position of the depth count is indicated by the surface echo very weakly only. It is preferable to determine the zero position by means of the backwall echoes of test blocks of known thickness. The "schnozzle" of the probe consists preferably of a low-absorption plastic material with satisfactory coupling through the coupling liquid even on rough surfaces, in contrast to metal.

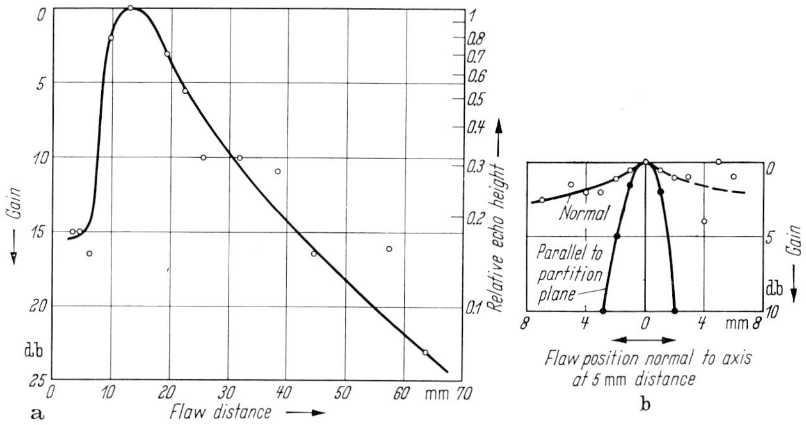

Fig. 2.44 Sensitivity curve in the field of a TR probe, design Krautkrämer, 4 MHz, measured in aluminium with flat-bottomed holes of 2 mm dia., coupling through thin layer of water. a) Gain in dB or relative echo height on axis as function of flaw distance; b) transverse to axis, normal and parallel to partition plane.

The sensitivity curve has the form of a ridge at the partition line of the two probes (Fig. 2.44). The sensitivity decreases rapidly with the distance. TR probes can, however, also be designed for greater testing depth by combining several transmitters and receivers alternately in one single unit (Kelvin and Hughes), which, however, fails to cover an unequivocal sensitivity zone immediately below the surface. Compared with single-probe operation they therefore offer no advantage.

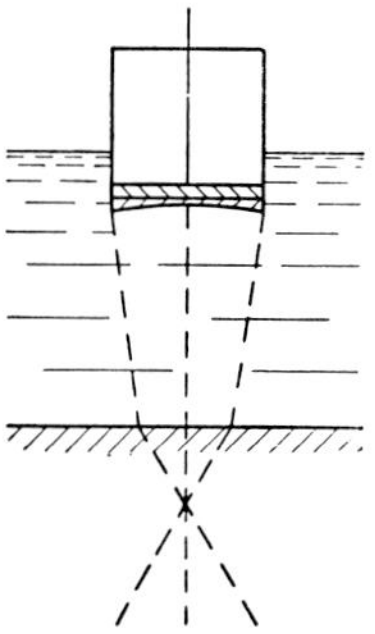

Fig. 2.45 Testing by the immersion technique with focused beam, schematic.

Occasionally focusing probes of special design are used to increase the sensitivity over a definite range for certain testing problems. For this purpose either a curved, ground, piezoelectric plate of ceramic material is used, or a curved layer with lens effect is cemented to the flat crystal plate. The latter method greatly increases the sensitivity immediately below the surface in the case of probes used according to the immersion technique (Fig. 2.45) where such a focusing layer is not subjected to wear. For testing by direct contact, curved transducer surfaces of barium titanate or quartz are suitably ground, or alternatively strips of quartz are assembled in the form of a cylinder (Fig. 2.46) for special testing purposes (round stock or forgings tested from holes). In the case of concave test surfaces and direct contact the sound beam would open wide, resulting in low depth sensitivity. This can be improved by inserting between the transducer and the test surface a lens-shaped body. This will produce a certain zone of disturbance which must be accepted, even if an absorbing material is used for the lens, such as vulcanized rubber which may contain fillers.

Special broad-beam probes (Fig. 2.47) are used for scanning large test pieces by the immersion technique, by means of which a track of up to 120 mm width can

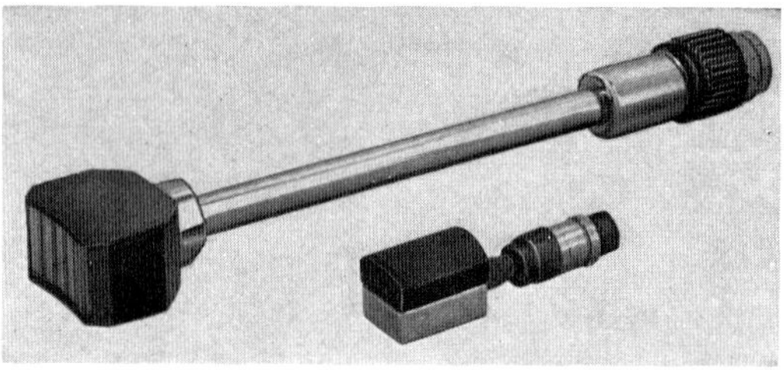

Fig. 2.46 Probes with cylindrical radiation surfaces, left concave with quartz strip mosaic for immersion tests, right convex cylindrical lens adaptor for testing from the inside of holes.

be covered in one run. These probes contain a number of crystals assembled so as to form long narrow rectangular oscillators. In aluminium and with 5 MHz they indicate flat-bottomed holes of 1.6 mm diameter and larger, at a maximum fluctuation of 15% of the echo height over a width of 120 mm. Such probes can also be used in combination with cylindrical ultrasonic lenses. At 10 MHz in aluminium, flaws of the above size could be indicated in the narrow focal zone at depths of 2 to 12 mm below the surface over a beam width of 75 mm ([10, Sec. 44]).

Conventional probes cannot be used at higher temperatures without taking certain precautions. Although they usually can withstand temperatures as low as approx. −20 °C, the maximum temperature may not exceed about 80 °C because of the usual cementing layer. Also the damping body, and in the case of barium titanate the crystal plate itself, cannot tolerate higher temperatures. For special probes quartz and lead niobate can be used (up to temperatures above 500 °C) and cast resins for the cementing layer and the damping bodies, some of which tolerate temperatures up to 350 °C. At still higher temperatures satisfactory damping is no longer possible. If the crystal plate becomes hot it may crack or spall. It is therefore usually preferable to couple via an intermediate piece, which can also be cooled. If the material used for this purpose is absorbing it has the advantage over metal or porcelain in that the multiple echoes returned from it are less disturbing (see also 3.115 and Fig. 3.237a). The above-mentioned heat-resistant cast resins may also be used for this purpose. Regarding coupling see 3.113.

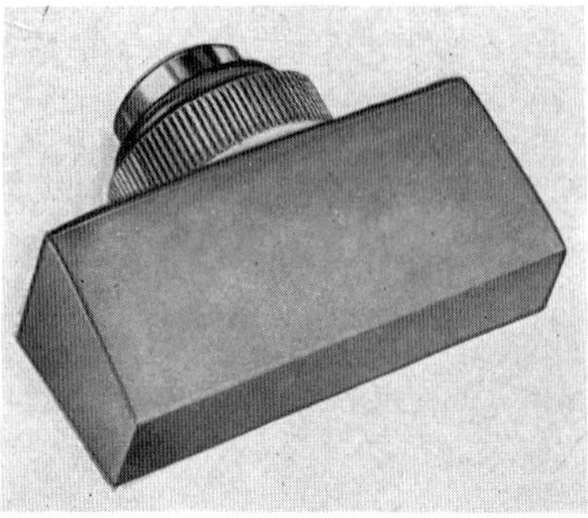

Fig. 2.47 Broad-beam probe for immersion technique (Curtiss-Wright Corp.).

2.332 Angle Probes

Refraction and conversion of wave modes are used for transmitting sound beams into test pieces at various angles to the surface; the relevant data are listed in Tables 5 to 8 in the Appendix for various contiguous materials and are characterized by their echo transmission.

In water over steel, i.e. when applying the immersion technique, any desired angle can be obtained in the test piece using both wave modes, by varying the angle of incidence between 0 and 27°. For contact testing it would similarly be possible to use a radiator for longitudinal waves mounted in a cup filled with liquid and with a bottom transmissive to sound. This arrangement has not proved to be successful in practice. Instead, rigid, wedge-shaped adaptors are used, Fig. 2.48, against which the piezoelectric transducers are pressed firmly, or to which they are cemented. Occassionally this wedge is designed as an adaptor which can simply be screwed to the normal probes (Réalisations Ultrasoniques), made for instance of perspex. However, if for accurate direction-finding of flaws the beam angle has to be known exactly, it is preferable to use angle probes which are supplied assembled for an angular range of 35 to 80° transverse waves with definite beam angles for a definite material.

a

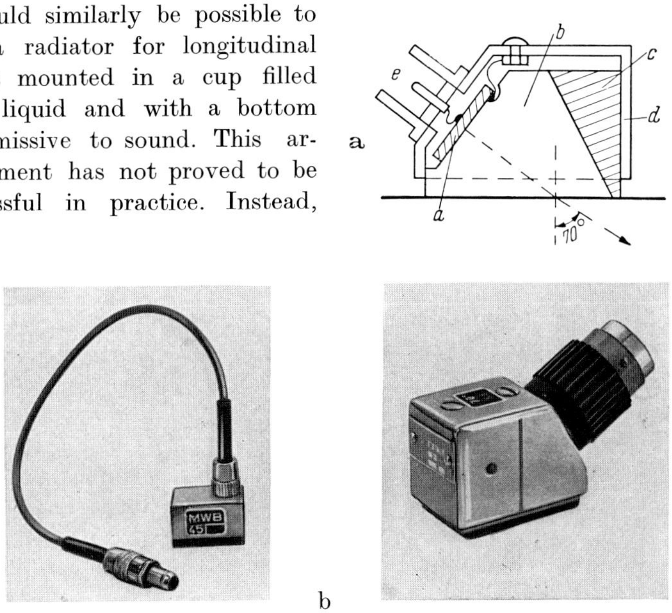

b

Fig. 2.48. Angle probes, design Krautkrämer. a) Crossection, schematic: *a* piezoelectric plate, *b* plastic wedge, *c* damping compound, *d* metal case, *e* plug; b) view of two different models for 2 and 4 MHz.

If the complete probe is housed in a protective case whose bottom edge is parallel to the beaming surface, the contact face, when much worn, can be ground repeatedly parallel to the metal edge and, whenever necessary, renewed by cementing on a new base without changing the beam angle. The exit point of the sound beam, from which the sound path and the sound angle is calculated for flaw-locating purposes (Fig. 2.48), can be permanently marked on the case.

The angular range up to nearly 90° in the test piece can be covered only if the sound at the entrance point is refracted away from the perpendicular, i.e. if the acoustic velocity in the wedge is smaller than in the test piece. If longitudinal waves are used in the test piece, which however will be done only in an emergency in the range of small angles in view of the always simultaneously present transverse wave at a different angle which can make interpretation of the echo ambiguous, according to Table A 1 (Appendix) many materials are on face value available for the wedge when testing in steel, e.g. besides plastics also metals such as copper, brass and lead. Usually, however, only the transverse wave is used for testing, which excludes all ambiguity in indication, while the sensitivity is high if one operates above the critical angle of total reflection for longitudinal waves. This requires that the wedge is made of a material whose longitudinal wave velocity is smaller than the transverse wave velocity in the test piece. In the case of aluminium and steel with $c_t = 3.1$ and $3.2 \cdot 10^3$ m/s, respectively, suitable plastics are available, such as perspex ($c_l = 2.7$) or polystyrene (2.4), which are therefore usually used. In the case of copper, however, with $c_t = 2.3$ the full angular range up to 90° could no longer be covered, nor in the case of grey cast iron with $c_t = 2.2$. Lead with $c_l = 2.2$ would be suitable for this purpose but according to [297] certain nylon grades with c_l from 1.69 to 2.60 are preferred. Soft rubber with $c_l = 1.5$ would also be suitable for this purpose.

Since most angle probes with perspex are supplied calibrated for steel, attention should be paid to the changed angle in the case of other materials, as given in Table 2.1 for some frequently used angle probes.

Table 2.1

Beam angle in steel	35°	45°	60°	70°	80°
Beam angle of transverse wave in					
Aluminium	33	42.4	55.5	63.4	69.6
Copper	23.6	29.7	37.3	41	43.4
Grey cast iron (mean value for lamellar cast iron)	23	28	35	39	41

In the case of 35° angle probes used on copper and grey cast iron there is present also a longitudinal wave at 57 and 55°, respectively. With these materials it is therefore preferable to use larger angles.

At the interface with the test piece part of the wave is reflected each time along the go and return path. The echo transmittance given in Tables 5 and 8 is a measure of the *efficiency*, which in the case of perspex/aluminium reaches its maximum because the acoustic impedances here differ least. For the same reason a wedge of lead would at first sight be more suitable for steel. However, the unavoidable liquid layer which must be applied during testing nullifies this advantage in practice. The loading of plastics with heavy-metal powders is also of little practical value besides introducing difficulties in uniform production.

Bradfield [51] has in this connection suggested the use of laminated wedges consisting of alternate layers of metal, such as steel or silver, and plastics such as araldite (a self-curing cement) (Fig. 2.49). Such wedges have the desired low acoustic velocity (approx. $2.5 \cdot 10^3$ m/s) combined with high acoustic impedance.

Even if the advantage of better matching is lost again due to the unavoidable oil layer when coupling to a surface which is not quite smooth, a heavy wedge-shaped body nevertheless has the advantage that the cemented-on piezoelectric transducer is better matched, which is particularly advantageous in the case of barium titanate.

Transverse waves can also be produced in the wedge itself, for instance by a firmly cemented-on Y-cut quartz. The plastic material with its high acoustic damping for transverse waves must then be replaced by a metal, preferably one with the lowest transverse wave velocity, e.g. copper. In the oil layer the wave naturally travels as a (steeper) longitudinal wave.

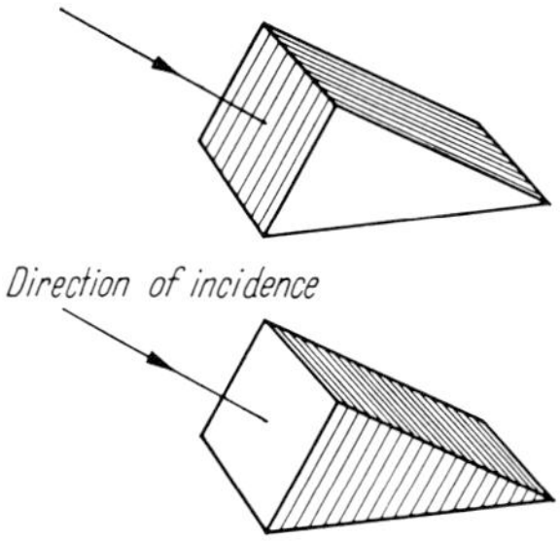

Fig. 2.49 Laminated wedges according to BRADFIELD.

LUTSCH and KÜHN [231] have investigated numerous combinations of materials and wave modes with a view to their suitability for pulse-echo testing by means of angle probes.

In most cases it is sufficient to damp the piezoelectric transducer by the wedge, also in the case of plastics, if no particularly high resolution is required. Otherwise it would be necessary to apply to the back an additional damping compound, particularly in the case of barium titanate which is otherwise difficult to dampen.

In the case of angle probes a special design problem is posed by the avoidance of interfering echoes immediately behind the transmitting pulse caused by the waves reflected at the interface which are then reflected back and forth in the wedge and in this way return to the transducer. This can be counteracted to some extent by using a wedge material with appreciable damping, such as perspex. Furthermore, the interference energy can be annihilated by sufficiently long transit paths of suitable shape, e.g. as shown in Fig. 2.50; for frequencies of about 2 MHz (as commonly used) and for lower frequencies this however results in somewhat unwieldy shapes. Space can be saved by using so-called anechoic traps in which the surface of the wedge-shaped bodies which reflect the waves are covered by layers which have low reflectivity and which strongly absorb the transmitted wave, such as fillings consisting of cast-resin compounds, cemented-on vulcanized

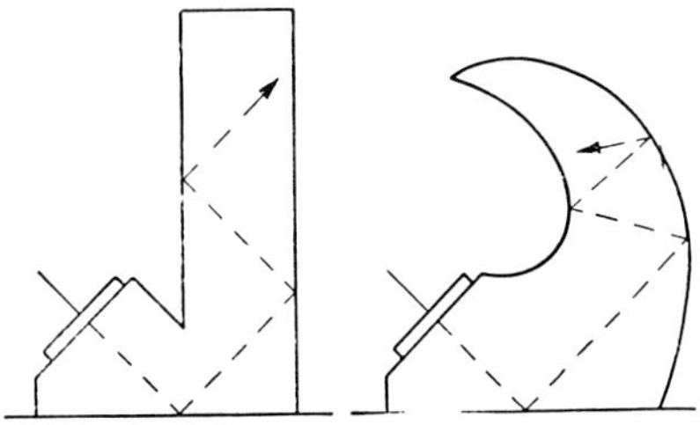
Fig. 2.50 Wedge shapes with long transits to reduce interfering reflections; on the right: Ultrasonoscope design.

rubber compounds containing fillers which increase the absorption, and so forth. In addition the rest of the reflected wave can be dissipated by deforming the affected surfaces into sawtooth or conically pointed shapes, or drilled holes filled with an absorbing compound. In the case of high gain these disturbances can, however, not be eliminated completely because a portion is always scattered back to the transducer directly from the contact point, particularly on rough surfaces.

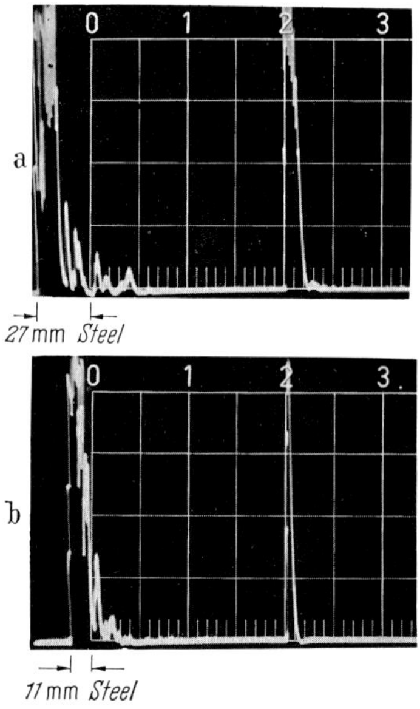

Fig. 2.51 Screen traces of angle probes with echo from a distance of 100 mm in steel. a) Angle probe for 2 MHz, 70°; b) 4 MHz, 70°, scale: 1 scale division = 50 mm steel.

Fig. 2.51 shows screen traces from barium titanate angle probes on perspex, indicating the zero shift and the zone of interference. Both the divisions and the scale zero were calibrated by using a special test body (see also 2.333). Because of the path in perspex the zero error is considerably greater than for normal probes, viz. at 2 MHz approx. 27 mm, and 11 mm in the case of the smaller 4 MHz probe. The length of the interfering zone depends on the gain used. To be able to adjust the gain reproducibly one can use the echo of a semi-cylinder as shown in Fig. 2.52b. The *standard gain* is then chosen so that the resultant echo just reaches its full height on the screen, or a definite height in mm. Flaw location requires a considerably higher gain. Therefore, in Fig. 2.51 the gain is set at 10 times the standard value.

If a given testing problem requires a beam angle smaller than 35° in steel, refracted

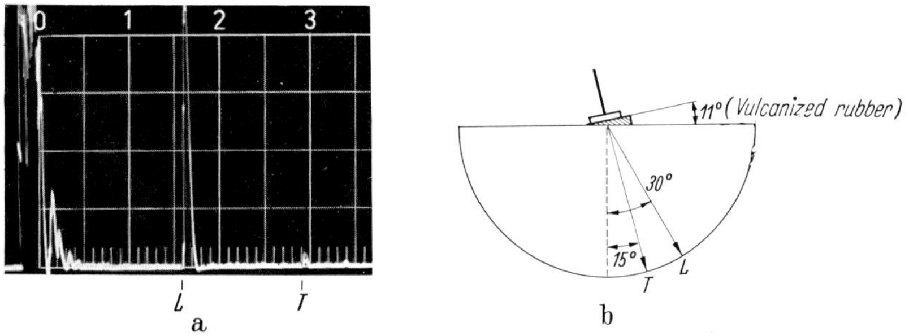

Fig. 2.52 Testing with beam angles of less than 35°. a) Screen trace showing the echoes of both the longitudinal and shear wave; b) probe placed on semicircular steel cylinder.

longitudinal waves have to be used. A disadvantage is the simultaneous appearance of a shear wave. As shown in Fig. 2.52a this shear wave is, however, very weak. In order to reduce the interfering zone to a minimum, a strongly aborbing material such as vulcanized rubber should be used for such probes in the case of flat wedges. Probes for this purpose are not as yet available in mass production.

Some testing problems require that the beam angle be adjusted continuously. Fig. 2.53 shows various possible solutions. In the case of the first design according to MESH [257] two plastic wedges are rotated against each other, one of which mounts the transducer. With equal wedge angles, any angle between zero and double the wedge angle can be obtained. The rotation changes the plane of incidence. The second design makes use of a plastic semi-cylinder with a cemented-on transducer mounted in a plastic block. In this design the plane of incidence remains constant but the beam exit point is shifted. In the third design, also the beam exit point remains practically constant.

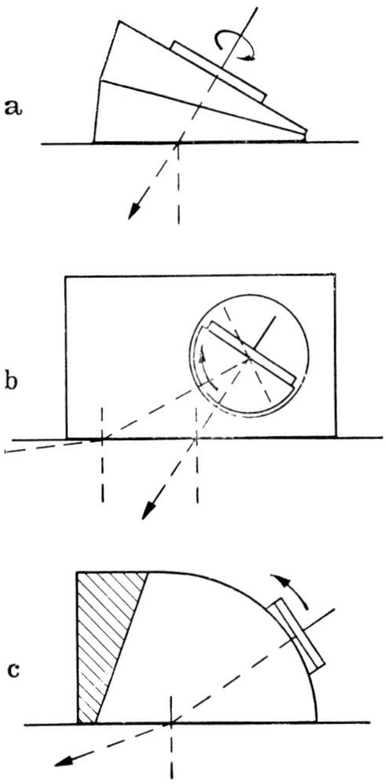

Fig. 2.53 Angle probes with continuously adjustable beam angle.

Fig. 2.54 shows a construction in accordance with the first and third solution, respectively. In the latter the transducer is shifted by means of a precision gear. The transducer case is filled with oil and sealed. This eliminates the cleaning and oiling of the sliding face which would otherwise be necessary after prolonged use. The angle is read through a window.

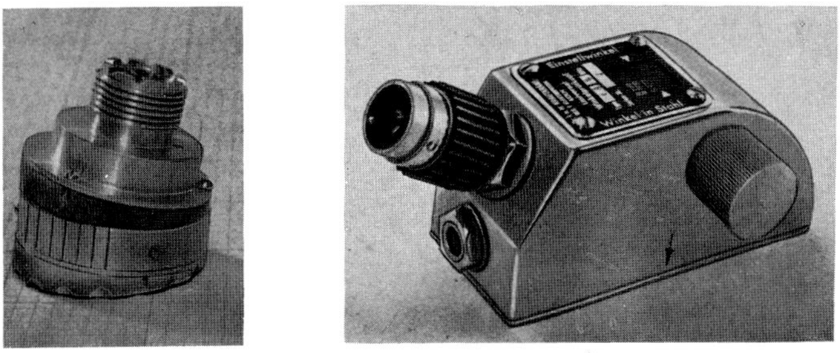

a b

Fig. 2.54 Adjustable angle probes. a) Design Ultrasonoscope (same system as in Fig. 2.53); b) design Krautkrämer (as in Fig. 2.53c).

A sound beam can be swung through small angles on either side of the perpendicular if the transducer is subdivided into individual units spaced close to each other, which receive the transmitting voltage at different phase shifts. Such a probe has been constructed by BRADFIELD [51]; it contains a switchable delay network by means of which the two angles of $\pm 4°$ and $\pm 8°$ can be introduced. The 2.5 MHz transducer consists of a barium titanate plate subdivided into strips by milled grooves. Using rotating switches and synchronized control of a CR tube it would be possible to map the zone covered in the test piece by applying methods similar to those used in radar technique.

This method permits very rapid switching on of selected angles. Devices as shown in Fig. 2.53b with rotatable beam are used for continuous scanning, in which the cylindrical insert unit with the transducer is swung back and forth by a motor or rotated continuously. Although this provides only scanning frequencies of approximately 10/s, this is sufficient, when using CR tubes with long after-glow, to produce an image.

For producing surface waves conventional angle probes are used, in which the perspex angle is chosen slightly greater than required for obtaining a grazing (with 90°) beam of transverse waves in the test piece. These probes therefore function properly only with a test piece of a given material.

When using angle probes on curved surfaces, interfering surface waves are frequently obtained (see also 3.112); this happens also on flat surfaces if the axial beam has an angle of 80° and more, so that the lateral beams at a larger angle already strike the boundary surface in the region of surface waves. On smooth surfaces these surface waves can be very strong but they can be recognized readily by touching their tracks with a finger dipped in oil because this strongly damps them. On the other hand, in the case of probes with a 35° angle, disturbing longitudinal waves, due to the divergence of the beam, are easily produced by lateral beams at angles smaller than the critical. These waves are propagated at large angles (60 to 90°) and unfortunately they cannot be distinguished so easily from transverse waves.

The least trouble by disturbing waves therefore occur at angles between 45 and 70°. As indicated by the curve of echo transmittance (Tables 5 to 8) all angles in this range give approximately the same sensitivity. This means that the directional characteristic of the transducer is not appreciably distorted. With an angle of 80° for the axial beam, the beams on the periphery with a smaller angle are at an advantage, and those with a larger angle at a disadvantage. The irradiation lobe is therefore strongly distorted towards smaller angles and its position depends on the angle of divergence of the transducer, i.e. on the size of the crystal plate and the frequency. Accurate measurements of the angle and direction finding, are therefore hardly possible.

Absorption by the wedge material causes a certain amount of distortion of the directional characteristic because the rays from different points of the transducer are not uniformly attenuated. The beam which strikes the interface is *attenuated transversely*. This also shifts the actual exit point towards the thin end of the wedge as compared with the penetration point of the axial rays.

Special probes as used for certain testing problems will be discussed together with these problems in Sec. 3.2.

2.333* Calibrating and Checking Methods for Probes

After manufacture, as well as after prolonged use, the characteristics of the probes should be checked. The most important factor is the *sensitivity*, i.e. the height of an echo trace on the screen under given conditions. The stability as a function of time of a given probe, which is used in combination with an instrument at a given adjustment, can be checked easily by means of any test body in which artificial or natural flaws produce echoes which are still within the modulation range, i.e. which produce deflections on the screenwhich are neither too small nor greater than the deflection range on the screen. This method can also be used for comparing probes of the same type. Suitable test blocks of simple, light and reproducible form have been manufactured from plastics such as perspex, which as a result of their damping, even at maximum gain and pulse intensity of a given instrument, still permit reliable deductions regarding the sensitivity to be made on the basis of the number of multiple echoes returned from a given depth. For instance, if the number of obtainable multiple echoes is given, this can be regarded as a sensitivity parameter for a given model of the probe and a given instrument.

Cylinders of 40 to 50 mm diameter and 20 to 100 mm long, have been suggested and used for this purpose. Such perspex standards are installed in some instruments or supplied with them. For use also on non-metallized probes, one face of the standard is made conducting by a silver coating; this has given better performance than a glued-on metal foil. The influence of non-uniformity in the production of the material or of ageing does not seem to be excessive; a disadvantage is however a pronounced temperature-dependence of the absorption.

This method can also be used for checking angle probes if they are placed on a semi-cylinder of plastic material, as shown in Fig. 2.52. In this case, naturally, only a longitudinal wave is transmitted in the test body.

This method cannot be used for comparing different probes or different instruments. For instance, two different probes placed on a test piece of steel may show behaviour precisely opposite to that on a perspex column because their matching may be different. In 1.84 the backwall echo of a thin plate has been mentioned as a suitable type of reference echo, which latter should be just outside the dead zone but if possible shall appear before the end of the near field. For angle probes we can choose a suitable wedge-shaped body, or better still, because suitable for any angle, a semi-cylinder as mentioned above, whose radius is smaller than the near field length. If the material chosen is steel, the most common material to be tested, the stated echo height furnishes a sensitivity parameter which is comparable for all models of probes and instruments and which can readily be checked in practice as long as the test is carried out on steel. In the case of probes for immersion testing it is, however, preferable to measure also the backwall echo of the plate by immersion testing. The material, as well as the thickness, is non-critical and therefore readily reproducible because its damping is of no importance at the small thicknesses involved, as long as the frequencies used are not too high (above 10 MHz) or the material grossly contaminated.

Since the plate echo is usually very large, the gain must be greatly *reduced* for the echo to fall into the modulation range. For the older instruments it is difficult to quote comparable and reproducible data concerning the required gain. This requires a *calibrated gain control* as described in 2.323. If the plate echo obtained with a given probe is then adjusted to the reference height by adjusting the calibrated gain control accordingly, a difference of, say 60 dB compared with the maximum gain may remain. Thus, a very much weaker echo can still be increased to the reference height, viz. 60 dB below the plate echo (= 1/1000). The numerical value of 60 dB is the sensitivity measure. This contains the transmitting energy, the sensitivity of the probe, and the gain of the whole instrument, but it makes no statement regarding the properties of the test body except its material and its surface condition. If in addition one specifies for the latter a uniform processing method, e.g. smoothing which was found to be superior to grinding, this supplies data valid for every instrument and probe and which furthermore are in agreement with practical experience.

If the sensitivity of a probe alone has to be given, such a probe should be regarded as a transducer of power, i.e. the power received as plate echo is referred to the transmitted power of the transmitting pulse. This requires that not only the voltage but also the impedance be measured by electronic methods. Any data concerning the sensitivity and referred exclusively to the voltages, are in agreement with data referred to powers only if the transmitter is matched optimally to the probe, and the probe in turn optimally to the amplifier. This, however, is possible only in the case of TR-operation, whereas in single-probe operation miss-matching must be expected because the output impedance of the transmitter is usually much smaller than the input impedance of the amplifier. Therefore, if it is intended to check a probe alone, only power sensitivity is comparable. In practice, however, determination of the combined sensitivity of instrument and probe will be found more useful.

A further important property is the *close-range resolution* or *dead zone* or interference zone; this refers to the distance at the beginning of the depth scale, given for instance in millimetres of steel, at which a given flaw echo cannot be amplified undisturbed as at long distance because of the trailing oscillations of the transducer or amplifier, or of jamming of the amplifier. This test therefore also covers both instrument and probe as a single unit.

As long as the trailing oscillations of the probe predominate, particularly in the case of probes with little damping, it is sufficient for a rough evaluation to read simply the length of the interfering zone on the screen. This presupposes, however, that a definite sensitivity setting has been agreed upon to be able to compare the evaluation for a given combination of both instrument and probe with that for any other arbitrary combination. For this purpose it is again preferable to use the plate echo of a steel plate with minimum thickness in relation to the near-field length of the probe, but in such a way that the echo is still outside the interfering zone to be measured. The plate echo is then first adjusted to the reference height (or, because the gain required for this purpose is usually very small, the gain is adjusted by means of the calibrated gain control to a value corresponding to 10 or 100-fold overmodulation by adjusting to 20 or 40 dB above this value). Using a normal probe the interfering zone can now be measured either with the probe coupled or free. In the first case the interfering zone depends largely on the surface quality and the pressure, particularly where the transducer is in direct contact. It is therefore preferable to measure this zone while the transducer is oscillating without making contact. Because it is practically impossible to excite them in this way, non-metallized probes then show almost no interfering zone. They should therefore be excited, but without being coupled acoustically. For this purpose they are placed on a dry metal surface, preferably dry, fine-mesh wire netting. In the case of protected probes and angle probes the difference is not considerable but here also it is always preferable to measure the interfering zone without coupling, i. e. dry. When coupled, this zone can only improve.

In view of the fact that strong interfering echoes are in practice more troublesome than a little *grass* behind the transmitting pulse, the interfering zone can also be evaluated according to the height of the interfering echoes, e. g. interferences exceeding 1/2 screen height up to 15 mm steel, above 1/10 screen height up to 30 mm steel. Naturally this presupposes that the amplifier has a linear characteristic. Since this is frequently not the case, particularly if the echoes are small, reliable and accurate measuring requires a movable measuring pulse, as shown for instance in Fig. 2.31. If the measuring pulse is shifted closer, interference with stray oscillations occurs, even if the latter are suppressed by non-linearity. The echo becomes periodically greater and smaller. The length of the interfering zone can be defined as the distance over which the echo first decreases by more than 1 dB (10%) as a consequence of such interference. In this way the dead zone can be measured even if no actual disturbances are discernible on the screen behind the transmitting pulse, either because the trailing oscillations of the probe, as a result of very effective damping, are in fact too small, or because they appear suppressed at this point as a consequence of non-linearity of the amplifier.

In some cases it is desirable to know also the true transmitted *frequency* of the ultrasonic pulse. This frequency can be measured by means of an interferometer according to Fig. 2.31, by bringing the test echo to coincidence with the plate echo. If both echoes are adjusted to about half screen height, strong interferences are then obtained during shifting. The distance in water, which can be read accurately between two or more maxima or minima, provides one or more half wave lengths (because of the go *and* return path in water) which can be used to calculate the frequency on the basis of the known velocity of sound in water (if necessary making allowance for the temperature). In certain circumstances the frequency at the beginning of the pulse can differ greatly from that at the end of the pulse (see 3.62, Fig. 3.239).

Because of the parallel-connected probe in the interferometer section, the frequency in this measurement may be slightly changed. It is therefore preferable to measure the echo frequency by placing the echo in its high-frequency form at the output of the high-frequency amplifier, on an oscillograph with large and accurately known sweep magnification, as Figs. 2.27a and b were obtained. This also gives the exact form of the pulse, permitting definition of the pulse width, e.g. as length in mm of steel, if both the build-up and the decay oscillations are considered from a definite height onwards, e.g. above 10% of the maximum amplitude. For the pur-

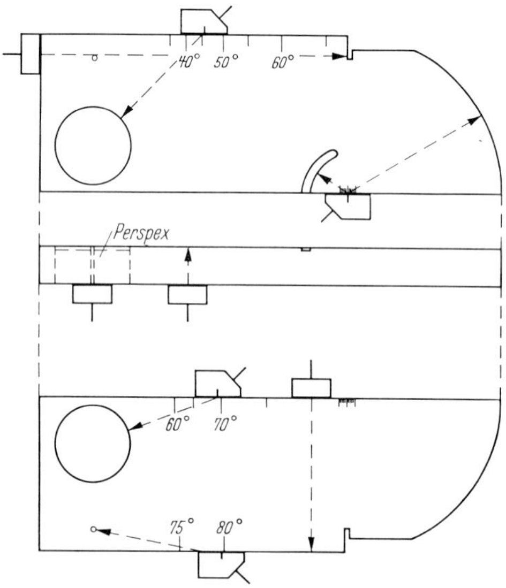

Fig. 2.55 Test block for calibrating the depth scale of an instrument with normal probes for longitudinal waves, with angle probes for transverse waves, for determining the beam exit point, and for measuring the beam angle on angle probes and for checking the stability of the sensitivity of normal probes placed on a perspex column.

pose of comparison these data are preferable to other definitions of the *long-range resolving power* (in contrast to close-range resolution) which have been tried, in which the echoes of closely spaced artificial flaws are used. In the latter case certain amplifier characteristics intervene which as a result of more or less intentional *trace cosmetics* may simulate resolution, i.e. separation of different echoes.

In order to measure the *directional characteristic*, the probe, with unchanged coupling conditions, is moved in a straight line across the test body containing a flat-bottomed pocket hole of minimum dimensions which acts as reflector. Coupling conditions of maximum stability are obtained by using the immersion technique and an adequate distance in water. This requires that the angle of divergence of the reflector characteristic of the flaw far exceeds that of the probe. Should this prove impossible, it is preferable to measure the lobe radiated into a semi-cylinder according to Fig. 2.52 by means of a movable probe placed on the shell in TR operation. The directional characteristic of the *echo* obtained by the first method is the square of the directional characteristic of the *radiation* obtained by the second method.

The radius of the semi-cylinder should be large enough to ensure that the measurement is made in the far field.

When measuring the *near-field length* of the probe, which is important when determining the size of a flaw, and which cannot be calculated reliably from the diameter and the frequency [207], it is necessary to measure the echo height of a plate, once as close as possible and again in the far field. For this purpose a calibrated gain control is recommended. The near-field length can then be calculated from equation (1.40) or according to Fig. 1.87 provided the measurements in the far field are not vitiated by the absorption of the material. However, since this is usually the case, materials of accurately known absorption should be used and the correction factor should be taken into consideration. This is possible with water. Normal probes with water delay lines and sufficiently large reflectors are therefore used. Their reflecting power is thereby cancelled out and so can be ignored. For angle probes one should use test bodies of very homogeneous metals, viz. light-metal alloys or high-quality steels whose absorption must be determined separately.

In order to check the deviation of the beam axis from the perpendicular to the radiation surface when using normal probes, which may happen occasionally in the case of faulty crystals, it is preferable to use the immersion technique and small reflectors which can be rotated excentrically around the perpendicular. If the probe were coupled directly to a suitable test body with an excentric flaw, the coupling conditions would vary excessively during rotation.

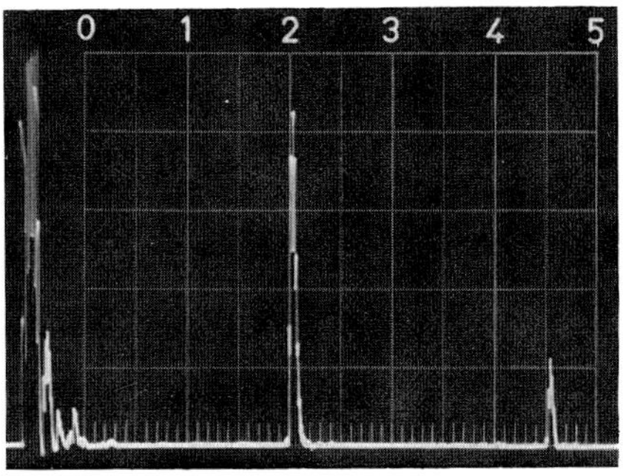

Fig. 2.56 Screen trace obtained after adjusting both zero point and distance of the scale of a pulse-echo instrument with angle probes, using the test block shown in Fig. 2.55, with 100 mm echo of cylindrical face, and 225 mm echo of a further reflection on the cylindrical groove.

When angle probes are used for accurate location of flaws, it must be possible to measure and check both the beam exit point on the probe and the beam angle; because of wear of the contact face of angle probes this check must be made more frequently than on normal probes. This is particularly important when testing welded seams. The International Institute of Welding, IIW, has therefore recommended the use of a special test block which is shown in Fig. 2.55. The beam exit point is determined by the reflection on a cylindrical face as described above. The centre of curvature is marked and indicates the beam exit point on the probe when the echo has reached a maximum. The beam angle is read on calibrated scales by tracing the maximum echo of the large cylindrical hole from the long, narrow sides of the test block.

For distance calibration and zero check with normal probes the dimensions 25, 100 and 200 mm are used. With angle probes the calibration of the scale and the zero check are made simultaneously as follows: if the beam exit point is in the centre of the cylinder, a first echo is obtained from a distance of 100 mm, and a further echo after reflection at the contact point and at the milled cylindrical groove of 25 mm radius around the centre. The second echo appears at 100 + 125 = 225 mm. By alternately expanding and shifting the screen trace relative to the scale, both echoes can be positioned correctly so that the zero point will be corrected automatically (Fig. 2.56). In this way the most important range for testing welded seams (250 mm) can be calibrated at the beginning, the approximate centre, and the end of the scale.

Except for minor changes this IIW test block has been taken over also by the German Standards Committee. Among these changes may be mentioned the replacement of the quarter-circle groove by two lateral saw cuts, with the result that the second echo in Fig. 2.56 no longer appears at 225 mm but at 200 mm [430, 271].

2.34 Instruments for the Pulse Transit Time Method[1]

The first pulse-echo instruments were put on the market in 1943, almost simultaneously by Messrs. Sperry Products Inc., Danbury, USA, and Kelvin & Hughes Ltd., London.

A few instruments of different manufacture are shown in Chapter 3. With the advances in electronics, these instruments, compared with the early days, have become much smaller and lighter while their performance has improved, e.g. with regard to sensitivity and resolving power. The use of transistors has led to a separate development series, viz. miniaturized instruments weighing as little as 10 lbs, while the larger instruments using valves still weigh about 40 lbs.

The latter are usually mains-operated. They incorporate a large number of electronic features which make them equally suitable for manual testing, use in automated installations, and as scientific measuring instruments in the laboratory: frequency range about 0.5 to 20 MHz, testing range 10 mm to 10 m in steel with correspondingly calibrated, accurate scale or electronic time markers, large CR tubes of at least 100 mm screen diameter and great brightness due to post acceleration voltages of up to 12 kV. Both the gain and the pulse energy can be controlled in several stages, frequently by means of precision controls, e.g. by stepping switches calibrated in dB. The amplifier characteristic as well as the amplifier gain as a function of the testing depth are variable. Where a monitor has not yet been installed, connections are provided for it as well as for other auxiliary instruments for use in automation and data processing. These instruments resemble the well-known CR oscilloscopes, but in view of their use as portable equipment they are usually stronger and easier to carry.

[1] See footnote p. 135.

The transistorized and miniaturized instruments use storage batteries which supply the necessary power of a few watts for approximately 4 to 12 hours. In some models exchangeable batteries are included to make continuous operation possible. Others contain both a battery and a charging unit. To save both space and power, CR tubes with screen diameters of only 50 to 70 mm must be accepted. This disadvantage can be compensated to some extent by installing a large magnifier lens (Krautkrämer, model USK 4 and 5). Incorporation of the numerous controls of the large instruments can be sacrificed because the miniaturized instruments are used exclusively for manual operation. Some of them, however, are already fitted with a simple go/no-go monitor (see 2.352).

Some of the more important manufacturers are:

Automation Industries Inc., Inspection Equipment Division (previously Sperry Products), Danbury, Conn./USA
Branson Instruments, Stamford, Conn./USA
Karl Deutsch, Wuppertal, Germany
Dr. J. and H. Krautkrämer, Cologne, Germany
Dipl.-Ing. P. Kretz, Zipf, Austria
Dr. Lehfeldt & Co., GmbH, Heppenheim, Germany
Magnaflux Corporation, Chicago, USA
Réalisations Ultrasoniques, Meaux, S. et M., France
Smith, Industrial Division, London, England (previously Kelvin & Hughes)
Sonatest Ltd., London, England
Ultrasonoscope Co. Ltd., London, England
VEB Funkwerk Erfurt, GDR
VEB Carl Zeiss, Jena, GDR

Data concerning Russian and Polish instruments may be found in [22] and [98], respectively. Finally, there are the instruments for the testing methods which include no radiator but use instead the magnetostrictive excitation of ultrasonic waves in the test piece itself, such as the Stalitron of VEB Funkwerk, Dresden, and the Ferrotron of Messrs. Dipl.-Ing. W. Kaule GmbH, Heidberg, Distr. Cologne. Externally these instruments resemble the conventional pulse-echo instruments (see Fig. 3.130) but they use a spark gap for generating the required high current pulses. All of them use separate coils for transmitter and receiver. The form and arrangement of the coils depend on the shape of the test piece and the desired wave mode. For example, for the detection of longitudinal surface cracks in bar stock, narrow, flat coils are used; these are adapted to the cylindrical test piece and are slightly inclined relative to the longitudinal direction. For further details see 3.251, testing of rod material. For other semi-finished products this method is still in the development stage.

Regarding special instruments for testing concrete, see 3.45.

2.35 Auxiliary Instruments for the Pulse Transit Time Method

2.351 High-precision transit time measurements

Measurements of the transit time, as described in Sec. 3.62, are used for wall thickness measurements and for determining moduli of elasticity. The usual accuracy when taking readings on the viewing screen with the aid of calibrated scales or electronic time markers is mostly inadequate for this purpose. The following methods are used instead.

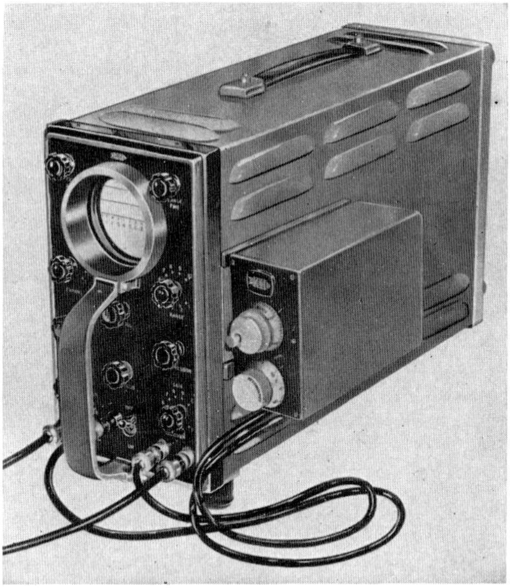

Fig. 2.57 Kelvin & Hughes Mark V flaw detector with thickness gauge attachment.

To measure an unknown transit time, a second probe with coupled variable delay line is connected in parallel (as shown in Fig. 2.31), and both echoes are brought to coincidence; this can be determined accurately by the interference fluctuations. The transit time is then deduced from the measured transit distance and the known velocity of sound in the delay line. Usually liquid delay lines are used in which a reflector can be shifted along a precision scale. Such a delay line is the depth and thickness gauge for the Mark V instrument of Smiths (Kelvin & Hughes, see Fig. 2.57), with a 25 mm liquid transit section, which thus can measure up to approx. 100 mm in steel. The control knob for shifting the reflector is directly calibrated in steel thickness. Messrs. Krautkrämer manufacture an open-type *Interferometer* (Fig. 2.58a) with a 200 mm transit section in which conventional probes can be mounted. This instrument can also be used for measuring the acoustic velocity in other liquids. According to [22] the Russian instrument USD 7 contains a built-in, variable liquid delay line based on the principle shown in Fig. 2.59. Finally, Messrs. Ultrasonoscope manufacture a dry delay line in the form of a nickel tube in which ultrasonic pulses are excited and received magnetostrictively. The transmitter-receiver coil can be shifted (Fig. 2.58).

A dry-type interferometer can also be operated with surface waves radiated and received by a cemented-on probe. The movable reflector consists of a knife-edge pressed dry against the surface (FIRESTONE [106]).

An interferometer of sound mechanical construction can reach and exceed an accuracy of 0.2% if the measurements are made carefully; for the following devices which are used to measure wall thicknesses and

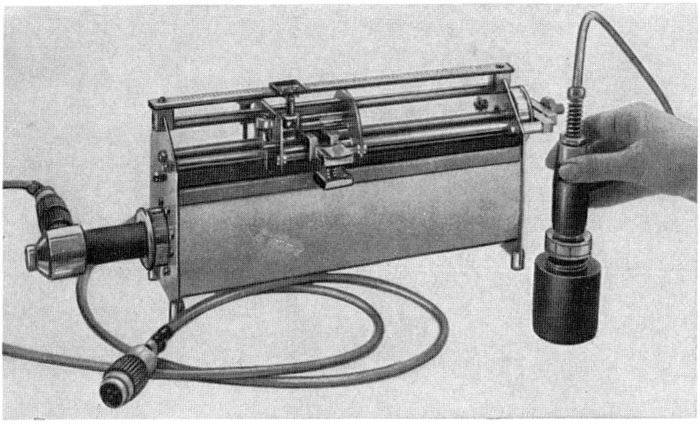

a

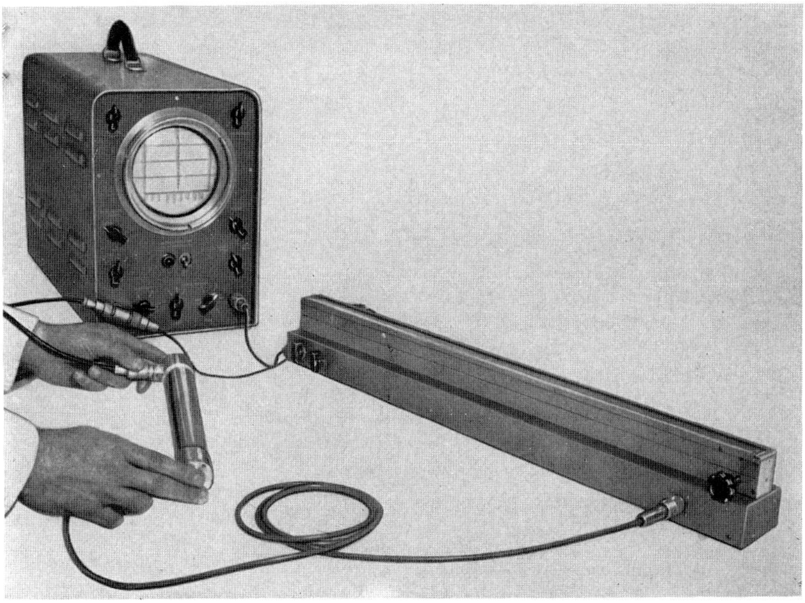

b

Fig. 2.58 a) Interferometer attachment, design Krautkrämer, with mounted normal probe and interconnected attenuator, a Y-cut probe being placed on the sample, both probes connectable to the instrument by a twin cable. b) Magnetostrictive delay line (Ultrasonoscope) with sample and pulse-echo instrument.

transit times, the accuracy is slightly lower, approx. 0.5 to 1%. According to KRAUTKRÄMER [200] it is advantageous to refer wall thickness measurements and transit times to a frequency measurement of the multiple echo repetition whose time intervals equal the transit time.

This *echo repetition frequency*, also called *travel frequency* because the transmitter pulse *travels* back and forth between the front wall and backwall, should not be confused with the pulse repetition frequency nor the ultrasonic frequency being used. The latter should merely be chosen as high as possible as compared with the echo repetition frequency in order to obtain echoes of minimum width from the wall, which are still clearly separated even in the case of thin walls, and which by their repetition sharply define a given frequency. The pulse repetition frequency should merely be low enough to leave enough time for the formation of an echo repetition between the individual transmitting pulses.

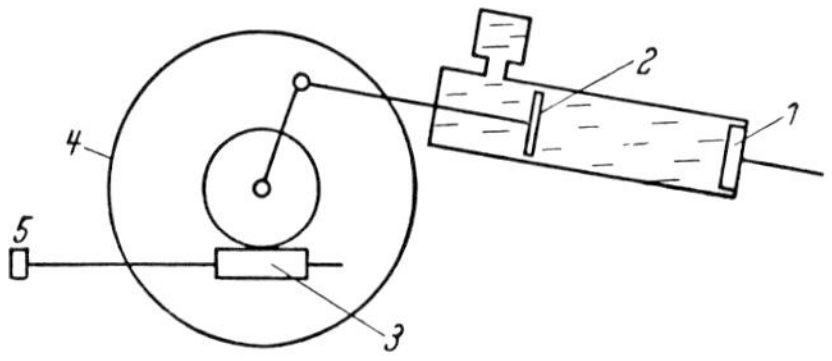

Fig. 2.59 Variable delay line of Russian instrument USD-7. *1* Transmitter-receiver quartz; *2* reflector; *3* precision gear and excentric for shifting the reflector; *4* scale; *5* control knob.

Fig. 2.60 shows the basic circuit diagram for a practical application of the method. A tuneable resonant circuit is connected to the output of the amplifier (behind the Video stage) and one of the leads to the deflection plates of the CR-tube. Fig. 2.61 shows the screen traces, above without, and below with connected resonant circuit. The transmitting pulse alone excites the resonant circuit according to its characteristic frequency; the damped oscillation is visible. If the multiple echoes from a given test plate are added when the probe is placed on it, each of these

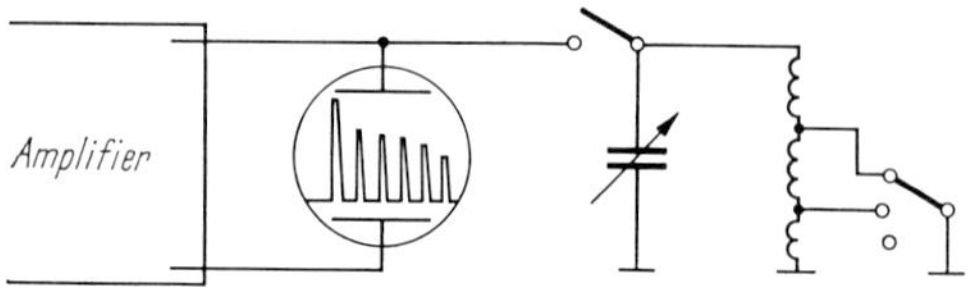

Fig. 2.60 Circuit of wall thickness gauge attachment according to KRAUTKRÄMER.

echoes excites the resonant circuit. In general these echoes will interfere with the oscillation because they do not arrive simultaneously. However, if the circuit is tuned to the repetition frequency of the echoes, each echo amplifies the action of the preceding echo and the voltage in the resonant circuit reaches a maximum. In this position of the variable capacitor the thickness of the material or the transit time can be read directly instead of the frequency, according to the calibration of the scale of the variable capacitor. Fig. 2.62 shows such a wall thickness gauge according to Krautkrämer, attached by means of plug and jack to the front plate of the instrument.

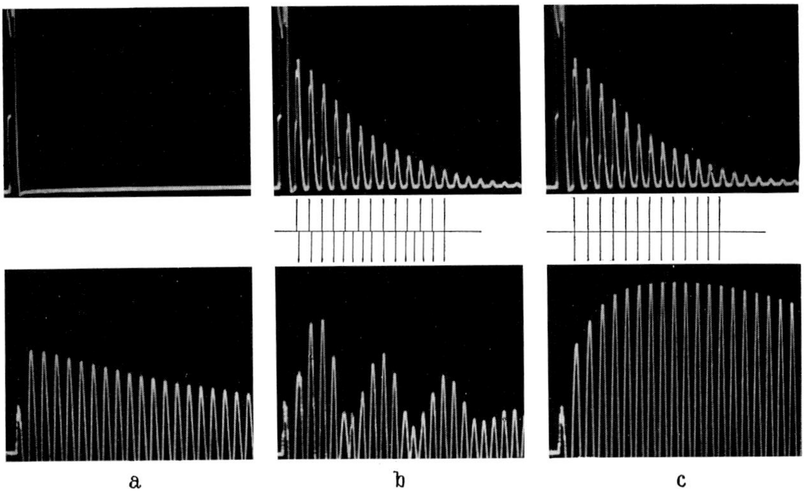

Fig. 2.61 Screen traces of wall thickness measurements with resonant circuit for echo repetition frequency, steel plate 9 mm thick, top resonant circuit switched off, bottom switched on. a) Probe not yet applied; b) probe applied, circuit not yet tuned; c) tuned to maximum oscillation.

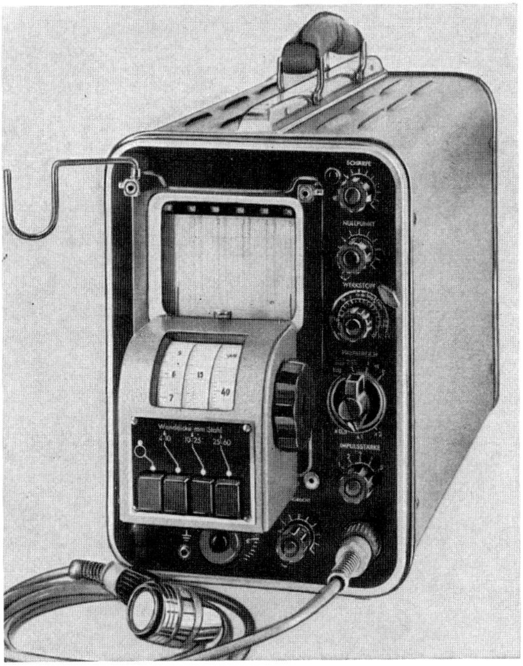

Fig. 2.62 Wall thickness gauge attachment, design Krautkrämer, mounted on USIP 10 instrument.

In the case of a steel plate 10 mm thick the transit time for the go and return path is 3.4 μs, and the frequency of the multiple echo repetition therefore 1/3.4 = 0.29 MHz. This is the frequency of the oscillatory circuit when tuned to resonance. To cover the thickness range from 4 to 60 mm, it should be possible to tune the circuit from 740 kHz to 49 kHz. For this purpose the coil of the resonant circuit is subdivided to give three measuring ranges: 4 to 10; 10 to 25 and 25 to 60 mm in steel.

If one arranges for the circuit to be excited by an echo only at the second, third, etc. oscillation, also resonance points are obtained so that a plate thickness of 60 mm produces resonance also at 30, 20, 15 mm, i.e. at 1/2, 1/3, 1/4 etc. of the actual thickness. Thicknesses greater than 60 mm can therefore also be measured by a higher resonance point provided the approximate thickness is known. The latter can first be determined approximately by means of the calibrated depth scale. For thicknesses below 60 mm the first resonance point gives the correct value if starting at large values.

Based on the design of the wall thickness gauge, Krautkrämer manufactures a transit time meter with which accurate measurements of the transit time of an individual echo can be made, even if no multiple echoes are available [275].

2.352 Electronic Data Processing

Visual evaluation of the screen trace is often too slow and too subjective. Evaluation of the screen data, viz. echo amplitudes and transit times in the form of electrical values which are independent of the remaining picture content, is therefore desirable and necessary for most recording methods (see 2.353).

It has therefore been suggested that photoelectric cells be mounted in front of the screen, either singly [77] or a whole series of them [35]. Purely electronic devices are, however, easier to adjust, offer greater possibilities, and leave the viewing screen free for visual observation.

In the simplest case a go/no-go or signal monitor can be used as an auxiliary instrument which as suggested by De Lano [73] indicates an echo automatically by means of an arbitrary signal as soon as it appears in a preselected transit time range, viz. the *gate*, and exceeds a preselected amplitude reading (Fig. 2.63). This gate (see Fig. 2.64) is usually indicated on the screen in the form of a step or a brightness change of the zero line. If several monitors are used, whose gates may also overlap each other, different ranges can be monitored separately.

Electronically the monitor consists of a gate amplifier getting the same voltage pattern as the CR tube, which however passes only the desired portion of this pattern through a transit time interval, viz. the gate. The gating voltage is synchronized with the repetition frequency of the instrument.

It is thus triggered either by the repetition frequency generator or the sweep voltage or the transmitting pulse (see Fig. 2.17). In the immersion technique which uses a variable water path to the object, a gate which depends on the transmitting pulse, is however a disadvantage: the zone of the test piece to be studied may vary its position relative to the gate. This difficulty can be overcome by using a circuit in which the first echo triggers the monitoring circuit, i.e. usually the entrance

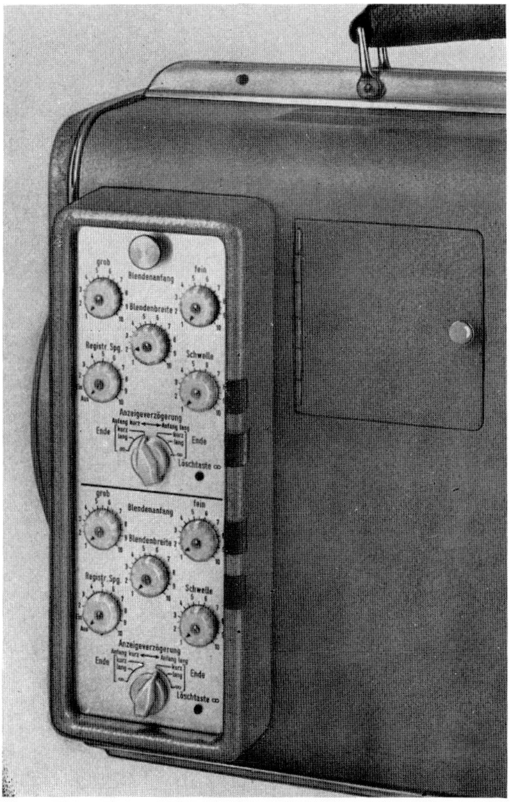

Fig. 2.63 Double monitor design Krautkrämer with two independent gates, used in both zones for alarm signals which announce the appearance or disappearance of a given echo, and with simultaneous recording by means of a go/no-go trace or proportional trace with rectified or pulse output voltage.

echo of the test piece (echo start monitor). Any change of the water path then only shifts the echo image of the test piece, together with the gate, a disadvantage which can still be remedied by the echo start circuit of the sweep voltage mentioned in Sec. 2.321.

The position and width of the gate is adjustable; the width can be varied from a few mm in steel upwards so as to be able to study also individual, narrow echoes separately from the remaining picture content. If only a go/no-go signal is required, the transmitted echo voltage is placed on a thyratron which actuates a relay as soon as the set ignition voltage is exceeded. This can then be exploited for actuating various, electrical signalling devices, e.g. acoustical such as ringing and hooting, optical such as lamps, and switching operations can be initiated which for instance stop the movement of the test piece in automated installations or which actuate a marking device for flaw indication, a paint spray gun, and so forth. Usually the monitoring relay is also fitted with a closed-circuit contact. This can therefore also be used for triggering a signal as soon as a given echo drops below an predetermined height, e.g. the backwall echo due to bad coupling.

In view of the unavoidable inertia of both the thyratron and the relays and their limited life, these devices are now replaced by circuits with semiconductor elements. These operate practically without delay and they can therefore indicate even a single pulse. However, delay-free response of the monitor is not always desirable for two reasons. Where automated testing installations operate at close proximity to electrical machines, interference by sparks cannot always be avoided. Such interference may cause faulty indication of the monitor. However, if the response is delayed so that only several pulses within the gate can take effect, most interference pulses will remain ineffective because they are usually of short duration and not synchronised. Similarly, the switching off of the monitor must frequently be delayed because the connected electromechanical signalling instruments are unable to respond to short monitor signals. It is desirable that both delays be optimally adjusted because unwanted delays naturally reduce the testing speed unnecessarily.

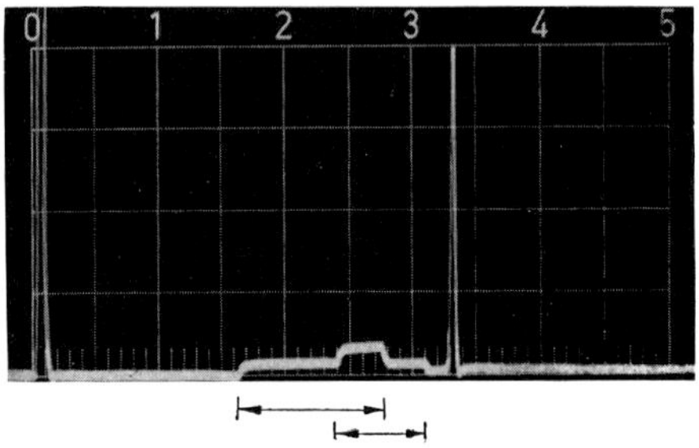

Fig. 2.64 Screen trace with two partially overlapping monitoring gates.

The output circuit of the monitor can also be modified in such a way that a voltage which is proportional to the echo height is obtained. Such an instrument is called a proportional or recording monitor because the voltage is usually used for recording purposes. It is not recommended that the pulse in the form as passed by the gate be used directly as output voltage because it is too short and consequently its frequencies are too high and its electric energy too low to operate conventional recording instruments. The pulses are therefore broadened artificially into triangular pulses and their duration is, instead of microseconds, a few milli-seconds. This pulse output voltage thus consists of a pulse repetition in the rhythm of the repetition frequency of the pulse-echo instrument, whose amplitude duplicates the echo height without relaxation (see Fig. 2.71).

This pulse output voltage cannot be used for operating high-inertia indicators such as measuring instruments with pointers, and recorders with low cut-off frequency. It is preferable to rectify this voltage and to filter out most of the ripple of the repetition frequency. This supplies the output DC voltage of the monitor which in fact also follows the amplitude fluctuations of the echo with a certain relaxation determined by the rectification. Depending on the time constant chosen this output voltage requires a certain number of single pulses before it can react to a given amplitude change (see Fig. 2.72). With rapid scanning, the use of the DC output thus implies reduced resolving power as compared with the pulse output.

The auxiliary instruments discussed so far convert the *echo height* into a voltage available for further evaluation. In addition the *transit time* which in general is a function of the distance of the flaw from the testing surface, or the thickness of the test piece, is of interest. Methods for converting the transit time into a voltage are described, inter alia, in Sec. 2.41 on instruments for pure transit time measurements. There is first of all the *integration method* in which a starting pulse initiates a charging or discharging process or the flipping over of a bistable circuit. The echo stops this process. The voltage reached, or the current which flows during the transit time, is a measure of the latter. There is also the *counting method* in which the initiating pulse starts a counter which counts the frequency-stabilized oscillations of an oscillator and which is then switched off again by the echo. The first method can be compared to the principle of an hour-glass and the second to that of a pendulum clock.

The transit time monitor of Krautkrämer produces, primarily, square pulses of constant height whose *duration* equals the transit time. By appropriate circuitry a pulse sequence whose *amplitude* is proportional to the transit time can be obtained from it. This is achieved by means of a capacitance–resistance circuit which integrates the current, or simply by means of a measuring instrument with sufficient inertia for ballistic measurements. In each case the transit time of each pulse is indicated without delay. However, if a commercial electronic precision timer is connected to the square pulse output, the device operates according to a counting method: the transit time is indicated digitally. Naturally, the eye is unable to follow the digital indication if the transit time changes too rapidly. This device can therefore be used to measure a transit time at a given moment and to store it, as in the case of point-for-point wall thickness measurements. Alternatively, it can determine a maximum and minimum over a certain length of time, as in the case of wall thickness measurements of pipes along a given circumference. Naturally this requires in addition suitable circuits. Digital indication furthermore offers the possibilities to print, to punch, or to record the data digitally.

Recording of the pulses in the case of the integration method requires very fast and therefore expensive recorders. For further processing in slower instruments, the means of the pulse amplitude can be formed. This provides a DC voltage which is proportional to the transit time and which follows rapid changes only after a certain response time.

It is advisable not to count the transit time from the transmitting pulse because its decay oscillations make it unsuitable for use as a starting pulse. There is in fact always the risk that with changing coupling conditions, individual decay oscillations may already terminate the transit time measurement. It is therefore preferable to produce a special, adjustable starting pulse which appears on the zero line of the screen as a small triangular pulse. Its position then enters into the calibration as a constant transit time. Instead of measuring the transit time between this starting pulse and the next echo, it is also possible to measure optionally the transit time between the following pulse and the next but one echo; this is desirable when testing according to the immersion technique or in the case of wall thickness measurements via fixed delay lines (schnozzles) as in the case of TR probes (see 3.61).

The shape of the echo pulse affects the accuracy of any transit time measurement. A certain minimum voltage is required to stop the measuring process, and small echoes are therefore ineffective. For larger echoes the whole rising front is, however, not normal to the zero line but, because of the high-frequency nodes, rises in steps as shown in Fig. 2.27. Any change in height may therefore shift the response threshold for the transit time measurement, more or less abruptly in increments of one wave-length. (In the case of full-wave rectification before the video stage of the amplifier, this skip would be one half wave-length.) Reliable measurement of the transit time therefore requires that both the echo height and echo shape remain as constant as possible between calibration and measurement. This applies to both methods of transit time measurements.

The methods described give the transit time of only one definite echo of the screen picture, not that of any other, simultaneously appearing later indications as obtained for instance when testing forgings. To record several transit times a method has been used which may be called *travelling gate method* [120]. As described above, the gate of the proportional monitor can be shifted manually as required by means of a control. This manual control can, however, be replaced for example by a servomotor, or alternatively, a periodic shifting voltage is produced which completely replaces the control, e.g. a saw-tooth voltage with a frequency considerably lower than the repetition frequency of the ultrasonic pulse. For instance, if this frequency is one hundredth of the ultrasonic repetition frequency and if the amplitude of the shifting voltage is just sufficient to shift the gate from the transmitting pulse as far as the right edge of the picture, one gate shift is equivalent to one hundred pulses. Should both the gate and the pulse be very narrow, equally spaced echoes could be indicated at one hundred discrete points next to each other, but not at intermediate positions. This therefore represents a discontinuous indication of the transit time. For evaluation purposes a recording system can be moved synchronously with the gate across the recording chart in such a way that the system records only when the gate indicates an echo. If the echo shifts slowly, it seems to jump on the recording. The pulse repetition frequency is limited by the size of the test object and the travelling gate frequency can therefore only be relatively low. Consequently only such transit time changes can be recorded faithfully as are still slow compared with the gating period. Suitable recording systems are spiral recorders or self-balancing recorders (see next Section).

In automated testing installations one frequently encounters the problem of storing the test data for a certain length of time, i.e. the echo height and the transit time, and to release them with a certain delay to be evaluated. This is for instance the case where the location of the flaw must be marked on the test piece by a paint spray gun and the test piece is inaccessible during the test, e.g. in a transit tank submerged in water. In this case the test piece can be marked only after it has passed through the testing installation. In simple cases a go/no-go signal must therefore be stored for a certain length of time, of the order of seconds. However, in most instances this delay does not remain constant but changes with the testing speed. Purely electronic storing of go/no-go signals is possible by using a chain of bistable circuit elements (shifting register), the monitor feeding the information to the beginning of the chain. With the motion of the test piece, and controlled by it via arbitrary, successively actuated switches, each element of the chain passes its information on to the next element until the last element actuates the marking device. Thus, the information travels in the chain, like the flaw in the test piece in the testing equipment. A given information must, however, be correlated to a given section of the test piece, i.e. the indication is scanned. Much more flexible is storage on magnetic tape. By this means it is possible to store not only the go/no-go signals of the signal monitor but also the amplitude-proportional voltages of the recording monitor or the time-proportional voltages of the transit time monitor. No scanning is required if in the case of variable testing speed coupling between the tape speed and the travelling speed of the test piece is acceptable. The pulse output voltages of the instruments mentioned are particularly suitable for storage on magnetic tape. The tape recording is then free of any lag.

2.353 Documentation Methods and Instruments

As described in the previous Section, the choice of suitable data processing instruments naturally depends on the desired evaluation of the test results. If only conspicuous visual indication which can be read more conveniently than the screen picture is required, it is sufficient for transit time measurements, e.g. wall thickness measurements, to connect a digital indicating instrument (digital short-time meter or digital voltmeter) directly to the transit time monitor. The distribution of flaws in a given test piece can also be conspicuously indicated visually by a lamp panel by the above-mentioned storing device. Alternatively the data can also be fed into computers or they can control automatic machine tools. Suitable documentation of the test results is, however, in all instances likewise desirable.

The documentation of all test data of a given test piece has no general rational solution. This would require that in addition to the three co-ordinates, at least some statement regarding the size of the flaw be recorded for every point of the three-dimensional test piece. Fortunately,

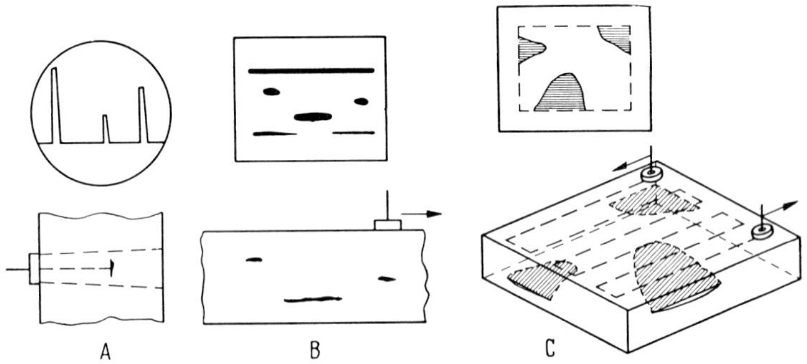

Fig. 2.65 A, B and C-scan presentation and scanning method.

several of these data can usually be omitted, e.g. if the shape of the test piece permits limiting the scanning to cross-sectional or laminary zones, as shown in Fig. 2.65. The usual screen picture, which is also referred to as A-scan, provides a one-dimensional description. To cover a given cross-section, i.e. a so-called B-scan, the probe must be shifted in one direction. Scanning in two directions provides a layer or C-scan. In the case of A-scan, the size of the flaw is defined approximately by the echo height; in the case of B-scan and C-scan the echo height, depending on the nature of the documentation process, can only be reproduced more or less partially.

Of the various documentation methods the *photographic* method will be discussed first. Using a CR tube, it is the most versatile and quickest as far as the testing process is concerned. These advantages are, however, frequently offset by the developing procedure which is still rather cumbersome.

A camera mounted in front of the pulse-echo instrument supplies the simple A-scan of a given test. Auxiliary photographic devices of this type are supplied by most manufacturers, which frequently also use polaroid cameras which produce finished prints after only a few seconds. As far as the test result for the whole test piece is concerned, a single screen picture is of little importance and it is at least necessary to take a series of pictures at different testing points. Cine cameras have also been used; they produce a most faithful document of the entire testing process but they are difficult to review and to evaluate.

According to a suggestion by Martin and Werner [246], the B-scan is derived from the A-scan in a simple way by photographing the viewing screen with a continuously but obliquely moving cine film. The echoes record ribbon-like mountain chains which, if correctly illuminated, also allow the recognition of features behind them. In this way both the position co-ordinates and the echo heights are recorded. This method is not yet being applied in practice. If the method shown in Fig. 2.67 is used, the peak-presentation on the screen is usually changed to dot-presentation by completely blackening out the time line through a bias of the modulator electrode of the CR tube (Fig. 2.17, voltage ⑤) and brightness-modulation at points of echo indications only, proportional to their height. The echo voltage is thus not placed on the deflector plates but on the modulator electrode. The photographic recording on a cine film moving synchronously with the probe gives a B-scan in the form of more or less blackened dots and lines. Since large echoes are also broader, they are not only blackened more but also appear broader on the record, thus providing a qualitative record of the echo heights. Long and narrow test pieces are particularly suitable for this recording method, in which the

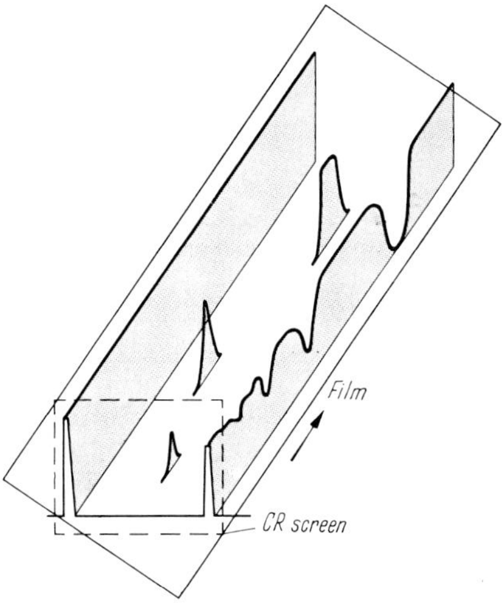

Fig. 2.66 Recording method according to Martin and Werner with slant-wise moving film, schematic, backwall echo with 3 flaw echoes.

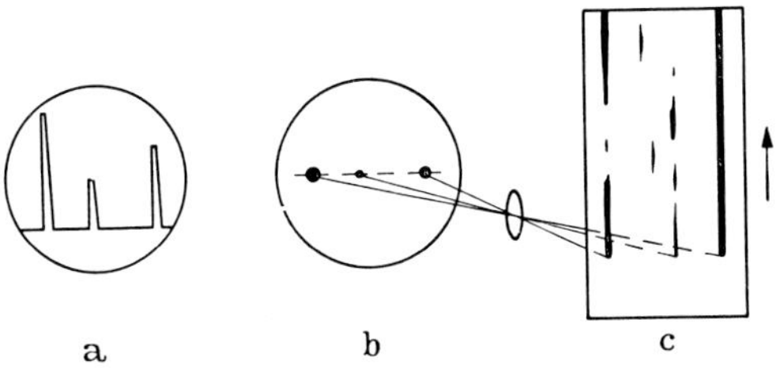

Fig. 2.67 B-scan recording method with intensity-modulated dot-trace. a) Trace with vertical deflection (A-scan); b) same picture with dot-presentation (bright dots on dark background); c) recording.

third co-ordinate is unimportant, e.g. rails (Fig. 2.68). The recordings can be made on cine film or highly sensitized paper which latter is used for instance in the rail-testing cars of the German Federal Railways (see 3.232). According to a suggestion by WERNER [383] the faithfulness of a B-scan, as shown for instance in Fig. 2.68, can be increased considerably if, in addition to the vertically beaming probe, several obliquely beaming

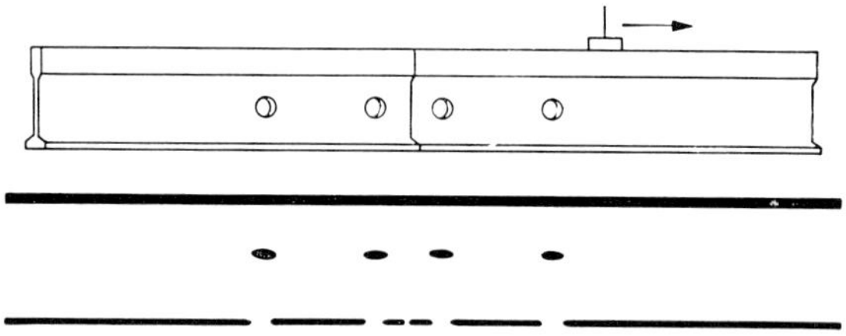

Fig. 2.68 Rail test and recording according to Fig. 2.67, schematic.

probes are used. In addition, a separate CR tube is used for each probe; its time base is orientated relative to the chart transport position and angle, as the beam axis is to the test piece. This for example would result in fishplate holes, which cannot be distinguished from small longitudinal flaws, on the basis of their indication in Fig. 2.68 being recorded as several short lines in the form of a polygon, i.e. resembling more closely the circular shape of the hole. Obliquely orientated cracks which in the simple testing method might be recognized only by the absence of the bottom echo, are made directly visible in this method by using additional obliquely beaming probes. Instruments using this method are not in regular production but are produced only as required.

For individual test pieces which are not too long it is advisable not to produce the B-scan on the recording chart first but directly on the viewing screen. For this purpose the (invisible) time base of the screen display (e.g. in Fig. 2.67) is shifted parallel to itself synchronously with the probe-shift. Usually the time base direction as well as the testing direction are orientated vertically, resulting in a single scanning process producing a picture as shown in Fig. 2.69. In this method the stationary film is exposed during the entire process.

For visual analysis of the screen trace the use of afterglow tubes of the same size as television picture tubes is recommended. An afterglow duration of 5 to 10 s is sufficient to study the picture after rapid scanning for an adequate time in a darkened room. In the case of image storing tubes, the so-called Memotron and the dark-trace CR tube, the picture persists considerably longer, practically infinitely. Both types of tubes, however, are manufactured only with effective screen diameters of up to approx. 100 mm.

VEB Carl Zeiss, Jena, supplies for the B-scan of a limited section of a test piece of approximately 200 mm length, a probe-guiding attachment for their Sonovisor pulse-echo instrument, which can be placed on a flat surface manually. The instrument can be switched over optionally to the conventional A-scan or to the *swing-section* scan. The position of the probe is transferred to the CR tube by means of a synchronously variable voltage. In a similar manner the instrument also produces *rotational section scans*. For this purpose either the test piece, e.g. round stock, rotates around its longitudinal axis while the probe beams into the test piece radially, or the probe rotates once around the test piece. In both cases the rotational movement is transferred synchronously on to the viewing screen by means of a voltage. There either the picture can be rotated electronically on the stationary screen, or the entire CR tube can be rotated once around its longitudinal axis. In either case the camera photographs a rotational section scan. A type of rotational section scan is also obtained with the Ultrasonic Weld Recorder by Krautkrämer (see also Sec. 3.281, Fig. 3.186). In this instrument the beam of an angle probe is swung mechanically through a given angular range. Synchronously, the time base of the CR tube is swung through the same angle and so doing produces a dotted-line recording of the flaw image in the selected cross-section of the test piece. In principle, this method is not restricted to tests on welding seams.

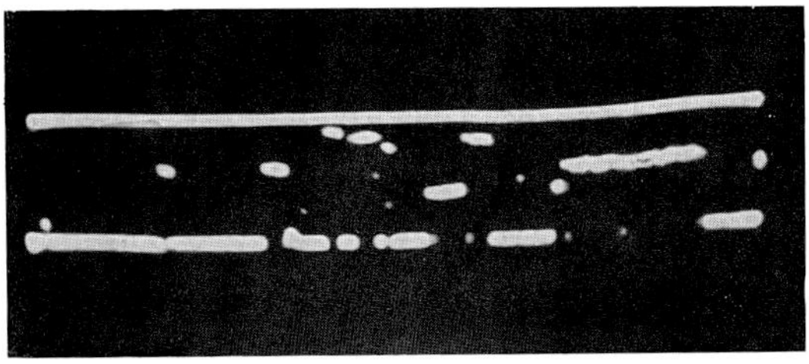

Fig. 2.69 B-scan of a 16 mm thick aluminium section with flaws (Electrocircuits).

Pictures in cross-section of large specimens, e.g. forgings several metres long, would require complex mechanical devices to shift the probe while the coupling conditions remain constant, if one wants to scan them continuously. According to Michalski [261] the problem is greatly simplified if the probe is placed by hand successively on previously marked testing points along the scanning track. Usually a discontinuous (scanned) composition of the cross-section where the individual test points are spaced a few centimetres from each other, is sufficient. First, the A-scan is used to check the coupling at each point. Then the camera of the B-scan instrument is actuated, whereupon the time base of the picture is advanced a fixed step. Fig. 2.70 shows pictures of this type obtained on a forging. This method can be used where a testing time of about one hour is acceptable.

A B-scan recording should be accepted only with reservation as being a true picture of the actual flaws. It should be kept in mind that the echo indicates only the position of the surface of the irradiated flaw and that the size of the flaw in the direction of the sound beam is only simulated in the cross-sectional picture by the finite width of the dots. Furthermore, the presentation of the flaw in the direction of the probe-shift appears broader because of the divergence of the sound beam. Consequently, flaws at longer distances appear longer than nearer ones. In addition, as always when using the echo method, the angular position of the flaw relative to the sound beam naturally plays an important role. But except where several flaws occur one behind the other in line with the sound beam, the degree of suppression of the backwall echo can be exploited for the evaluation.

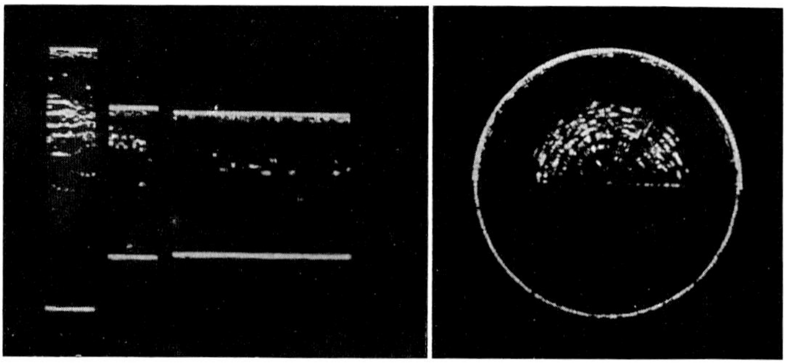

Fig. 2.70 Longitudinal and cross-sectional picture of a forging (KRAUTKRÄMER).

The recording of a C-scan according to Fig. 2.65, requires that the section of the time base of the A-scan to be studied be cut out by a monitor. In the case of thin specimens, or if the actual depth is of no interest, the entire picture contained between transmitting pulse and bottom echo is placed as control voltage on the modulator electrode of a CR tube. The composing of a C-scan for visual observation on the viewing screen, as in the case of a television picture, is only possible with an image storing tube in view of the slow, mechanical scanning motion of the probe (Fig. 3.200). A photographic picture can then be obtained by photographing in the usual way the image storing tube after scanning. If ordinary CR tubes are used, the photographic picture must be recorded while scanning. The relative movement in two co-ordinates between probe and specimen on the one hand, and luminous spot and film on the other, is determined essentially by the specific testing problem and the geometry of the specimen. Systems using this principle have been installed only in rare cases because direct recording is preferable to photographic recording.

In the case of photographic recording the testing speed is limited by the feasible scanning speed with constant coupling conditions, and by the pulse repetition frequency. The latter manifests itself by a picture as shown in Fig. 2.69 being resolved into individual points at high scanning speed, which correspond to the individual pulses. If the speed is excessive, the scanning grid becomes too coarse in relation to the flaws to be detected. The repetition frequency can be increased only with due regard to the thickness of the specimen if delayed echoes are to be avoided. In the immersion technique repetition frequencies of 1000 Hz and scanning speeds of up to 1 m/s can be used, corresponding to one pulse per mm which is quite adequate. The only problem which still remains is the mechanical movement of the probe.

Direct recording methods and instruments use either moving recording systems which produce deflections at right angles to the movement of the strip chart, or stationary recording pens which merely record a dotted line. Moveable systems have a mechanical cut-off frequency which in the case of pointer and ink recorders is far below 100 Hz; those using a moving stylus and wax paper have a maximum cut-off frequency of some 100 Hz. In the case of the *light-spot recorder* (by Hartmann & Braun, Frankfurt, and similarly by Honeywell) which produces a directly visible record on sensitized paper using a strong UV light beam and a mirror system, the cut-off frequency is some 1000 Hz. With the ink-jet recorder *Oscillomink* (by Elema, Stockholm, and Siemens & Halske, Karlsruhe in Germany) recording speeds above 1000 Hz can be obtained on ordinary paper. This instrument was used in Figs. 2.71 and 2.72. The cut-off frequency of the recorder usually limits the testing speed of the method applied.

Optimal resolution and maximum speed are obtained with the pulse recording method: the pulse output voltage of the recording monitor is placed directly on the recorder. At a repetition frequency of 130 Hz the instrument therefore records 130 peaks/s whose height is proportional to the echo height. This requires a substantially higher cut-off frequency of the recorder to ensure that the peaks do not flow together. Fig. 2.71 shows a recording obtained by scanning according to the immersion technique. The test specimen contained holes at right angles to the sound beam, with different spacings and diameters.

The first two recordings at slow scanning speed and low repetition frequency show the influence of the probe on the resolution: whereas a 6 MHz probe of 12 mm diameter has optimal resolving power because the holes are close to the end of its near field, a diameter of 20 mm is unsuitable because the test is then carried out inside the near field. In the first case spacings of 5 mm can no longer be resolved: the resulting interference falsifies both the position of the flaw and the echo height. With the broader sound beam it is already impossible to resolve 10 mm, and the remaining indications are distorted. It is therefore imperative to choose first the most suitable sound beam. The other pictures show, for the 12 mm probe, the influence of the repetition frequency at increased scanning speed. At 200 mm/s the low repetition frequency of 130 Hz barely suffices to record the position of the flaw and the echo height. The recording system of the jet-type recorder shows the individual pulses still clearly separated, but begins to fail at 500 Hz. Due to its inertia transients occur, resulting in the peaks of the pulses flowing together. This recording system, nevertheless, would still permit a scan-

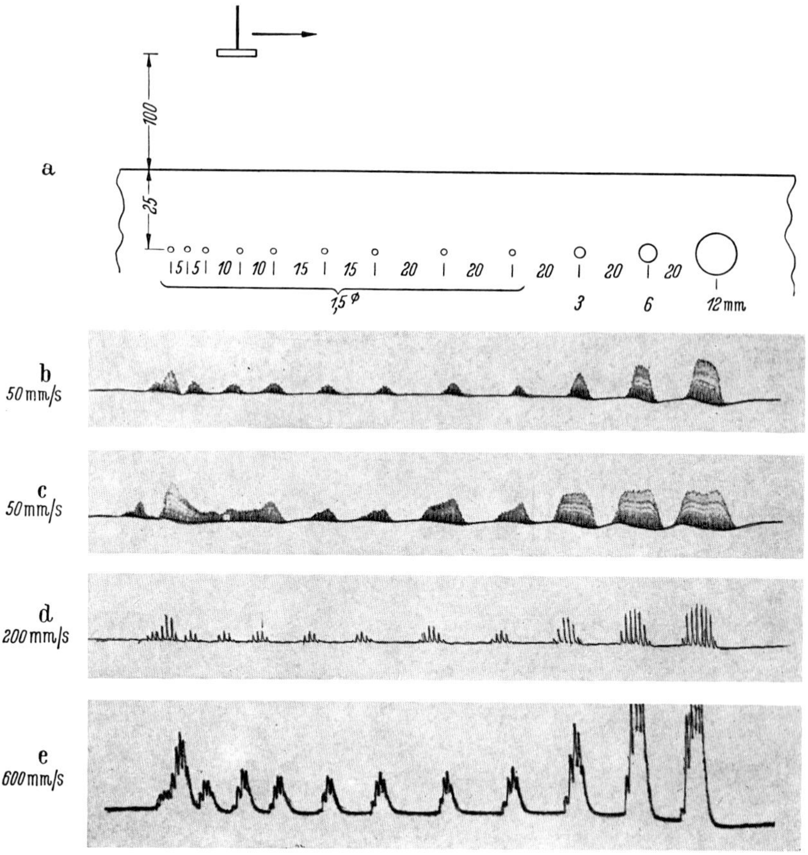

Fig. 2.71 **Direct recording of pulses proportional to echo height (with Oszillomink of Elema – Siemens & Halske). a)** Test piece; b) to **d)** repetition frequency 130 Hz; b) and c) scanning speed 50 mm/s, **probe in b) 12 mm**; in c) 20 mm dia.; d) scanning speed 200 mm/s; e) scanning speed 600 mm/s, repetition frequency 500 Hz.

ning speed of 1 to 2 m/s which also would permit a further increase of the repetition frequency without the resolution of the 10 mm spacings being lost. Since at present still faster recording systems are not available, this probably represents the limit of direct recording in which the echo height is still proportional to the indication.

Fig. 2.72 shows proportional recordings with the DC output of the proportional monitor for moderate demands in respect of both resolution and speed. The voltage curve no longer contains high frequencies and is therefore also suitable for recorders with low cut-off frequency, e.g. below 100 Hz. However, at a scanning speed of 200 mm/s the resolution is then already insufficient. The time constant of the rectification then becomes just as disturbing as a too low cut-off frequency of the system.

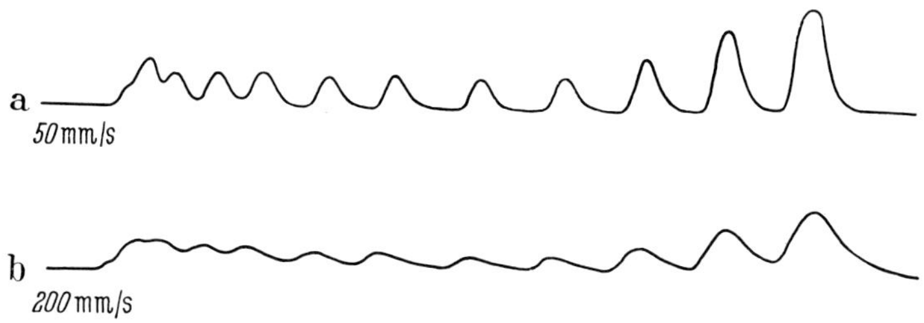

Fig. 2.72 DC recording proportional to echo height. a) Scanning speed 50 mm/s; b) scanning speed 200 mm/s.

Fig. 2.73 compares various go/no-go recordings of the same scanning process with mechanically actuated recording systems, using a monitor and relay. The response threshold has been set just a little above the small echoes which are therefore not recorded. The simulated larger flaw is, however, indicated. In a) and b) the relay places a constant direct voltage and an alternating voltage, respectively, on the recording system. In c) and d) a different recording system was used whose stylus is lifted periodically from the recording chart, e.g. in the case of wax paper with cold or heated stylus. None of these systems offer special advantages

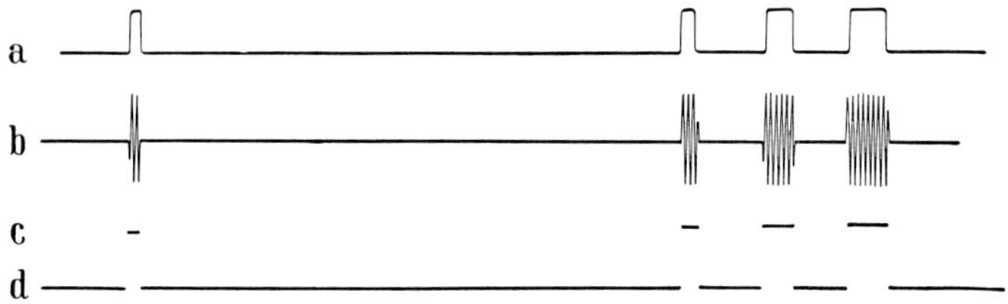

Fig. 2.73 Go/no-go recording via monitor and relay. Scanning speed 50 mm/s. a) Relay places a direct voltage on recording system (Oszillomink); b) ditto with 50 Hz alternating voltage; c) recording system using wax paper and heated stylus placed on chart intermittently, positive recording; d) ditto, negative recording (stylus raised during echo indication).

regarding resolution or speed and they differ only from a practical point of view in respect of legibility. The speed is either limited by the relay which fails to respond in the case of very short indications of less than approx. 10 ms even if the inertia of the relay is very low, or by the inertia of the recording system.

Practically inertia-less recorders are those using stationary recording tips on electrosensitive paper, e.g. electrochemical or electric discharge recording papers. Such chart papers are obtainable in the trade under different names, e.g. Teledeltos, Belipa, MP paper (for spark recording), Alfax, and so forth (for electrochemical recording). In the case of the former the heat effect when a current flows from the electrode to the metallized paper is exploited, and in the latter the discolouration by electrochemical processes in a saturated and humidified paper is utilized. The required voltage is usually from a few volts to 100 V. These instruments therefore record continuous lines as shown in Figs. 2.73c and d, when the voltage is switched on and off. To some extent these recorders can also be used however for proportional recording because in the case of some chart papers the intensity of the discolouration is a function of the voltage placed on the system. Since in this case no mechanically moving parts nor a monitor relay are required, both the resolution and the speed are determined primarily by the repetition frequency: at high recording speeds the line dissolves into dots which correspond to the individual pulses. The upper limit depends largely on the uniformity of the recording trace, i.e. the quality of the chart paper. For instance in the case of some electric discharge recording papers contamination by ash occurs during continuous operation which interferes with the clear recording of short breaks in the line of the recording of individual dots.

The problem to be solved is the recording of the results of an ultrasonic test by means of the direct recorders described. When scanning a long specimen, e.g. a rod, pipe or rail in the longitudinal direction, the speed of the chart feed of the recorder is usually determined by the scanning speed. The recording thus reveals the position of a given flaw in *one* co-ordinate, viz. the longitudinal direction of the specimen, in the form of a go/no-go trace or proportional trace. This solution is acceptable in such simple cases as do not require a more exact statement of the position of the flaw. This method requires only a simple recorder with narrow strip chart and fixed recording system.

The so-called x-y recorders (self-balancing recorders) would make it possible to simulate on a stationary sheet of chart paper the scanning movement of the probe in two co-ordinates, as in the case of the C-scan in Fig. 2.65; in practice this would, however, be too slow. For disc-shaped specimens such as turbine discs the answer is a type of gramophone record scanning combined with a suitable recording system as shown in Figs. 3.79 to 3.81. Both the specimen and the recording chart rotate, while the probe and the recording system are shifted slowly in the same sense, either rectilinearly or along an arc as in the case of a gramophone record.

A C-scan in rectangular co-ordinates, e.g. in the case of sheet metal, can be recorded by using a larger number of recording points simultaneously next to each other as in Figs. 2.74, 1.106 and 3.108.

In the case of the pulse-echo method, however, this is very costly because each recording point requires a complete testing equipment, from probe to monitor. This system is therefore preferred for testing according to the intensity-transmission method which requires less instrumentation. Particularly suitable are recorders using electro-sensitive paper because their recording tips can be mounted at a distance of only a few mm from each other, as for instance in the case of the 42 point recorder by Siemens & Halske using metallized paper.

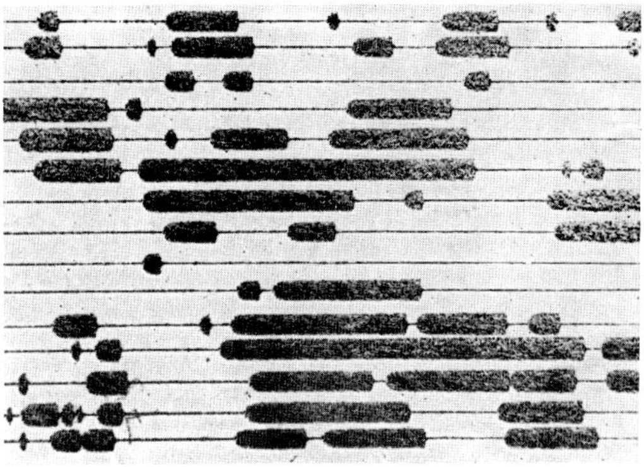

Fig. 2.74 C-scan of a sheet with flaws. Section of approx. 110 · 180 mm, scanning speed 50 mm/s, method according to Fig. 2.73b, recording system with cold stylus on wax paper using 200 Hz alternating voltage.

Frequently spiral recorders for electrochemical chart paper are used for C-scan presentation, e.g. the Helix recorder of Messrs. Alden, Brockton, Mass./USA. In this system the strip chart is stretched over a cylinder having a raised metal spiral, e.g. a wire, which is fixed to its surface in a pitch extending over the full width of the chart. A straight metal bar presses the chart down against the spiral. If the cylinder with the spiral turns, the contact point where the current passes from the bar through the paper and into the cylinder, travels from one end of the chart to the other. The rotation of the spiral cylinder is coupled to the scanning movement of the probe which for instance scans a band-shaped specimen transversely to its direction of feed. If both the recording chart and the test piece move uniformly, a C-scan consisting of closely-packed lines is obtained. The spiral described is not suitable for rectilinear back and forth movement of the probe, i.e. for scanning of the test piece along a zig-zag line; this can be achieved by a different design using two contra-rotating spirals with one half pitch each over the full length of the cylinder. During the first half turn of the cylinder the contact point then travels from left to right, and travels back again during the second half turn.

In combination with the travelling gate method for the measurement of transit time (Sec. 2.352), the spiral recorder can be used for recording a B-scan. Synchronously with the rotation of the spiral cylinder the gate is moved along the time base. As soon as an echo enters the gate, the signal blackens the contact point reached by the rotating spiral at that moment. GOLDMAN and AUGER [120] obtain the B-scan recording of a forging in this way.

Documentation methods include also the printing and punching methods favoured for automated testing installations. These methods require that the test result be first presented digitally and they are therefore particularly suitable for digital measurements and thickness readings (see Sec. 2.352) and for supplying data concerning the length and number of flaws in sheet and strip metal (Sec. 3.24). Some relatively inexpensive and handy instruments, as for instance the Kienzle printer, can print up to 14 digits about 5 times per second. Manufacturers of electronic data processing instruments can, however, supply even more efficient instruments should they be required.

2.36* The Shock-wave Method

This pulse-echo method uses particularly short pulses, but because of its limited testing depth can be used only on thin specimens. It was mentioned first by SPROULE [334] who used a special form of exciter voltage, viz. a step-function voltage. An instrument was constructed according to this principle by Ultrasonoscope.

This method uses piezoelectric crystals of a thickness such that the transit time of a pulse in the crystal exceeds the forward and return transit time in the specimen. For instance, a 20 mm thick quartz plate (transit time 3.5 μs for a longitudinal wave) can be used for testing approximately 10 mm steel (transit time there and back 3.4 μs). Such a transducer is backed by a damping body to reduce reflections to a minimum. If coupled to a specimen and if a step-function transmitting voltage is applied, Sec. 1.103 states that a square wave is radiated (Fig. 2.75). For reception of the echo SPROULE uses a separate receiver which is much thinner than the transmitter and which is mounted in front of it and separated by a spacer (Fig. 2.76). The receiver is in contact with the test piece. The radiated square wave passes through the receiver and produces in it a voltage of very similar shape (Fig. 2.77). The backwall echo of the specimen, owing to reflection on the sonically softer material, has undergone a phase reversal and consequently, on its return path to the receiver, cancels the receiving voltage, reducing it almost to zero, depending on the attenuation to which it has been subjected. Thus, the receiving voltage has the form of two opposite, successive trapezoids whose base is equal to double the transit time in the test piece. The low frequencies are then cut off in the amplifier so that only the differentiated voltages appear as short pulses on the viewing screen. Of these, the first pulse, pointing upward in Fig. 2.77, plays the role of the previous transmitting pulse, while

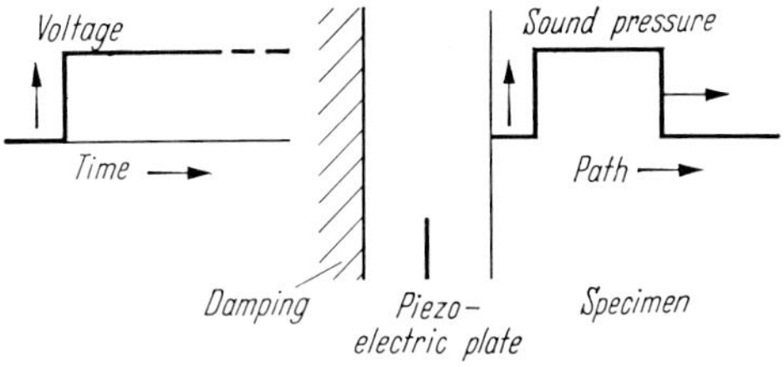

Fig. 2.75 Step voltage on thick piezoelectric plate produces a square pressure wave.

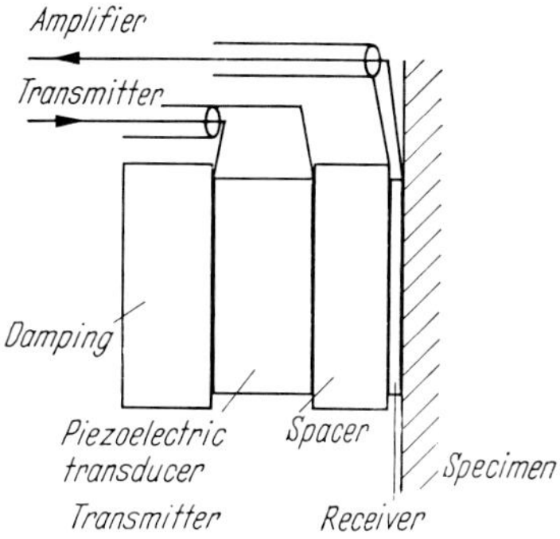

Fig. 2.76 Probe according to SPROULE for the step voltage method.

the second pulse represents the backwall echo. Flaw echoes, if present, appear between them. Only this section is placed on the viewing screen because the rest is only a repetition with the phases reversed, and possibly intermixed with the multiple echoes of the first group of pulses.

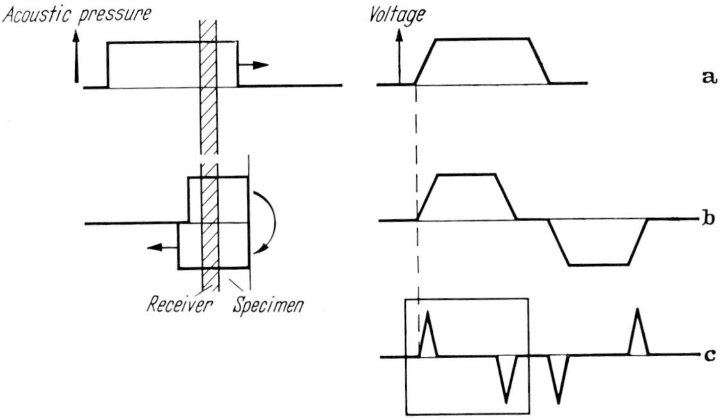

Fig. 2.77 Receiving voltage on probe according to Fig. 2.76, a) Transit of a square wave; b) reflected wave passing through simultaneously; c) the same after reduction of frequency band with the corresponding screen portion.

The step voltage of Fig. 2.75 can also be replaced by a square voltage of sufficient duration. The sloping edge generates a square wave of opposite phase which falls into the masked portion.

Alternatively the transmitter can be used simultaneously as receiver; this, however, requires an amplifier with very short dead time to be able to exploit the high resolving power. In the case of SPROULE's probe this is less critical because transmitter and receiver are separated by a spacer.

If a very short DC pulse is placed on the transmitting oscillator instead of a step voltage, it radiates two opposing acoustic pressure pulses as in Fig. 1.112, and in the case of imperfect matching also a succession of pulses whose amplitudes first increase and then decrease. The first pulse can then also be used as in the case of the conventional pulse-echo method. The only difference then is the testing range of a few mm, limited by the transit time in the oscillator. Here the characteristic frequency of the oscillator is far below the transmission range of the amplifier.

Using a pulse duration of 0.1 μs the resolution in steel is theoretically approx. 0.3 mm. This requires a minimum amplifier band width of 10 MHz. In practice, using still shorter pulses and wider frequency bands, it has been possible to resolve still shorter spacings. With shorter pulses, however, the sensitivity decreases because the receiving voltage is proportional to the area of the pulse, and because in addition the noise level of the amplifier increases with the band width.

Without rectification the echo pulses, depending on their phase (compression or tension pulses) appear on the viewing screen pointing upwards or downwards. It is thus possible to distinguish whether a given echo has been reflected on a sonically softer or sonically harder interface. Any cutting-off of higher frequencies in the echo, e.g. by absorption or by frequency-dependent reflection, furthermore manifests itself by a characteristic distortion: the echo pulse is broader and contains several oscillations instead of a single peak. In this case the pulse thus contains more information concerning the specimen and the reflection than when using the conventional method.

In addition to measuring the thickness of thin walls and detecting flaws at close range, the method has been used for testing glued joints (see 3.292), and experimentally also for measuring hardness depth (see 3.61).

2.37* Frequency Modulation Method

2.371 Principle

The frequency modulation method, like the pulse-echo method, permits determination of both the intensity and the transit time of a reflected wave. It is interesting to note that in the case of both ionosphere sounding and the testing of materials, the FM method was the precursor of the pulse-echo method, although the former is by no means easy to understand. SOKOLOV in 1941 proposed that this method be used for nondestructive testing, but it was soon superceded by the pulse method and to-day plays only an unimportant role.

The method uses continuous waves whose frequency, however, is varied periodically, rising linearly with time and decreasing again according to a saw-tooth pattern. Before the next rise there should be an interval. This is explained on the frequency-time diagram in Fig. 2.78. Starting at time 0 with frequency f_0 the transmitting frequency f_s rises linearly as far as the frequency f_1. It is assumed that the probe radiates all frequencies uniformly. Reflected by a flaw or the backwall, an echo wave then arrives at the probe after the transit time t there and back, which has the frequency f_0 at the moment when it arrives, followed by a frequency rising up to f_1.

Numerical example: $f_0 = 10$ MHz, $f_1 = 15$ MHz, frequency rise therefore 5 MHz. Rise time $T = 340$ µs, equalling the transit time of a longitudinal wave in 1 m steel there and back. Followed by a transmitting interval of 1660 µs, this together furnishes a period of 2000 µs or a repetition frequency of 500 Hz. After 136 µs the echo wave of a flaw 400 mm distant arrives at the probe, having the frequency 10 MHz if the transmitting frequency has already risen 136/340 = 0.4 of 5 MHz, i.e. 2 MHz. The difference between the frequency of the two waves is constantly 2 MHz. A flaw at 800 mm depth would produce a wave whose frequency would always be 4 MHz below the transmitter frequency.

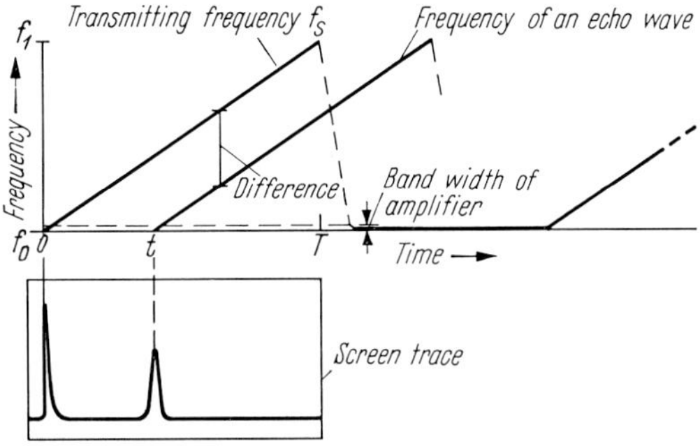

Fig. 2.78 Frequency modulation method for measuring intensity and transit time of an echo wave.

In this case the probe transmits and receives simultaneously. The total voltage, transmitting as well as receiving voltage, is placed on an amplifier with narrow frequency pass band, e.g. for a band about frequency f_0 or also a higher frequency. Consequently at time t_0 (or at a later time) a strong signal is received as the transmitting frequency passes through. A further signal is obtained at the time of arrival of the same frequency in the echo wave. The result is a screen trace similar to that obtained with the echo method, if, as shown, the luminous spot of a CR tube is deflected horizontally and synchronously with the frequency variation and at right angles to it with the output voltage of the amplifier, either as a high frequency trace or a video trace.

The simple method, however, is practically only suitable for high frequencies, otherwise the dead time of the amplifier, because of overdriving, becomes too great and the transmitting frequency cannot be suppressed outside the signal time at the high transmitting voltage used. Erdman [85, 86] has proposed a considerably more complex system which is set forth in Fig. 2.79. It is intended for tests by the immersion technique, in which the path through water is irrelevant as far as the reception of echoes is concerned. The shortest transit time of an echo which is of interest is much longer than the rise time. The frequency of the echo wave is not amplified directly but is first superimposed on to a second, likewise linearly modulated frequency. If it changes *in the same sense* as the transmitting frequency, e.g from lower to higher values, the difference between echo frequency and heterodyne frequency remains constant. For the design of the amplifier at low ultrasonic frequencies, it is, however, more advantageous to use a heterodyne frequency which changes *in the opposite sense*. The sum then remains constant, a frequency higher than the difference. A narrow-band amplifier tuned to the sum then produces a signal only if this frequency is contained in the mixture. This is the case only if the heterodyne voltage starts its sweep simultaneously with the arrival of the echo wave. To be able to cover different transit times, it would be necessary to vary the start of the heterodyne frequency. If this change is made by hand the test piece could be scanned for echoes layer by layer, but where the entire testing depth is displayed on a CR tube this testing depth would have to be shifted automatically, i.e. synchronously with the deflection of the luminous spot.

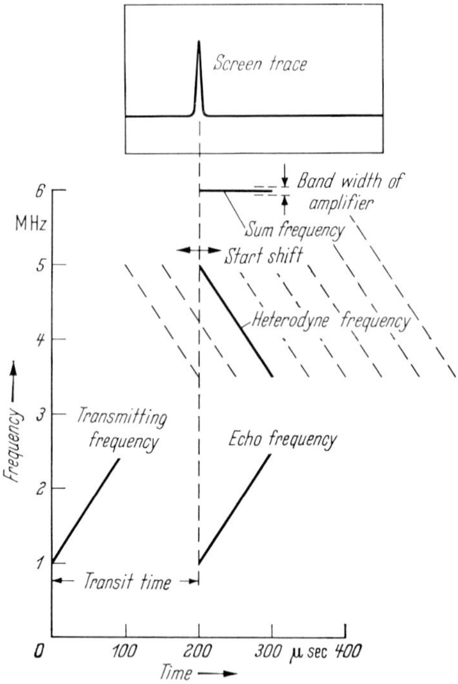

Fig. 2.79 FM method according to ERDMAN with heterodyne amplification, below, frequency diagram with numerical example; above, screen trace. The heterodyne frequency changes in a sense opposite to that of the transmitting frequency and has a delayed start. Together with the echo frequency it produces a constant sum frequency which, however, falls into the pass band of the amplifier only if both frequencies start simultaneously. For display on the screen the start shift is synchronised with the luminous spot in the form of a saw tooth time function.

Such an instrument thus has a high repetition frequency for the transmitter wave trains, and a much lower repetition frequency for the time shift of the heterodyne voltage, e.g. 1000 Hz and 30 Hz, respectively. This still results in a stationary picture on the screen.

As in the case of frequency-modulated VHF radio reception, the ultrasonic FM method likewise has a more favourable signal-to-noise ratio. According to ERDMAN who has investigated and applied this method, the practically attainable resolving power should also be better than that of the pulse-echo method.

2.372 Instruments for the FM Method

Branson manufactures small, portable, battery-operated instruments with acoustic indication, for testing rails (*Audigage Rail Flaw Detector*, Fig. 2.80). This instrument operates according to the principle shown in Fig. 2.78; if the frequency rise of the transmitting voltage is adjusted to only a few thousand cycles per second, the resulting differential voltage will always be audible. An amplifier which lets through the entire audible range thus produces during the rise time a low note for a given echo wave from shallow depth, and a higher note for a more distant flaw. If a loudspeaker or headphones are connected to the output, a noise is heard in which at first the repetition frequency predominates. To prevent the latter from disturbing unduly, a very low frequency is chosen, for instance 50 Hz or even lower, so that it produces a background hum. Depending on the transit time of the echo waves, this noise is then accom-

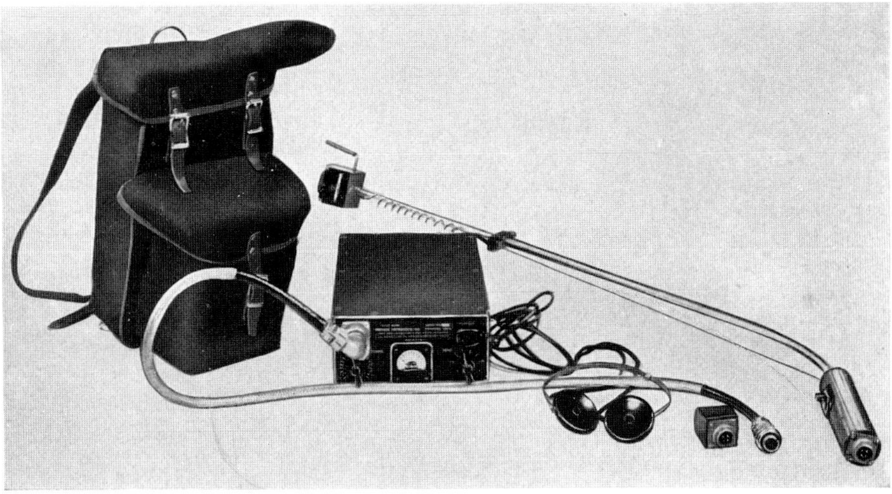

Fig. 2.80 Audigage Rail Flaw Detector by Branson.

panied by lower or higher chirping sounds which are more or less pronounced, depending on the intensity of the echo waves. A trained ear can deduce from it both the position of the flaw and the intensity of the echo if the instrument is used for testing simple and uniform specimens.

2.4 Transit Time Method

2.41 Pulse Methods for Pure Transit Time Measurements

Pure transit time methods are derived from the IT methods by simply disregarding the intensity readings, as long as they do not drop below the minimum value required for the measurement as such. Seen in this light, a wall thickness measurement with a pulse echo instrument is already a pure transit time measurement. Similarly, the methods described in Sec. 2.352, where the transit time supplies electrical data, convert a pulse echo instrument into an instrument measuring transit time. The instruments listed below therefore are pulse-echo instruments without CR tubes but with digital or analogue indication of the transit time. The fact that in the case of wall thickness measurements errors are easily introduced if the height of the backwall echo is not kept constant, is partially responsible for these instruments only recently having found wider application.

The General Electric Company, Schenectady, USA, has developed the *Ultrasonic Micrometer* (Fig. 2.81) used for measuring transit times in air and claimed to have an accuracy of 0.1%. This can be achieved only by compensating all possible effects of temperature and humidity on the speed of sound in air. A reference transit time section of constant length in air, which is placed next to the transit time section to be measured, is used for this purpose. Using a probe resembling a slide gauge, it is possible to measure distances which can be indicated digitally; alternatively the instrument can also be used for controlling machines, e.g. for contactless monitoring of finished sizes when working with automatic machine tools.

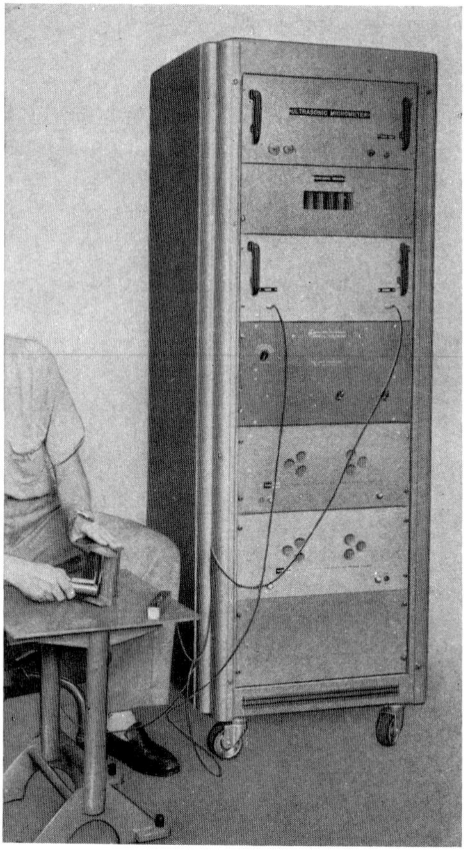

Fig. 2.81 Ultrasonic Micrometer, a dry-type transit time meter of high precision (General Electric). On the left can be seen the measuring gauge in use and next to it the reference delay line.

Using this principle, various wall thickness meters with pointer instruments have been designed, one of the first constructions being Sperry's *Ultrasonic Gage* (Fig. 2.82) in the form of a small and light model for battery operation.

Steinkamp has developed a transit time meter according to the integration method used for testing concrete [351, 79], manufactured by Phywe Göttingen (see also 3.45).

A special method for measuring transit times is the *sing-around method*; as the first ultrasonic pulse method, this had already been proposed and used in 1941 by Hiedemann et al. [142]. In this method the echo of a pulse triggers the next pulse and so forth. The repetition frequency of the pulses which in the case of the conventional pulse-echo instruments is preset, in this case is self-regulating and becomes approximately equal to the corresponding transit time of the pulse in the test piece. By measuring this frequency, e.g. by comparing it with a standard frequency generator, it is thus possible to determine the

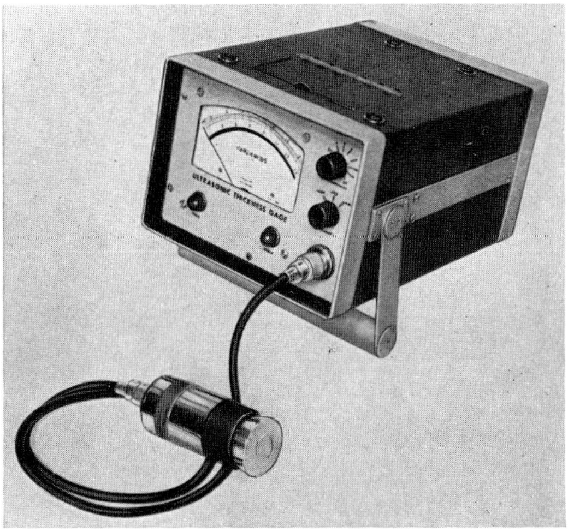

Fig. 2.82 Transit time, alternatively, thickness meter, Ultrasonic Gage Model UT-2, by Sperry.

transit time, and, given the thickness of the specimen, the acoustic velocity. The method can therefore be used for measuring acoustic velocities or thicknesses. The change of the repetition frequency at constant thickness of the specimen can of course be used to deduce indirectly the presence of a flaw.

Numerical example: In a section of steel 100 mm thick the transit time is 34 μs. The repetition frequency therefore becomes 1/34 MHz, i.e. approx. 30 kHz, which is already outside the audible range. In smaller thicknesses it is still higher.

Since frequencies can be measured with very high accuracy, it would seem that this method gives very accurate absolute values. In reality, however, this is not so because of the unavoidable zero error of the transmitting pulse as explained in Fig. 2.83.

A certain time elapses between the reception of a given echo pulse, its amplification, the triggering of the electric transmitting pulse and the actual start of the transit time of the ultrasonic pulse; this is the zero error by which the measured time exceeds the transit time. Consequently also the measured repetition frequency is too low. Since the start of the pulse is defined the less accurately, the smaller the damping of the crystal (see also Fig. 1.108), the error may depend on the damping and thus on the coupling of the crystal. However, even if the crystal is strongly damped and the gain is high enough so that the first oscillations of the pulse can already be used for triggering the next transmitting pulse, a certain residual error is unavoidable. For accurate measurements, the method must be applied to two different, known thicknesses in order to eliminate the error or to determine it once and for all, provided the same probe is used under identical conditions of material and surface.

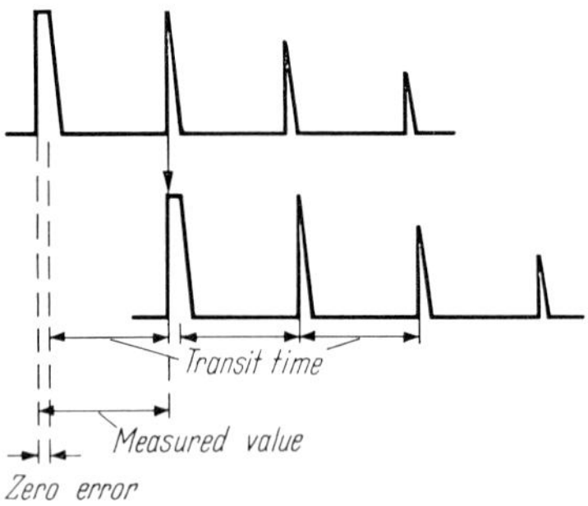

Fig. 2.83 Principle of sing-around method for measuring the transit time and its systematic error.

To be able to initiate the sing-around at all, a pulse would first have to be triggered by hand. A simpler solution is provided by a multivibrator circuit with a time constant so large that, without echoes, the repetition frequency is very low, corresponding to transit times which far exceed the range which is of interest here. The arriving echoes raise the repetition frequency to the value to be measured.

Instruments according to the sing-around method are not yet in regular production. The method is used primarily for scientific purposes and has been applied, inter alia, by Schmauch [324] and Lutsch [240] for determining acoustic velocities in metals and sea water. Dory [76] mentions a special circuit with blocking oscillator which can be used for this purpose.

2.42* Phase Measuring Method

The phase method uses continuous waves of constant frequency. To measure the transit time, the phase of the echo wave is compared with the phase of the emitted wave. If the transit time interval there and back in a given plate is less than one wave length, it can be determined unequivocally on the basis of the phase difference between zero and 2π, by which the receiving voltage is delayed. In the case of greater thicknesses the measurement becomes ambiguous. To avoid errors by a whole number of wave lengths, the approximate thickness concerned must therefore be known. Since also it is not difficult to use very low frequencies for this purpose, this method is particularly suitable for measuring thicknesses or acoustic velocities of strongly absorbing materials, such as rubber and plastics. In practice, however, this method is limited to just such materials because multiple echoes impede the measurement. It was mentioned by HATFIELD and used for measuring thicknesses in rubber [135].

Separate transmitters and receivers are used. For phase measurements any device known from electronic engineering may be used, e.g. an electrostatic CR tube, the transmitting voltage and the amplified receiving voltage being placed on the two pairs of deflecting plates. Depending on the phase difference, the well-known straight lines, ellipses or circles are produced. It is preferable, however, to use an electric phase compensator, and the CR tube for zero indication only.

3 Applied Ultrasonic Testing of Materials

3.1 General Testing Technique

3.11 Coupling

3.111 Condition and Preparation of Surface

In any ultrasonic test the shape and roughness of the surface is of decisive importance. On the one hand these factors often limit the sensitivity of the method applied making it necessary to first prepare the surface. On the other they have a decisive influence on the wear of the probe used for continuous and routine tests if in direct contact with the specimen. The surface conditions therefore greatly influence the economics of testing.

All methods make uniform surface conditions desirable for reliable flaw evaluation. In the case of direct contact where the probe is pressed against the specimen covered by a thin film of coupling liquid, foreign particles or layers are very disturbing because they can considerably vary the thickness of the liquid film, and thus its transmission between different test points (Fig. 1.17). It is therefore absolutely necessary to remove any dirt, loose scale and sand, for which rags, cotton waste and steel brushes are required. Often it is more effective to use a scraper, particularly in the case of loosely adhering layers of rust or paint which form air gaps with the base, which may completely prevent the penetration of sound. In some cases a hammer or grinder may be used, preferably a rotating emery disc with flexible backing which adapts itself to the surface to be treated. Care must be exercised when using rotating grinding wheels to prevent the creation of slightly concave spots, resulting in bad or erratic coupling. If large surfaces have to be treated, as in the case of automated testing, blasting with sand or steel pellets gives best results.

Uniformly and strongly adhering films such as thin oxide layers or even paint, may not necessarily interfere and are often preferable to an unevenly cleaned surface.

Where the surface can be dressed mechanically, it is more important to obtain a uniformly curved shape than high surface quality with an irregular shape. High surface quality is less important for the commonly used frequencies because a surface roughness of less than approx. 1/10 wave length, i.e. of the order of 0.1 mm or less, contributes only relatively little to an increase in sensitivity. On the contrary, polished flat surfaces are often awkward to test because the probes stick due to suction, and therefore cannot be slid along easily. Furthermore, the echo attains its maximum value on such surfaces slowly only, viz. after the liquid has escaped from the narrow coupling gap. In the case of contact tests on test blocks a smoothed surface is therefore preferable in view of the better reproducibility of the echoes.

A roughness of more than 1/10 wave length difference in height impairs the coupling markedly. The acoustic pressure in axial direction is reduced and greater lateral scatter occurs. This also impairs the beaming accuracy and increases the risk of lateral reflections simulating flaws along the axis. Roughness of a uniform pattern, such as turning grooves, can strongly amplify the lateral radiation at certain angles, like an optical diffraction grid, resulting likewise in possible locating errors. Finally, very rough surfaces act on the sound beam like frosted glass on light: the beam becomes diffused and is scattered in all directions, making position fixing impossible.

3.112 Curved Surfaces

Most test surfaces are cylindrical, and of these convex surfaces are better for contact making than concave surfaces. On a convex, cylindrical surface the commonly used flat probe has a reduced contact face in the shape of a narrow rectangle, which enlarges the angle of divergence of the sound beam in the plane normal to the axis of the cylinder, as shown in Fig. 3.1. In the plane at right angles to it and along the axis of the cylinder the angle of divergence remains unchanged.

This reduced contact face also reduces the sensitivity proportionally, as shown in Fig. 3.2 on the echo of a test plate with cylindrical contact face.

If angle probes with plastic material are used the contact face can easily be adapted to an ordinary curved surface, either by grinding the plastic adaptor accordingly, or by inserting and attaching a preformed adaptor, using oil or cement. An exchangeable adaptor makes the angle probe more versatile but it slightly reduces the sensitivity and increases the number of interfering echoes as compared with a cemented-on or suitable ground contact face. After rough-shaping with a file or grinding disc, the surface of the probe can be trued on the test piece itself by inserting coarse emery cloth and rubbing it in. It is by no means absolutely necessary to polish the surface of the plastic adaptor.

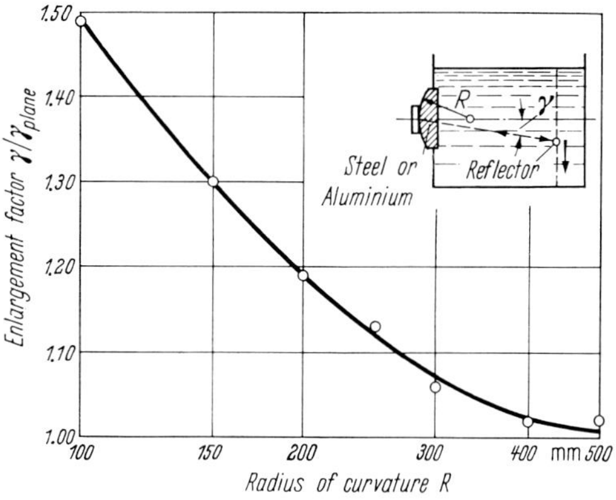

Fig. 3.1 Enlargement of the angle of divergence of a probe in contact with a cylindrically curved surface, mean values from measurements on steel and aluminium with metallized 2 MHz quartz probe, coupled through thin plastic foil and light oil. The enlargement of the angle is referred to the angle of divergence for a flat surface and can be used for all angles of divergence for conversion purposes, both for the directional characteristic of a transmitter and for the sensitivity characteristic in echo-pulse operation, furthermore in any type of material. The measurement was made in the distant field in water.

Even if, as indicated in Fig. 3.3, the apex of the curvature is placed at the sound exit point, the angles of the peripheral rays may easily exceed the permissible sector: steeper angles may produce interfering waves in the form of longitudinal waves, while flatter angles produce surface waves. If, according to Fig. 3.4, the axis of the curvature of the cylinder is located in the plane of incidence (e.g. tube in longitudinal direction), the lateral divergence of the beam is increased. In the case of large angles, e.g. 70° and larger, this may

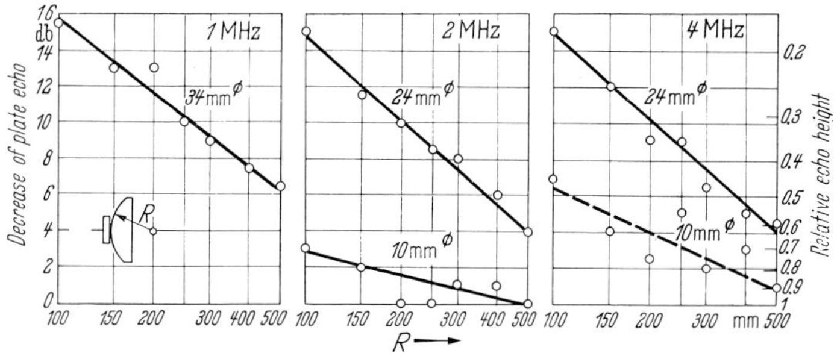

Fig. 3.2 Drop in sensitivity on cylindrically curved surface, indicated by the decrease of the echo on a plane backwall, in decibels as a function of the radius of curvature, measured with metallized quartz probes on steel coupled through 0.3 mm thick Vulkollan foil and light oil.

likewise result in the appearance of interfering surface waves which leave the probe at an angle to the forward direction on both sides.

In order to avoid such disturbing waves it is advisable in the case of surfaces with high curvature not to adapt the probe too perfectly and to be satisfied with a smaller contact face. This face also increases the angle of divergence of the sound beam, acting like a diaphragm, but it avoids the disturbances caused by peripheral rays.

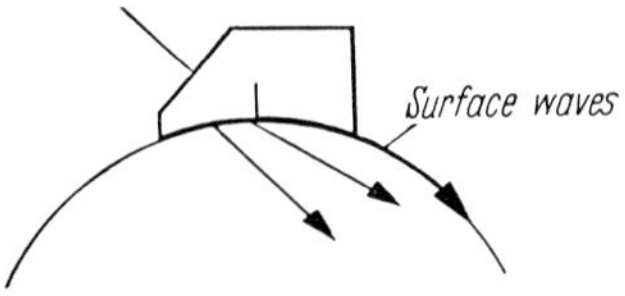

Fig. 3.3 Angle probe on curved surface.

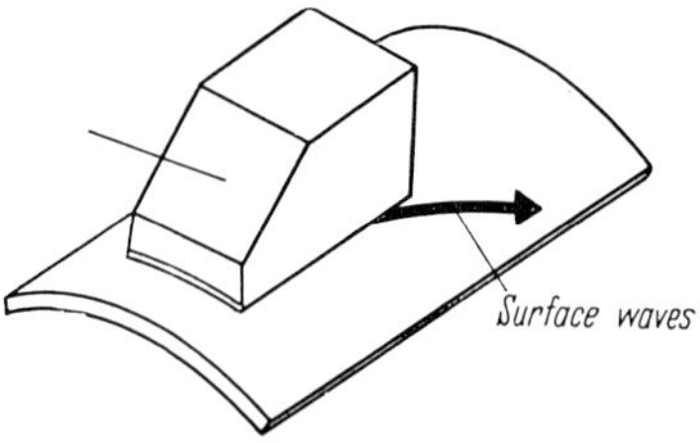

Fig. 3.4 Angle probe on cylindrical surface, axis of curvature in plane of incidence.

If the contact face is small it is difficult to guide the probe. This can be improved by attaching adaptors or supports which slide or roll on the surface. It is also possible to use a perfectly matched contact face as guiding face, and to limit the sound beam by sawing lateral slots into the plastic body parallel to the probe surface until the interfering waves have disappeared.

Fig. 3.5 shows another possibility for avoiding disturbances on curved surfaces: the sound is beamed focused, e.g. by using a strip mosaic.

If flat, normal probes are used on concave surfaces, which latter should be avoided wherever possible, the sensitivity is very low because the centre of the probe does not make contact, nor can this difficulty be over-

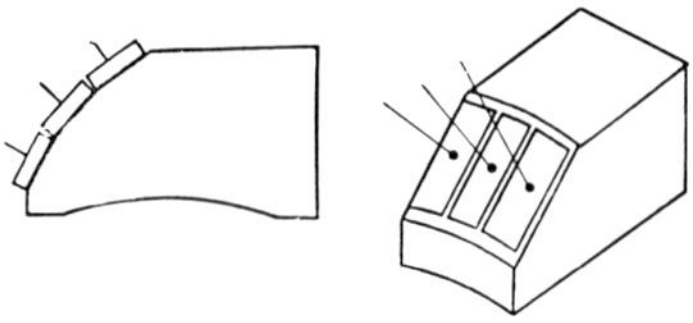

Fig. 3.5 Probes with strip mosaic for adaptation to curved surfaces as shown in Figs. 3.3 and 3.4.

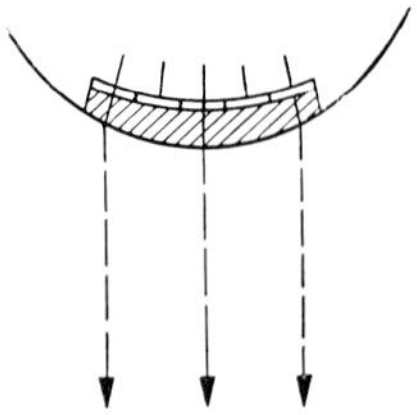

Fig. 3.6 Standard probe for concave surfaces, using strip mosaic and adaptor.

come by the couplant used. It is necessary to use special designs, e.g. rectangular adaptors which in combination with a focusing arrangement of several crystals compensate the curvature by a lens effect, as indicated in Fig. 3.6. Also mosaic assemblies consisting of small, spring-mounted crystals have been used on curved surfaces.

3.113 Coupling Media

Attempts to compensate for the effect of a curved or rough surface by means of a coupling medium have met with little success because all liquid coupling media have a much lower acoustic impedance than the materials of most test pieces. This applies also to liquids containing metal powders in suspension, and to mercury which latter must be excluded, if for no other reason than its cost and toxicity. Of all suitable liquids glycerine still has the highest acoustic impedance. By far the most generally used couplant is oil and for contact tests usually an oil of medium viscosity, grade SAE 30. On smooth surfaces and for measuring, oil of low viscosity or even diesel oil is preferable, and on rough surfaces oil of higher viscosity.

For testing on vertical walls and overhead, a non-dripping couplant is preferable. Grease and petroleum jelly can be used for this purpose but they are expensive and unpleasant to handle; a water-soluble paste such as stiff sizing is preferable.

A suitable paste can readily be prepared on site with cold water and methyl cellulose (wallpaper paste). Since the dried-up residue is difficult to remove, glycerine or a substitute can be added to prevent drying. Corrosive action on metal surfaces is reduced by adding a soluble phosphate such as trisodium phosphate.

Easy cleaning of test pieces, probes and hands, which latter are invariably affected, by the mere application of water is always desirable. Therefore a concentrated sugar solution, which is even cheaper than some oils, is often used. Compared with oil, ordinary water has the disadvantage that it does not always wet satisfactorily, which is very important for good coupling. However, if it wets well, perhaps by adding a wetting agent, it is a very useful couplant if used either as a stationary layer on horizontal surfaces or as constant flow of water between probe and surface.

The latter method was first mentioned by TIMMERMANS, for probes used in medical therapy [366]. In the case of angle probes the liquid can be brought directly to the contact point through a small hole in the plastic wedge.

If a quartz probe, whose contact face is unmetallized and unprotected, is used for testing metal, the sensitivity on rough surfaces can be increased considerably by applying a couplant which contains water and is therefore electrically conducting. This results from the fact that the quartz plate now has an electrode in close proximity which brings it to full excitation. This is an advantage when testing at some depth, but not necessarily always when testing close to the surface. In the latter case the stronger interfering echoes may disturb which are less strong if oil is used, because with oil the quartz plate is excited fully only at the points of actual contact with the metallic test piece. At the free points the effective voltage placed on the quartz plate is reduced. This results in less acoustic energy being radiated into the thicker layers of oil where the disturbing zig-zag reflections originate. For tests on smaller specimens with curved surfaces, it is therefore often preferable to use an unprotected probe and oil coupling, provided the resultant wear can be tolerated. On the other hand, a couplant containing water makes it possible to use also unmetallized probes on non-conducting surfaces.

From a theoretical point of view it is interesting to note that thin metal foils, e.g. copper foil 20 μm thick, in an oil layer considerably increase the transmission between the transducer and the flat metal surface (FIRESTONE [107]). This effect is explained by the improved matching due to the increased, effective acoustic impedance of the whole coupling layer.

Highly viscous materials, such as mixtures of wax and oil and vegetal resins can be used for coupling normal probes for transverse waves (Y-cut quartz plate). On smooth and flat surfaces it is more practical to press the dry transducer against the specimen, using for instance a clamping device or a heavy weight. The coupling can be further improved by rubbing in the quartz plate, applying a slight rotary motion under pressure. In the laboratory the probe can also be stuck on, e.g. by applying sticky wax and heat; instead of a complete probe one can use only a quartz plate, which is metallized at the back and has a soldered-on lead, because the damping of the cemented layer is usually sufficient to produce short pulses. This method is also commonly used for accurate attenuation measurements of plates (see 3.63), also in the case of X-cut quartz plates. For this purpose the use of salts with low melting point and strong supercooling of the solidification point, such as salicylic acid phenyl ester obtainable in the trade as "Salol" (for medical purposes). For permanent connections self-curing cements such as Araldite, etc. can be used. Some of these can even withstand temperatures above 300 °C.

In addition, for liquid coupling on hot surfaces, high boiling-point cylinder oil (up to 300 °C) or silicon oil can be used, although this is very expensive. No satisfactory liquid couplants for temperatures above 300 °C are known. Satisfactory results have been obtained with bitumen, Mircogel grease (Shell) and Midland silicone Ms 550. These couplants are being used successfully on probes fitted with a coupling adaptor of heat resistant plastic material, and where very short coupling periods for recording the test result or measuring result on a luminous screen are sufficient. The time interval between two testing or measuring points is used for cooling both the probe and the coupling adaptor. In this way it has for instance been possible to make point by point measurements with suitably equipped TR probes to determine the wall thickness of corroded pipes at temperatures of 550 °C and upwards [354]. For testing hot specimens, metal adaptors can also be used; these are kept cooler than the hot test piece by applying a continuous flow of coolant, at least at the point of contact with the probe.

Using a cooled metal adaptor (schnozzle) it has also been possible to transmit ultra-sound into liquid metal. The liquid metal must, however, wet the adaptor, which is not always easy to achieve. On cast iron LEHTINEN [334] has used an adaptor made of stainless steel and coated with borax.

According to another suggestion by FARROW [93] hot specimens can be tested by inserting between transducer and test surface a spacer which consists of fusable material, resulting automatically in liquid coupling. No practical applications of this principle have as yet been reported. Regarding probes for higher temperatures see 2.331.

It is rather remarkable that on hot surfaces coupling by means of water still permits transmission of sound in spite of the vapourization, e.g. when testing sheet metal with water jets (see 3.241). Even in the case of incandescent metal transmission of sound has still been observed. It has not yet been determined whether the effect is based on local cooling of the surface under 100 °C, or on sound transmission through the thin layer of steam. It must also still be established whether the transmission of sound is sufficiently uniform for testing.

3.114* Checking of Coupling

Uniform coupling at all points of a given specimen is very important for quick and reliable evaluation of the readings. Occasionally this can be checked by means of a backwall echo. An experienced operator can also check the coupling stability by means of the screen display with its varying, small indications (grass). For this purpose the zero line should always show a little "life". When angle probes are used the quality of the coupling can with a little experience also be deduced from the sliding resistance when shifting the probe, e.g. deterioration in the presence of foreign bodies, or "seizing" if there is not enough couplant.

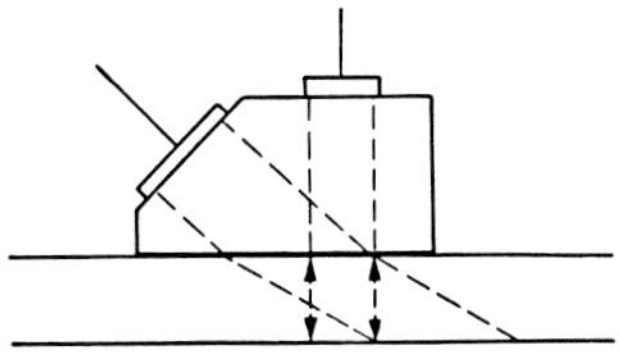

Fig. 3.7 Coupling check with angle probe on plate, using separate transducer.

Electronic devices have therefore been adopted for controlling and measuring. Devices for automatic gain control, mentioned in Sec. 2.35, exploit the backwall echo. Measuring is made possible by utilizing an equivalent electric circuit of the probe as in Fig. 2.33.

Another solution has been described by LUTSCH [238]. On a crystal transducer with only moderate damping at the back, the intensity of the trailing oscillations depends largely on the degree of coupling. If therefore one measures their amplitude by connecting immediately behind the transmitting pulse a gated monitoring amplifier, the output signal of the amplification can serve as a measure of the degree of coupling.

According to a suggestion made by VAN VALKENBURG [370] the degree of coupling of an angle probe on sheet metal as shown in Fig. 3.7 can be checked by means of a second TR crystal which beams through the plastic body normally into the sheet metal, producing a series of multiple echoes. The height of the echoes or the length of the echo sequence can also be converted into a go/no-go indication which actuates a signal.

3.115 Coupling through Intermediate Layers

Wear, and insufficient constancy of the degree of coupling, are the reason for the disfavour into which direct contact of the transducer has fallen. Direct contact makes wear of the transducer unavoidable because the probe, during scanning, cannot always only be placed on and taken off again. Sometimes it must be shifted because any change in the flaw echo while shifting the probe provides valuable information on the flaw concerned for the examiner. He can observe the disappearance and re-appearance of echoes and their change with depth. Particularly when used on cast, rolled or forged, rough surfaces of steel or iron covered by very hard and angular scale, the probe is severely eroded. This makes continuous, automated testing by direct contact impossible. Spacing layers consisting of liquids or plastics cut down the wear but if the pulse-echo method is used, an increase in the number of interfering echoes must be accepted.

The screen traces shown in Fig. 3.8 demonstrate the effect of spacing layers as a function of their thickness. A layer of 0.1 mm already greatly reduces the sensitivity compared with direct contact and considerably broadens both the transmitting pulse and the echoes because with the only moderately damped probe the reduced coupling reduces the damping. Since the length of a 3 MHz wave in oil or water is approx. 0.4 mm, the 0.1 mm layer constitutes a 1/4 wavelength layer. The go and return path of a zig-zag reflection corresponds to a transit time difference of half a wavelength, and results in a cancelling interference. In the case of a layer of double the thickness (c) one therefore obtains by additive interference, approximately the same echo height as in case a. The interfering oscillations behind the transmitting pulse and echoes have, however, increased.

A 1 mm layer in case d already produces a very indistinct picture which would make indication of a flaw in the test plate practically impossible. In addition the echo height is low so that the gain had to be increased. As shown in Fig. 3.8 e the interfering reflections from the coupling layer can be greatly reduced, according to a suggestion by Martin and Werner [250], by adding to the coupling layer, a layer of an absorbing material. In this case Vulkollan was used which, if serving as coupling layer, has the added advantage of high abrasion resistance. The gain, however, has to be increased still further, the same echo height as in the case of direct contact being reached only at a tenfold gain.

If thicker spacing layers are used the surface echo and its multiple echoes become separated from the transmitting pulse. The screen display again becomes clearer and the first surface echo plays the role of the transmitting pulse as in the case of direct contact. It is merely necessary to choose a water transit section of sufficient length for the second surface echo already to appear behind the first backwall echo of the test piece, i.e. at least 1/4 of the thickness of the specimen in the case of steel and water.

A weakly damped probe as in Fig. 3.8 has the disadvantage that its pulse is relatively broad. With thin test pieces, effectively damped transducers should therefore be used for the immersion technique. In the case of quartz transducers this reduces the sensitivity, which in the immersion technique and compared with testing by direct contact has in any case already been reduced to less than 1/10th, as can be seen when comparing the backwall echoes and the gains in Figs. 3.8a and f. For the immersion technique it is therefore preferable to use highly sensitive and effectively damped transducers, e.g. lithium sulphate. Fig. 3.9 shows the same screen trace as in Fig. 3.8f obtained with such a probe. The gain was only 1/10th of that used for direct contact with a quartz transducer.

As a substitute for direct contact testing three possibilities are thus available, each having certain advantages and disadvantages:

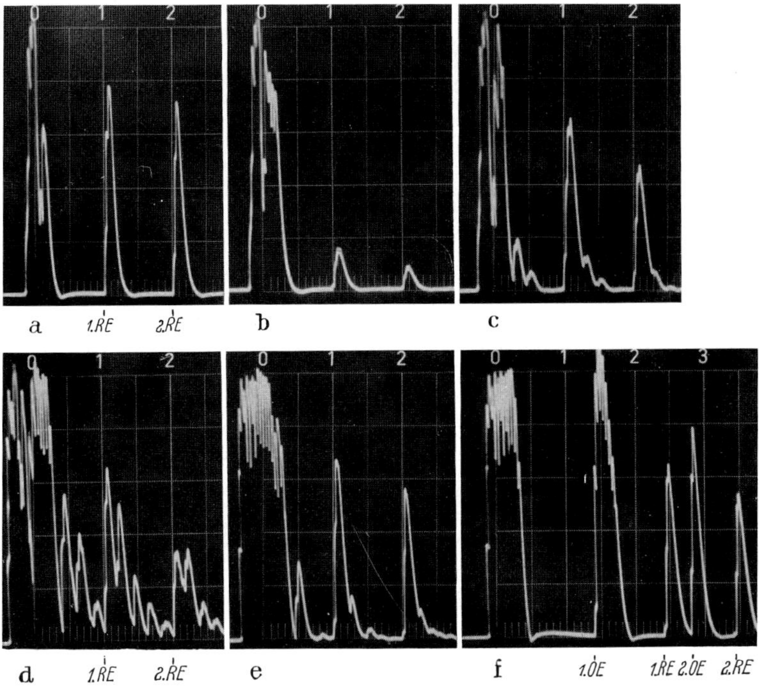

Fig. 3.8 Coupling with increasing layer thickness d (oil or water), quartz probe 4 MHz, moderately damped, on 20 mm steel plate. Calibration: 1 scale division = 20 mm in steel. RE = backwall echo, OE = surface echo. a) Direct contact, $d < 1/100$ mm; b) $d = 0.1$ mm; c) $d = 0.2$ mm; d) $d = 1$ mm, gain compared with a to c, approx. 3 times higher (plus 10 dB); e) $d = 1$ mm, but with inserted Vulkollan foil, gain 10 times higher (+ 20 dB); f) coupling by immersion technique, $d \approx 6$ mm, gain same as in e).

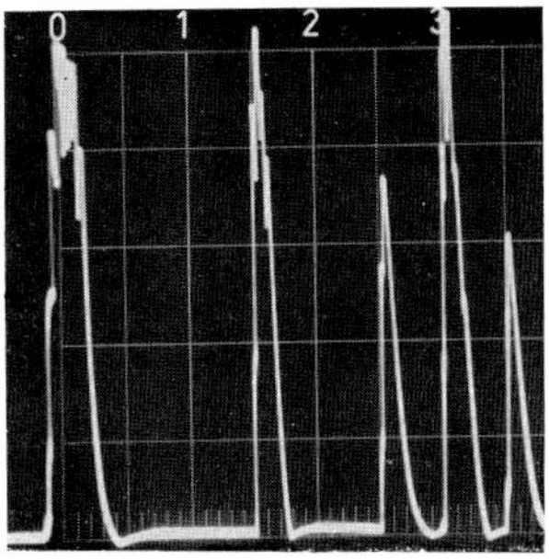

Fig. 3.9 Same test as in Fig. 3.8f, but with lithium sulphate probe, gain 1/10th that of Fig. 3.8a (− 20 dB).

1. Protective layer in front of transducer plate, fixed or exchangeable, not completely wear-resistant, can therefore not be used without further question for continuous testing. Fixed protective layers, once worn, are not readily repairable. The pulse, however, is broadened only moderately. *Examples:* Cast-on synthetic resin layers, possibly containing admixtures of hard substances, or with supporting rings of metal to reduce wear, glued-on or sprayed-on plastic layers such as Teflon or glued-on contact faces on hard crystals such as quartz or sapphire, which latter have given better service than steel. Loose protective layers require a second liquid coupling film, which usually results in pulses which are broader, and therefore un-

suitable for thin test pieces, but conveniently exchangeable by the operator. If the layer is absorbent, the thickness is not critical.

2. Water gap, width without absorbing layer critical, better with absorbing layer, requires device for constant spacing, therefore less suitable for testing by hand than for continuous, automated testing, no wear, pulses broadened.

3. Water transit section or immersion technique, interfering multiple echoes between probe and surface determine minimum width, device for constant spacing, therefore more suitable for continuous, automated testing; pulses not broadened, therefore suitable also for thin specimens.

The first-mentioned method, with a protective layer in the form of an endless belt moving between probe and surface, is also used for continuous, automated testing. Since, when using this device for testing, e.g. heavy plate, particles of scale may enter the space between belt and probe and produce wear, a closed construction as suggested by Messrs. ACEC [418] is more suitable.

Fig. 3.10 shows a practical example of coupling by a water gap, viz. a tester

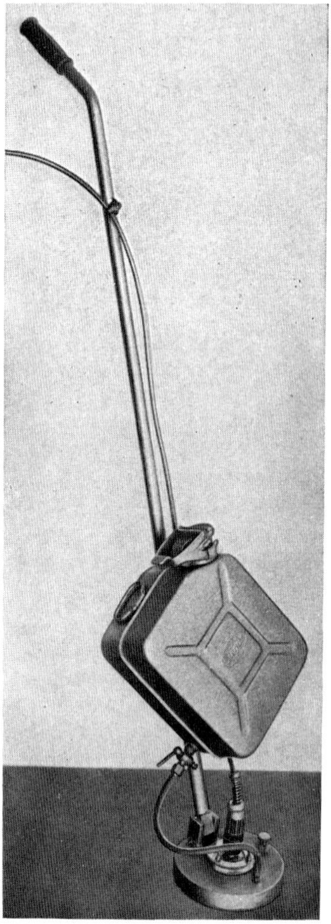

a

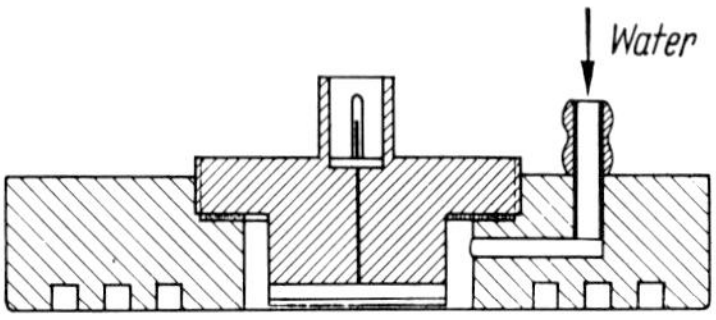

b

Fig. 3.10 Plate tester, design Krautkrämer, photograph and schematic cross-section.

for heavy plate which can be shifted continuously by hand. The screen display is shown in Fig. 3.11. If one does not wish to observe instead the sequence of multiple echoes of a given test plate, but directly the flaw echoes, some of which may be close below the surface, it is advantageous to use a TR probe with a water gap by inserting the probe for instance in a device as shown in Fig. 3.10. The water gap of a few tenths millimetre between the plastic adaptor of the TR probe and the test surface hardly increases the surface echo.

For single-probe operation and thin test pieces it is preferable to use a water transit section, as shown in Fig. 3.12, which consists of a pipe nipple mounted in front of the probe and fed by a constant flow of water which is discharged through the gap between adaptor and specimen. With this method the mount should be guided over the specimen in such a way that the sound beam enters the material at right angles.

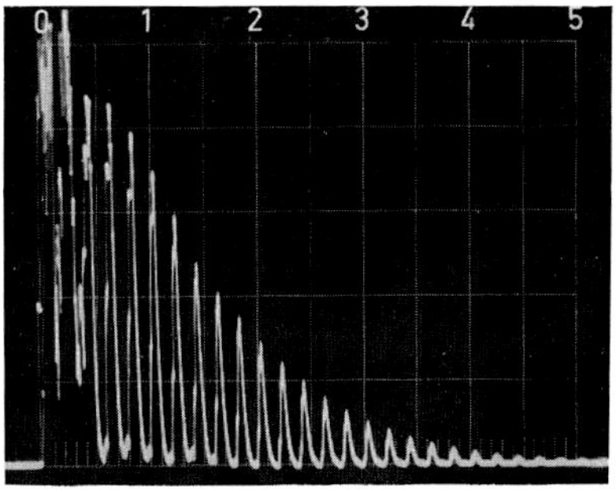

Fig. 3.11 Screen trace of a flawless plate 10 mm thick, tested by water gap coupling (plate tester of Fig. 3.10).

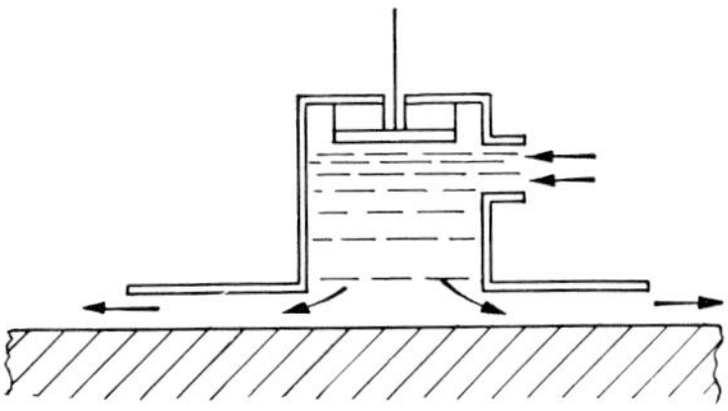

Fig. 3.12 Method of coupling and guiding the probe by means of a transit section with water cushion according to ERDMAN.

For continuous testing it is preferable to couple such a device to the specimen from the bottom instead of from the top because the transit section will then always be filled with water and the transducer coupled to the specimen immediately, only enough water being required to produce a small flow. With a stronger flow of water this method can, however, also be applied from the top or on a vertical wall; before starting, however, it is necessary to expel the air.

If, as shown in Fig. 3.12, the pipe nipple for the transit section ends at the exit side in a large plate, and if water is fed at sufficient pressure, a water cushion is obtained along which the probe can slide without being in mechanical contact with the surface (ERDMAN [85]).

If the water is discharged from the pipe at high speed, a jet is produced by means of which contactless coupling of the probe to the specimen can be effected over a distance of 100 mm and more. This is important in cases where during rapid, automated testing the equipment might be damaged by an uneven surface or by projecting parts of the test piece, e.g. in automated testing of heavy plate. This method of coupling is, however, unsatisfactory when applying the echo method because the flow of water at the contact point produces too many disturbing echoes behind the surface echo, even if the jet is smooth. For sheets this method is therefore used only in sound transmission by applying water jets on both sides [188] (see also 3.241).

The wheel probe by Sperry (Fig. 3.13) is a combination of the endless plastic belt and a liquid transit section. It consists of a plastic tyre completely filled with coupling liquid under pressure. This tyre is rolled over the test specimen. The probe, attached rigidly to the shaft, is positioned a few centimetres from the surface of the tyre. It can also beam obliquely into the specimen and produce transverse waves in it. The angle between the plane of incidence and the rolling direction of the probe can be adjusted to 0°, 45° or 90°.

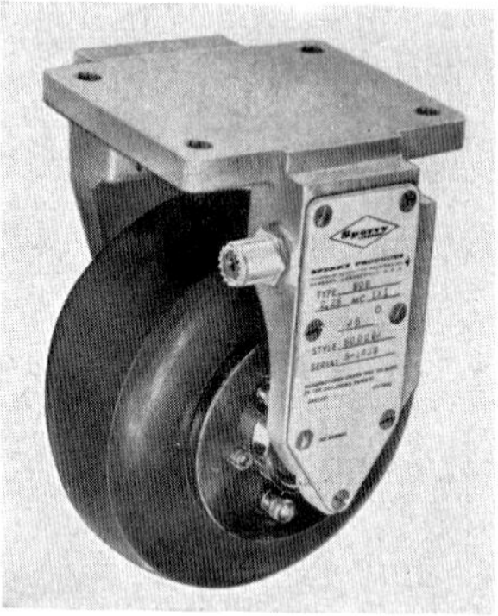

Fig. 3.13 Sperry wheel probe.

Coupling by means of the immersion technique, i.e. with the test piece completely immersed in liquid, was already in use thirty years ago during the first tests involving sound transmission. Today it has found much favour again in automated testing installations using the echo method, particularly for testing light-metal plates, sheets and sections for aeroplane construction, where testing reliability and speed justify the large demand on space and the high costs of this method. Installations of this type used in American plants are shown in Figs. 3.63, 3.109 and 110. Here the probe is moved in two horizontal directions, either by hand or by remote control, according to a fixed scanning programme. A manipulator permits remote control of the distance between probe and test piece, and adjustment of the beaming angle. If the surface is corrugated the probe is preferably rolled across the specimen in a small carriage in such a way that the beaming angle always remains normal to the surface. Significant advantages are uniform and non-abrasive coupling as well as simple transition from normal beaming to oblique beaming without exchange of probes.

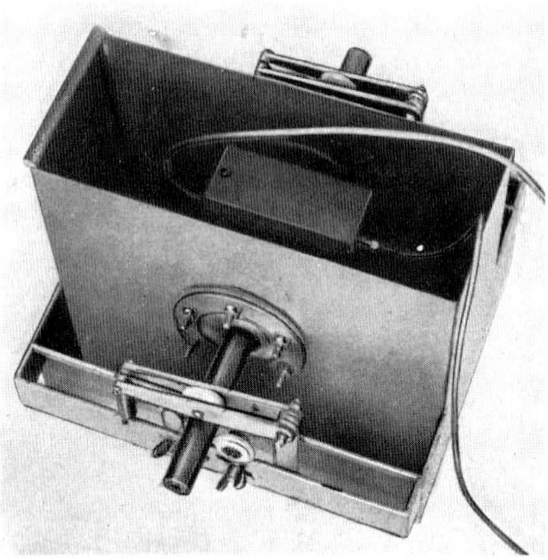

Fig. 3.14 Transit tank with sealed windows for testing round stock and tubing by the immersion technique.

The immersion technique is occasionally also used for testing complex sections manually, e.g. light-metal forgings for aeroplane construction. For this purpose a pipe nipple is mounted in front of the probe, whose free end can be shaped to match the shape of the specimen and to ensure reproducibility and uniformity of spacing and direction of beaming.

For tests by the immersion technique long and flexible test pieces such as sheets and wires are bent and passed through a short tank. To avoid the costs of a large tank for less flexible material, pipes and rods can also be tested by passing them through a short test tank with two windows and with rubber seals which match the shape of the specimen, as shown in Fig. 3.14. After inserting the specimen, the water level in the tank is rapidly brought to the required level by a pump.

In the coupling methods discussed, viz. contact without and with protective layer, water gap, water transit section and full immersion, the cost of a given testing method increases according to its position in the sequence mentioned, but usually at the same time also the economy and the testing reliability. The choice therefore depends largely on the nature and the importance of the testing problem and on the costs involved. Practical examples will be discussed in Sec. 3.2.

3.12 Ultrasonic Frequency and Type of Probe

Even without taking into account the special probes used for specific testing problems, the number of probes listed by the manufacturers is rather bewildering. A few brief directives will therefore be given to facilitate selection.

For testing fine-grained materials by the contact method it has been found that a testing frequency in the range from 2 to 5 MHz is an optimal compromise between the demands for high resolution and great testing depth. The corresponding wave lengths from 3 to 1 mm in steel permit under favourable conditions, detection of flaws of approx. size 0.5 mm and larger, i.e. sizes where the designation *flaw* usually begins to be applicable. With these frequencies, the most common diameter of the standard probe for *daily use* is 20 to 25 mm.

Using this standard probe a skilled examiner will be able to solve a great many problems. When, however, skill alone cannot give the answer, other frequencies will have to be used: where scattering in the material in the form of grass masks the display on the screen, lower frequencies such as 1 and 0.5 MHz may have to be used, although in general this lengthens the close-range interference zone by a factor of 2 and 4, respectively, while proportionally reducing the detectability of small flaws. Even lower frequencies may have to be used to make penetration at all possible in materials with strong acoustic attenuation, such as castings, plastics and wood. Frequencies above 10 MHz are more rarely required because excessive sensitivity to minute flaws is by no means always desirable, and particularly also because these thin crystals, when used in the direct contact method, are not very resistant even if fitted with a protective layer. This high frequency range is mainly reserved for indirect coupling where even fragile crystals such as lithium sulphate can be used.

Diameter of probe and frequency determine the form of the sound beam which in the case of the standard probe can be characterized by a near field in steel of 30 to 130 mm and an angle of divergence of 10 to 3°. A long near field means long range, i.e. high sensitivity for small flaws at great depth if the attenuation of sound in the material is neglected. The length of the near field determines the decrease in sensitivity with distance: to bring this decrease to a minimum the length of the near field should where possible be not less than approx. 1/3 of the maximum flaw distance, as shown in Fig. 1.88. In the case of large specimens this condition cannot be fulfilled because, although the length of the near field increases with the square of the diameter of the probe, the standard probe constitutes a practical limit since most test pieces lack sufficiently large contact faces. On the other hand, higher frequencies, owing to the strongly increasing attenuation, are ruled out.

Thus, while for long ranges probes of maximum diameter are used, the smaller probes of, e.g., 10 mm and less at frequencies from 2 to 15 MHz, are used only for testing ranges up to 100 mm. Compared with the larger probes, the smaller probes in this range have the advantage of more accurate lateral flaw location because of their narrower beam in the near field. They are used perforce where the coupling surface of the test piece is too small for the larger probes.

Accurate lateral flaw location usually makes a large angle of divergence undesirable. However, when the problem is the detection of smooth, obliquely orientated flaws which might easily be overlooked completely if a pencil-like beam is used, and if the specimen cannot be scanned for such flaws by oblique beaming at all possible angles, it is preferable not to attempt an exact flaw location and rather to use a wide-angle beam, e.g. a 10 mm dia. probe at 2 MHz with an angle of divergence of 20°. For the immersion technique one can also use special probes with uniform sensitivity over a sector of ± 45° and more, which can be achieved by using concave radiators.

The recommendation of a definite frequency and a definite probe which have been used successfully with a definite instrument for solving a given testing problem, does not necessarily lead to similar favourable results when an instrument of different manufacture is used; it is therefore always advisable first to dry out the most suitable probe. The reason for this is that *a particular* instrument with probe may, for instance, have a substantially higher sensitivity at 0.5 MHz compared with that at 1 MHz than the other instrument. Thus, while in the case of the first instrument a given test should preferably be carried out at 0.5 MHz, the results in the case of the second instrument may be better when using 1 MHz. At both ends of the frequency range, viz. the high and the low, the amplification of the instrument or the sensitivity of the probes usually decreases. Unfortunately no standardized data concerning this point are as yet available.

The neglect to consider the frequency dependence of the sensitivity of a given instrument has led to the common error of trying to deduce directly from the echo heights of a given specimen, the frequency dependence of the attenuation in the test piece at different frequencies. Even without changing the control adjustment on a given instrument, the switching over of frequencies and the exchange of probes may introduce characteristics of the instrument which can be taken into consideration only by using a calibrated gain control and referring the echoes to the reference echo of the test plate and by making an appropriate allowance for the distance dependence according to Sec. 1.84.

3.13 Interference Effect of Boundaries, Complicated Sound Paths and Screen Displays

The conversion of wave modes on oblique reflection at boundaries of the test piece sometimes results in the basically quite simple testing technique becoming very complicated, and interpretation of the screen picture more difficult. The principles of wave propagation discussed in Section 1 will therefore be applied to a few frequently occurring cases.

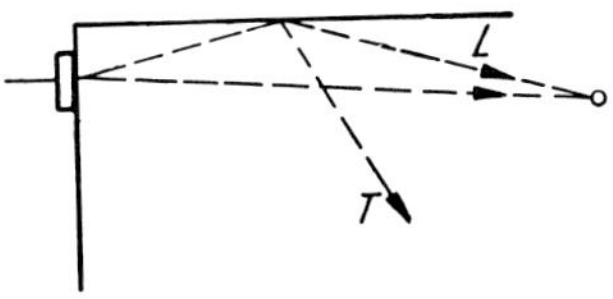

Fig. 3.15. Interference by lateral boundaries.

Disturbances of normal propagation already occur if the peripheral rays of the lobe strike a lateral boundary as in Fig. 3.15. This affects both the sensitivity and the direction of the original beam and additional echoes are produced by split-off transverse waves.

3.131 Effect on the Sound Field by Boundaries Parallel to the Beam Axis

The reflected longitudinal wave interferes with the direct wave and disturbs the original pattern of both the acoustic pressure and the sensitivity, as indicated in Fig. 3.16 by measurements of the echo height of a small flaw in comparison with its undisturbed echo height.

Instead of actually measuring the echo height of a small reflector face in steel at various distances from the lateral wall, the pattern of the acoustic pressure on the smoothly ground backwall was recorded by means of a small receiver, and the squared values plotted in Fig. 3.16 as echo height.

The most troublesome disturbance is the strong decrease of the sensitivity close to the wall, making it difficult to detect small flaws in this zone, such as incipient cracks. In such cases one makes the usual mistake and moves the probe as close as possible to the edge. According to Fig. 3.16 this is wrong: for flaws in the distant field the sensitivity becomes the smaller, the closer the probe is to the edge. The result is still worse if the probe projects partially over the edge, because then also its maximum sensitivity decreases as the remaining contact face. The probe diameter should be chosen as large and the frequency as high as possible. For a given probe and a given flaw distance there is always an optimal distance between probe and edge which gives maximum sensitivity and which may have to be determined with the aid of artificial flaws, such as lateral saw cuts. However, close to the lateral wall the sensitivity is always much

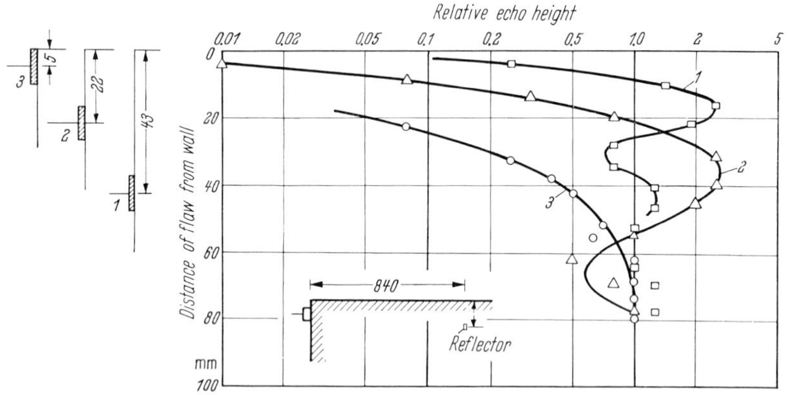

Fig. 3.16 Influence of a plane lateral boundary on the longitudinal sound field; relative echo height of a small flaw plotted as a function of its distance from the wall, measured at a distance of 840 mm in steel, for 3 distances of a 10 mm dia. probe at 4 MHz.

lower than without the distance effect; such flaws are therefore better located by one of the methods illustrated in Fig. 3.17, which are much more suitable for size estimation.

The cause of the reduced acoustic pressure close to the lateral wall is the phase skip of the reflected longitudinal wave by half a wave length. The nearer the angle of incidence is to 90°, the closer to unity will be the coefficient of reflection and the more completely will the reflected wave cancel the direct wave. This skip occurs also in a transverse wave which oscillates parallel to the plane of incidence and whose sensitivity along the wall is therefore likewise reduced. This skip disappears only if the plane of oscillation is parallel to the wall in which case the wall increases the acoustic pressure to twice its value.

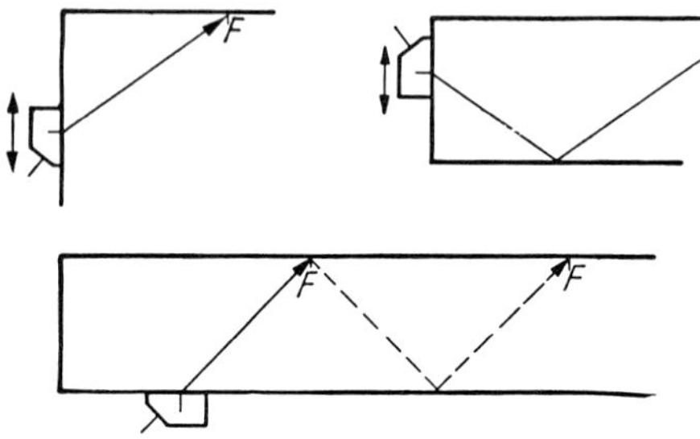

Fig. 3.17 Method for locating flaws close to the surface.

According to Fig. 3.16, the influence of the wall distorts the directional characteristic of the probe so that it has a shape which is no longer axially symmetrical. The cross-section through the lobe under consideration passes through maxima and minima, of which however the greatest maximum no longer lies on the axis but moves away from it as well as from the wall by a distance which is the greater, the closer the probe to the edge. This disturbance can be described vividly by imagining that the original sound beam close to the wall is forced away from it so that it bends, this deflection being the greater the more the beam is forced towards the wall. With such a beam normal flaw locating is therefore no longer possible.

A lateral wall also influences the backwall echo which is greatly reduced near such a wall. However, the larger the diameter of the probe, the more the probe averages the maxima and minima which in general are therefore less pronounced in the backwall echo than shown in Fig. 3.16.

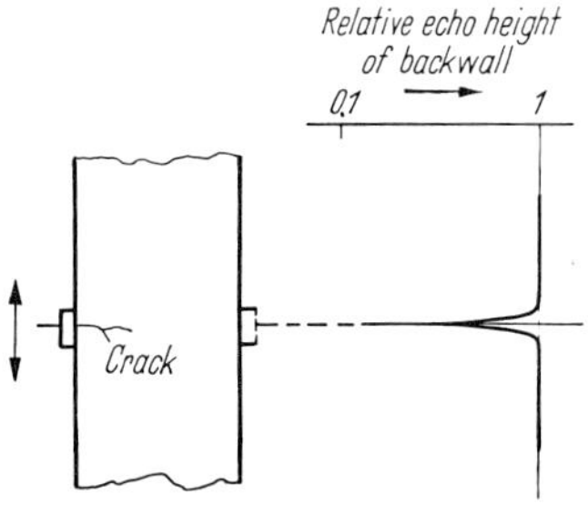

Fig. 3.18 Detection of crack by disturbance of backwall echo, reduction of echo height, schematic.

Occasionally the sidewall effect can be useful, viz. for detecting a crack parallel to the axis of the beam as shown in Fig. 3.18, e.g. if for some reason or other the crack cannot be irradiated at right angles. The backwall echo (or in the case of straight sound transmission the measured value) reaches a minimum if the crack is exactly in the axis of the beam. It then distinctly separates the beam into two laterally bent lobes. If the crack is not too short in relation to the thickness of the specimen, it may lie at the front or the backwall or in between without this making much difference. For good results in this test, probes with a small diameter and low frequencies should be used.

A transverse wave is similarly influenced if it oscillates normal to such a crack surface, but no indication is obtained if it oscillates parallel to it.

So far the disturbance caused by a single sidewall has been discussed. In the case of a plate, however, a second wall is added. For a wave in the plate the disturbance caused by the one wall can be compensated again by the other wall at certain points. Over longer distances and in the case of thin plates, the longitudinal wave is nevertheless strongly damped and only the parallel-oscillating transverse wave can be used, as was already shown in 1.65, Fig. 1.31. Surface waves of high amplitude can travel along the narrow edges of test pieces, and similarly plate waves along strips. Apparently the lateral edges do not interfere and even increase the sensitivity.

If the lateral faces are not flat but for instance cylindrical, as when round stock is tested longitudinally, the focusing effect of the laterally reflected waves is added. This effect is particularly strong if the sound is radiated into the cylinder in the axial direction. The wave which is reflected all around the periphery, can, under certain conditions, produce much higher acoustic pressures along the axis than the direct wave, so that interferences with this wave are no longer of any consequence. This has the effect that the sensitivity along the axis and at greater distances is, in the case of long cylinders, higher as compared with unimpeded transmission. The pattern of the acoustic pressure as a function of the distance is however not uniform because also minima are produced by the interferences of waves reflected a different number of times; this makes it very difficult to estimate the size of small flaws.

If the influence of sidewalls is neglected, this can frequently lead to wrong results for test blocks with artificial flaws. In the case of the pulse-echo method the minimum distance between the beam axis and a sidewall required to avoid disturbing influences can be estimated as follows: The path with sidewall reflection is longer than the axial beam. If the path difference exceeds approx. 4 wave lengths, the first 4 oscillations of the pulse will not be disturbed. In the case of short pulses,

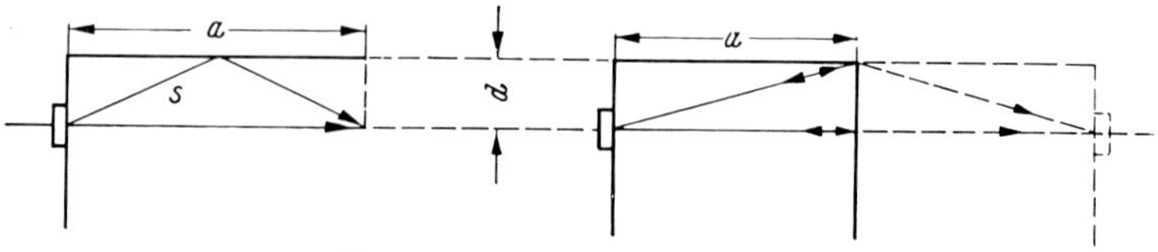

Fig. 3.19 Minimum distance d of a probe from an edge, to eliminate interference by the sidewall in steel, a) for small flaws along the axis, b) for backwall echo.

i.e. instruments and probes with a wide frequency band, it is already possible to distinguish the maximum in this undisturbed zone of the pulse from the disturbed zone following it. According to Fig. 3.19a this requires that

$$2s - a > 4\lambda$$

or approximately

$$\frac{2d^2}{a} > 4\lambda$$

and, e.g., for steel

$$d > 3.5\sqrt{\frac{a}{f}}\ \text{mm} \quad (\text{frequency } f \text{ in MHz}).$$

This applies to the sensitivity along the axis, whereas for the backwall double the length a should be inserted, according to Fig. 3.19b:

$$d > 5\sqrt{\frac{a}{f}}\ \text{mm}.$$

For an undisturbed backwall echo the distance from the wall should be longer than for the echo of a small flaw on the axis. Numerical example: in order to obtain an undisturbed backwall echo from a depth of 100 mm with 1 MHz, the probe should be at a distance not less than 50 mm from any sidewall. The angle of divergence of the sound beam, i.e. the diameter of the probe, is in this case irrelevant.

3.132 Secondary Echoes Produced by Split-off Transverse Waves

Transverse waves split off as shown in Fig. 3.15 leave the sidewall at an angle of approx. 33° to the vertical in the case of steel, and, according to Fig. 1.20 and Table 1, nearly independent of the angle of incidence of the longitudinal wave, provided this angle already exceeds 70°. In the case of grazing incidence the amplitude of these waves is small, on the other hand at steeper incidence the amplitude of the incident lateral radiation of the probe is smaller. For given values of probe diameter, frequency and distance from the edge, the transverse wave therefore reaches a maximum at a certain distance as shown schematically in Fig. 3.20. This maximum moves closer and becomes stronger if the probe is moved closer to the edge.

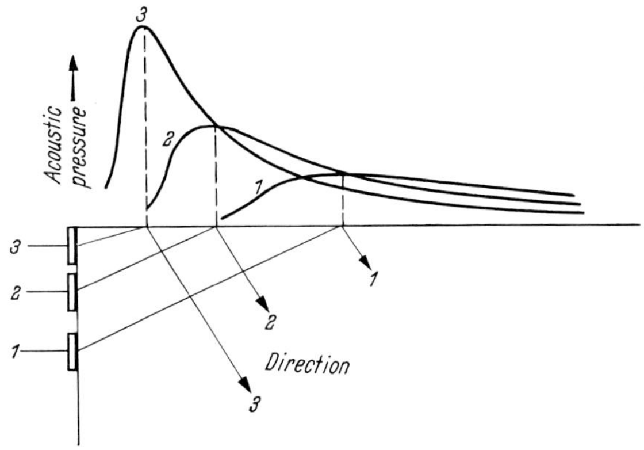

Fig. 3.20 Distribution of acoustic pressure of split-off transverse wave, calcultated for various distances between probe and edge.

If this transverse wave is reflected directly back to the probe as shown in Fig. 3.21a, this hardly interferes because the probe is insensitive to it (see also Fig. 1.59). However, if, e.g., the wave is reflected at an edge back into its own path, it is partially transformed into a longitudinal

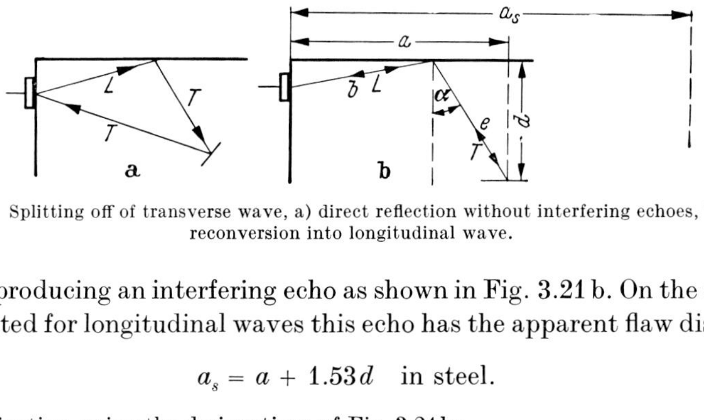

Fig. 3.21 Splitting off of transverse wave, a) direct reflection without interfering echoes, b) mode reconversion into longitudinal wave.

wave, producing an interfering echo as shown in Fig. 3.21b. On the screen calibrated for longitudinal waves this echo has the apparent flaw distance

$$a_s = a + 1.53d \quad \text{in steel.}$$

Derivation, using the designations of Fig. 3.21b:

The transit time is composed of the time over distance b at wave speed c_l, and the time over distance e at speed c_t

$$\frac{a_s}{c_l} = \frac{b}{c_l} + \frac{e}{c_t}.$$

However, in the case of grazing incidence

$$b \approx a - d \tan \alpha .$$

Furthermore $e = d/\cos\alpha$, and for the critical angle α, $\sin\alpha = c_t/c_l$. Thus generally

$$a_s \approx a + d\sqrt{\left(\frac{c_l}{c_t}\right)^2 - 1}\,. \tag{3.1}$$

The error in this approximation is less than 1% for waves with angles to the axis up to 10°, i.e. for all cases encountered in practice.

To avoid a wrong interpretation of such echoes, as can be expected in the examples of Fig. 3.22, the apparent position of the flaw should be irradiated at distance a_s from other directions, or the test from the same position should be repeated by using a more sharply focused beam. If the echo now becomes smaller, this points to a possible interference phenomenon. Echoes in the form of a *grass mound* are frequently obtained with rough internal surfaces of holes or threads as shown in Fig. 3.22c. The real reason for this phenomenon is readily demonstrated by the fact that the mound comes closer if the probe is shifted towards the edge or even slightly over it.

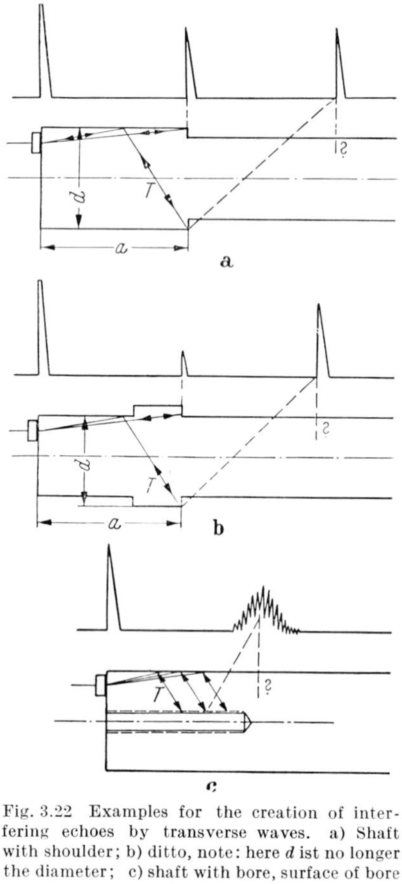

Fig. 3.22 Examples for the creation of interfering echoes by transverse waves. a) Shaft with shoulder; b) ditto, note: here d ist no longer the diameter; c) shaft with bore, surface of bore rough or threaded.

If the sidewalls are parallel (plate, rod, cylinder) the transverse wave can also travel between the walls along a zig-zag path and produce multiple interfering echoes. According to Fig. 3.23 the transverse wave, when it strikes the wall, is partially reflected as a transverse wave at an angle of approx. 33°, and partially retransformed into a longitudinal wave reflected at a grazing angle. If the test piece concerned is narrow enough, the longitudinal wave, after reflection on the backwall, can again return directly to the probe. The echo obtained in this way has, however, only half the delay shown in Fig. 3.21b. This echo will therefore appear only $0.76d$ behind the backwall echo. At the next reflection the reflected transverse wave is again split, resulting in a further secondary echo shifted $1.53d$. In this way a sequence of secondary echoes is obtained in slender test pieces behind every backwall echo and flaw echo, as shown schematically in Fig. 3.24. In the case of rods of rectangular cross-section this sequence consists of two telescoped sequences corresponding to the two different cross-sections.

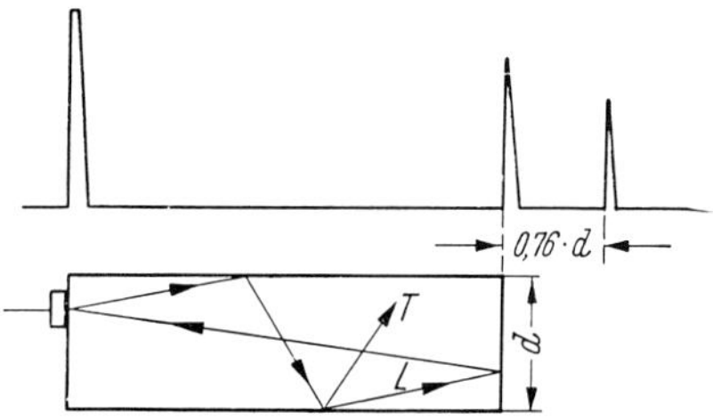

Fig. 3.23 Secondary echoes in a slender cylinder (steel).

If such test pieces give no indication of flaws, the secondary echoes cannot be mistaken for flaws because they appear only behind the end echo. However, if flaw echoes are present, the secondary echoes cause confusion and they may give the impression that there are more flaws than are actually present.

For very long and slender test pieces the secondary echoes may be more pronounced than the backwall echoes and they may finally be all that remains, appearing in the form of a "beard" (bell-shaped sequence of closely packed echoes), if the end echoes themselves have already become very weak.

Secondary echoes appear as a long sequence of considerable height only if the conditions for reflection are good at all points owing to a smooth surface. If, however, in the case of a given specimen these echoes are comparatively badly distorted in spite of a good surface, this points to elongated flaws in the specimens which, while still passing the direct longitudinal wave, suppress the oblique transverse waves.

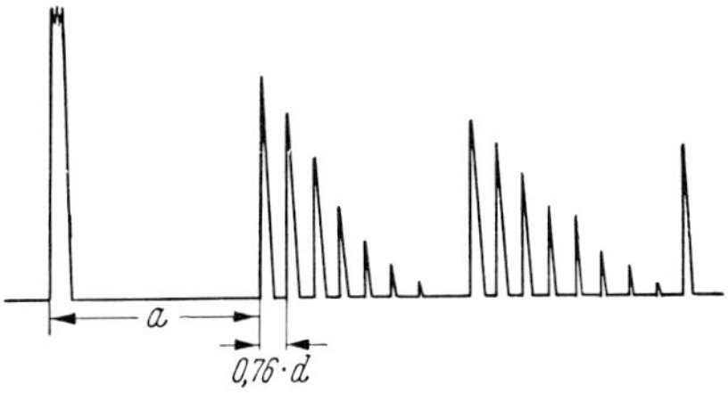

Fig. 3.24 Schematic screen trace of a specimen (plate or round stock or square section) with $d : a = 1 : 6$, with multiple backwall echoes and sequences of secondary echoes (steel).

3.133 Triangle Reflections

In a solid cylinder or a sphere, the peripheral rays of a normal probe making an angle of 30° with the axis may produce reflections in the form of a triangle as in Fig. 3.25. The angle of divergence of a plane probe used on small-diameter round stock, or even more so on a sphere, is particularly wide and the triangle echo therefore very pronounced, as shown in Fig. 3.27. In addition to this reflection in the form of an equilateral triangle, there occurs also a triangle reflection with wave conversion according to Fig. 3.26. Both types of interfering echoes appear behind the first backwall echo, at the following apparent distances:

triangle wave without conversion: $a_s = 1.30d$,
triangle wave with conversion: $a_s = 1.67d$ for steel,
$= 1.78d$ for aluminium.

Fig. 3.27 shows the screen trace of 40 mm steel round stock at 4 MHz.

Derivation: according to Fig. 3.25, in the equilateral triangle with side s, we have

$$\frac{s}{2} = \frac{d}{2} \cos 30^\circ,$$

and the total sound path $3s = 3d \cos 30^\circ$. Of this, however, only half can be taken because the screen is calibrated in distance and not in echo path there and back. Therefore, irrespective of the material

$$a_s = \frac{3}{2} d \cos 30^\circ = 1.30\, d. \tag{3.2}$$

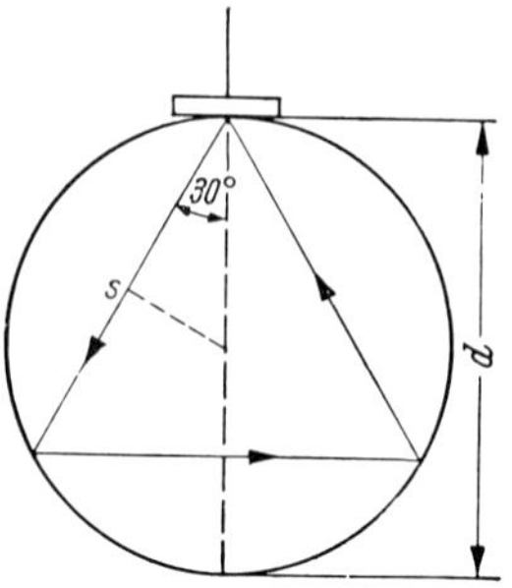

Fig. 3.25 Triangle reflection in round stock without mode conversion.

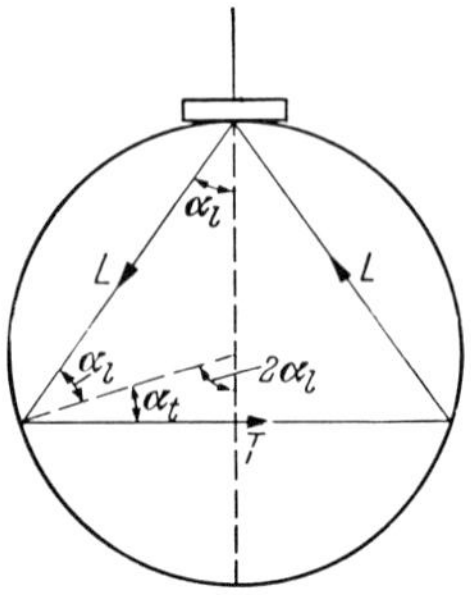

Fig. 3.26 Triangle reflection with mode conversion.

From Fig. 3.26, and using trigonometry it follows that

$$\alpha_t = 90^\circ - 2\,\alpha_l$$

and from the law of refraction

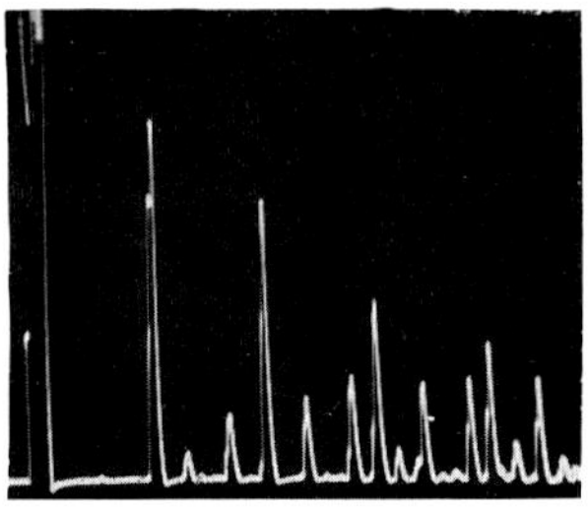

Fig. 3.27 Screen trace when testing round steel (40 mm).

$$\frac{\sin \alpha_t}{\sin \alpha_l} = \frac{c_t}{c_l}.$$

Therefore

$$\sin \alpha_l = \frac{1}{4}\left(\sqrt{8 + \left(\frac{c_t}{c_l}\right)^2} - \frac{c_t}{c_l}\right)$$

and the apparent flaw distance

$$a_s = d\left(\cos \alpha_l + \frac{1}{2}\frac{c_l}{c_t} \sin 2\,\alpha_l\right). \tag{3.3}$$

Calculating the angles we get for

steel: $\alpha_l = 35.6^\circ$, $\alpha_t = 18.8^\circ$

aluminium: $\alpha_l = 36.5^\circ$, $\alpha_t = 17.0^\circ$

from which the above-mentioned values for a_s may be calculated.

Echoes of multiple triangle cycles appear behind the second backwall echo, where they complicate the screen picture.

As in the case of all echos created by peripheral radiation and imperfect contact, the height of the triangle echoes fluctuates considerably with the degree of coupling and the spreading of the couplant. They interfere with the detection of flaws if the direct flaw echo in front of the first backwall echo is not used but instead, e.g., the W-echo shown in Fig. 1.50. According to Figs. 1.48 and 1.49 a zone of high sensitivity occurs a little beyond the axis owing to the focusing effect of the cylindrical surface. Therefore larger flaw echoes usually appear between the first and the second backwall echo, where also the triangle echoes are located.

In the case of round stock thinner than approx. 20 to 30 mm, the interfering zone behind the probe often masks the direct flaw echo. It is then preferable to use a TR probe.

3.134 61° Reflection

Sometimes a reflection of the longitudinal wave is obtained in a steel specimen at a boundary inclined at 61° as shown in Fig. 3.28. This is accompanied by conversion to a strong transverse wave. If simultaneously reflection on a lateral wall occurs, strong echoes from apparently great depth are obtained.

Derivation: From the conditions

$$\alpha_l + \alpha_t = 90^\circ$$

and the law of refraction

$$\frac{\sin \alpha_l}{\sin \alpha_t} = \frac{c_l}{c_t}\,.$$

the angle α, which at the same time is an angle of the prism, is given by

$$\tan \alpha_l = \frac{c_l}{c_t}\,.$$

The corresponding values are for

steel: $\alpha_l = 61^\circ$, $\alpha_t = 29^\circ$,
aluminium: $\alpha_l = 64^\circ$, $\alpha_t = 26^\circ$.

If the entrance point of the beam in Fig. 3.28 is shifted, the apparent echo path, i.e. the transit time, remains unchanged; at first glance this may seem surprising because this also changes the travel distances for the longitudinal and transverse waves. However, the longer path at the higher longitudinal velocity exactly balances the shorter path of the slower transverse wave, as shown in Fig. 3.29. The longitudinal portion of the path along *2 — 2* is longer by a than along the path *1 — 1*, while the portion of the transverse wave is shorter by b. The transit times along these paths are a/c_t and b/c_l, respectively. From the triangle it follows that

$$a : b = \sin \alpha_l : \sin \alpha_t$$

and from the law of refraction

$$a : b = c_l : c_t\,.$$

Therefore

$$\frac{a}{c_l} = \frac{b}{c_t}\,.$$

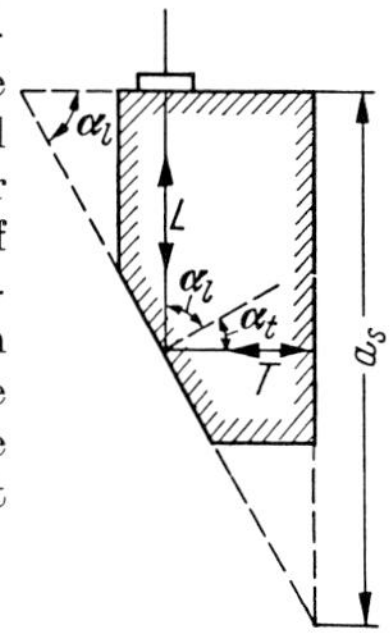

Fig. 3.28 Reflection accompanied by 90° deflection and mode conversion in 61° steel prism (64° for aluminium).

If the cross-section of the test piece in Fig. 3.28 is supplemented so that the indicated triangle is obtained, the transit time of the echo is identical for all beam entrance points along the shorter base. The apparent distance of the echo equals the longer perpendicular.

Table 1 in the Appendix indicates that the product of the two reflection coefficients during the conversion along the go and return paths is approximately unity.

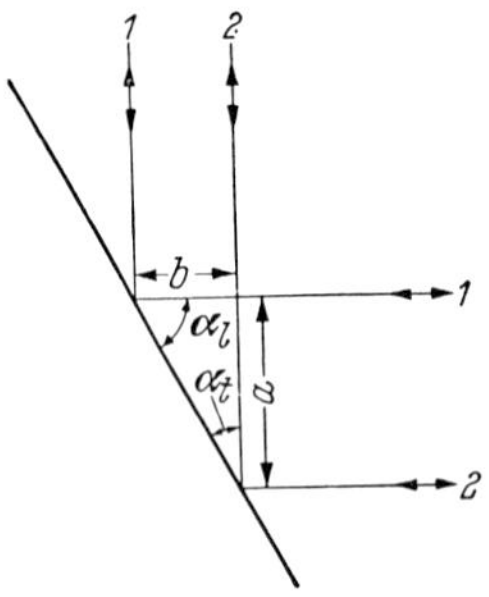

Fig. 3.29 Conditions for mode conversion in a 61° steel prism.

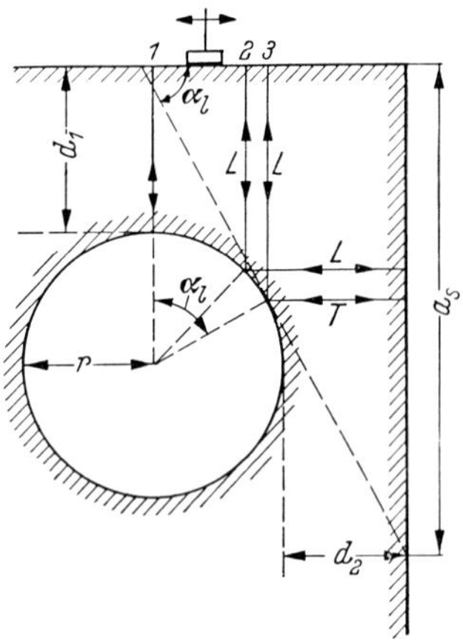

Fig. 3.30 Interfering echoes when checking a cylindrical hole for incipient cracks.

The waves of the same mode which occur during this process, but are reflected away unfavourably, are very weak. This device therefore represents an almost loss-free converter from one mode into the other, with 90° deflection. One can also begin with a transverse wave, beamed for instance by a Y-cut quartz into the perpendicular wall on the right in Fig. 3.28, assuming that its direction of oscillation is parallel to the direction of incidence. In the case of aluminium the *efficiency* is still greater.

A practical example of such a reflection is the testing of a cylindrical hole near a right-angled corner in a test piece as shown in Fig. 3.30, e.g. when checking a high-pressure pump cylinder for the presence of incipient cracks on the internal wall. In addition to any flaw echoes the following echoes will occur:

1. Echo of hole at distance d_1.

2. Echo from sidewall after a 45° reflection via longitudinal waves. At this point the split-off transverse wave produces no interfering echo because it is diverted at an unfavourable angle and disappears. The echo appears at the distance

$$d_1 + d_2 + 2r\,(1 - \sin 45°) = d_1 + d_2 + 0.568\,r$$

irrespective of the material.

3. Echo as above after 61° reflection; the apparent distance is calculated by the formula

$$d_1 + d_2 \tan \alpha_l + r\left(1 - \tan \frac{90 - \alpha_l}{2}\right) = d_1 + 1.82\, d_2 + 0.742\, r$$

for steel.

If, e.g., $d_1 = d_2 = r$, the echo distances are as 1 : 2.57 : 3.56. Naturally, in addition to any flaw echoes, other echoes can also occur depending on the shape of the specimen, e.g. backwall echo between hole and lateral wall, and multiple echoes of the above.

3.135 Screen Pictures when Testing a Plate

At first glance the screen picture of a plate as in Fig. 2.16 shows nothing remarkable. In the case of a flawless plate the multiple echoes follow each other at the distance of the plate thickness without intermediate echoes, provided the gain is not too high.

The height of the echo does not decrease, as is often erroenously assumed, simply according to an exponential function as a result of attenuation but for various additional reasons. Firstly, the path of the rays can be visualized as being repeatedly reversed, as in Fig. 1.37, so that each multiple echo can be regarded as the backwall echo of a plate of multiple thickness. In the near field of the probe the backwall echo of a given plate decreases only slightly with the thickness, but more rapidly in the distant field, inversely with the thickness (see also Sec. 1.84). To the attenuation according to an e-function, must be added the disturbance introduced by the probe on the front of the plate with each reflection of the wave. The probe absorbs a portion of the incident wave. Consequently the reflection at the contact point is smaller than at points around it; phase shifting, which depends on the design of the probe, may also occur. As shown in Fig. 3.31, a long sequence of echoes may therefore show an irregular decrease of the echo height, similar to beats, showing minima and maxima, whose position shifts if the coupling is changed slightly. Such a sequence of echoes is not very suitable for quantitative evaluation, e.g. for attenuation measurements. For this purpose it is preferable to couple via a water transit section, a condition which is uniformly and quantitatively determinable.

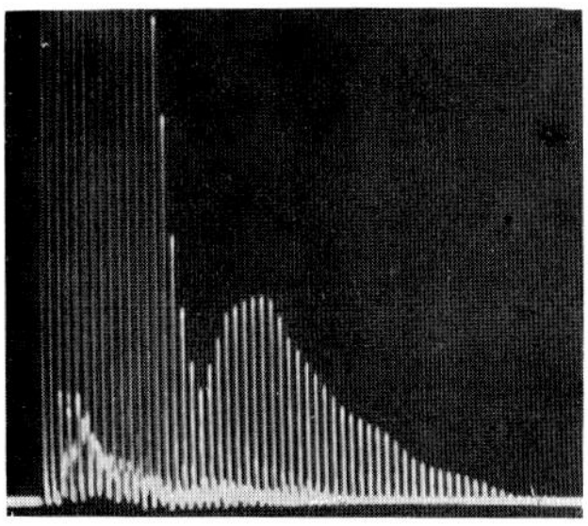

Fig. 3.31 Screen picture of a long series of multiple echoes obtained on a flawless plate in a contact test.

If the plate contains a small flaw which is not big enough to markedly mask the backwall echo, its echo appears in the same position behind each multiple backwall echo. The echo height however, changes, but not in the same way as the backwall echo. For in the case of the small flaw, according to Sec. 1.84, the wave structure in the near field of the sound beam makes itself felt. The point of maximum sensitivity is reached at the end of the near field while in the distant field the echo decreases inversely with the square of the distance. This explains the screen picture shown in Fig. 3.32, which, while showing the different behaviour of flaw echo and backwall echo, also depends on the size, frequency and design of the probe.

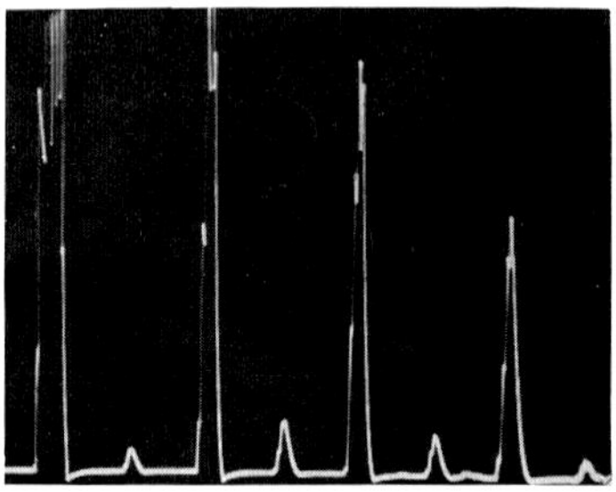

Fig. 3.32 Screen picture of a plate with small flaw.

Sometimes the screen picture is further complicated by multiple echoes which follow the flaw echo. As shown schematically in Fig. 3.33, this sequence of flaw echoes may in certain circumstances also extend behind the first backwall echo where it is superimposed on further sequences of flaw echoes, resulting in a very complex picture. This portion of the picture is however of little significance for the evaluation.

However, this case occurs rarely only because these multiple flaw echoes decay rapidly unless the flaw concerned is flat, smooth, and at right angles to the axis of the beam, and comparatively near. According to Sec. 1.84 the ratio of two successive echoes of a small flaw in the form of a circular disc is determined by

$$\frac{H_n}{H_{n-1}} = \frac{F}{2\,a\,\lambda}$$

(F flaw area, a flaw distance), calculated on the assumption that the distance is much greater than the near field length of the flaw; it can be assumed that this condition is fulfilled if for the ratio H_n/H_{n-1} values of less than 0.5 are calculated. This relationship can be used for determining the sizes of artificial flaws. In order to obtain measurable multiple echoes, a higher frequency (smaller wave length) can be chosen, provided the damping of the sound, which has been neglected here, permits this.

The screen picture of a plate looks slightly different, as shown in Fig. 3.32, if the flaw does not consist of a small, limited discontinuity which reflects the sound completely, but of a layer with a certain transmittance, which therefore reflects incompletely. Examples of this nature are accumulations of finely distributed inclusions in a given plane of a sheet, which are partially transparent like a curtain, imperfectly welded laminations as frequently encountered in light metals, furthermore also shrink fits and platings, where even a flawless bond may have a certain reflection power due to different acoustic impedances. This then need not necessarily constitute a defect and the resultant echoes are therefore called layer echoes.

The various sequences of layer echoes, as produced by each backwall echo in a manner similar to that shown in Fig. 3.33, need not decrease uniformly but may show characteristic maxima whose positions depend on the coefficient of reflection of the layer concerned. Such an echo picture is shown schematically in Fig. 3.34, as well as the formation of the individual echoes, each designated by three indices. Since the pulse when it reaches the layer is split each time into a transmitted and a reflected portion, it breaks up into an increasing number of partial pulses as the number of multiple echo reflections increases. The three indices of such a partial pulse indicate how often it has passed through the entire plate or the two sections respectively above and below the layer. Nearly all echoes are then composed of several components with equal transits. In the case of the echo marked 210 the total number of transits is 6, namely 3 of type 210 and 3 of type 121. They are shown next to each other above the screen plate. Each of the six components is found again in the diagram of the pulse paths under the screen picture. With increasing echo distance the number of components participating in a given echo is greatly increased so that this echo can become higher than the previous echo of the same sequence, although the individual partial pulses themselves are smaller [125, 272]. Fig. 3.34 indicates that the echoes of a given sequence – the indices within a given sequence are identical except for the first index – first increase in height and decrease again only after they have passed through a maximum. The envelope of each echo sequence including the envelope of the backwall echoes passes in its further progress through alternating zeros and maxima – not indicated in Fig. 3.34.

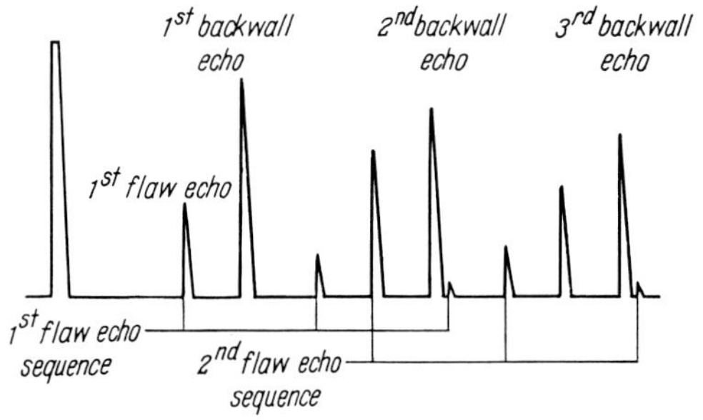

Fig. 3.33 Schematic screen trace of a flaw in a plate showing multiple flaw echoes.

By making the simplifying assumption that at the surface of the plate facing away from the probe, loss-free reflections occur, and that we are dealing with a plane sound wave, and thus are operating entirely in the near field of the probe, the relative height of the echoes with the indices M, N and Q can be calculated as follows

$$H_{M,N,Q} = R_0^{M+N-1} R_1^{N+Q} (1 - R_1^2)^M \times \sum_{\mu=0}^{M-1} \left\{ \binom{M+N}{N+\mu} \binom{M+Q-1}{Q+\mu} \left(\frac{R_1^2}{1 - R_1^2} \right)^{\mu} \left(-1 \right)^{\mu} \right\}, \tag{3.4}$$

where R_0 is the coefficient of reflection at the coupling point of the probe, R_1 the coefficient of reflection at the layer, both being referred to the amplitude.

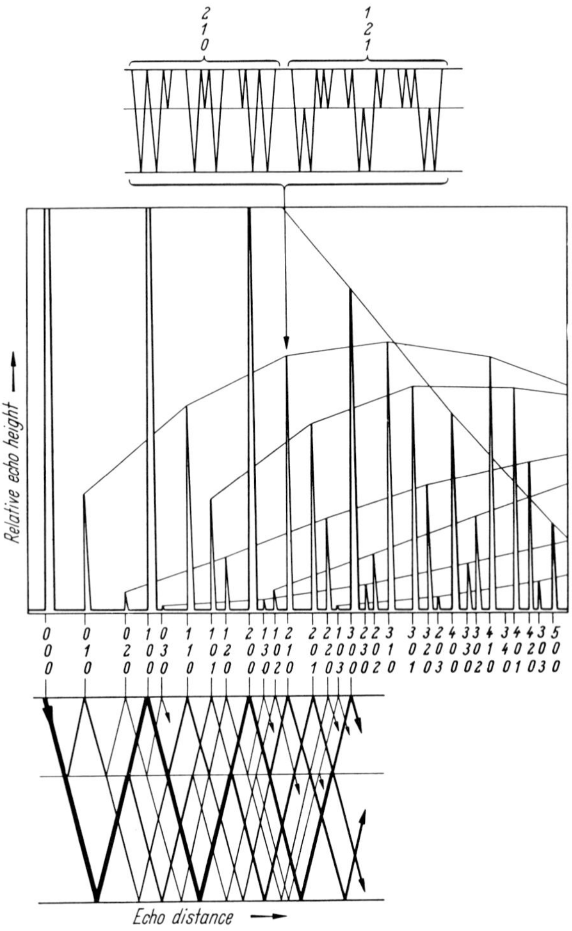

Fig. 3.34 Calculated screen picture of a plate with a partially transmissive layer. Multiple echoes of backwall shown in bold lines. Coefficient of reflection at layer 0.2, at coupling point 0.9. The echoes belonging to a given sequence are connected by curves for clearer indication of their change in height. Below: pulse splitting at layer; above: example of an echo composed of several partial pulses.

Eq. (3.4) does not apply if the layer is approximately in the centre of the plate, because in this case the echoes $H_{M,N,Q}$ are superimposed on each other in such a way that except for the backwall echoes only a sequence of intermediate echoes remains, each of which being located in the centre between two backwall echoes. Depending on the phase differences which occur, very different screen pictures as well as pronounced interference maxima and minima of the individual echoes can be obtained on one and the same layer as a function of its position. At certain layer positions one again obtains alternating zeros and maxima within the envelope of the sequence of backwall echoes and layer echoes. Further details concerning theoretical and experimental investigations of such layer echoes are found in reference [272].

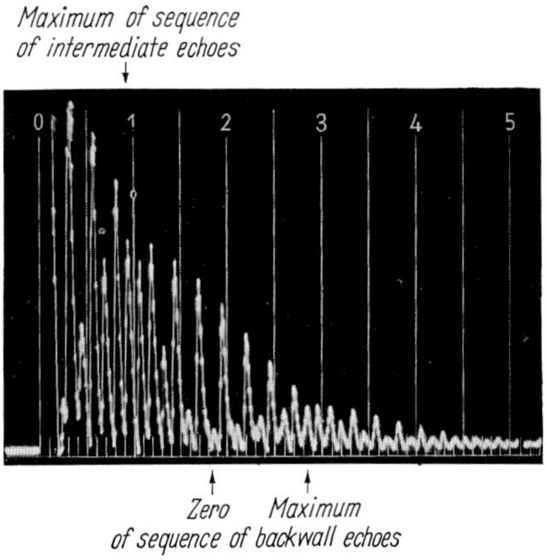

Fig. 3.35 Screen picture of a long series of multiple echoes obtained on a plate with semitransmissive layer (finely distributed inclusions), approximately in the centre of the plate. Coefficient of reflection of layer approx. 0.1.

This summation effect of the partial pulses can serve for deducing the presence of weakly reflecting layers from the increase of the intermediate echoes behind numerous multiple reflections of a given plate, the reflecting layer being hardly visible before the first backwall echo. Furthermore, the position of the maxima can give information regarding the coefficient of reflection of the layer and thus, where applicable, the quality of a bond. As an example, Fig. 3.35 shows a screen picture of a sheet with finely distributed inclusions in the centre which correponds to a coefficient of reflection of the layer of approx. $R_1 = 0.1$. The first maximum of the sequence of intermediate echoes is clearly visible, likewise the first zero and the subsequent maximum in the sequence of the backwall echoes. – In evaluating screen pictures of this type it is, however, necessary to take account of interfering echoes whose causes are described below.

If the gain is high enough, interfering echoes appear behind the multiple backwall echoes also in the case of a flawless plate, which are already faintly visible in Fig. 2.16. These disturbing echoes are shown more distinctly in Fig. 3.36 on screen pictures of steel and aluminium, respectively. Their position thus depends on the material. According to [125] and [172] these interfering echoes are produced by multiple backwall echoes which have travelled through the plate along their single or repeated paths as transverse wave. The sound beam of a probe for longitudinal waves does not transmit a strictly plane longitudinal wave but also obliquely travelling longitudinal waves as well as transverse waves of low amplitude, as shown in Fig. 1.59 for a very small probe. A wave incident obliquely on the backwall is, however, converted partially into another mode, although at the small angles concerned this is very weak. The probe also receives echoes of obliquely incident transverse waves because the transmitting and receiving characteristics are always identical. Therefore, a first interfering echo is produced by a wave which on its outward path passes through the plate as an oblique longitudinal wave,

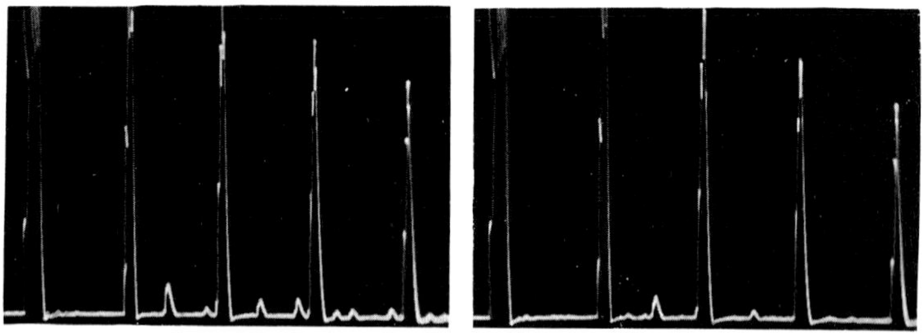

a b

Fig. 3.36 Screen pictures of flawless plates of steel (a) and aluminium (b) at high gain.

and on its return path as a transverse wave, producing a longitudinal-transverse (LT) *echo*. This, however, is also the transit time of a transverse-longitudinal (TL) wave. The next is a transverse-transverse (TT) wave whose apparent echo path is c_l/c_t times the plate thickness d. Generally the apparent echo path for a combination of m longitudinal paths and n transverse paths is determined by

$$0.5\,d\left(m + n\,\frac{c_l}{c_t}\right).$$

For the first two paths one thus obtains

for steel:	LT + TL 1.41 d	TT 1.82 d,
for aluminium:	1.51 d	2.04 d.

As shown in Fig. 3.36, the TT wave in the case of aluminium is invisible because it is masked by a multiple backwall echo.

These echoes should not be wrongly interpreted as flaw echoes, e.g. when testing sheets. Owing to the above-mentioned summation effect their height may at first increase in a lengthy series of echoes.

3.136 Interfering Echoes through Surface Waves

Surface waves are frequently produced unintentionally. Whenever a probe is coupled to a solid they are radiated unavoidably, but usually they are very weak compared with the longitudinal or transverse waves. This however, is no longer the case if the sound beam is no longer sharply defined, i.e. in the case of a small d/λ ratio, as in the case of probes of exceptionally small diameter, incomplete contact, and probes for low frequencies, below say 1 MHz.

Using a 0.5 MHz normal probe, it is for example possible to obtain on the polished face of a large forging or casting, large and pronounced interfering echoes which are produced by surface waves at the edges of the specimen or the periphery of the ground face. Higher frequencies can still be damped by merely touching the surface with an oily finger, and this can be used for distinguishing such interfering echoes from true echoes. At frequencies below 1 MHz this, however, is already more difficult, even if the palm of the hand is used. If one does not want to use considerably larger probes, which naturally require correspondingly larger coupling faces, specially designed probes can overcome this difficulty; subdivided transducer plates as shown in Fig. 2.39 do not radiate the surface waves in the contact plane uniformly in all directions but in the shape of a four-lobed directional pattern. By rotating this probe about the contact point, interfering echoes can be distinguished from true echoes. For reason of interfering surface waves, low frequencies should be used on non-polished surfaces. Mill-rough surfaces damp the interfering wave quickly and merely produce a little grass.

Incomplete contact is moreover frequently unavoidable, e.g. on round stock. On small diameters strong surface waves are radiated even if higher frequencies are used. The remaining longitudinal waves can then be entirely suppressed by completely dry coupling at slightly higher pressure, thus exploiting the original interference effect for testing by means of surface waves (3.14).

In the immersion technique boundary waves correspond to the surface waves, which can also produce interfering echoes. These waves are likewise propagated in all directions from the point of incidence of the sound beam, and, compared with the useful sound, they are the stronger, the smaller the d/λ ratio of the point of incidence. On a surface which is not very smooth, the interfering grass of the boundary wave may greatly impair the resolution of flaws close to the surface. Boundary waves between solids have so far not given any noticeable trouble.

3.14 Testing by Means of Transverse, Surface and Plate Waves

When testing curved plates or pipes, *transverse waves* which are propagated along a zig-zag path are frequently used (Fig. 3.37). Compared with longitudinal waves their chief advantage here is that if incident at angles greater than 33° in steel (30° in aluminium) they are totally reflected without being split. In such specimens they can therefore travel long distances provided the roughness of the surface is small compared with the wave length so that losses by scatter reflections do not occur. The effect of surface roughness, however, decreases as the angle of incidence becomes larger. In addition the amplitude decreases only according to the law of distance (divergence of beam) and the attenuation of the material for transverse waves.

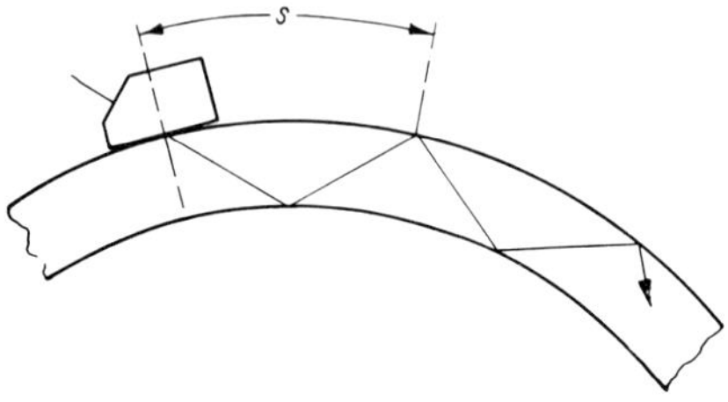

Fig. 3.37 Propagation of a transverse wave along a zig-zag path by total reflection.

When the zig-zag method is used the whole cross-section of the test piece can be scanned if the probe is shifted through the *skip-distance* *s* (Fig. 3.37). In this way both surfaces can be checked for incipient cracks, and the entire cross-section for other defects. A backwall echo, as in the case of sounding normal to the surface, is obtained only at a limiting edge on which the zig-zag path is incident at right angles (Fig. 3.38). If the probe is moved back and forth across this edge, angle reflection produces alternately echoes of the bottom or the top edge. In accordance with the divergence of the beam, these echoes reach a maximum and then disappear again, i.e. they pass through envelope curves with a more or less pronounced maximum (Fig. 3.38). For short sound paths in thick

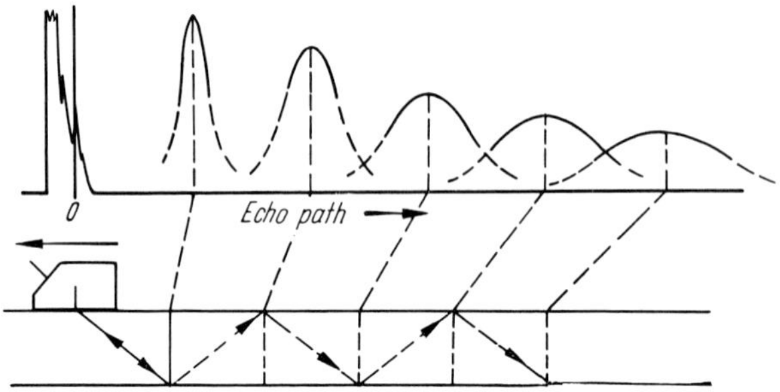

Fig. 3.38 Edge echoes in a plate and their envelope curves, schematic.

plates only one echo at a time is visible, while for longer paths or thinner plates the envelope curves are broader, overlap, and one has from an edge (Fig. 3.39) just as from a flaw several simultaneously produced echoes, in accordance with the zig-zag paths of different inclination. This may make it difficult for the inexperienced examiner to interpret and locate flaws because he is accustomed to viewing the echo traces while the probe is stationary. If, however, a dynamic testing technique is applied by steadily moving the probe back and forth while observing the screen trace (which requires some skill and dexterity) it is easy to co-ordinate each echo the maximum of its envelope curve, which facilitates interpretation.

With longer paths and thin cross-sections, the echoes along the various zig-zag paths form a dense echo group, as shown in Fig. 3.40 on an incipient crack in a pipe. In this case exact flaw location as well as differentiation between several closely spaced flaws is difficult.

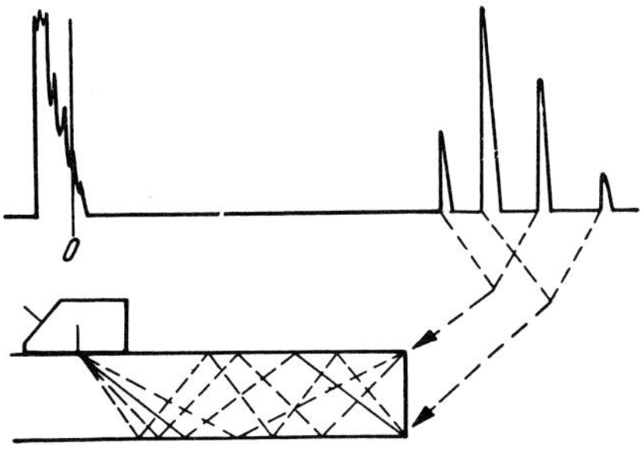

Fig. 3.39 Edge echo along different zig-zag paths.

For tracing the zig-zag path and the origin of echoes the finger-tip test can be used: if one touches, with an oily finger, the reflection point of an obliquely incident transverse wave, or for that matter also an edge, the echo height, in the case of steel, may fluctuate by as much as one third, in the case of longitudinal waves, however, only very little, and in the case of vertically incident transverse waves, not at all.

Flaw location by means of the zig-zag method, is facilitated if one marks on the viewing screen the reflection points of the two surfaces along the associated sound paths, e.g. by means of movable pointers. Since this method of flaw location is particularly important for testing welded seams, this is discussed under that heading (Sec. 3.28) in greater detail. In some cases (Fig. 3.41) the reflection points are

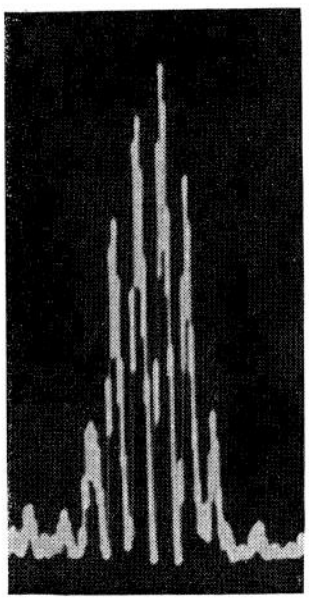

Fig. 3.40 Echo of a flaw with zig-zag waves in pipe.

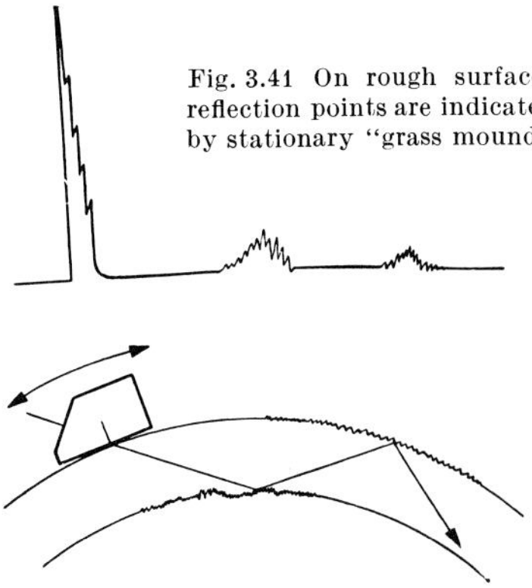

Fig. 3.41 On rough surfaces reflection points are indicated by stationary "grass mounds".

indicated automatically if the surface is a little rough. "Grass mounds" appear at these points on the viewing screen, which, if the probe is shifted, maintain their position while small echoes travel over them continuously. If for example a flaw echo reaches the maximum of its envelope curve exactly at the midpoint between two such points, the flaw is located halfway between the faces of the specimen, and its distance from the probe can be calculated; its position is therefore completely determined.

In order to check the sensitivity of the angle beam or zig-zag test, it is frequently found convenient to use the edge of a rectangular block as in Fig. 3.39, or often simply a piece of sheet with one straight edge. According to Fig. 1.29b, the echo height in the case of angle reflection can, however, be used as a reference echo only with caution: in the case of steel, total reflection occurs only between 33° and 57°, but very little reflection for instance at 60°. This is also important when checking the angle of the sound beam: in the case of a 60° probe, the peripheral rays of the beam are reflected strongly at 57° and at the usual adjustment for maximum edge echo, they therefore shift the apparent beam angle to values smaller than 60°. This angle can accordingly be measured more accurately on a hole drilled normal to the beam axis and parallel to the surface of the test piece. This also applies to larger beam angles.

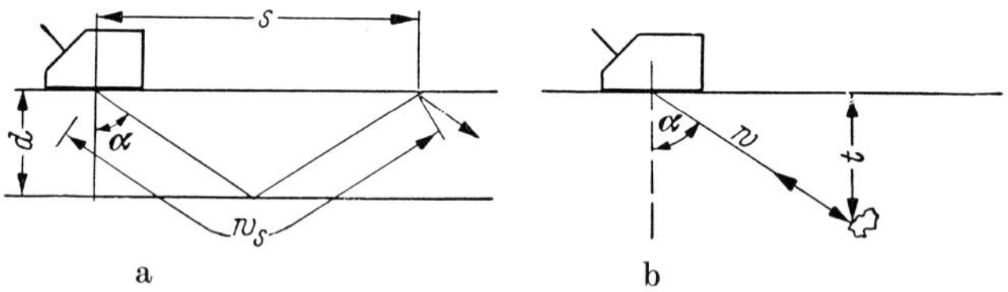

Fig. 3.42 Relation between skip distance s, sound path w, beam angle α and flaw depth t in a plate, (a) with reflection, and (b) without reflection.

In order to calculate the location of the flaw when the oblique or zig-zag method is applied, the following simple formulas are used. According to Fig. 3.42a the skip distance in a flat plate of thickness d is

$$s = 2d \tan\alpha \tag{3.5}$$

and the sound path corresponding to a full skip distance

$$w_s = \frac{2d}{\cos\alpha}. \tag{3.6}$$

Finally, the depth of the flaw in the case of an arbitrary, rectilinear sound path w is according to Fig. 3.42b

$$t = w \cos\alpha. \tag{3.7}$$

The corresponding factors for a few commonly used beam angles are

α	35°	45°	60°	70°	80°
$2\tan\alpha$	1.4	2.0	3.5	5.5	11
$2/\cos\alpha$	2.4	2.8	4.0	5.8	11.5
$\cos\alpha$	0.82	0.71	0.50	0.34	0.17

Since the skip distance provides a vivid picture of the sound path, the factor $2\tan\alpha$ is marked on some probes to facilitate calculation on the basis of sheet thickness.

In pipes both the skip distance and the correlated sound path are increased by a factor f_s and f_w respectively, which depends on the pipe diameter D and the wall thickness d. Fig. 3.43 gives these factors as a function of the ratio d/D and the above-mentioned angle. Where the tangents of these curves are vertical the inside wall is no longer touched. In the case of round stock and tubing Fig. 3.44 shows that only a certain maximum depth d (or wall thickness d of pipe) can therefore be covered: this is determined by

$$d/D = 0.5\,(1 - \sin\alpha)\,.$$

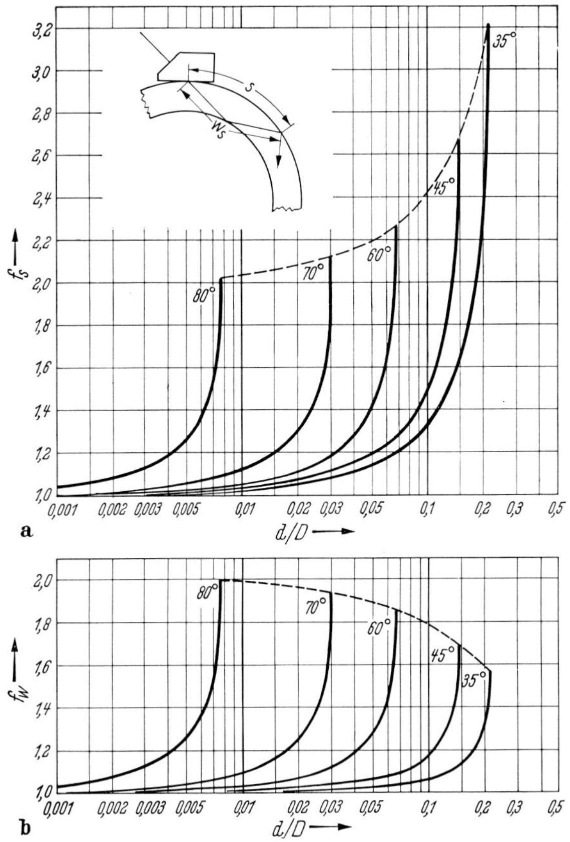

Fig. 3.43 Zig-zag waves in the wall of a pipe in a circumferential direction. Ratio of skip distance (a) and sound path (b) in the pipe to the values in a plate of equal thickness, plotted as a function of the ratio of the wall thickness to O. D.

For the above-mentioned angles one obtains

$$d/D = 0.21 \quad 0.15 \quad 0.067 \quad 0.030 \quad 0.0076\,.$$

Since for oblique transverse waves in steel only angles above 33° can be considered for practical purposes, cylindrical specimens can be tested only to a depth of 0.22, i.e. approximately one fifth of the diameter.

Since for the smallest angle of the transverse waves we have $\sin\alpha_{\min} = c_t/c_l$, the maximum testing depth quite generally is

$$\frac{d}{D_{\max}} = 0.5\left(1 - \frac{c_t}{c_l}\right),$$

which, for aluminium and copper, gives slightly greater values, viz. 0.25 and 0.26 respectively. If, theoretically, the wave still barely grazes the internal wall of a thick-walled pipe, the sensitivity is nevertheless already zero as a consequence of the side-wall effect. Therefore, when one is checking for small internal flaws, one can no longer apply the calculated critical thicknesses.

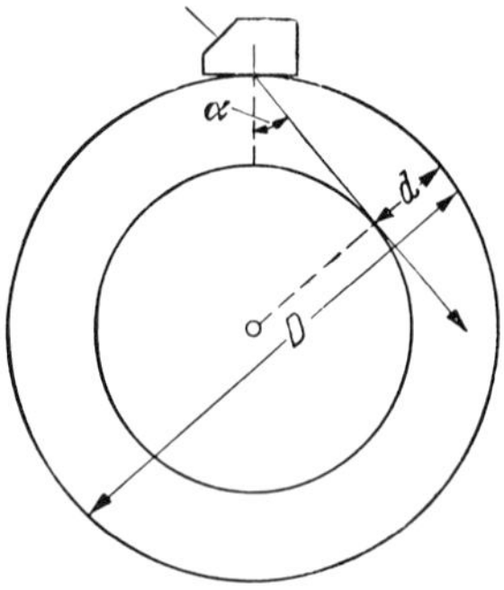

Fig. 3.44 Maximum penetration depth for round stock or alternatively when thick-walled pipes are tested at given beam angle α.

In a flat plate the direction of the zig-zag path, i.e. its projection on the testing surface, is rectilinear and agrees with the longitudinal direction of the casing of conventional probes, making allowance for manufacturing tolerances. If one extends this direction by means of a ruler, its edge passes through the projection of a flaw on the surface which can then be used for its location. This no longer applies in the case of a test piece whose thickness transverse to the direction of the probe changes, e.g. a wedge or a turbine blade. In this case the zig-zag path curves towards the thicker side, which makes flaw location more difficult. Here one can fall back on the finger-tip test to determine the direction.

Occasionally transverse waves are used on pipes or solid cylinders, which are beamed into the specimen obliquely to its axis. Their reflection points on the surface are located on a spiral to which the longitudinal direction of the probe is a tangent. This track is therefore less difficult to visualize for flaw location.

In the testing of wedge-shaped specimens, e.g. eccentric pipes in the direction of their circumference (Fig. 3.45), the wave may return along its own path because

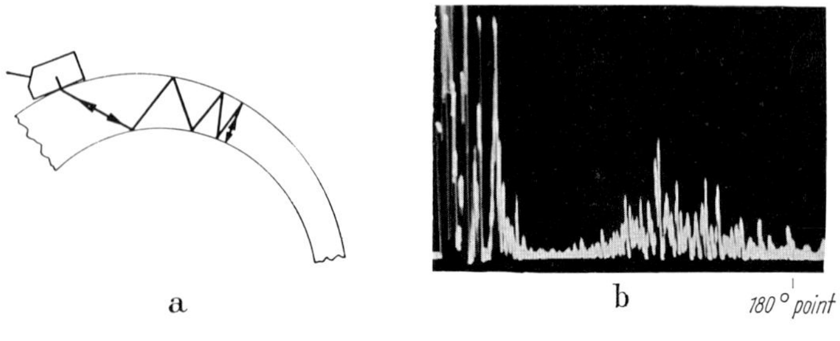

Fig. 3.45 Interfering echoes in the case of an eccentric but otherwise flawless pipe, by reversal of steeply incident zig-zag waves.

the angle of incidence decreases with each reflection if the sound is beamed in the direction of the thinner section. Since this involves an angle smaller than that of total reflection, the wave is at the same time strongly weakened by split-off longitudinal waves. This may prevent the detection of flaws beyond the thin section. The difficulty can be overcome by using large incident angles.

Tests by means of *surface waves* are of no great importance because many detectable flaws can also be found directly by visual inspection or by cheaper methods, such as magnetic particle tests or penetration tests. Furthermore only very uniform and smooth surfaces, finished machine components or rolled and extruded pieces, particularly of light metal are suitable for this purpose.

As indicated in Fig. 3.46, the wave also follows a curved surface and travels with little interference over edges if rounded with a radius greater than the wave length. But even a sharp, projecting edge still fails to reflect them completely. A weak wave travels over it and according to [48] the reflected wave reaches a maximum only in the case of a projecting knife edge.

Favourable in this connection is also that the surface wave is not subjected to splitting and mode conversion at an edge if incident obliquely. Consequently, an incipient crack starting normal to an edge of the specimen, as on the turbine blade in Fig. 3.76, can be determined reliably at any beam angle directed into the corner formed in this way, e.g. also when beaming close to the edge. The wave, as shown in Fig. 3.78, can be permitted to travel also on a narrow edge of the specimen, whether this edge is rounded or of rectangular cross-section. The sensitivity on this edge is reduced merely in accordance with the smaller contact face of the probe. On a rounded edge the plastic wedge of the probe can be suitably ground in for better coupling and guidance.

a
b
c

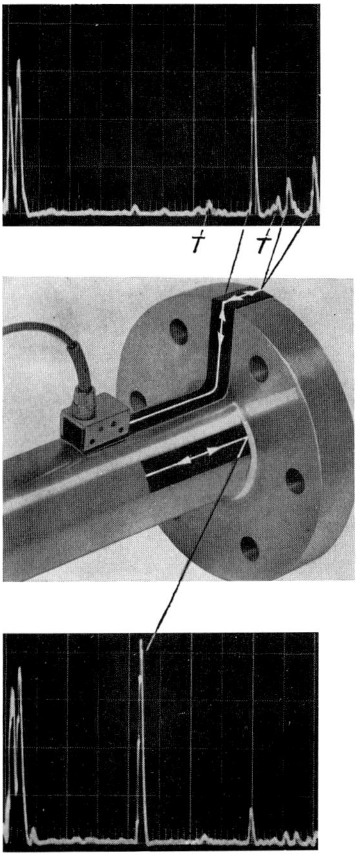

Fig. 3.46 Checking a machine component by means of surface waves for incipient cracks, frequency 3 MHz, depth of crack approx. 0.3 mm. *T* interfering echoes by split-off transverse waves according to Fig. 3.47.

Like all other waves, the surface wave is attenuated by the absorption of the material and scattering at the grain boundaries. In addition, it is also attenuated by layers of foreign matter, such as oil and dirt. Therefore the coupling liquid should be limited to the contact point as far as possible. Slight damping by means of an oily finger, which is much more pronounced than in the case of the reflection point of a transverse wave, can be used to trace the path of the wave on the surface of the specimen and thus to find the location of the flaw. Cleaning rags and oily fingers are therefore indispensable when using the surface wave technique.

At a re-entrant edge (Fig. 3.47) a complication arises: the wave is partially reflected, partially it continues, and partially it is converted into a transverse wave which, if the specimen is shaped as shown in the drawing, can give rise to an interfering reflection. This also happens at a groove sawn into a specimen for testing purposes and at incipient cracks which a portion of the wave thus bypasses. This can be demonstrated by applying the touch test: the echo of the transverse wave in Fig. 3.47 can be damped together with the echo of this edge only by touching the track *before* the edge concerned, but no longer behind the edge. The reverse, viz. disturbance of a transmitted transverse wave by conversion into a surface wave and back, can also occur, e.g. in the testing of shafts according to Fig. 3.48a, if the beam strikes the radius of the fillet. If there is any doubt, use the finger-tip test.

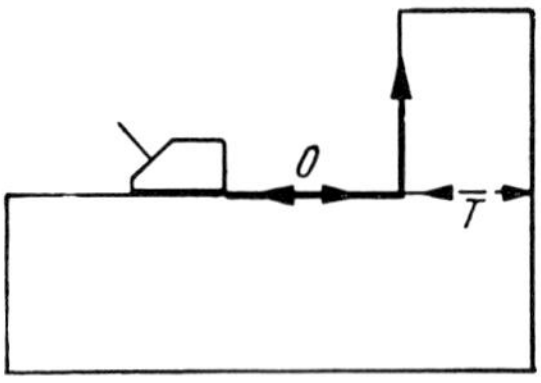

Fig. 3.47 Conversion of a surface wave into a transverse wave and vice versa.

As far as the detection of flaws is concerned, it can be stated quite generally that elongated incipient cracks, provided they do not start in a surface at an edge, should be irradiated at right angles where possible. If they are long enough, their length can be determined by means of a sharply collimated beam as in Fig. 3.50. However, the depth of the crack determines the height of the echo to only a very limited extent and is an unreliable measure. Since the entire oscillation process decays rapidly with depth, cracks measuring fractions of a wave length already reflect very strongly, but at greater depths, no longer proportionally. Since the wave length at 4 MHz in steel is 0.75 mm, a scratch 0.1 mm deep can still be indicated. The height of the echo is an unreliable measure of the depth of the crack for yet another reason: only empty, even if very fine, incipient cracks produce a reliable reflection. However, if they are filled with polishing or drawing compound, as for instance in the case of hardness cracks on a shaft ground after quenching, failures may result.

In contrast to the penetration method, sub-surface flaws can also be discovered. Thus, according to [48], cracks can approach the surface to within a little more than one wave length and still be indicated.

Since a knife edge pressed dry against the surface also produces an echo, an adjustable delay line for interferometry can be constructed in this way.

The "grass", which in the presence of coarse grain or very rough surface makes the location of a flaw impossible, can also be used as a quantitative measure of one of these two quantities if the other remains constant, e.g. on turbine blades.

In this connection should also be mentioned the possibility of using surface waves for measuring layer thicknesses on the basis of their velocity, e.g. in a hardening layer or plating, for determining texture and for checking surface layers for faulty bonding (cf. Secs. concerned).

Using surface waves, RASMUSSEN [298] was able to detect the minutest incipient cracks on the surface of tensile test specimens and he could thus predict the fatigue break.

Of the three possibilities for generating surface waves, viz.:

1. Surface wave probe (conversion of longitudinal waves via plastic wedge, 1.64),
2. Y-cut quartz, 7 : 1 format with liquid contact (1.101),
3. Standard probe with dry, rectilinear contact (3.136),

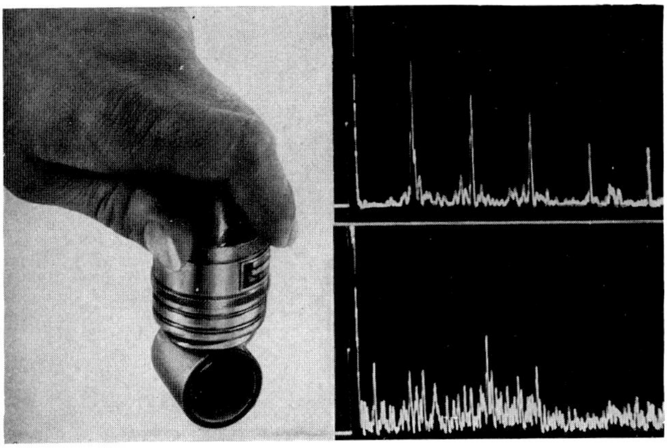

Fig. 3.48 Testing round stock and similar specimens with a bright surface for cracks by means of surface waves and dry contact of a normal probe, screen displays of specimens without and with crack (hardened bushings).

the first is the most commonly used because it is largely independent of the shape of the test piece.

The optimal effect, however, depends on the material of the test piece. If the latter has a transverse velocity c_t which differs by more than approximately 5% from that for which the probe has been designed, either no waves at all or oblique transverse waves are produced in the test piece, depending on whether the velocity is greater or smaller.

The second method is hardly ever used. The third can be very useful in certain problems of which Fig. 3.48 illustrates an example [123]. The surface waves which radiate laterally in both directions from the narrow linear contact area, produce on a sound specimen (round stock, tube, wire) a series of multiple echoes. Smaller flaw echoes which may be present between these multiple echoes can be recognized more readily if the specimen is rotated; the flaw echoes then wander among the stationary circumferential echoes. If the specimen is rotated rapidly, the flaw is indicated by strong flickering of the trace at the position of the flaw which can readily be distinguished from the stationary picture produced by a sound section (Fig. 3.128).

This method can be applied on bright surfaces with a radius of curvature up to approx. 20 mm. On small specimens care should be taken so that the circumferential surface wave is not accidentally damped by contact with the hand.

For the third method one can also use a *Y*-cut quartz plate. If the direction of oscillation in this case is parallel to the cylindrical axis of the specimen, also pure transverse waves are radiated along the surface which can be distinguished from the surface waves by their different acoustic velocity. In this way it is possible to produce Love waves, which e.g. are more sensitive than surface waves for testing the quality of a bond because they are stopped completely at a detached layer with a separation distance of less than one half wave length [129].

With surface waves the pulse method is usually used. If in a special case one wants to work with a separate receiver, any of the above-mentioned generating methods can be used. In addition there is available, for point by point scanning of the sound field, a point-shaped probe (Ultrasonoscope) or a probe according to NAUMANN [274]. The latter consists of a carbon, graphite or metal rod in light contact with the surface. On a metallic specimen this contact acts like a carbon microphone for ultrasonic frequencies, connected via a bias of a few volts to the usual amplifier of a pulse-echo instrument. Ultrasonic waves with components normal to the surface, such as surface and plate waves, are indicated with high sensitivity.

Concerning testing technique with surface waves see also [107, 67, 264, 373, 374].

Plate waves. The testing of plates over long distances by means of transverse waves reflected along a zig-zag path has already been described at the beginning of this Section. Certain peculiarities to which attention should be paid when using this method on thin sheet, will now be pointed out.

Fig. 3.103 shows schematically the pattern of such a reflected beam. At the beginning the zig-zag path is still clearly distinguishable. However, after a few reflections, the divergent beams overlap so that the entire sheet is affected by the oscillatory motion. In the case of thin sheet it cannot be avoided that this overlapping already begins directly under the probe. Such waves which in a plate leave no zone free of sound are generally called plate waves.

If the angle of propagation is unfavourable, the overlapping of several reflected beams results in cancellation by interference as shown in Fig. 1.32. Table 9 (Appendix) gives the favourable angles of propagation for steel plate at which no cancellation occurs. Apart from the material, these optimal angles also depend on the thickness of the plate and the frequency of the wave. This explains the phenomenon that some plate-wave echoes have a different form from that of the usual echoes: they are broader and consist of a large number of high-frequency oscillations

(Figs. 3.114 and 3.115). This "melting away" of the plate wave pulse is the more pronounced the longer the transit path and the steeper the branch of the curve in Table 9 for the corresponding plate thickness.

In practice plate waves are used both in reflection and transmission. The angle probes used for excitation should preferably have an adjustable angle of incidence.

The echo method using plate waves is, however, more suitable for qualitative than quantitative analysis when used as go/no-go signal, for the following reasons: the echo height is difficult to reproduce because the front end of the plastic contact face of the probe immediately damps any wave just produced, like an oily finger tip. For the same reason the echo height in the case of surface wave probes is affected by any small change in the distribution of the coupling liquid, slight undulations of the contact face and surface, and the pressure exerted by the operator on the probe.

A further reason why plate waves are largely unsuitable for quantitative determinations of the size of the defect on the basis of the echo amplitude results from the fact that the wave reflected from the defect, depending on its shape, can be split into different wave modes, and furthermore the great diversity of the shape of the defects, which preclude any non-ambiguous definition of "flaw size".

Influences resulting from coupling can largely be eliminated by using liquid transit sections (sheet test 3.242). It is also possible to apply complete immersion (pipe test 3.26 and bonding test 3.29) in which case, however, the plate wave is strongly damped by the continuous radiation of longitudinal waves into the liquid.

Since plate waves and rod waves are used exclusively for testing sheets and rods or wires, the testing technique will be discussed in greater detail in 3.242 and 3.25.

3.15 Determination of Shape and Size of Flaws

The difficulties of this problem were fully discussed in 1.84. The practical possibilities are summarized in the following.

The "size" of flaws – depending on whether this concerns "large" or "small" flaws – is determined by very different methods. "Large flaws" (where the flaw is larger than the cross-section of the sound beam at the location of the flaw) in an otherwise sound specimen are scanned in order to determine their projected contour on the surface of the specimen (see Fig. 3.49). This dynamic scanning method determines the "extent of the flaw", to be regarded here as its size. The size of "small" flaws (area of flaw smaller than cross-section of sound beam) can be determined only by measuring the maximum echo amplitude produced by the flaw (static determination of size of flaw, see also Sec. 1.84).

Examples of the determination of the extent of large flaws are incipient cracks in heavy shafts and columns, the extent of laminations in sheets, and so forth.

If the probe is moved from the unaffected zone over the flaw, the echo rises from zero to a constant maximum value (Fig. 3.50) if the area of the flaw is normal to the sound beam. In this rare case, and on the further assumption that no lateral surfaces disturb the sound beam, the echo height reaches half its maximum value when the axis of the beam touches the edge of the flaw. In this case the cross-section of the beam influences only the steepness of the echo front. Nevertheless, it is preferable to work with a beam of almost parallel rays, i.e. if possible in the near field of a probe of maximum size, or in the distant field of a probe with minimum angle of divergence.

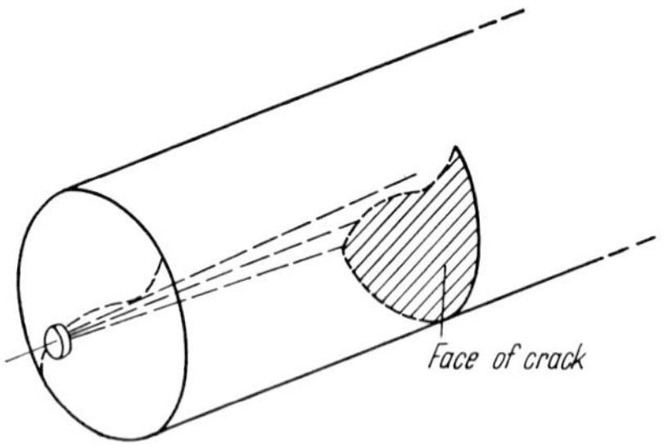

Fig. 3.49 Large flaw normal to beam axis.

A large flaw of arbitrary shape and orientation (oblique crack, shrinkage cavity) can still be scanned in the same way provided it is

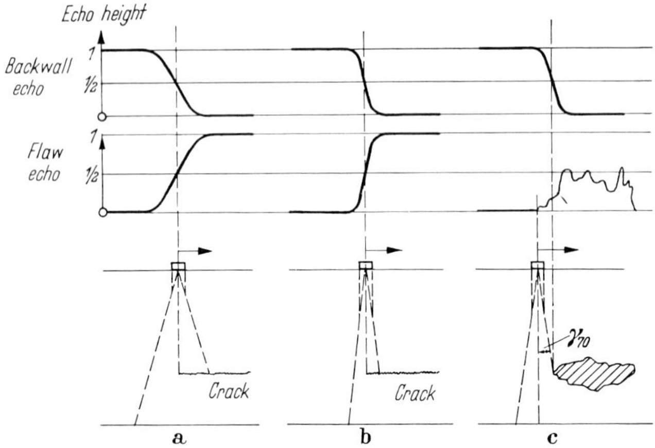

Fig. 3.50 Behaviour of flaw echo and backwall echo during the scanning of a large flaw; schematic.

possible to obtain a backwall echo without interference from lateral walls. In this case the backwall echo is reduced to approximately half its value if the beam axis touches the periphery of the flaw (Fig. 3.50c).

If the flaw is elongated, so that only its longitudinal extension normal to the beam axis is still large compared with the diameter of the beam, only this dimension of the flaw can be determined by the method described.

If the backwall echo is not utilized, the contour of an arbitrarily shaped flaw can be determined only approximately (Fig. 3.50c). The contour line at which a small echo of the flaw first appears when the probe approaches the flaw from the flawless zone is traced on the surface at high gain. Generally this contour will be too large and it can be corrected to its true size, to a first approximation, by taking half the diameter of the sound beam at the distance of the flaw. The beam diameter is preferably determined on the basis of the angle of divergence for 70%, γ_{70}, instead of the larger value γ_0. The result is slightly influenced by the gain used and also by the shape of the flaw, viz. spherical or areal (see also [163]). In exactly the same way one can measure by means of angle probes of 70 to 75° the depth of surface cracks, or the distance of cracks from the surface in the case of large internal cracks (plate-sized cracks on forgings, Fig. 3.51). Since here the best attainable accuracy is only a few millimetres, only large cracks can be scanned in this way. Eq. 3.7 with a correction for γ_{70} is used. In such cases the echo is produced by the wave being diffracted at the edge of the flaw; it is always very weak compared with the mirrored reflection, so that a high gain must be used. Where possible, the depth is measured from both sides, and averaged.

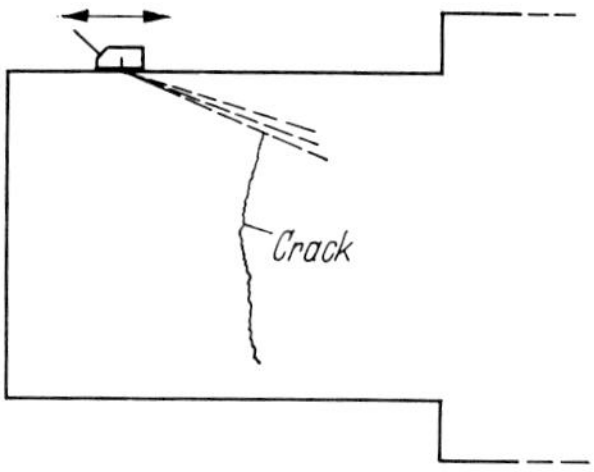

Fig. 3.51 Determination of distance from surface to crack (large shrinkage crack in forging).

Obliquely orientated flaw surfaces, when scanned, produce weak, strongly fluctuating and sometimes split echoes which move over the screen (travelling echo). This provides information on the direction of the crack.

In the case of *small flaws* the height of the echo during scanning does not remain constant over a given shifting distance of the probe and evaluation by geometry therefore fails. In the case of flaws resembling a circular disc normal to the beam, the maximum echo height according to 1.84 can be used for estimating the size of the flaw if compared with the reference echo of a thin plate (cf. [227] which also gives corrections for curved testing surfaces). The formerly used rule of thumb:

$$\text{flaw echo} : \text{backwall echo} = \text{area of flaw} : \text{cross-section of beam}$$

is completely unreliable.

If measurement according to 1.84 is impracticable, e.g. because of sidewall interference, the only way out is usually comparison with artificial flaws in a similar specimen, which resemble the suspected shape of the flaw as closely as possible, in the form of a blind hole with flat or spherical bottom (inclusions and pores), drill holes normal to the beam axis (elongated inclusions), saw-cuts (surface cracks), etc. For certain forms of the specimen and position of the flaws, calibration curves of both echo height and size of artificial flaws may also be plotted in this way. In view of the variegated shape of natural flaws it can, however, not be expected that such comparisons furnish anything more accurate than an order of magnitude.

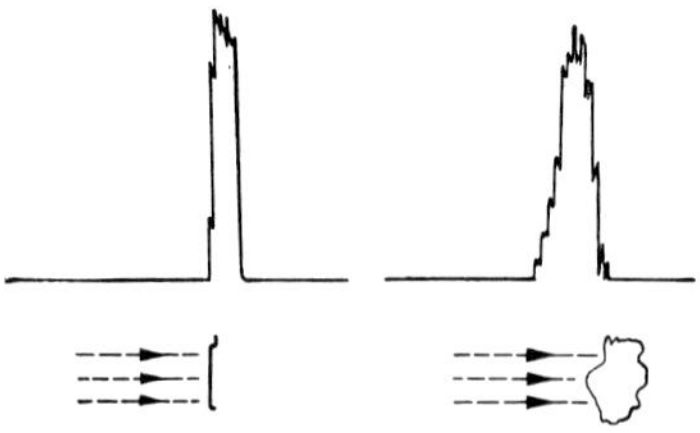

a b

Fig. 3.52 Flaw shape and echo shape, a) laminar flaw irradiated normally, b) irregular roundish flaw.

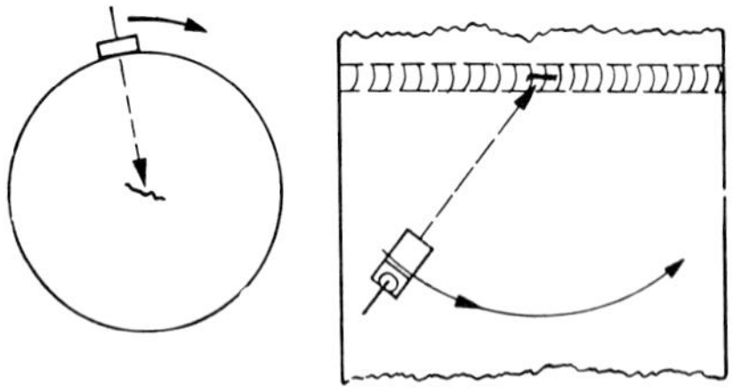

a b

Fig. 3.53 Change in the direction of irradiation a) on cylindrical specimens with core defect, b) on a welded seam.

Some information on the shape of the flaw is given by the shape of the echo (Fig. 3.52) as well as the change of the echo if the direction of irradiation is changed. A steep rise of the echo, even if the total echo height is small, usually indicates a laminar flaw irradiated almost perpendicularly. With video presentation of the echo on the CR screen, the steepness of the rise is readily indicated by the distance of the first high-frequency nodes: if the echo is produced by a laminar flaw, the maximum echo height is already reached after 2 to 3 nodes. In the case of a flaw not irradiated at right angles, or spherical flaws, the rise is more gradual. If the flaw is of irregular shape, the echo is often complex and changes its shape rapidly during scanning, which may, however, also point to several closely spaced flaws.

The direction of irradiation can be changed, e.g., in the case of core defects in cylindrical specimens, or on faulty welded seams (Fig. 3.53). Whereas a laminary flaw (crack and smooth bonding defects) as well as a linear flaw (slag streak and undercutting) produce a sharply orientated reflected beam and give a clear echo only with perpendicular irradiation, this does not apply to spherical flaws (pores and slag) (Fig. 3.54). This behaviour is the more definite the higher the frequency.

When making such comparisons, it is of course necessary to keep distance and sensitivity as constant as possible. Care should therefore be taken when comparing the echo of a flaw with straight beam and with angle beam testing to avoid a wrong interpretation.

In order not to overlook accidentally flaws irradiated unfavourably during rapid testing, very much higher sensitivity is used during scanning than during the subsequent analysis of a given flaw. To obviate changing the adjustment of the instrument, probes with built-in sensitivity control have been made available to save time.

Changing the ultrasonic frequency is another promising method for analysing the nature and shape of a flaw. This has been pointed out by KNORR and RICKEN, on the basis of the fact that when the size of flaws is determined according to the principles of Sec. 1.84, a lower frequency

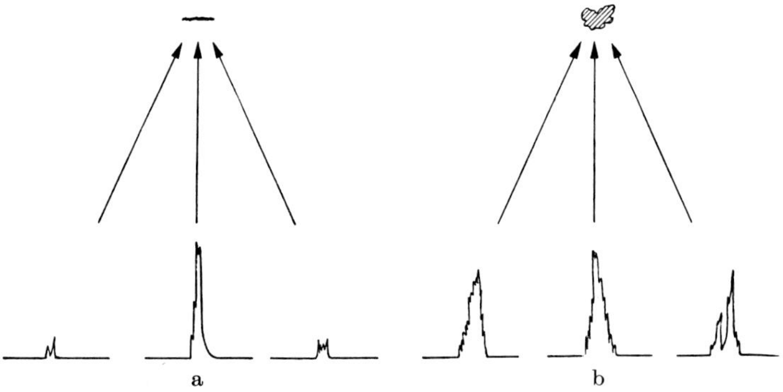

Fig. 3.54 Change of echo height and echo shape when the direction of irradiation is changed, a) on laminary or linear flaw, b) on roundish flaw.

gives a value more in keeping with the actual size of the flaw than a higher frequency [182]. Any deviations from the ideal, normally irradiated circular disc reduce the measured size of the flaw the higher the frequency used.

According to GERICKE [112, 113], additional information can be obtained on the size, nature and shape of a flaw by using more sophisticated equipment at different frequencies. With the aid of an additional frequency analyser the wave reflected by the flaw can be checked for changes of the frequency spectrum. This requires that the transmitted wave contains a frequency band of maximum width, i.e. the transmitting pulse should be as short as possible. Instead of a frequency band, one may also radiate simultaneously from the transmitter, two different frequencies spaced as widely as possible from each other, and compare the corresponding echoes. This is GERICKE's two-frequency method. It also permits simple determination of the size of the flaw.

3.16 Disturbances by Extraneous High Frequency and Ultrasonic Sources

To eliminate internal disturbances of the instrument, only the corresponding service manuals can be of assistance. For external disturbances however, there are remedies of general validity.

Since the frequency range of the amplifier is practically that of radio receivers, radio interference, which manifests itself in the loudspeaker by crackling, rattling, etc., may also appear on the fluorescent screen where this optical phenomenon is also called *crackling*. These interferences are caused by the sparking of electrical machines, transmitted to the ultrasonic instrument either through the mains or through the air. A powerful short-wave transmitter in close proximity can also cause interference, the radio programme producing spurious disturbances on the fluorescent screen. Ultrasonic instruments with broadband amplifiers are more sensitive in this respect than instruments with narrow band. In the case of ultrasonic transmission testing these disturbances manifest themselves by an instable zero of the instrument.

Individual interfering pulses do not interfere with the visual observation of the fluorescent screen, and even stronger crackling hardly interferes with the test. For automated testing installations with monitors or recording instruments this may, however, prove troublesome. If a monitor operates without delay, i.e. if it responds to a single pulse entering the gate, an interfering pulse will not be distinguished from a true echo, resulting in a false alarm. This can be remedied to some extent by using a very narrow gate because this reduces the probability of a single interfering pulse entering the gate at the same moment. It is, however, preferable to delay the response of the monitor so that it responds only to several successive pulses in the gate, which in the case of disturbances would occur only in rare cases. Naturally this limits the testing speed in rapid automated testing.

Another possibility for nullifying the effect of interferences on automatic evaluation devices of testing installations is the use of an interference suppressor. This instrument receives the radio interferences by means of an aerial and blocks the evaluation device connected to the pulse echo instrument for the duration of such interference. Naturally this also suppresses "true" flaw indications recorded simultaneously with the interferences.

To overcome this shortcoming another approach has been made. Using an auxiliary instrument "flaw signals" are fed into the evaluation device of the testing installation only if, e.g., three successive transmitting pulses produce an identical flaw echo in the monitor gate. This, on the one hand, prevents a single interfering pulse from reaching the evaluating device, while on the other hand a flaw occurring simultaneously with a disturbance is evaluated in the normal way. If in addition the pulse repetition frequency of the pulse-echo instrument used is increased, this avoids the otherwise necessary reduction of the testing speed to ensure the same, reliable flaw recognition.

If several pulse instruments with repetition frequencies which are not identical, are operated in close proximity, the pulses are transmitted from one instrument to the other along electrical circuits and travel across the viewing screen. It then becomes necessary to synchronize the repetition frequencies of the instrument, e.g. if several are operated in one testing installation. Regarding the necessary, simple changes in the circuits, it is best to consult the manufacturer.

If electrical interferences are not already suppressed at the source, they can still be suppressed on their way to the amplifier. For this purpose interference suppressors consisting of filtering chokes and capacitors are on most instruments already interposed at the connection to the mains. In difficult cases, additional external filters can be installed.

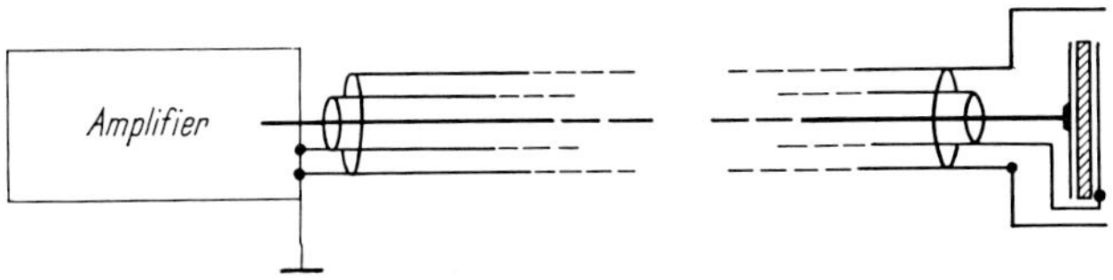

Fig. 3.55 Probe and connecting cable with double shield.

The installed filters can only suppress interferences arriving via the mains but not interferences transmitted through the air to the probe and the test cable which acts as aerial. Probes with unprotected front are more sensitive to these interferences than probes with earthed metal layer in front of the transducer crystal. If also this type of probe proves unsatisfactory, the only effective remedy is usually double shielding of the probe and the cable as shown in Fig. 3.55. In this case the earth electrode of the crystal is not, as usual, connected to the metal case and the shield of the concentric cable but is connected at the amplifier input to the instrument chassis via a second, internal shield of the cable.

If the disturbances are very stubborn, particularly in the case of testing installations where a long cable connection between probe and pulse-echo instrument is unavoidable, the above-mentioned means for suppressing interferences may prove inadequate. Frequently there then remains another remedy: instead of single probe operation, separate transmitting and receiving probes can be used with a preamplifier connected between the receiving probe and the pulse-echo instrument, which amplifies the echo signals so that they are raised well above the noise level at the input of the instrument. At the same time the gain on the instrument is reduced accordingly. This method is, however, fully effective only if the preamplifier is mounted in close proximity to the probe, using a short connecting cable between probe and preamplifier. This arrangement avoids the possibility that the connection between probe and preamplifier can act as receiving aerial for electric and magnetic interference fields. The length of the connection between preamplifier and instrument is less critical.

Interfering ultrasonic waves, in addition to audible sound, are produced during most machining operation on test pieces, as for instance by hammering, cutting or grinding, which frequently makes simultaneous ultrasonic testing impossible. These spurious ultrasonic signals appear on the viewing screen as crackling. The cause is nondirectional interfering sound with wide frequency range and arbitrary wave modes.

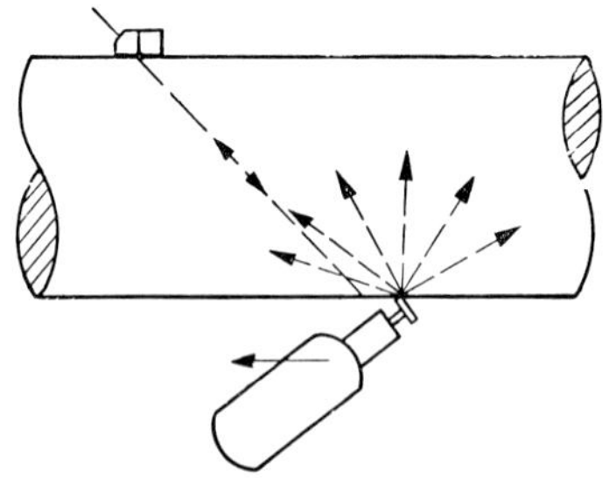

Fig. 3.56 Hand grinder as source of ultrasonics.

Occasionally this can be put to good use: for instance, in order to determine accurately the point of incidence in a large forging of an oblique transverse wave by means of which a fine, invisible surface crack has been located, a small, high-speed portable grinder as shown in Fig. 3.56 can be used. Strong waves are radiated in all directions from the small contact area with the specimen; this includes also transverse waves, which are indicated on the screen by crackling along the entire time base, the indication reaching a maximum the moment the grinding wheel touches the specimen on the axis of the sound beam.

Rapid automated testing is frequently made difficult by such "body" sound. Rotating steel brushes used for cleaning the surface should be applied at a sufficient distance from the probes, e.g. on rails preferably at several metres. Other sources of interference are the guiding devices of the probes on the specimen. At guiding speeds above 0.5 m/s they should preferably be made of plastic and not of metal.

3.17 Organisation of the Test, Staff and Training Problems

Where the same testing problems on identical or at least very similar specimens occur frequently, it is recommended that the head of the testing department work out a test specification and that the tests be carried out by a trained examiner. From complaints and experience gained in destructive tests, the suspected nature, size and position of flaws will be known, on which the non-destructive test then concentrates to eliminate any unnecessary effort. The specification should cover: designation of specimen, possibly with sketch, instructions whether and where the surface should be prepared, couplant, setting of instrument with probe for each testing procedure, together with indication of testing track and suspected position of flaw, reference to possible echoes which should not be confused with flaw echoes. In the case of mass tests, the examiner can, as a rule, be relieved of the necessity of preparing individual reports; on the evidence of the flaw echoes he can quickly make his own decision whether a given specimen should be rejected or not. In the case of more costly test pieces, sorting out of doubtful specimens is advisable; these are then submitted to the more experienced head of the testing department for decision.

For mass tests involving identical specimens it is essential to check the testing equipment regularly at the selected adjustment. This should be done by means of a test sample which has the same dimensions and properties as the specimens to be tested. In order to obtain flaw sizes and flaw shapes which can be used for checking the adjustment of the instruments, artificial flaws are incorporated in the test sample which, as regards size, shape, position and orientation, closely resemble the natural flaws to be detected. On the strength of these checks which should be made periodically during the mass tests, the examiner feels more confident that the sensitivity remains constant during his tests.

If judgment of the specimen on the basis of the ultrasonic indication alone is not possible, or if experience in evaluation is as yet insufficient, additional non-destructive tests can be applied, e.g. spot tests with X-rays or γ-rays. The ultrasonic test then plays the role of a rapid and inexpensive preliminary test. With greater experience, the ultrasonic test then frequently develops into the only test applied, e.g. on welded seams.

Routine tests using only normal probes, e.g. on plate or rod material, demand the least experience. Often a training period of a few hours is sufficient if the examiner has good powers of apprehension and a certain dexterity in manipulating the probe without excessive wear and tear. No higher school education is necessary. More experience is required when working with transverse, surface and plate waves, e.g. for testing complex specimens, such as shafts, pipes and especially welded seams which require more experience and some training, at least the study of a manual of testing methods, a course, or apprenticeship with an experienced examiner. In addition, a certain amount of technical training, knowledge of elementary mathematics and a good capacity for visualizing objects and processes in space is needed. Before being promoted to the position of unassisted examiner of welded seams and of more expensive test pieces, the acquisition of a thorough knowledge of materials is indispensable, preferably an examination for technicians in the field of production, furthermore also qualities of character such as diligence and thoroughness, to an even greater extent than for other testing methods. Independent application of these ultrasonic methods for many different and newly developed tests presupposes at least the study of physics and mathematics as given at a technical college, and in addition long practical experience (see also [198]).

Valuable mass-produced articles and single specimens are usually judged on the basis of a written test report. This presupposes suitable forms on which the required data can be filled in with minimum effort, using abbreviations and symbols, but covering the observations as completely as possible. In this preliminary report it is not yet advisable to speak of flaws or flaw echoes, but of indications or intermediate echoes, to avoid any hasty judgment of the specimen concerned. It is the duty of the examiner to submit a maximum of data on a given indication, viz. changes of both shape and size of the echo during scanning and sounding from different directions. This should enable the head of the testing department to determine the position, nature and size of the flaw, but he cannot, without consulting the designer, decide on the usability of the test piece with due consideration of the stress to which it will be subjected.

When complex specimens are to be tested, particularly pieces which are not readily accessible from all sides, the test should be planned by consulting a drawing. This makes it possible to select in advance the most suitable probes, especially angle probes, and echoes of bores and edges as well as expected detour echoes can be predicted. Since drawings are not always in perfect agreement with the specimen, indications should be carefully checked as to whether they might not result from the special form of the specimen, e.g. holes drilled subsequently, which may have been plugged by pins, or on parts which have been shrunk on in order to bring a part which accidentally has been turned too small, to the required size. Frequently also the regularity or symmetry of certain indications leads to the conclusion that they most probably are not caused by flaws.

3.18 Testing Installations and Evaluation of Test Results

Parallel with the gradual mastering by testers of "orthodox" methods of manual testing in the course of the years, went the development of continuous and automated testing installations (cf. [295]). The purpose of these installations is to relieve the examiner not only of the often tiresome guiding of the probe, but also of the constantly required, and in the case of mass tests exhausting, subjective decision making by observing fleeting screen displays. A testing installation should evaluate the test result "objectively". Naturally, this requires that the program, according to which the installation arrives at the decision "good" ("acceptable") and "bad" ("reject"), is first worked out on test blocks or test pieces containing flaws of known size, or on the basis of an adequate fund of experience. Test blocks, as already mentioned in Sec. 3.17, are used for general adjustment of a testing installation in the widest sense and for checking these adjustments. Suitable test blocks will be discussed in their relationship with the various testing problems. If no, or unsuitable, test blocks are used for adjusting a given testing installation, this may put the entire consequent test in doubt.

In tests carried out by hand the examiner can make immediately the decision: "good", "bad", "doubtful", or "specimen should be rechecked".

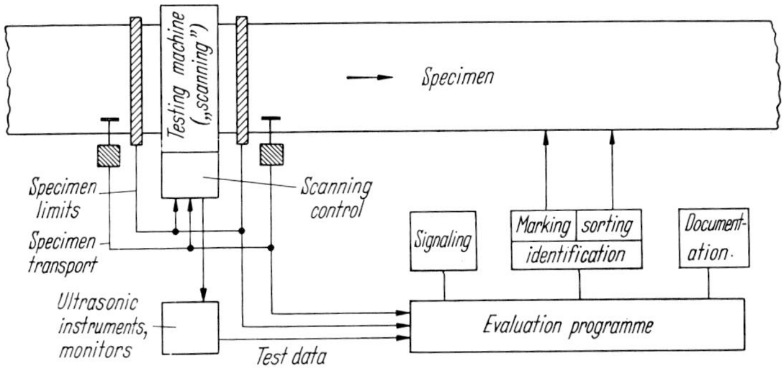

Fig. 3.57 Block diagram of an ultrasonic testing installation comprising: testing machine, ultrasonic instruments, evaluation device and specimen transport.

In the following the possible evaluation devices which, in the case of continuous and automated testing installations process the test data and make decisions, will be briefly summarized. Fig. 3.57 shows schematically the elements of an ultrasonic testing installation: the "testing machine" which scans the specimen, the ultrasonic instruments and monitors, the evaluation device, and the conveyor for the specimens.

The evaluation device, based on a more or less complex program of data processing, can make provision for

signalisation of flaw,
identification of defective specimens or
documentation of test result.

These 3 groups cover several variants:

A given flaw indication can either be announced simultaneously with its appearance, by an arbitrary optical or acoustical warning signal, or by a flaw display of limited duration. This flaw display can either be realised, for instance by an image storing tube (see also Sec. 2.353), a lamp board, or luminous numerals.

Defective specimens can be identified either by marking or sorting. The test material can be marked either with paint, mechanically by grinding, or by spot magnetization. The identification marks can either simultaneously indicate the position of the flaw, or be of a general nature applied at an arbitrary spot on the specimen. The specimens can be sorted either by being ejected into various containers or troughs, or they can be shunted by means of controlled deflecting gates and separate conveyors to various processing stations.

The documentation of test results can take various forms (see also Sec. 2.353). In addition to the recording of test data according to length or area by direct writing recorders, film recording is also used in some cases. Recently increasing use has been made of printers with digital presentation of the test result. Mention should also be made of the possibility of recording the received test data either on punched tape or on magnetic tape, although these methods have not yet found much favour in practice. It is characteristic of this group of documentation methods that the decision concerning a given specimen is made elsewhere and that the test result recorded on a strip chart, a printed, or film strip, must still be transferred to the specimen. This type of evaluation is therefore frequently combined with a signalling or marking method.

The simplest program for use with the above-mentioned evaluation methods is the setting of a threshold at the signal monitor. This requires classification of the flaw indications on the basis of their amplitude by means of the monitor relay, according to two groups: "good" and "bad". Recording by means of direct writing recorders would give a go/no-go display. If recording alone is to be used, it is advisable to record the readings by means of a recording monitor as a function of their amplitude, which greatly increases the decision making power of the statement of the document obtained.

With increasing testing speeds it became necessary to compress the data of the test results because daily evaluation of mile-long charts or film strips is found acceptable only in some special cases. On the other hand the requirements concerning the processing of test data became more diversified, so that mere evaluation by a simple "go/no-go" program proved increasingly inadequate. Both circumstances led to the appearance of more complex evaluation programs. A solution is provided by counting flaws or flawed sections, followed by "grading". This grading of test results, which at first glance looks more complex, has in addition to compression of the data material, the advantage in that its implementation permits many variants. For instance, this method of grading can be combined with the marking of the specimens (e.g. by using different colours), with sorting into several grades, and a flexible system of recording or printing devices. A few practical examples will be discussed in detail together with the various testing problems.

The following general remark seems justified: in most testing installations the specimen is scanned in the longitudinal direction and the test results obtained are co-ordinated with the longitudinal datum concerned, e.g. testing of billets, rods, pipes, sheets, strips, rails, etc.). To facilitate the above-mentioned compressing of test results, the specimen is generally subdivided in its longitudinal direction into so-called "evaluation sections". These are subdivided into "sub-sections". Grading is then realised by, for instance, regarding the number of defective sub-sections in the correlated evaluation section as the grading number. This number can be recorded digitally by a printer, separately for every evaluation section. Alternatively, the testing zone corresponding to the evaluation section can be marked by a colour allocated to the grading number concerned. In addition, all defective sub-sections can be added and used for sorting into a given number of grades, by specifying various limiting numbers.

These few directives of a general nature already show the great flexibility offered by the various evaluation devices in combination with a specially prepared evaluation program (cf. [122, 204]).

3.2 Flaw Detection on Metallic Specimens

Systematological difficulties are encountered when an attempt is made to classify the many testing problems discussed in this and the following two Sections 3.3 and 3.4. While in this Section an attempt is made to group the tests according to the shape and the method of manufacturing the *specimens*, the discriminating factor in the next Section is the *material*. Strict division, however, is neither possible nor practical, so that the subject index may have to be consulted. Furthermore, the sequence is frequently arbitrary.

Unless stated otherwise, the method concerned is always the pulse transit time method.

3.21 Heavy Forgings

In view of the high manufacturing costs of such steel forgings as rotors for generators and turbines, the tests are started as early as possible during the manufacturing process and are repeated frequently and with increasing accuracy, right to the acceptance test.

In the case of *ingots*, the test is controversial. First of all, large ingots with diameters of several feet cannot always be penetrated by sound. On the other hand, testing at, for instance, 0.25 MHz is often not practical because of the poor concentration of the beam and the inaccuracy of location, the main object being the determination of the extent of primary and secondary piping. With the usual probe diameters this, however, requires at least 0.5 MHz. In special cases the coarse grain of the cast structure can be reduced by heat treatment already of the ingot. High-alloy steel usually has insufficient transmittance, even in the smaller ingots. Another argument against the test is the fact that shrinkage cavities which are not in contact with the atmosphere, and therefore hardly oxidized, can be welded together completely during the subsequent forging.

The test is carried out in the direction of the smallest dimension, i.e. transverse to the axis, along a few longitudinal tracks, which if necessary can be prepared by grinding.

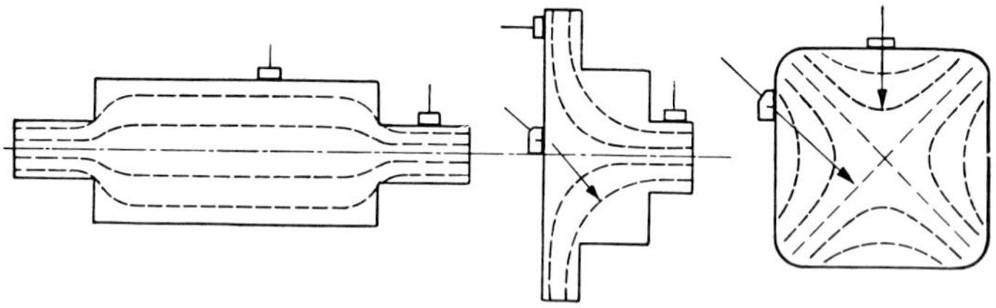

Fig. 3.57a. Fibering of large forgings and testing technique.

On *forging blanks* tests are interspersed as often as possible between the individual forging and annealing operations, should the specimen cool off during the intervals. Here a frequency of 0.5 to 1 MHz is used because the grain of the forging at that stage is usually still rather coarse and 2 to 5 MHz can be applied only after quenching and tempering. A few surface tracks are freed from scale by grinding or simply with a hammer. In addition, the face where top or base have been cut from the block can be used for coupling in a longitudinal test.

The testing technique depends on the pattern of the forging fibre, as shown in Fig. 3.57a for a few examples. Since many flaws, such as inclusions and cracks extend by preference in a direction parallel to the fibre, the sound should be beamed as nearly as possible at right angles to this direction. In the case of long forgings for turbine or generator rotors, the longitudinal test is therefore not very informative because most flaws will produce hardly any echo, but certainly will if tested in the transverse direction. Furthermore, the long distances in a longitudinal direction are a disadvantage. If a longitudinal test should produce no end echo, this does not necessarily point to the presence of flaws because it can also be the result of the coarser structure in the middle zone, or the side wall effect near the shell. Only large tension cracks, so-called cold shuts, are determined preferably from the face because they are orientated transverse to the axis. They can, however, also be located from the shell with angle probes of 45° and larger (Fig. 3.51). In the transverse test they absorb the bottom echo without, however, producing any distinct flaw echo.

Types of flaws which can already be determined on the blank are:

1. Flake cracks (hydrogen shatter cracks, frequently in combination with segregation zones), segregation cracks, slag cracks.

2. Non-metallic inclusions (deoxidation products such as oxide of silicon, aluminium or calcium, or slags from the surface of the bath), furthermore, but more rarely:

3. Forging cracks (on surface when forged at wrong temperature), forging tears (cavities), cold cracks.

4. Foreign bodies (furnace bricks, incompletely fused pokers or sheets).

Pure segregation is not indicated or only very weakly. For the same reason a Baumann or sulphur print, which indicates segregations, cannot be used for comparison with the ultrasonic test result.

According to Beckmann and Spiegelberg, non-metallic inclusions such as sulphide slags and fine alumina cannot be detected reliably by ultrasonics [42].

Should earlier, preliminary tests of the forging blank have revealed serious flaws, an attempt can be made to eliminate these flaws by a repeated, thorough forging, which, however, will succeed only in the case of cracks free of slag. Alternatively, depending on the position of the flaws, the specimen can be used for producing differently shaped or smaller forgings than originally planned. In the case of a square block for a crank shaft, the flawed section can possibly be positioned to fall into the cut-out between two cranks. In the case of forging cracks, the decision regarding the further use of the specimen can be based on a determination of the penetration depth according to Fig. 3.51.

On a *worked forging* the main test is carried out as long as it is still compact, i.e. before cutting fillets, conical transitions, grooves and numerous steps. If the surface prior to quenching and tempering has not been cut too rough, and especially if cut uniformly, it can generally be used for testing without further turning because the sharp burrs of the coarse turning groove are removed by oxidation during quenching and tempering. The thin layer of scale can then readily be removed by flame-scarfing. Preferable, and to be recommended in the case of more valuable specimens, is further turning until a maximum roughness of only a few tenths of a millimetre is obtained. To ensure uniform echo evaluation, the surface of the most important sections should be as uniform as possible but need not be very smooth. A roughness of a few microns, as recommended in the USA for testing turbine and generator rotors (ASA 125 [404]), is regarded in Germany as excessive. The coupling medium used is oil, SAE 20 to 30, cellulose paste, or also sugar solution with a slight admixture of hydrochloric acid.

The highly stressed parts of the specimen, in the case of rotors therefore, the barrels, are scanned completely, i.e. over the entire length and 360° of the circumference. This can be done either by hand on a stationary specimen by turning it once only through 180°, or on a suitable turning device as shown in Fig. 3.58. A cross-section as shown in Fig. 2.70 provides a good general picture of the distribution of flaws, from which it is often possible to deduce their origin, nature and importance even if fine details of the complete screen picture are not given. Such a picture covers the flaws of only one given plane in cross-section or longitudinal section. Automatic, complete recording of the echo indications has been realised by GOLDMAN and AUGER in an installation at General Electric

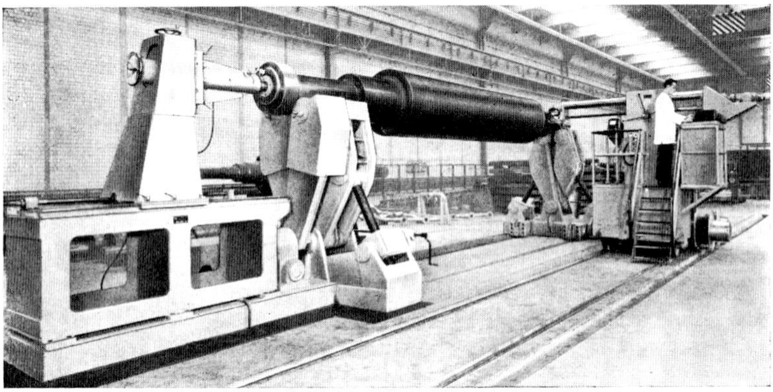

Fig. 3.58 Testing a large forging. The probe holder is mounted on an arm of the testing car. For coupling, a constant flow of oil from a large supply tank is used. Ultrasonic instrument, monitors and film recording device are placed on the test car which travels alongside the forging (works photo BBC, Baden/Switzerland).

[119, 120]. This installation uses direct recording on a five-fold spiral recorder. The amplitude of both the flaw echo and the backwall echo are recorded further a B-scan with position of the flaw echoes according to the travelling gate method (see 2.352). This shows up particularly well the so-called *travelling echoes* which are important for analysing the nature of the flaw (see below). Also recorded are the reference co-ordinates for the testing point. COOK and WALKER describe a similar installation using direct recording [69]. Since compared with the long testing time required for a larger forging the time for developing a film is of no great consequence, photographic recording of a B-scan with simultaneous recording of amplitudes can be envisaged. Such tests have proved successful in the case of the installation shown in Fig. 3.58 [267]. RICHTER and LINKE [309], using a Krautkrämer cross section recorder (see 2.353), have designed an automated installation for testing forgings by the immersion technique.

In the *interpretation of readings* obtained on forgings, one of the main difficulties is to distinguish between less dangerous, non-metallic inclusions and genuine cracks because both types of flaws can produce very similar indications. It is then not enough merely to record the indications according to echo height and flaw depth, but additional information must be obtained from the screen picture, particularly from its change as the probe is shifted, as will be described in the following.

Inclusions usually occur in large numbers and of all sizes in a given zone of the specimen, in the core or also in an annular zone. The screen picture shows many, densely packed echoes of different size, and the zero line between echoes is rarely free of indications (Fig. 3.59a). Cracks

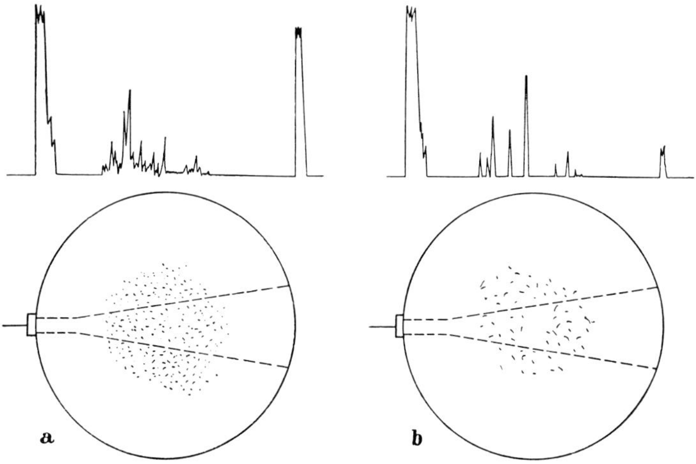

Fig. 3.59 Differences between the indications of inclusions and cracks, drawn schematically and exaggerated for greater clarity. a) Inclusions; b) flake cracks. The echoes of the more distant flaws, because of divergence and attenuation of the sound beam, are rather weak.

usually occur at more regular, greater distances, or also singly and are of more uniform size. Although they are often orientated with one axis of their area in the direction of the fibre, they can assume various angular positions around this general direction, from completely tangential to radial. Consequently they reflect more or less favourably, and larger and smaller echoes are obtained from such a cracked zone; however, in contrast to inclusions, the echoes are usually clearly separated. The zero line between echoes remains free even at higher gain (Fig. 3.59b). Furthermore, the backwall echo in the presence of cracks is usually more strongly attenuated. Since high resolving power is desirable and the differences at higher frequencies are more pronounced, frequencies up to 5 MHz are used.

If the probe is moved in the longitudinal direction, the indications of both types of flaws change in the same way, their height fluctuating rapidly. Differences appear, however, in the circumferential direction which are explained in Fig. 3.60.

A single flaw of approximately cylindrical shape travels during scanning in the circumferential direction, into the sound beam and at first produces a small echo which then quickly reaches a maximum while approaching still closer. In the reverse sequence it then decreases in a similar way. A tangential crack behaves similarly, but the echo increases still more abruptly. A radial crack however, when entering the sound beam, already produces a large echo at a greater distance. When it comes closer, it again decreases to zero, and conversely when leaving the sound

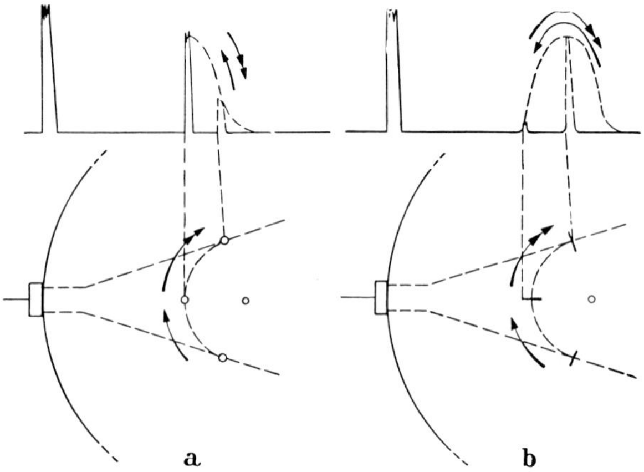

Fig. 3.60 Travelling echoes which appear when a rotor is scanned in the circumferential direction. The envelope of the travelling echo in the case of cylindrical flaws and tangential cracks (a) differs from that obtained in the case of radial cracks (b).

beam. A crack with a position intermediate between tangential and radial produces a line of travel which, when it enters the beam, shows a pattern different from that followed when it leaves the beam. Such *travelling echoes* thus point to cracks not orientated tangentially. In the case of inclusions, because of their clustering, a single echo can rarely be observed in this way. On echoes which can be observed separately, however, IVENS could in this way obtain stronger evidence of cracks and predict their position as confirmed in the majority of the specimens after they were cut up [208].

For a conclusive analysis of a given forging its history is taken into consideration: it is well known that cold cracks can certainly be avoided if the heat treatment is sufficiently slow, but for reasons of economy one stays as close as possible to the critical limit. The probability of cold cracks therefore depends on the nature of the treatment. Finally, it is known that cold cracks occur preferentially in the region of the main piping (Fig. 3.61) which determines the critical zone in the forging. It is always in the barrel, while the thin ends of the shaft, because of their smaller diameter, are usually free of cold cracks.

Practical experience in the USA, particularly at the General Electric Company, Schenectady, New York, has led to a more statistical acceptance specification [293, 294, 404], see also [265]. Irrespective of their positions in the forging, all indications are counted and sorted according to size (size = height of echo in per cent of the echo of the bore, which in contrast to German practice is customary in the USA on all rotors). The size versus number characteristic is entered in a diagram which specifies a lower and a higher acceptance limit (Fig. 3.62). In addition, the travelling echoes from all indications having an envelope according to Fig. 3.60b, as being particularly suspect, are entered in a second diagram with narrower acceptance limits. Depending on the position of these two characteristics, the specimen concerned is either accepted outright, or accepted depending on the outcome of a tensile test on up to six trepanning samples removed from six strategically placed spots, or rejected outright.

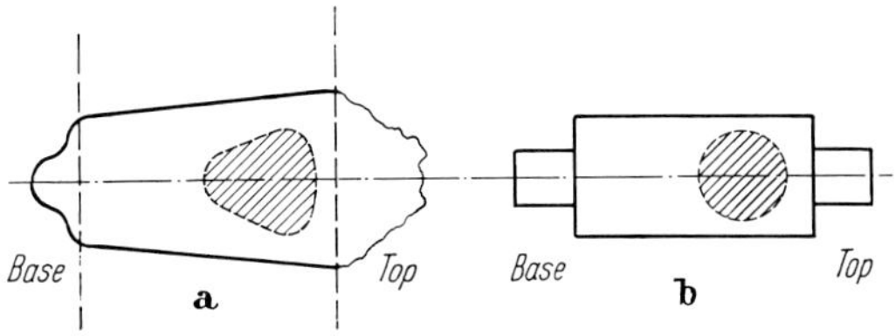

Fig. 3.61 Position of segregation zone in ingot (a) and of corresponding zone in forging subject to cold cracking (b).

According to Fig. 3.60, the travelling echoes are preferably observed in a sound beam with greater divergence. The American specification therefore recommends probes of 1 MHz and 25 mm diameter. The test piece, against whose very finely machined surface the quartz is pressed with a simultaneous flow of oil, rotates slowly so that the flaw indications can be recorded by the observer watching the screen picture, as regards nature, size and number. According to another suggestion, the incident sound beam of longitudinal waves is inclined approximately 5 to 10° to the perpendicular for detection of the travelling echoes, and especially for better recognition of incipient cracks in the central bore of large rotors [267].

The American method, which in respect of the empirical determination of the acceptance limits is based on experience gained on approximately 1500 rotors for turbines and generators, can therefore not be applied to forgings of different shape. The classification according to echo height must already be changed in the case of specimens with other outside diameters or diameters of the bore. This would make it necessary to compute the reference echo according to Fig. 1.47. The change in echo is of course particularly marked if instead of the bore, the backwall of a solid cylinder is used (see also 1.75).

Furthermore, in the case of a short, thick forging, a preferential orientation of cracks or inclusions as in long rotors can by no means be expected, nor can they be evaluated according to the same pattern.

In Germany the Association of German Ferrous Metallurgists (see Rauterkus [302]) has proposed a table for numerical characterization of ultrasonic tests on forgings, according to nature, size, quantity and position of inhomogeneities. Intentionally no attempt was made to specify the testing technique. The result therefore remains largely subjective, as hitherto.

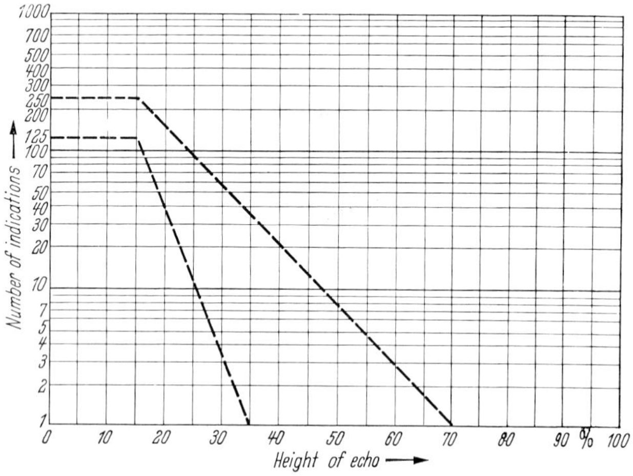

Fig. 3.62 Graph of number versus size for echo indications obtained on rotors for turbines and generators, with narrow and wide acceptance limits, according to RANKIN and MORIARTY, General Electric Co., Schenectady, USA.

On large forgings much too little attention has so far been paid to quantitative law of distance of the echo amplitude and the attenuation of sound, the latter serving both as a characterizing quantity of the structure and as an interfering quantity when judging the size of flaws on the basis of their echo height.

To classify the latter, consider a numerical example: Usually the gain of the pulse-echo instrument is adjusted so that the backwall echo has full screen amplitude. Let us consider a rotor in which the distance to the bore at the stub is 200 mm and at the barrel 500 mm. According to IVENS [165] the attenuation in forged carbon steel and low-alloy steel can exceed $20 \cdot 10^{-3}$ dB/mm at 2 MHz. Table 10 in the Appendix shows for a value of 30 and a distance of 200 mm a reduction of the echo to 25%, and for 500 mm already to 3%. If both echoes are brought to the same height, the amplitude at the stub is increased 4 times, but at the barrel 33 times. At the barrel the zone at a depth of 200 mm is therefore tested at $33/4 \approx 8$ times greater sensitivity than at the stub. Apart from any actual differences between stub and barrel, uncritical testing therefore produces a considerably more unfavourable picture of the barrel.

Using a gain control calibrated in decibels, the total attenuation can thus according to [20] be measured quantitatively, from which together with the thickness a mean attenuation coefficient can be calculated [206, 182, 279]. Since in fact the attenuation may decrease going from the outside towards the inside, this may not yet give the true value at all depths, but the mean value at least precludes that very gross errors are made.

Concerning the testing of forgings, see also [74, 164, 193, 244, 41], regarding geometrical influences in this connection [330, 177, 196, 197], and specifically regarding the determination of flaw sizes, reports [279, 182, 193, 186].

In the case of *steel drop forgings*, their usually more complex form and oxidized surface make testing more difficult. Most flaws can also be determined more easily in the initial material (billets, rods, sheets, bars). For light-metal forgings, particularly for airplane construction in the USA, the immersion technique is used. The excellent surface permits detection of the minutest flaws. In the case of more complex specimens the probe is guided under water by an exchangeable pipe spacing support, whose front edge can be suitably shaped to match a curved surface, thus permitting reproducible coupling. Fig. 3.63 on the other hand, shows a mass test with a probe manipulator for testing larger numbers of more simply shaped specimens, or for testing only a few specific points on such pieces. A complete test is never possible, nor hardly ever required.

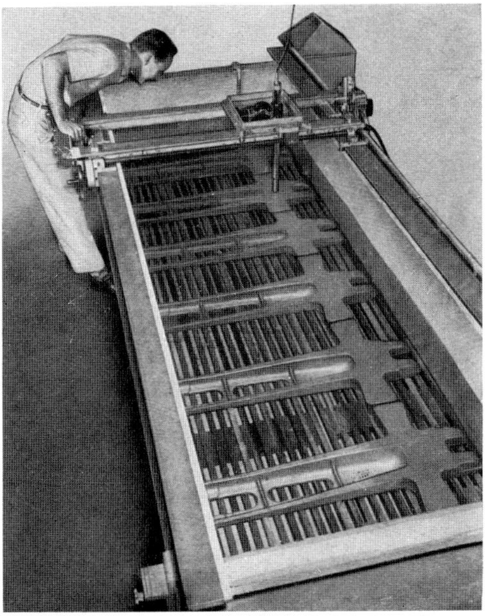

Fig. 3.63 Testing aluminium forgings by the immersion technique (works photo Douglas Aircraft Co., Santa Monica, Calif., USA).

On *finished forgings* it is less important to detect manufacturing defects than to observe flaws which are already known but which did not result in rejection taking account of the stresses during operation, or to check the specimen for new defects which appeared while in service, so-called endurance failures or fatigue cracks. On cold cracks it can for instance be observed that they already grow after a short time and without being specially stressed while in use.

Since the shape of specimens is often unfavourable for continuous checking, this is sometimes taken into account in the design stage; of this the generator rotor shown in Fig. 3.64 is an example [265]. To be able to test the internal structure including the zone under the slots conveniently, four cylindrical grooves into which a convex ground quartz probe can be fitted were machined into the body. Because of the pronounced divergence it is preferable to use a focusing probe provided the interfering echoes near the surface, and caused by the intermediate pieces, can be tolerated.

The testing of finished rotors from the internal bore is discussed in reports [296, 300].

Well-planned testing for fatigue cracks presupposes experience with identical or similar specimens. The examiner should furthermore be aware of the stressing and as far as possible also of the pattern of the fibres of the specimen concerned, to enable him to determine the test procedure in advance with the aid of drawings so that the sound beam can be directed as far as possible at right angles to the face of any cracks.

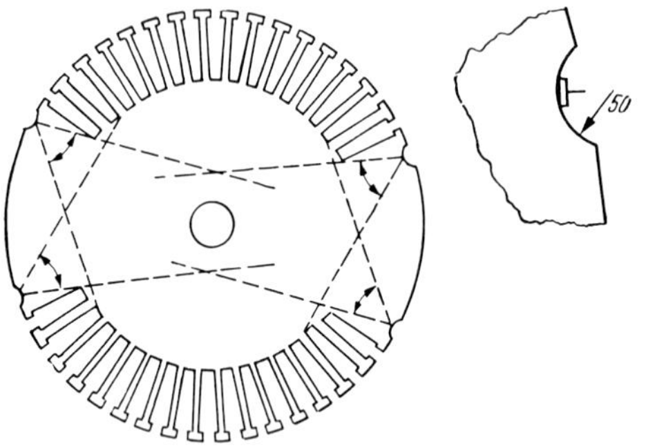

Fig. 3.64 Section through generator rotor with 4 grooves according to Westinghouse for inspecting the internal cross-section.

Crankshafts or *crankpins* are subject to fatigue cracks in the fillet, which proceed at an angle of approximately 45° to the axis. Accordingly, Fig. 3.65 shows that tests with standard probes are less suitable than angle probes. If a bore in the pin prevents application of this method, the bore can also be used as reflector. This, however, greatly reduces the sensitivity. Calibrating for reference purposes is possible on the free edge which reflects 100 % at 45° beam angle. Occasionally such cracks proceed

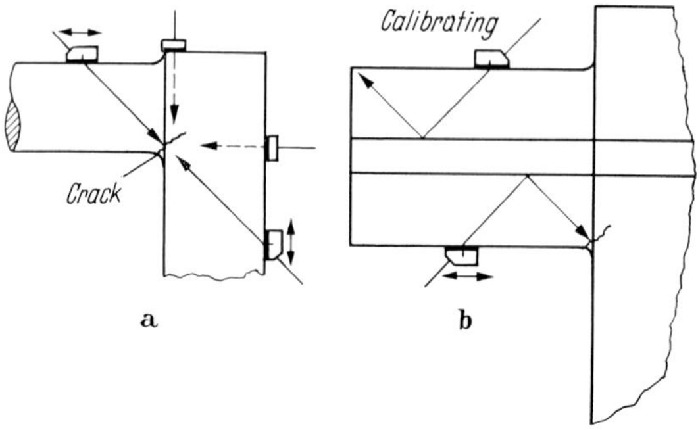

Fig. 3.65 Testing for fatigue cracks on crankshafts and crankpins, a) without bore, b) with bore.

obliquely relative to the axis of the pin, owing to additional torsion. They are then detected more easily from the flat face of the cheek (Fig. 3.66), whence the beam can likewise be directed obliquely to the surface of the pin. Previous experience with cracks of this type is very valuable and avoids unnecessary scanning. Compared with the magnetic powder method the ultrasonic test offers certain advantages because it is not absolutely necessary to dismantle the bearing of the connecting rod, and because it is possible to determine approximately the depth of the crack, preferably after calibration on a similar specimen.

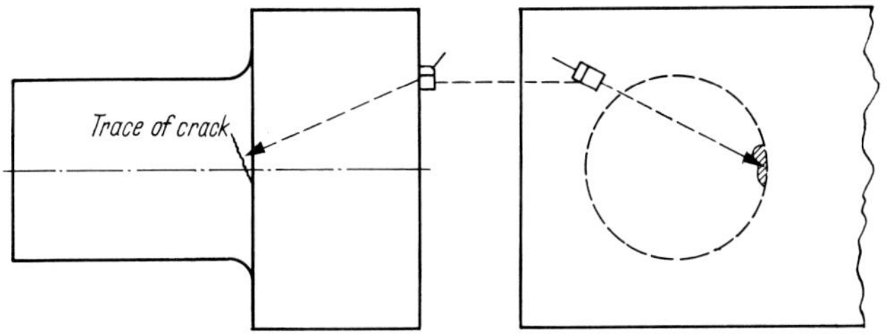

Fig. 3.66 Oblique fatigue cracks on crankpins (trace of crack on surface not in circumferential direction).

In the testing of heavy machinery, oil-filled oil holes are frequently encountered. They produce not only the expected echo from the front wall but also a backwall echo. Because of the lower acoustic velocity of oil, the backwall echo appears behind the front echo at a distance equal to four times the bore diameter; it is surprisingly strong due to the focusing effect of the front wall (see also 1.75 and Fig. 1.52).

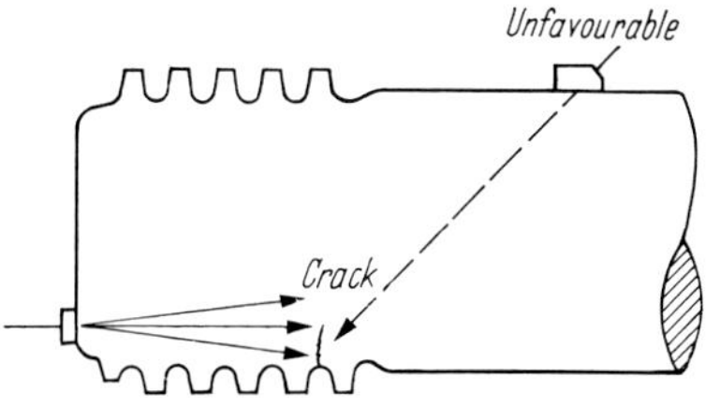

Fig. 3.67 Crack test on columns, pump rods, etc.

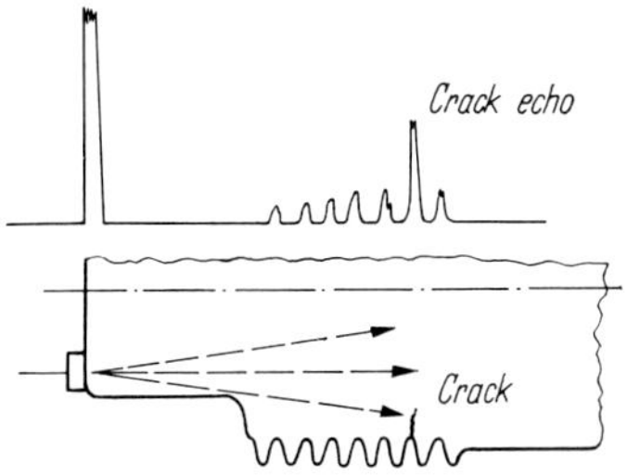

Fig. 3.68 Crack test on thread in the shadow of a sound beam, above schematic screen picture.

Supporting columns of heavy presses as well as pump rods are subject to fatigue cracks in the thread (Fig. 3.67) which start at the bottom of the thread and proceed at right angles to the axis. Usually they can be readily detected from the end face if a normal probe is applied near the edge. If this also shows the threads, these can be identified by their regularity. This, however, makes it more difficult to detect smaller incipient cracks. In this case the optimal angle of divergence of the sound beam is found by testing a reference specimen with a saw cut at the base of a thread. Testing in an oblique direction is in this case less favourable because of the strong indication of the threads and should be considered only if the face is inaccessible.

Satisfactory test results are also obtained in the case of reduced ends of pump rods as shown in Fig. 3.68, from which the thread could no longer be irradiated directly. The screen picture showed the perfectly regular echoes of these threads, from which the additional crack echo could be clearly distinguished at one point. This was indubitably due to diffraction of the wave at the point of reduction.

Retaining rings, consisting of austenitic (non-magnetic) ring cylinders to protect the ends of windings on generator rotors, are subject to fatigue cracks (Fig. 3.69), which sometimes start at arcing points caused by

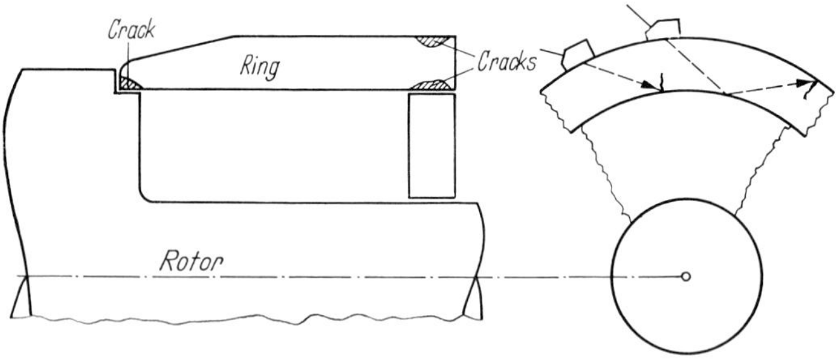

Fig. 3.69 Testing a generator retaining ring.

stray currents. These cracks can be easily detected, using angle probes of approximately 45°. At the conical end the probe should be shifted while inclined at an angle to the edge, so as to irradiate the internal edge. If the material has been worked sufficiently during forging and cold straining, these components can, in general, be readily penetrated by sound. Sometimes, however, they contain zones with coarser structure which can be very difficult to penetrate; this makes flaw detection with 2 MHz transverse waves very difficult, forcing the examiner to use 1 MHz.

The rings are shrunk on to the rotor and a supporting disc and they are therefore subjected to considerable stresses. If they are pulled off, previously definite crack indications may disappear. They must be caused by fine cracks which transmit sound unless dilated. The tests should therefore be carried out on the shrunk-on component.

These components are furthermore subject to inter-crystalline corrosion; the finely branched cracks clearly visible in the etched microsection, *cannot* be detected reliably with transverse waves at frequencies up to 4 MHz.

3.22 Worked Parts of Machines

No testing directives of general validity can be given here in view of the many different shapes and manifold testing problems. Examples at random sequence will be discussed in as far as they refer to typical or particularly important cases.

Screws, bolts and rivets. Manufacturing defects of pressed parts of this type are internal separations transverse to the axis, so-called overdrawing cracks, especially at the head (Fig. 3.70). The test can be made from both ends using a normal probe of 2 to 5 MHz whose diameter should not exceed that of the test piece. Testing from the head is preferable provided there is no interfering embossing. An even curvature of the contact face does not interfere. In the case of mass tests it is recommended that the probe be mounted on a table with the crystal on top, and to press on the oil-coated test piece. Other manufacturing defects are longitudinal cracks in the core and on the surface; these, however, are the result of defects in the initial material and they can therefore be detected more easily at that stage (see also 3.25).

Fatigue cracks occur as incipient cracks in threads and at the transition from the head to the shank. The former are found as shown in Fig. 3.67. The latter (Fig. 3.71) are located using normal probes; this can be done better from the shank than from the head where these cracks, if they are small, are difficult to distinguish from the always

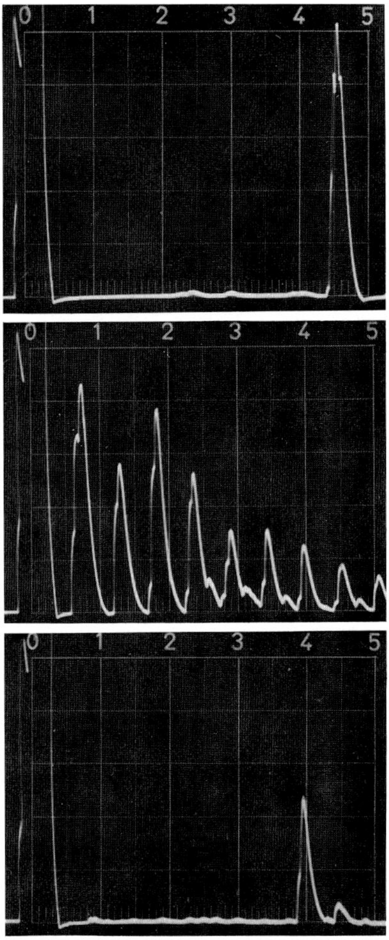

a

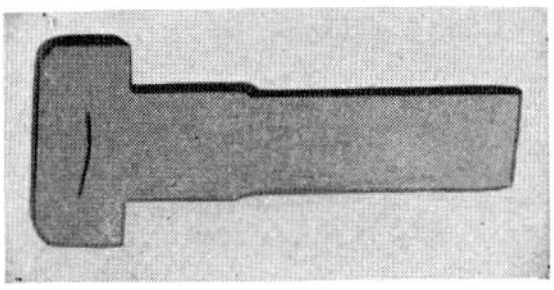

Fig. 3.70 Testing an extruded screw for cracks in the head. a) Crack in polished cross-section made visible by the magnetic powder method; b) screen picture of a sound screw tested from the head, 4 MHz, testing range 50 mm; c) ditto of screw with flaw; d) ditto tested from base. In both cases the flawed screw is infallibly-distinguished from a sound screw.

present echo of the bottom face of the head. Angle beam testing from the smooth shank is also satisfactory. Bolts with a bore, whose external surface when installed is no longer accessible, can also be tested obliquely from the inside by means of special probes with a diameter of a few millimetres.

Re. incipient cracks of rivet holes, see 3.291.

In *quenched work pieces* stress cracks occur which need not necessarily be caused by flaws in the initial material. They appear on the finished article, e.g. tools for presses and die blocks, where they do not always penetrate to the surface. The critical zones should therefore be scanned with normal or angle probes. Fig. 3.72 shows an example for small parts, e.g. steel balls of 12 mm diameter.

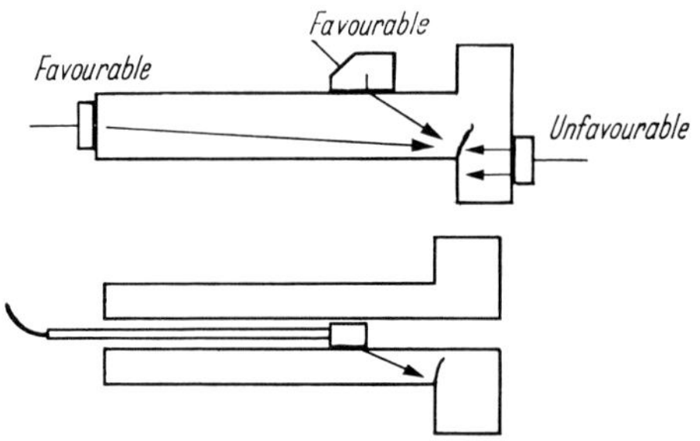

Fig. 3.71 Testing for fatigue cracks on bolts.

This is an example of the so-called "brush" technique with the pulse-echo method, in which one no longer observes the detailed echo picture in order to sort out flawed specimens according to flaw echoes, but instead the height and length of the echo sequence obtained with the specimen at a large testing range. Flaws as well as differences in structure influence the damping of the sound and thus the shape of the echo "brush". Once the nature of the defects and their influence have been established on the basis of a larger number of preliminary tests, this method can be used successfully for rapid mass sorting, even by untrained examiners. On small, simply shaped parts the position of the testing point has little influence on the result, and in the case of balls as shown in Fig. 3.72 none at all (see also Fig. 3.214).

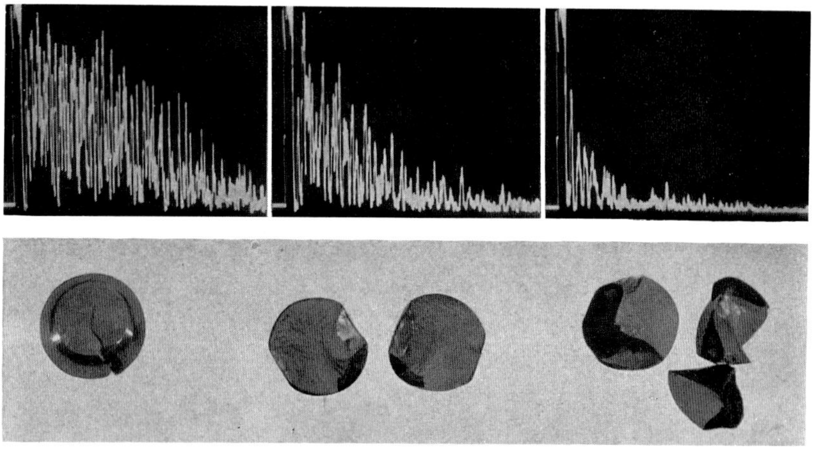

Fig. 3.72 Testing 12 mm steel balls for flaws in the initial material and quenching cracks, standard probe 4 MHz, 10 mm diameter with plastic protective cover, testing range 250 mm. Left, sound ball, burst during pressure test at 17.9 tons, centre, ball with small flaw, broke at 8.2 tons, right, ball with large flaw, burst at 2.6 tons and broke at 5.2 tons (Söding & Halbach, Hagen).

On larger and more complex components, such as bolts, leaf springs or helical springs, quenching cracks on the surface are detected by one of the various wave modes, depending on the position of the cracks, using directed echo sounding; examples are shown in Figs. 3.48, 3.73 and 3.74.

Turbine blades for water, steam and gas turbines, can be of very different material, shape and manufacture. Particularly successful have been tests on gas turbines. Cast steel blades for Pelton wheels are mentioned in 3.32.

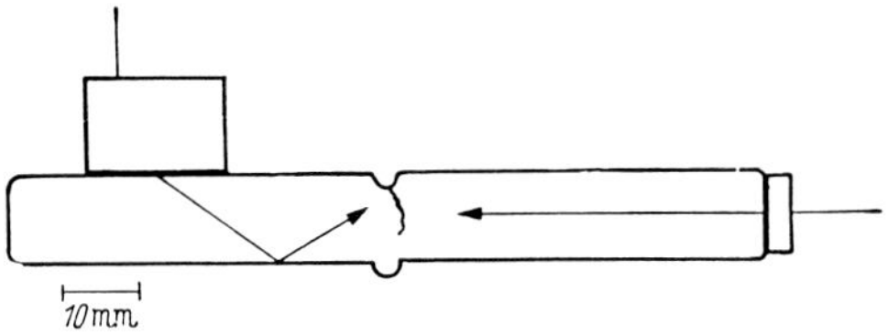

Fig. 3.73 Cross-section through a leaf spring for railway cars, with quenching crack. Testing with small angle probe or normal probe, surface waves unfavourable due to roughness.

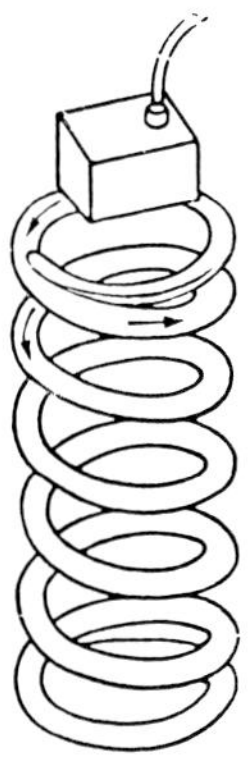

Fig.3.74 Testing a bright helical spring for quenching cracks, using surface waves, according to [264].

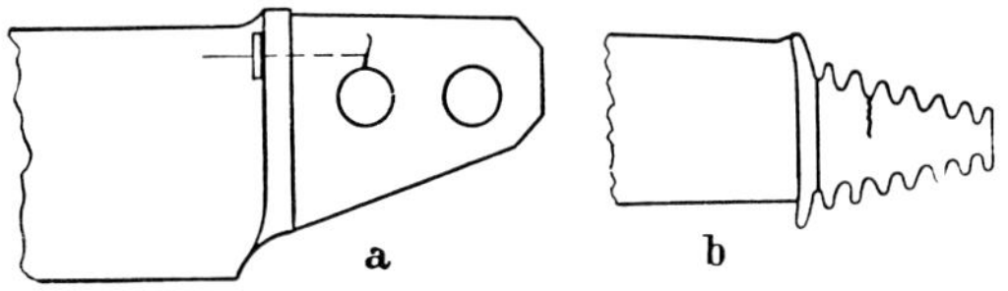

Fig. 3.75 Cracks in base of blades, in design (a) possibly detectable while assembled, in design (b) (fir-tree base) very difficult.

Blades for steam turbines usually are made of magnetic material, and can therefore also be tested by the magnetic powder method or other methods for crack detection without dismantling. Ultrasonic tests, carried out as described below on gas turbine blades, are often hampered by severe corrosion along the leading edge. Deposits on the surface can be removed by blasting with fly-ash. This produces a sufficiently smooth surface for finding fatigue cracks by testing from the end of the blade using surface waves. The blades need not be dismantled for the test, even if assembled in closely spaced bucket rings.

Components for gas turbines, such as turbine blades, compressor blades and bucket rings, all of which are highly stressed, are tested very carefully, beginning with the raw material. The costs for testing play only a secondary role, which is understandable if one takes into consideration that a broken blade in a jet propulsion engine may cause the loss of an entire jet plane, quite apart from the risk to human life.

Manufacturing defects differ greatly according to the method of manufacture, viz. drop-forging, milling from the solid, or precision casting. The initial material for the two first-mentioned manufacturing methods, viz. rods, may contain the usual longitudinal defects (3.25). In the case of the highly heat-resistant NiCrAlTi alloys (*Nimonic*), incipient transverse cracks may also occur. The sections, cut into short lengths, are therefore tested from the smooth end faces using small probes and high frequencies.

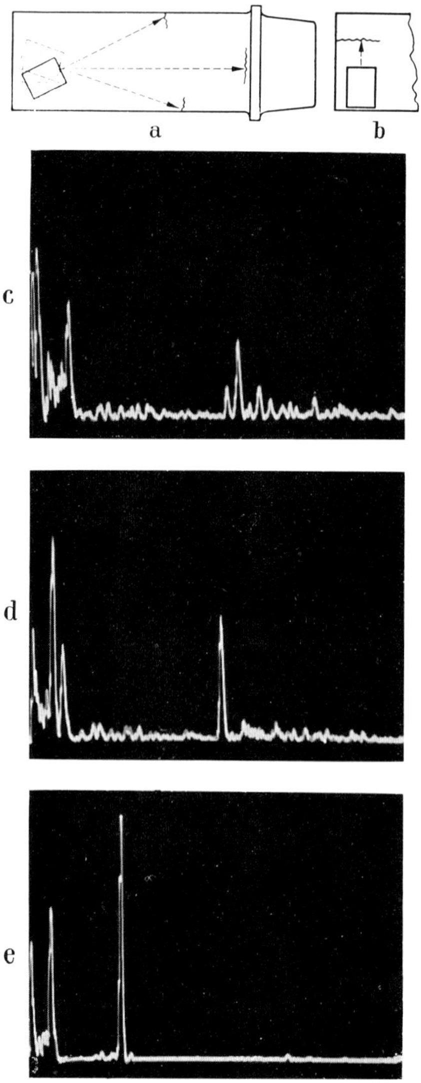

Fig. 3.76 Testing blades with surface waves. a) and b) positions of probes; c) screen picture showing incipient crack at transition from blade to base; d) screen picture at same testing direction on sound blade; e) screen picture showing incipient crack on the edge.

Fatigue cracks can occur as incipient cracks along both edges of the blade, at the transition from the blade to the base, at the tip of the blade, and finally also in the base. The complex shape of the base usually makes testing in the assembled state very difficult. Whereas an incipient crack, as shown in Fig. 3.75a, may in some cases still be detectable with special probes, the method fails in the case of blades with "fir-tree" bases as in Fig. 3.75b. At all other points, however, the test as shown in Fig. 3.76 is quite feasible, provided the material is not too coarse-grained and the surface free of corrosion and deposits. The test is made from the convex side of the blade, using surface waves from 2 to 5 MHz, as shown in Fig. 3.76a and b. At the right angle, usually formed between incipient edge cracks and the edge itself, surface waves are reflected favourably. Cracks at the transition to the base and longitudinal cracks at the tip of the blade should be irradiated perpendicularly where possible. The edge at the base always produces a strong echo in front of which at a short distance a crack echo would appear.

For mass tests it is advisable to use devices which quickly position the probe in a definite, reproducible position. Fig. 3.77 shows such a device according to RASMUSSEN [297] and LUND [230].

Sometimes access to the surface of a blade is very difficult. The sound can then be transmitted into the blade from an edge as shown in Fig. 3.78, either as a surface wave along the coupling edge, or as a transverse wave of 45 to 60° for testing the opposite edge and the tip of the blade. In spite of the small contact face, which can still be improved by grinding a matching groove into it, the sensitivity is remarkably high. Using special probes, it is possible in this way to mass test bucket rings while installed.

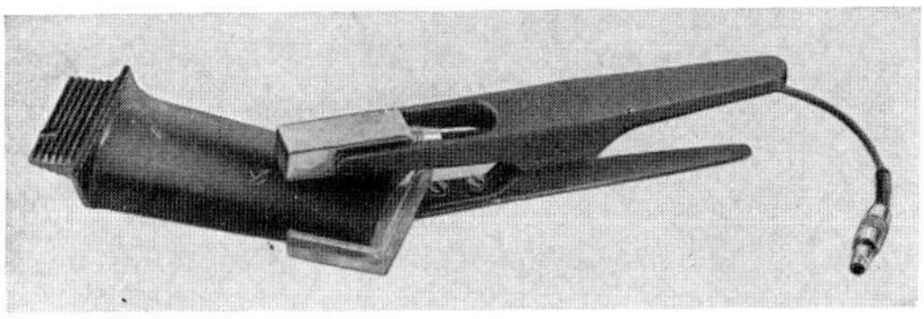

Fig. 3.77 Probe for surface waves with holder according to LUND ensuring reproducible coupling according to Fig. 3.76a.

In Nimonic the velocity of sound is almost exactly the same as in steel. In other materials used for blades, however, it is different, so that wedge angles and material-for the probes must be chosen correctly for surface waves. Copper alloys in particular, as used for some compressor blades, have very low values of c_t so that wedge materials with c_l values lower than perspex or ordinary polyamide qualities must be used. According to RASMUSSEN a special grade of nylon mark 6.6 is suitable.

Even if the propagation of surface waves is impeded by corrosion and deposits, this does not always preclude a test. It is then still possible to use transverse waves from the edge as shown in Fig. 3.78, or alternatively from the surface of the blade along a zig-zag path.

Coarse crystallization, as already known from the manufacture of forged blades in Nimonic, hamper the test considerably. Since the edge at this stage frequently does not yet show coarse grain, testing by means of surface waves along the edge according to Fig. 3.78, is still promising. In the case of grain diameters of the order of centimetres, also lower frequencies are no longer feasible.

Hitherto the opinion has frequently been expressed that recrystallization is not a disadvantage in operation. STÄGER and MEISTER [349] have found, however, on Nimonic 80A (with approx. 19 Cr and 75 Ni) that both acoustic velocities decrease with increasing grain size, and therefore also the modulus of shear and Young's modulus. Furthermore, fatigue tests showed a considerable influence of grain coarsening. Elimination of recrystallized blades thus seems advisable, and for this the ultrasonic test offers as a possible criterion, either the attenuation of the sound or its velocity. The fir-tree base of the blade is best suited for such measurements.

Also the *turbine discs* for gas turbines are checked carefully for manufacturing defects. Since the finished shape is rather complex, the test is usually carried out at an earlier stage with parallel surfaces as shown in Fig. 3.79. This arrangement is particularly suitable for automated testing by the immersion technique, since the test is required to be as complete as possible. This can also readily be combined with flaw recording. A further advantage for mass testing is coupling without wear.

The forging defects, at least those in the highly stressed thin parts of the disc, are located favourably for testing. Using the immersion technique, also obliquely orientated flaws can be detected simply by tilting the probe. Fig. 3.79 shows such a simple arrangement. The rotation of the disc is synchronized mechanically or electrically with that of the recording disc. The probe moves either continuously or in steps in the radial

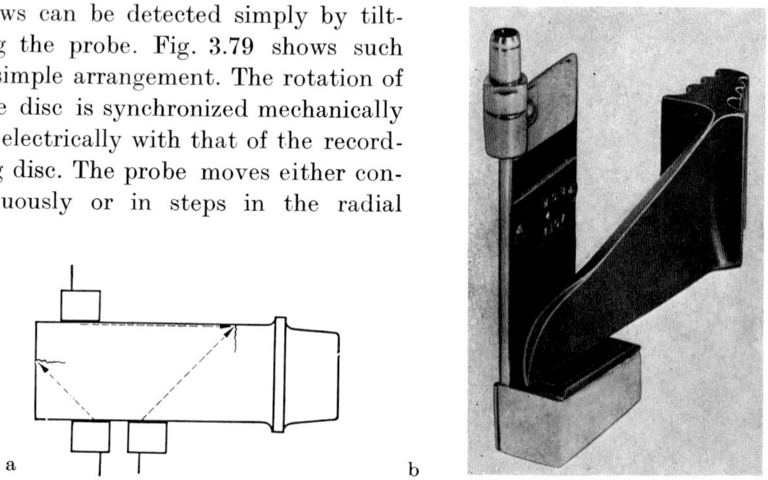

Fig. 3.78 Testing blades from the edge, using surface or transverse waves. a) Method; b) view of special probe, design Krautkrämer.

direction, or along an arc like the pick-up arm of a record player. The recording system goes through the same motion, possibly on a changed scale. The recording can take either the form of a go/no-go indication with interrupted trace, or a full trace is recorded with deflections

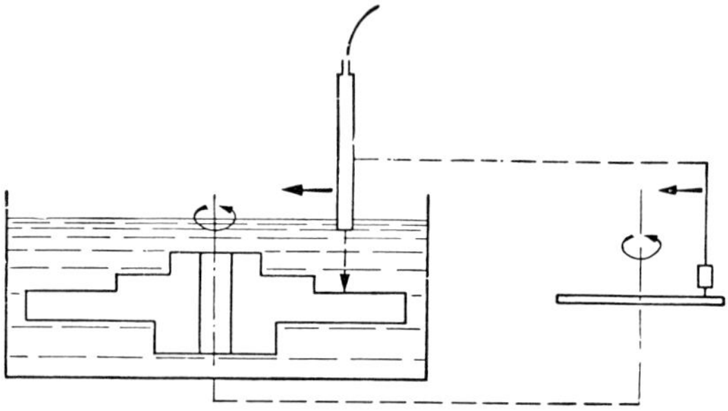

Fig. 3.79 Checking blanks of turbine discs by the immersion technique with turntable recorder, schematic.

which latter can also be controlled so that they are proportional to the height of the echo. In the first simple case, using electrosensitive paper and a fixed stylus without fast moving components, recording speeds and thus also testing speeds of the order of 1 m/s can be realized. In the second case the speed, in accordance with the cut-off frequency of the recording system used, becomes slower (cf. 2.35).

Unless the depth of the flaw can be stated, the recording still remains unsatisfactory because only flaws which later will still be present in the

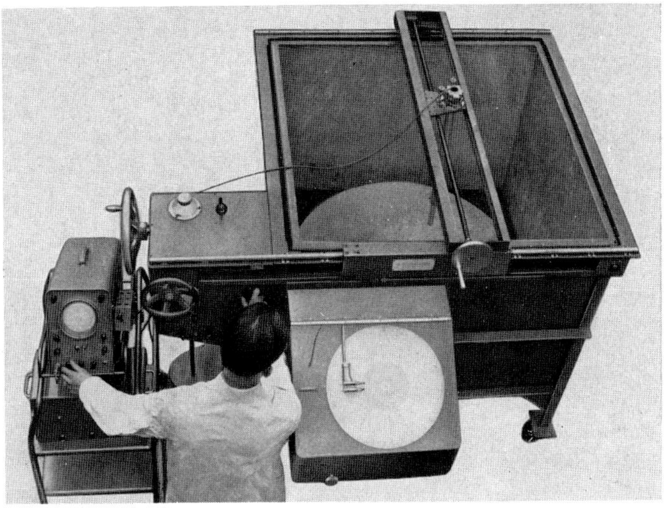

Fig. 3.80 Installation for testing turbine discs using the immersion technique (Ultrasonoscope)

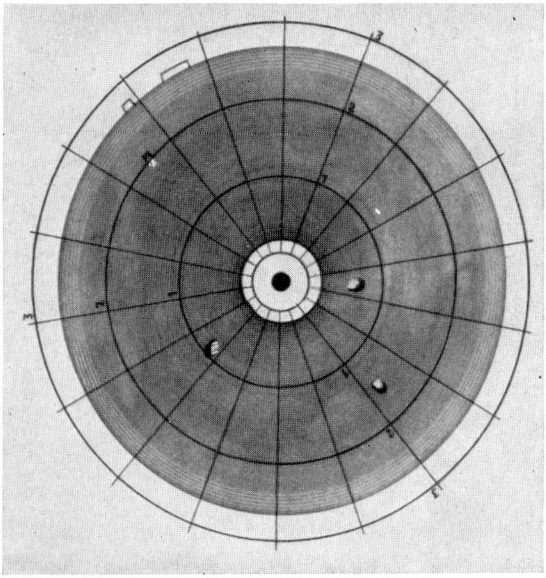

Fig. 3.81 Recording of a turbine disc showing four flaws (Ultrasonoscope).

finished specimen are of interest. No practical solution has yet been found for recording the three position co-ordinates. Frequently therefore one still relies on observation of the viewing screen, assisted by flaw warning by means of monitors, as well as B-scan display.

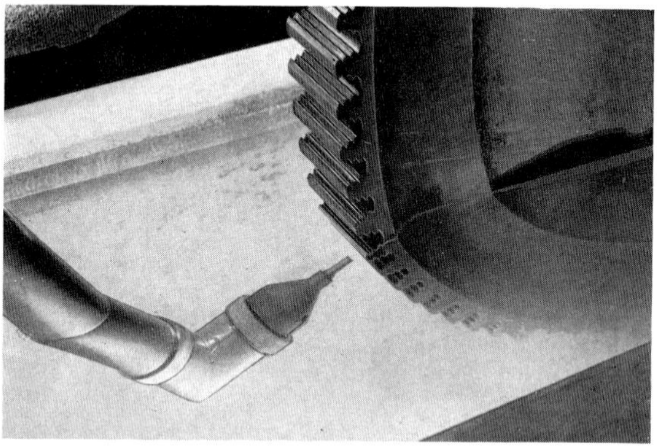

Fig. 3.82 Testing a turbine disc for jet engines for fatigue cracks in the blade mounting (Electrocircuits).

Fig. 3.80 shows testing equipment by Ultrasonoscope, and Fig. 3.81 the recording of a turbine disc produced by it with proportional trace. Regarding other testing installations, see also [337, 290]. Fatigue cracks in turbine discs occur at the rim in the mounting for the blades. The shape in these zones is rather complex. For certain flaw positions the immersion technique can be applied, using an accurately masked beam of high frequency, as shown in Fig. 3.82 (cf. [56]).

Automated installations have been built in the USA also for this purpose, in which every disc of the completely assembled rotor with blades is scanned under water [84].

3.23 Railway Material

Separate treatment of these testing problems, which individually should be classified under other Sections, seems justified in view of the extent and the importance of ultrasonic testing in railway engineering. Many of these applications can, however, also be applied to similar testing problems encountered in other branches of industry.

3.231 Axles

Manufacturing defects consist primarily of inclusions in the core which, if they are not very densely packed or, worse still, are accompanied by crack-like defects, do not impair serviceability. They are readily detected by transverse tests, either already in the blank using 1 to 2 MHz, or in the finished axle using 2 to 5 MHz. In order to detect reliably also flaws such as over-forgings and piping cracks, which frequently reflect directionally, tests are carried out along a few longitudinal tracks.

In Germany, these tests are optional for the manufacturer; the German Federal Railways (DB) have thus far demanded an acceptance test by means of ultrasonics only in exceptional cases, e.g. in the case of cranked axles for certain types of locomotives and plates for building railway bridges. In other countries, other components such as wheel tyres and discs (France) are occasionally also checked for manufacturing defects.

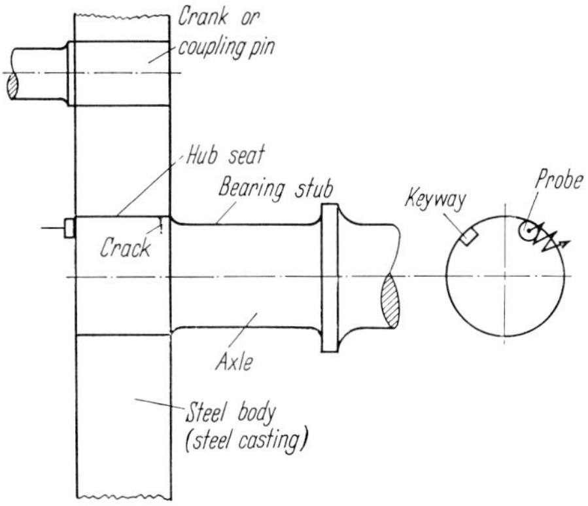

Fig. 3.83 Crack test on axles of steam locomotives.

As for all railway material made of steel, the main purpose of testing axles is the determination of fatigue cracks. In the case of *steam locomotives* with wheels on axles with inside bearings as shown in Fig. 3.83, the test according to [245] is particularly simple and reliable because the cracks almost invariably occur at the hub seat as shown. Since the front faces are directly accessible the test can be carried out on the locomotive ready for service. After removing any dirt or loose paint and grinding off any burrs around punched numbers, the edge is coated with heavy oil and scanned with a 2 MHz probe. If the front face of the axle and the wheel body are flush, the probe can during scanning be moved along a zig-zag track, passing slightly over the edge. A backwall echo may be obtained through the wheel body which coincides with the transition from hub seat to bearing stub. This can be used as reference echo at full gain. Fatigue cracks almost invariably appear 20 to 30 mm in front of this echo, rarely coming from the zone of the bearing stub. The depth of vertical incipient cracks can be determined fairly accurately from the height of the echo using a calibration curve; not, however, in the case of oblique cracks. In the case of small echoes, one therefore checks whether the end echo of the axle has not perhaps been much attenuated, which would point out a larger, obliquely orientated crack. If readings are obtained from greater depths of the axle, which cannot be explained as secondary echoes caused by the splitting off of transverse waves according to 3.132, it will be necessary to carry out transverse and oblique tests.

Checking the axles of an express train steam locomotive from both ends takes less than 30 min. The German Federal Railways record the results of such periodical tests on a special report card for each axle, particularly the depth and circumferential length of a given indication. Under favourable conditions incipient cracks with depth of a few millimetres can already be detected, although such small defects are less important because long experience has confirmed that the risk of a shaft breaking exists only with cracks of greater depth (cf. [248, 427, 325]).

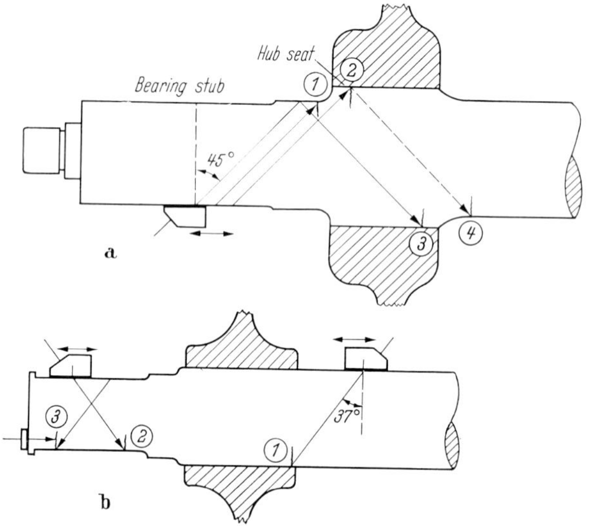

Fig. 3.84 Examples of axles with outside bearings of the German Federal Railways. a) Axle of electric locomotive, b) of goods truck.

Usually less convenient to test are the axles with external bearings for *tenders, electric locomotives and railway trucks* (Fig. 3.84). The front faces of the axles are of smaller diameter than the hub seats, are some distance away from the latter, and sometimes leave little space for coupling the probe, especially if the axle has a bore and keyways and threaded holes. In this case it is advisable to test with angle probes from the bearing stub as shown in Fig. 3.84a, either with a direct beam (flaws ① and ②) or with reflection (flaws ③ and ④). The test can also be carried out on locomotives standing by, as it is only necessary to remove the cover of the axle bearing to make the axle stub accessible from the bottom. In order to cover the entire circumference it is of course necessary at one stage to move the locomotive a little [249].

Where experience has shown that in the case of railway truck axles (Fig. 3.84 b) the cracks mainly occur in the bearing stub, as in the USA, these axles can simply be tested from the front face. For this purpose Sperry has constructed a small automotive truck in which the examiner travels alongside the train from axle to axle and tests without moving from his seat (3.85). A special design of the probe with 6 separate transducers makes it possible to cover the entire circumference of the axle. These probes radiate longitudinal waves at an angle of approximately 10° to the axis of the axle. An electromagnet holds the probe in position during the test. Flaw echoes actuate an alarm device.

For cracks in the hub seat this method is reliable only in the case of larger flaws. In Germany, where cracks at this point also occur, angle probes as shown in Fig. 3.84b are used with 2 MHz and 37°, and at the three positions shown in the drawing. Although the surface of the shaft between the wheels is sometimes badly corroded, cracks in the hub seat which are only a few tenths of a mm deep can be detected reliably after the axle has been cleaned with a scraper and a steel brush. In the case of incipient cracks in the bearing stub, which can already be detected when only 0.1 mm deep provided the surface is very good, an attempt is then made to remove them by turning, as far as this is still permissible.

Hollow axles (Fig. 3.86a) can, under favourable conditions, still be tested from the front face or from the bearing stub, using several zig-zag reflections. The external surface of the axle between the wheels is frequently inaccessible unless dismantled. Recourse can then be taken to testing from the bore using a special angle probe, provided the surface is not too rough [25].

Where it is unconditionally required that the hub seat be tested from the end, larger flaws can be detected relatively reliably with a normal probe (1 to 2 MHz) with sufficiently wide beam angle. For axles of American Diesel locomotives probes with longitudinal waves and small angles (15 to 24°) have proved successful for this purpose (Fig. 3.86b). The longer interference zone of these probes can be tolerated in view of the greater flaw distances. Another solution is illustrated in Fig. 3.86c. Here the railway administration decided to machine a conical surface on the front face to facilitate testing. All critical points can then be scanned by a probe with suitably ground quartz plate in one revolution.

In view of the large number of truck axles, automated testing installations prove economical. Fig. 3.87 shows a test bench designed for this purpose and used by the German Federal Railways in several of their repair workshops.

Automation begins with the hydraulic lifting of the rolled-in wheel set. It starts to revolve, the probes are coupled by a flow of water, and the sets are then scanned one after the other. The angle probes for the bearing stubs have several crystal plates connected in parallel to be able to cover all possible flaw positions simultaneously without shift in axial direction. A flaw is indicated on the signal board in the centre of the yoke by a red light signal at the point concerned. Before scanning the hub seat by means of the angle probes, the backwall echo is first checked by means of normal probes, in order to determine whether there are no serious defects

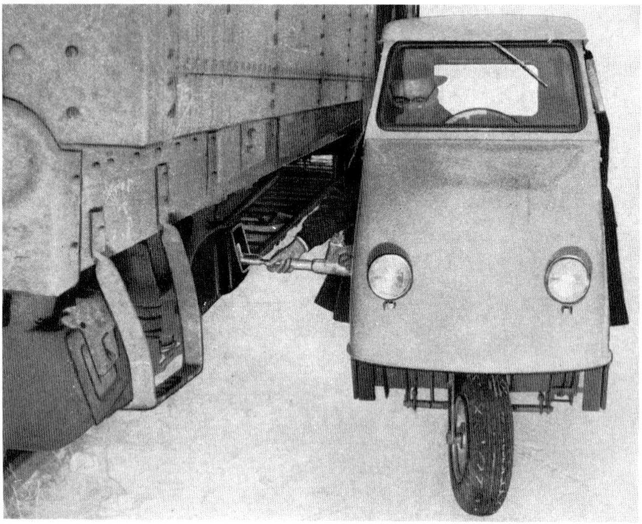

a

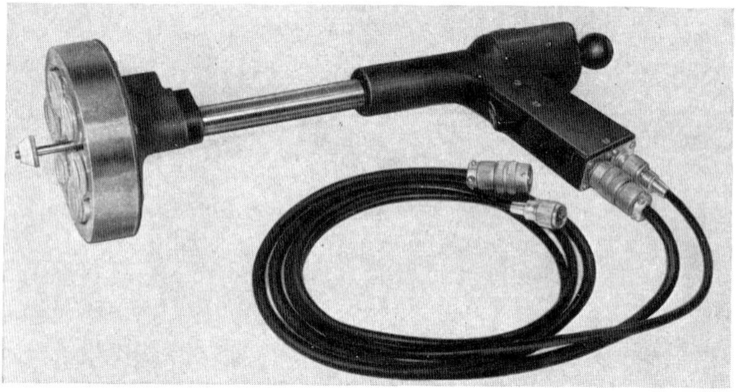

b

Fig. 3.85 Sperry axle car, a) automotive vehicle during testing, b) special probe used.

in the core which would make oblique testing impossible. Only then can the oblique test be made. The whole test lasts approximately one minute. The test result is kept on display clearly visible by means of red and green lamps until the next wheel set is rolled in.

If axles of railway coaches are to be tested on which the roller bearings on the bearing stubs are usually not removed because the risk of a crack developing there is small, the two outside probes can be raised.

In general the shrunk-on wheel body does not affect the result of any tests on axles, this being one of the great advantages of ultrasonic testing. It should, how-

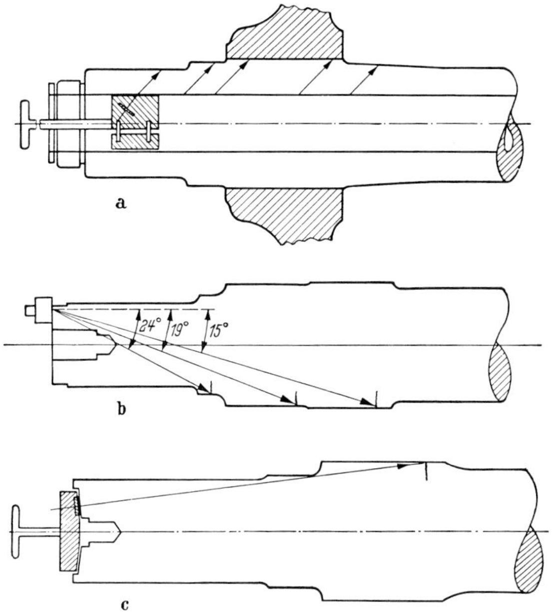

Fig. 3.86 Axle tests with special probes. a) Hollow axle for German electric locomotive, internal angle probe; b) axle for American Diesel locomotive, probes for longitudinal waves at 15, 19 and 24° according to Sperry; c) axle with external bearing (schematic) and conically machined front face using matched normal probe (Swiss Federal Railways).

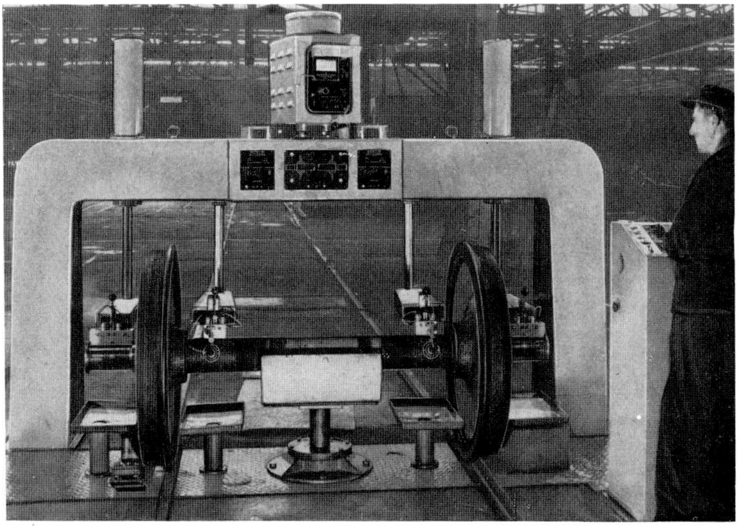

Fig. 3.87 Automated test bench of the German Federal Railways for wheel sets.

ever, not be overlooked that the wheel body is partially transmissive to sound entering through the seat. Therefore echoes are sometimes obtained from the wheel body with both wave modes, reflected at its boundaries or also from flaws in the steel casting. In doubtful cases a higher frequency (4 to 5 MHz instead of the usual 2 MHz) can be used for which the shrink fit and the steel casting are less transmissive, resulting in interference echoes becoming less distinct than true echoes. The possibility can also not be excluded that weak echoes may be produced by irregularities of the shrink fit. However, a trained examiner usually can distinguish them reliably from echoes of incipient cracks, provided they are not too small (exceeding 2 mm).

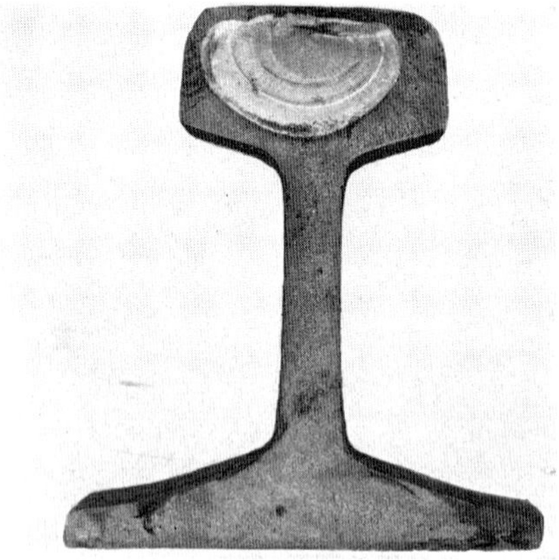

Fig. 3.88 Shatter crack (transverse crack in rail head).

3.232 Rails

Manufacturing defects in rails usually consist of rolled-out shrinkages, especially in the transition zone from the head to the web, and of impurities consisting in elongated, non-metallic inclusions. So-called cold cracks in the head of the rail are also encountered. Usually they are not orientated like the transverse crack in Fig. 3.88, but in the longitudinal direction of the rail. This, however, depends on the rolling method. Using normal and oblique irradiation from the tread of the rail, as is customary for operation defects, such longitudinal flaws would produce no reliable indication. Therefore, when testing new rails, the sound is in addition also transmitted from one side of the rail head; this can be combined with the above-mentioned test from the tread using a rail testing bench similarly to Fig. 3.89. One difficulty arises from the fact that cold cracks sometimes form only a few days after cooling. A test made in the production cycle after straightening, where its application would be most convenient after the rail has passed through the roller bed, would thus be unreliable. Experiences covering periods of some length are not yet available.

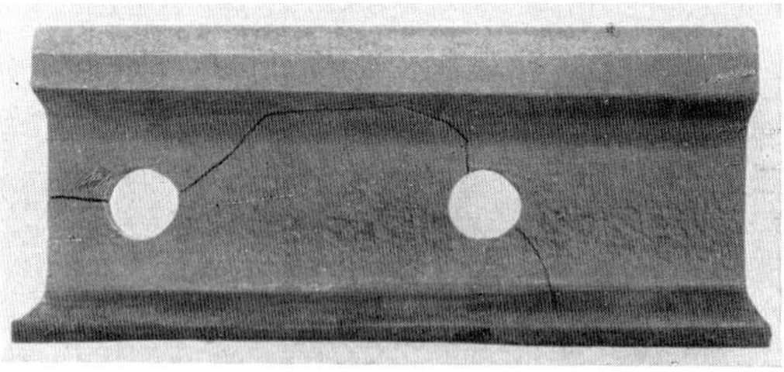

Fig. 3.89 Cracks at fish-plate bolt-holes.

On rails while in use, transverse cracks and inclusions, even elongated ones, lead to so-called shatter cracks in the rail head (Fig. 3.88) which are particularly dangerous because they frequently occur in rails at short intervals, so that pieces of rail can break out. Similar transverse cracks start at wheel burns where wheels skid during starting, e.g. in front of signals, leading to thermal cracking as a result of overheating. True operation cracks are the incipient cracks at bolt holes of fish-plates, i.e. fatigue cracks produced by the impact stress of the fish-joint. These may likewise cause a piece of the rail to break out, resulting in serious accidents. Depending on the shape and the material of the rail, the flaws encountered in various railway systems can differ greatly regarding position and frequency, for which the testing method should make allowance. In England, shatter cracks are rarer because the rails used are less hard. In the USA, transverse cracks from the edges of the head are also observed in addition to shatter cracks starting in the centre of the rail head; this is not observed in Germany.

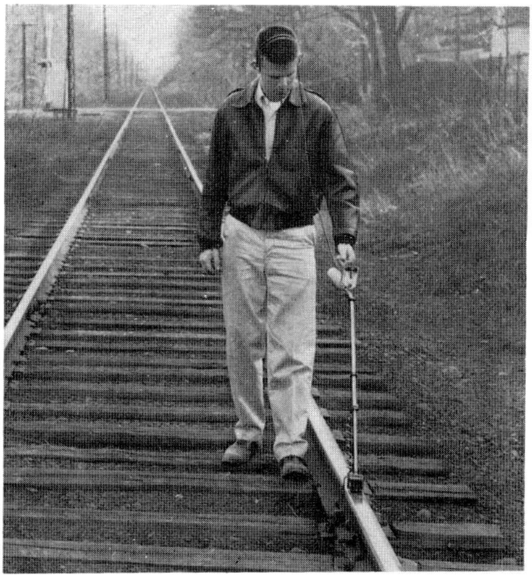

Fig. 3.90 Audigage Rail Flaw Detector in use (Branson Instruments) transistorised design. The electronic unit and the batteries are housed in the handle.

Rapid and relatively inexpensive testing for larger defects is possible with the frequency modulation instruments described in 2.372, in the literature often wrongly called resonance instruments. Fig. 3.90 shows an instrument in use. Every change of the sound in the head phone is caused by an anomaly in the rail, which in addition to genuine flaws, may also be the result of reduced reflection due to corrosion at the bot-

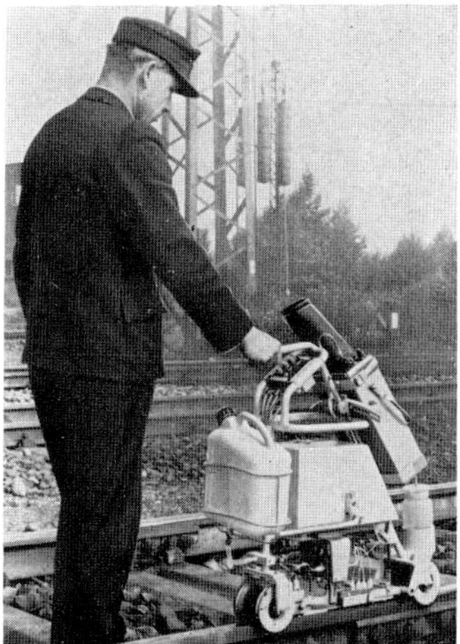

Fig. 3.91 Rail testing instrument in use at the German Federal Railways (Federal Railways, Central Office, Minden).

tom, attenuation caused by inclusions which by themselves may not yet be serious, and so forth. An experienced examiner can correctly diagnose larger defects and detect incipient cracks exceeding approximately 1 cm in length at fish-plate bolt holes. Incipient cracks in the foot of the rail, if they do not reach the web, cannot be detected with any of the ultrasonic testing methods used in practice, but they are usually spotted by visual inspection.

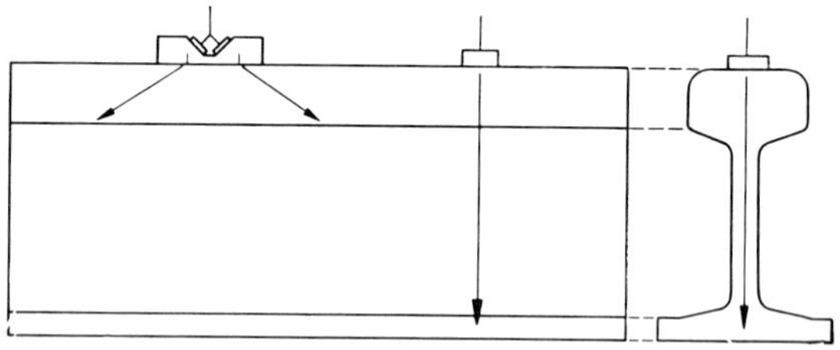

Fig. 3.92 Probe arrangement for testing rails with the rail tester of the German Federal Railways.

Here the pulse echo method has given the best results. Fig. 3.91 shows a rail testing instrument designed specifically for this purpose. It contains a battery-operated miniaturized pulse-echo instrument – usually with a built-in monitor –, connected to a vertical-beaming 4 MHz TR probe and a 2 MHz twin angle probe (likewise designed as TR probe). A flow of water, supplied from a small tank which forms part of the test equipment, is used for coupling. As shown in Fig. 3.92, the rail is scanned from the tread. The vertical-beaming probe detects incipient cracks at fish-plate bolt holes, laminations in the head of the rail and cracks in the web. Transverse defects are indicated by the twin angle probe as travelling echoes. A beaming angle of 75° was chosen because the transverse defects to be detected – mostly shatter cracks – usually are inclined at angles of 10 to 20°. The two beams of the twin angle probe pointing in opposite directions ensure that these flaws are detected reliably in both possible directions of inclination.

Fig. 3.93 explains the screen picture obtained with some typical rail defects. The viewing screen shows the simultaneous echoes of the three probes. Characteristic for all defects of appreciable size with one component in the longitudinal direction is the absence of the bottom echo.

If a miniaturized instrument with monitor is used, the gate is set for the zone between the entrance point of the beam of the perpendicular radiator (rail surface) and the bottom echo from the foot of the rail. In this way the transverse defects detected by the twin angle probe, as well as any laminations in the rail head, fish-plate bolt holes and incipient cracks starting from such holes and detected by the perpendicular radiator, are indicated acoustically. The signal produced by a sound fish-plate bolt hole draws the attention of the examiner to the viewing screen where, by observing the echo trace, he will in due course recognize any incipient cracks starting from fish-plate bolt holes. The testing speed therefore should be appropriately reduced when passing over a fish-joint.

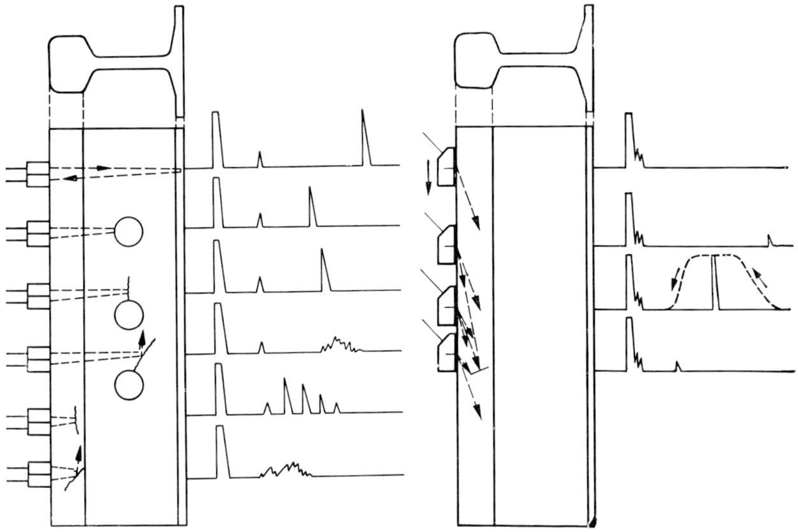

Fig. 3.93 Indications of various rail defects by perpendicular and oblique beaming.

At the German Federal Railways a *single* examiner operates the instrument. He requires, however, two look-outs if the test is carried out while there is normal traffic on the track concerned. Apart from operating the instrument, the examiner is also required to make reports. All defects found are classified according to size and position in two groups, of which the flaws belonging to the first group require immediate elimination because they constitute a pressing danger. The testing efficiency is on the average 6 km track per day when checking both rails; it depends, however, very much on the traffic density and the frequency of defects.

Based on the experiences gained with such portable rail-testing instruments, the Federal German Railways have designed an ultrasonic rail-testing car powered by its own Diesel unit (Fig. 3.94) [247, 383, 78] and installed in the body of a standard rail bus. The car in front contains the testing equipment while that at the back serves as a living-room for the personnel. The probes are mounted in a test rack installed under the car (Fig. 3.95); they can be raised hydraulically, separately or together with the entire rack. In addition to the probes according to Fig. 3.92, a pair of 35° radiators according to Fig. 3.96 was mounted and likewise connected in parallel. Each of them receives the pulse of the other after a bottom reflection, and in addition also the echoes from fish-plate bolt holes, obliquely orientated incipient cracks at fish-plate bolt holes, and transverse cracks in the foot provided the latter extend to a point under the web. This naturally furnishes considerably more information.

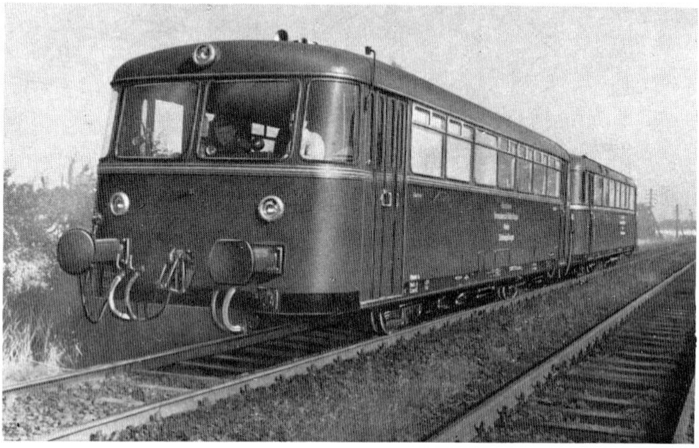

Fig. 3.94 Ultrasonic rail-testing car of the German Federal Railways (Federal Railways Central Office Minden).

The indications are displayed on 6 pulse-echo instruments each one of which is assigned to one of the normal, the 70° and the 35° angle probes on both rails respectively. Using the method described in 2.353 and pre-

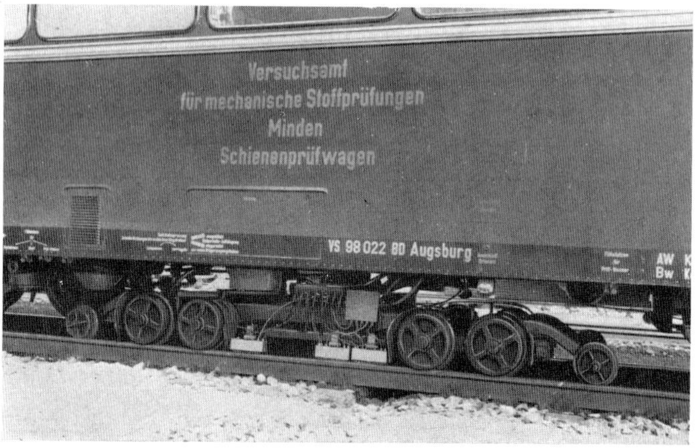

Fig. 3.95 Probes mounted on rail-testing car (Federal Railways Central Office Minden).

sented in Figs. 2.67 and 2.68, the results are recorded photographically on 35 mm strip film (Fig. 3.97). The chart feed is coupled to the velocity of the car in the ration 1 : 100. Since the position of the flaw is not marked on the rail, provision is made by means of accurate metre marks and simultaneously recorded kilometre marks, for the position of the flaw to be found afterwards when evaluating the strip. For this purpose, an additional echo sounding instrument with airborne sound has been installed whose sound beam is directed against the sleepers and possibly also against the foot of the rails. Thus the sleepers can be counted by the simultaneously recorded indications of the airborne sound beam which also shows any changes of the foot of the rails, e.g. weld beads, as well as lost nuts of the rail ties.

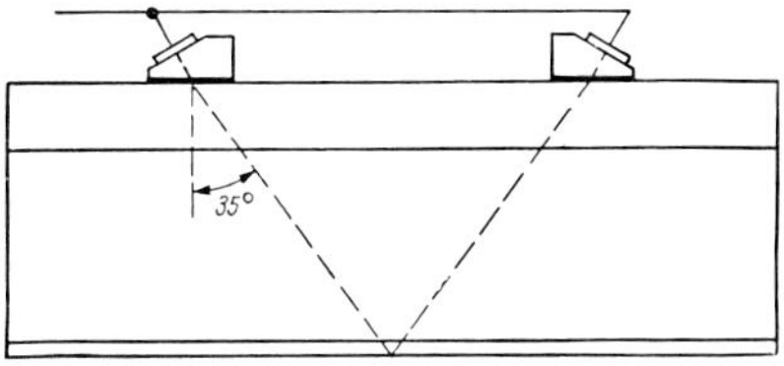

Fig. 3.96 Pair of 35° angle probes mounted on rail-testing car, in addition to the probe assembly according to Fig. 3.92.

In order to obtain a sufficiently dense pulse sequence along the rail, the repetition frequency has been stepped up to several thousand cycles per second, all instruments being synchronized accordingly. At a testing speed of 15 m/s (corresponding to approx. 55 km/h) this furnishes a pulse spacing of about 5 mm, which is still acceptable. The usual testing

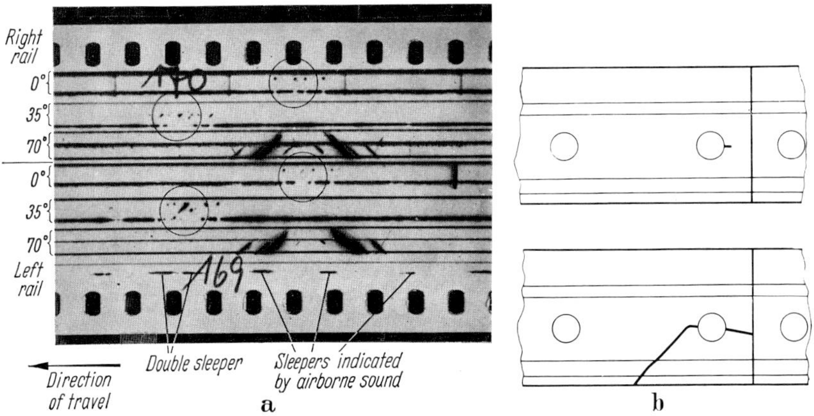

Fig. 3.97 Recording diagram (a) of rail-testing car at two defective fish-joints, showing reconstruction (b) of incipient cracks based on recording. The evaluated points of the normal (0°) and the 35° radiators are marked by circles (German Federal Railways Central Office Minden).

speed of approximately 20 to 30 km/h furnishes slightly better recordings, but maximally 70 km/h have already been reached.

At such high speeds plastic contact shoes have again proved successful; these are replaced every few hundred kilometres. The consumption of water for the average daily testing distance of 100 km is a few thousand litres which are carried along in the car.

Old rails, which are overhauled in the workshops and welded together to full lengths for re-use, are preferably first subjected to automatic testing by ultrasonics. Stationary rail testing benches (see Fig. 3.98) were designed specifically for this purpose and large numbers of them

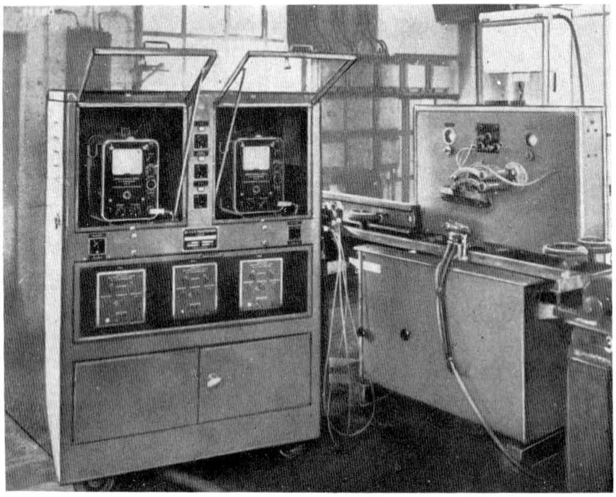

Fig, 3.98 Stationary rail testing bench at a rail depot of the German Federal Railways.

have been in use for several years. Basically, the same method is applied as for testing rails on the track, with the simplification, however, that the fish-joints are disregarded because they are invariably cut off.

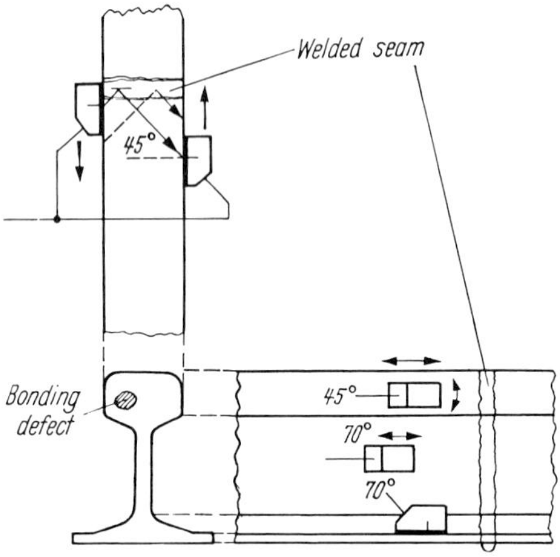

Fig. 3.99 Testing welded seams of rails.

The test procedure is as follows: the rail is transported on a roller bed through the test bench in an upright position. Frequently the test bench follows immediately after the planing machine in which the tread of the old rails is machined. The approaching rail actuates a contact roller which controls the positioning motion of the probe assembly – consisting of two angle probes beaming at 75° in opposite directions, and a normal probe. Any defects in the rail head or the web actuate a position-true colour marking device directed against the web by means of auxiliary monitors. When the end of the rail is reached the probe assembly is lifted off automatically and returned to its initial position. The testing speed is usually 0.8 m/s, maximally approx. 1 m/s has been reached.

Welding in the workshop involves cutting and butt welding. On the track also oxacetylene welding is used. In both cases it is desirable to check the welded seam. Since automatic welding machines in the workshop, once adjusted, produce reliable and flawless welds, ultrasonic tests on a number of welds are made only as an initial check of the adjustment. Fig. 3.99 shows the method introduced successfully at the German Federal Railways. Since the most dangerous defects when cutting and butt welding are clear separations normal to the longitudinal axis, which cannot be detected reliably with the angle probes used in the above technique and even then only in the middle zone of the head, web and foot, two parallel-connected 45° angle probes for 2 MHz applied to both lateral faces of the rail head are used. An ordinary 70° angle probe as used in normal testing of welded seams, is sufficient for the web and foot. As a consequence of the wedge-shaped profile of the foot, it is necessary to place the probe first on the edge in a longitudinal direction and then on the inclined section, obliquely in the middle zone. In all instances it is necessary to shift the probes back and forth over the seam and at the same time to swing them through a small arc.

Finally, the *points* of the tracks can have defects which can also be detected by ultrasonics. At the German Federal Railways the point locks are checked for fatigue cracks. The points themselves cannot be tested because they are made of hard manganese steel whose coarse cast structure is not penetrable by ultrasonics.

3.233 Miscellaneous Railway Material

In addition to the routine tests on shafts and rails as discussed above and applied also by foreign railways, in Germany *porcelain insulators* for the contact wires and *spring-clamping bolts* for coaches are regularly tested according to a specification by ultrasonics. In view of the similarity of the problems encountered in the case of these components, the reader is referred to 3.41 and 3.22 (bolts). *Wheel bodies* for trucks are sometimes checked for fatigue cracks according to Fig. 3.100 (a). Since the rough surface of these steel castings cannot be smoothed, only larger incipient cracks of say 10 mm depth can be found reliably; penetrating cracks, however, can be found without difficulty. 60° angle probes and 2 MHz are used after the surface has been cleaned with a steel brush and a viscous oil or paste applied.

In some organization in the USA when truck wheels cast in one piece with the tyre are overhauled, the tyres are also tested for fatigue cracks [see Fig. 3.100 (*b*)].

Other railway organizations occasionally also check the *forged tyres* for locomotives for manufacturing defects and fatigue cracks.

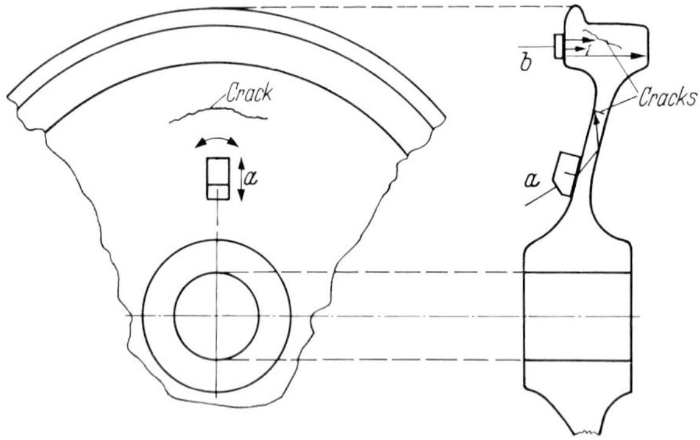

Fig. 3.100 Fatigue crack test on truck of cast steel, *a* in wheel disc, *b* in tyre.

Elongated inclusions in the circumferential direction can lead to transverse cracks, like similar defects in rail heads, causing pieces to break out. IRSID has designed a testing device for this purpose using the immersion technique, as shown in Fig. 3.101 [35]. Sound of 2 MHz frequency is beamed into a lateral face. Flaw echoes exceeding a certain minimum height are counted by means of monitor and register, a photoelectric scanner ensuring that the counter is switched on only if the wheel turns. The number of defects provides a sufficiently reliable measure of the quality. In addition, a normal or oblique beam applied to the tread of the wheel can be used for detecting operation defects.

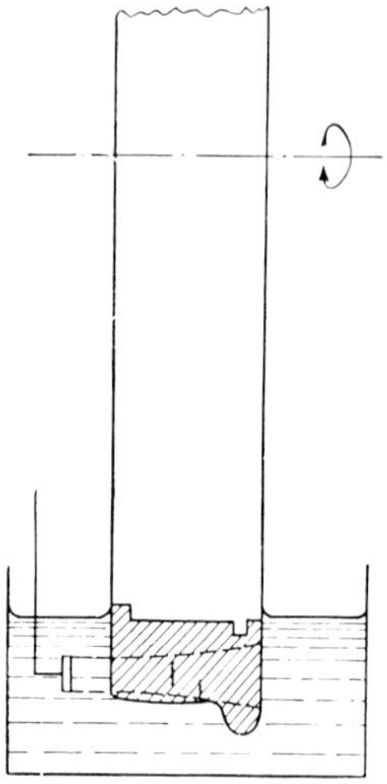

Fig. 3.101 Principle of testing tyres by the immersion technique according to IRSID.

Shrink-fit tests (cf. 3.29) on wheel tyres have so far shown little promise because the tread surface used for beaming into the shrink fit is not uniformly smooth, and especially because it is not parallel to the shrink fit. A further difficulty arises from the absence of a backwall echo for reference purposes. This would make it necessary to use an adjustable probe for the immersion technique and to take care that water cannot enter an open shrink fit.

Other occasional tests used in railway engineering present no special problems and they are therefore discussed in the Sections concerned, viz. *plate* tests for railway bridges and fire boxes (3.241), testing *welded seams* on railway bridges (3.281), tests of *bearing boxes* (3.29) and determination of *wall thickness and corrosion* on fire boxes (3.61).

3.24 Plates

When plates are tested ultrasonically this rarely concerns fatigue cracks. These testing problems will therefore first briefly be discussed. Where operation defects are not the result of manufacturing defects, they always occur as incipient cracks normal to the surface. This applies for instance to corrosion fatigue cracks in the case of caustic embrittlement, cracks at rivet holes, or fatigue cracks in flanges, rims, etc. If the direction of propagation of the cracks is known approximately, they can be easily found by means of zig-zag transverse waves, and if the surface is good, also by means of surface waves. Regarding cracks at rivet holes, see also 3.29, and regarding corrosion and thickness determination on plates, see 3.61.

The testing of plate for manufacturing defects is very diversified, which is not surprising in view of the many different uses made of plate in industry, and the resultant varying significance of a given plate defect, the wide range in plate thickness from 1 mm to more than 100 mm, and the diversity of the defects according to their nature, shape, position and size. Consequently in this field all the known ultrasonic testing methods find application to a greater extent than in almost any other situation. Classification into medium and heavy plate for thicknesses above 2 to 3 mm and sheet for thicknesses less than this seems practical in view of the different problems involved, the demarcation is, however, fluid.

3.241 Medium and Heavy Plate

If at any stage during the production cycle the slab, as the preliminary to the manufacture of plate, is available in the cold state, it can be tested in order that in this way any serious plate defects may already be eliminated. This test, however, is controversial because on the one hand flaws in the slab, such as enclosed small shrinkages, can be forged together during rolling, and because on the other hand, segregations which in the slab are still closed may be opened up during rolling [356]. Furthermore, new defects may be introduced on plate in the form of laminations at the top and sides, so that testing of the finished plate cannot be circumvented. Slabs are therefore first tested for continuous primary piping, and subsequently preferably on a statistical basis by means of which pieces with excessive indications are eliminated.

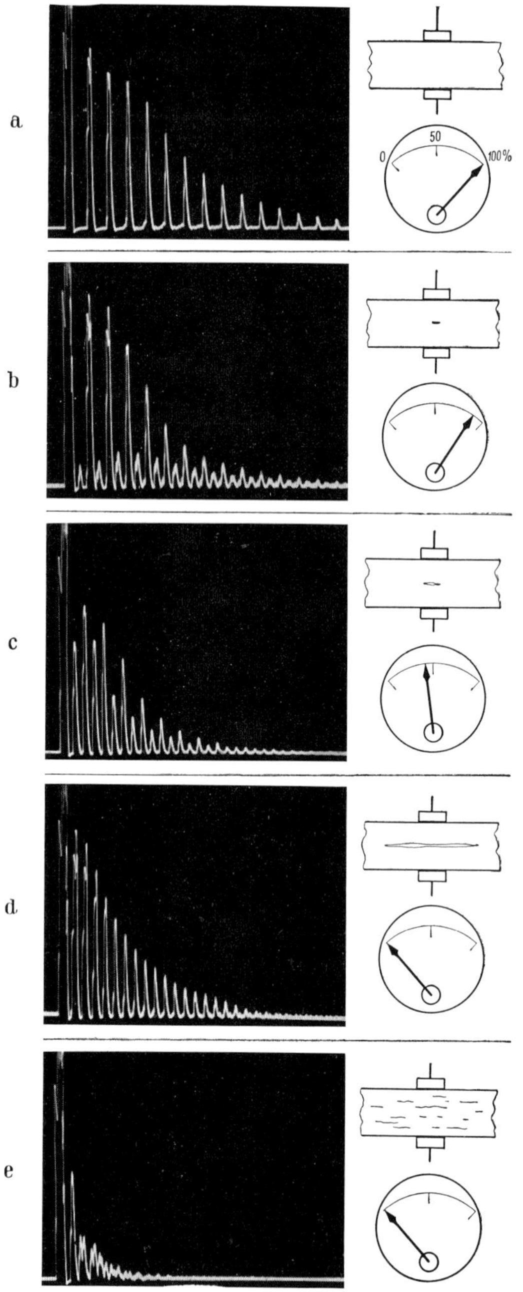

Fig. 3.102 Plate test using the pulse echo method and intensity method with straight sound transmission, showing various defects in 15 mm plate.

The surface is cleaned by flame-scarfing or roughing and then scanned at various points by means of normal probes of 2 MHz, using a liberal application of oil, water or paste. In the case of automatically flame-scarfed surfaces, the quality is sufficiently good for continuous scanning with water-gap coupling according to Fig. 3.10. A continuous slab testing installation has been described by Silber [335].

Coarse and medium plate may contain defects showing all transitional stages, from the curtain-like finely distributed inclusion layer which is partially permeable to ultrasound, to compact inclusions foliated singly in a layer or in several layers, to gaping laminations with no mechanical cohesion. Since they originate from piping, true laminations usually are located at half-plate thickness. Their extension in the plane of the plate largely depends on the rolling process. A slab rolled not excessively in both directions furnishes heavy plate in which top and secondary piping extend funnel-like and ribbon-like through the middle zone, whereas other defects show no preferential direction of extension. The extreme case on the other hand consists of strips which may contain flaws extending for several metres in the rolling direction; these may, however, be only a few millimetres wide. The testing method should make allowance for this.

For a plate thicker than approximately 10 mm, whose multiple echoes in the pulse-echo method are therefore so widely separated that flaw echoes can still be observed between them, Fig. 3.102 shows screen pictures obtained with the pulse-echo method and the intensity method by straight sound transmission. Contact testing with a probe of approx. 4 to 5 MHz has been chosen, whose near-field length considerably exceeds the plate thickness.

The flawless plate furnishes a long echo sequence and an intensity which is adjusted to 100% (a). A flaw (b) with an area considerably smaller than the area of the radiator produces small intermediate echoes, while the intensity drops slightly. Because of the unavoidable coupling fluctuations, this drop in intensity cannot be regarded as a reliable indication of a flaw. For both methods, the indication becomes more distinct if a smaller probe is chosen, but only as long as its near-field length does not become small compared with the plate thickness. A flaw (c) whose area is not much smaller than the area of the radiator produces echoes which are comparable with the still visible backwall echo, while the intensity drops markedly. A pronounced lamination (d) produces an echo corresponding to that of a plate of half the thickness, because the lamination usually is in the centre. In the case of a gaping, i.e. air-filled lamination, the echo sequence may again be very long. Usually, however, the flaw obliterates a portion of the echo sequence, especially if the flaw is filled with slag. In this case only a short echo sequence of half the plate thickness is obtained. In the case of straight sound transmission, zero intensity clearly indicates a separation. In the case of a multilaminary defect (e) the various flaw echoes interfere with each other. In addition, the sound is then usually attenuated considerably. With straight sound transmission the indication here also is zero.

If in the case of the pulse-echo method the flaw indication is not observed but only the disappearance of the long and regular echo sequence of the flawless plate, the lower testing limit for this method is reached at a plate thickness of approximately 2 mm for frequencies around 5 MHz (i.e. double plate thickness equals approximately 3 wave lengths). There is no upper testing limit. On the other hand, the straight sound transmission method has no lower limit; practically, however, an upper one which depends on the smallest flaw size to be detected.

In addition to the two methods mentioned, it is basically also possible to test by means of zig-zag transverse waves according to Fig. 3.103. It was found that particularly favourable results can be obtained if the frequency and the beaming angle in relation to the plate thickness are chosen in such a way that the cross-section of the plate is completely filled by the sound waves reflected back and forth (so that they form a plate wave). This method was tried out first with frequencies above 1 MHz for sheet, and has produced satisfactory results also for plate above 10 mm, using 0.5 to 1 MHz. On sound plate one still obtains a

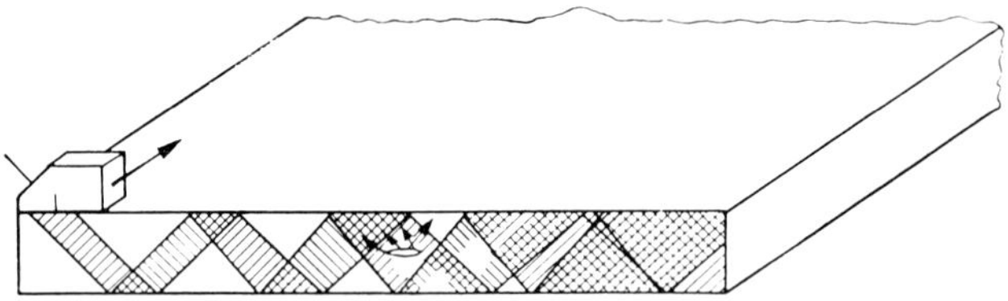

Fig. 3.103 Testing plate with zig-zag transverse waves.

distinct edge echo over a width of 4 m. Adjustable angle probes are used for this purpose, the angle being determined empirically for optimal indication of the edge. Since the three methods respond differently to the various types of defects, they have proved to be more or less successful also in practice for testing plate according to different requirements. The pulse-echo method furnishes the most complete information, but only if the plate is scanned completely point by point, which, owing to the time required, can be considered only in exceptional cases, automation moreover being possible to only a limited extent. The intensity sound transmission method is reliable in the case of complete laminations (cases d and e, Fig. 3.102), but less so at points with clusters of inclusions (cases b and c), particularly where this concerns many small inclusions occurring predominantly in the centre plane. These, however, can be detected readily by plate waves using the echo method; the viewing screen then shows a "beard" of stray echoes whose position and width correspond fairly accurately to the flawed area. Provided the affected zones are not too wide, and the inclusions not too coarse, the wave is still strong enough even behind this zone to indicate other flaws and also the edge so that a display of the tested strip is obtained on the viewing screen. In the case of complete laminations, particularly smooth laminations in an otherwise sound plate, the indication is limited mainly to the point of incidence at the edge of the flaw. Its width is then no longer recognizable and the end echo disappears. The attenuation of the wave can be partially compensated electronically by a variable gain of the instrument which increases with distance.

In the case of testing in plate mills which, up to the present, has mostly been done by hand, the evaluation is statistical, i.e. the plates are tested along strips or according to a grid. For a plate of 4×10 m containing few defects, and a strip distance of 200 mm, the testing time is, for example, 20 min, i.e. 1/2 min per square metre. If a larger lamination is encountered, its contour is traced and recorded in a report form. Otherwise merely a code number is entered for the echo height relative to the bottom echo along the scanned strip, e.g. 1 for small readings, 2 and 3 for readings of the order of the bottom echo, or greater. The theoretically possible case that a greater lamination would just fall into a mesh of the testing grid while the rest of the plate would be sound, is practically impossible: a flaw never occurs alone, and tests using grids of different density and different orientation have nevertheless led to practically the same overall evaluation of a given plate.

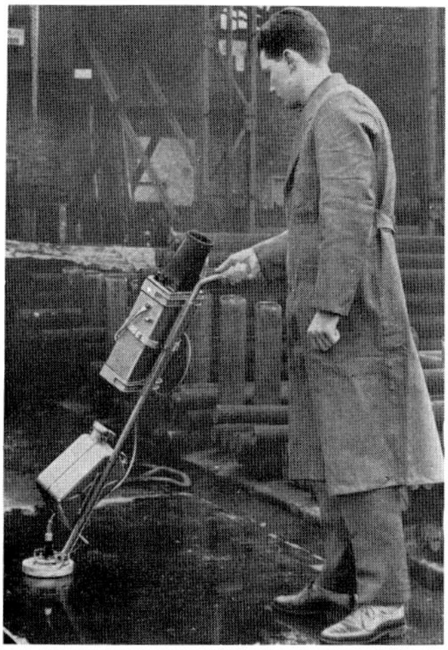

Fig. 3.104 Testing heavy plate with the plate tester and battery-operated miniaturised ultrasonic flaw detector (design Krautkrämer).

This method of testing is suitable only for plate, whose utilization does not require closer examination at certain points. If for instance boiler plate is required, the user will find it desirable to have such points tested accurately where for instance tubes are to be welded in, specifying the maximally permissible flaws. A similar procedure is adopted for instance by the German Federal Railways for the acceptance of gusset plates for railway bridges on which cross-pieces are welded on edgewise. At such points, because of the welding and the transverse stresses produced by the cross-piece, a given flaw is far more serious than on an unencumbered plate. The test specification should make allowance for these requirements. Quite generally, the edge zones should be checked more critically if the plate is to be welded without being trimmed.

As far as the wear and tear of probes when testing by hand is concerned, this can represent a considerable expenditure; in this respect best results have been obtained with coupling by means of a water gap and a plate tester according to Fig. 3.10. Guiding such an instrument along straight tracks and simultaneously observing the viewing screen which frequently may be several metres away, is very tiresome for the examiner. This can be remedied in two ways. Either a miniaturized instrument is mounted directly on the shaft of the plate tester (Fig. 3.104) in such a way that the examiner directly faces the viewing screen, or the flaws are indicated by means of monitor and signal, while the instrument is installed separately. In the case of plate thicker than 20 mm, the alarm can be triggered directly by the intermediate echoes of a normal probe; in other cases a TR probe in the plate tester can be used, flaw echoes being indicated automatically also in plate as thin as 5 mm.

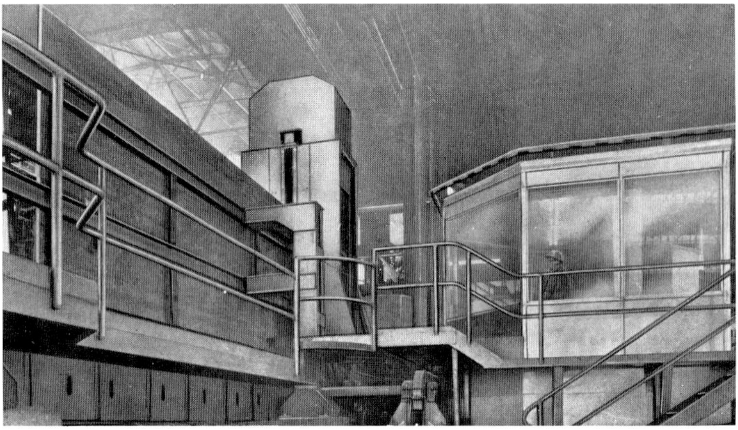

Fig. 3.105 Testing installation for heavy plate of the Hüttenwerke Oberhausen using ultrasonic instruments supplied by Lehfeldt. A plate is just leaving the testing installation in the towerlike structure (left), on the right is the cabin with the control and indicating instruments.

Automated testing installations not only save time but they also furnish permanent records. A testing installation for heavy plate [148] (Fig. 3.105) tests plates already cut which leave a steel shot descaling device in upright position, and which uses sound transmission with frequency-wobbled ultrasound of 2 to 3 MHz.

To prevent cross-interference from one pair of probes to the next, three different frequencies are used in turn. A multigraph of Messrs. Hellige is used for recording; this records straight lines if no flaws are present, and ribbons of constant amplitude at points with flaws (Fig. 3.106). Ten pairs of probes spaced 300 mm apart are used.

The probes operate with a water transit section and are pressed hydraulically from both sides against the entering plate. A hard metal ring at the contact point seals off the water space. Since it takes a certain time for the water space to be filled after the probes have been applied, the whole probe assembly first travels a certain distance together with the plate. By shifting the probe assembly up and down during scanning, it is also possible to test along zig-zag paths instead of straight tracks. At the relatively low plate speed of 3 m/min (limited by the descaling process) this mechanical shifting of the probes can still be realised satisfactorily.

Another coupling method – likewise for sound transmission – has recently found practical application. In this case the plate is tested on the production line during its normal transit through the roller bed. The ultrasonic waves radiated from the bottom by the transmitting probes are coupled to the plate through free water jets approximately 60 mm long, while the transmission from the plate to the receiving probes mounted on top is effected by means of accurately juxtaposed free water jets approximately 130 mm long [188]. This method of testing by means of a comb of free water jets prevents wear of the probes and largely avoids damaging the testing equipment by projecting spills and turned up ends

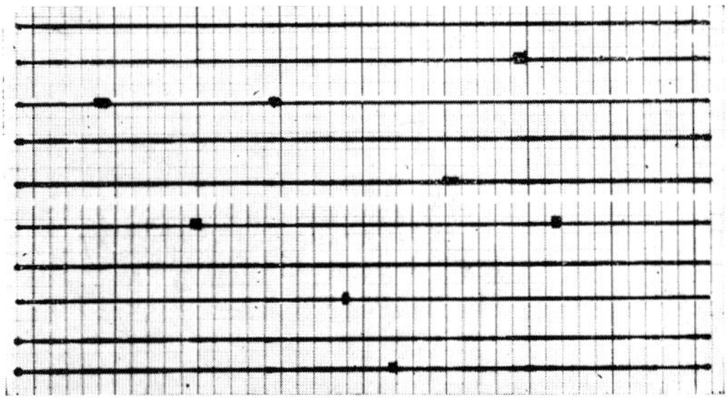

Fig. 3.106 Recording of a heavy plate with small defects, obtained in the installation of Fig. 3.105 (go/no-go recording with Hellige recorder on wax paper with heated stylus).

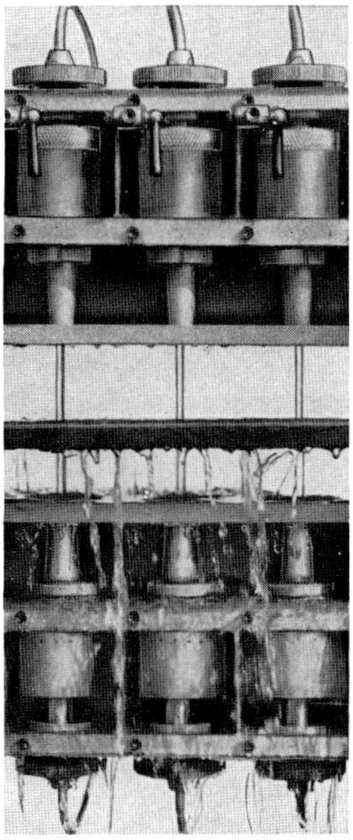

Fig. 3.107 Section of an installation for testing heavy plate, using free water jets (Krautkrämer).

of the plate. Although theoretically completely uncut plates can be tested in this way, in practice continuous tests are only carried out on precropped plates. Fig. 3.107 shows a section of an experimental installation which clearly indicates the testing principle. In order to prevent cross-interference from one test point to another with certainty, they are spaced 100 mm apart. Should in practice a greater density of testing lines (usually 50 mm) be required, the test points should be staggered in two rows.

The method of linear testing applied as "whole panel test" which has been described has of course a statistical character: with a water jet of approximately 8 mm diameter and the test points arranged in single rows spaced 100 mm, 8% of the total plate surface has been tested, and in the case of lines spaced 50 mm, 16%.

The large numbers of test points (generally 60 to 80 with the usual plate widths of 3 to 4 m) requires a special evaluating device for presentation of the test result. Fig. 3.108 shows the simplest method for data presentation: the "C-scan" of a plate, obtained by closely spaced testing graphs on a multigraph metallized paper recorder. Every line is assigned to a test point; the longitudinal direction of the recording is related to the longitudinal direction of the plate according to a given scale, usually 1 : 20.

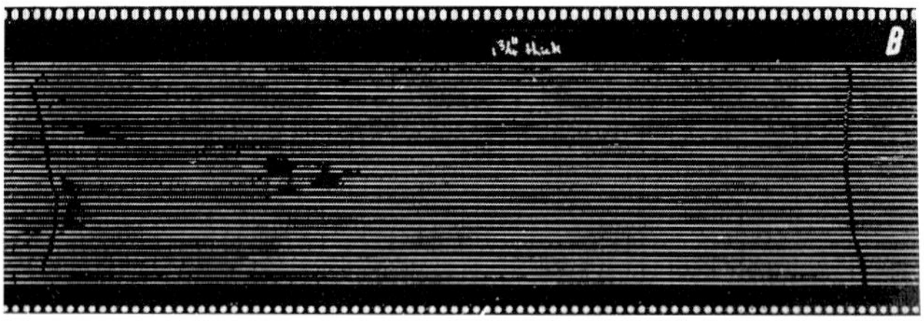

Fig. 3.108. Recording of a heavy plate with laminations, using the testing method shown in Fig. 3.107 (go/no-go recording on electric discharge chart paper).

In the reproduction of test data as C-scan on a uniform scale one obtains for plates with maximum length of approximately 30 m, lengths of recording strips of 1.5 m which must then be analysed in order to judge the quality of the plate and to decide how much must be cut off at the shears as waste. Since, according to the technical terms of delivery for plate tested ultrasonically, the flaws to be watched already start at sizes of 10 × 10 mm, – corresponding to a recording length of 0.5 mm – the presentation scale for the C-scan cannot be compressed still further in order to obtain a more general picture. Attempts were therefore made to obtain a more concise recording. Printed pictures which present the test result classified, using numbers or symbols, have therefore recently been proposed and are already partially in use.

As an example a so-called "graded C-scan" will be explained briefly: each testing track is divided longitudinally into 10 mm sections and every 10 of these sections are combined in one recording section. If a recording section contains at least one flaw, a number is printed at the corresponding point of the recording chart. This states the maximum number of faulty connected 10 mm sections in the 100 mm in question. It furnishes position-true number fields; the individual number characterizes the "gravity" of the flaw in the co-ordinated recording section.

A further step has been taken towards automating the testing of heavy plate by means of this multiple sound transmission installation: the decision as to how the cuts at the shears should be placed so that all important flaws are cut off, is made by an electronic computer. The latter is therefore fed with the entire test information. Naturally it makes its decision on the basis of a predetermined programme which enables it to print the co-ordinates for the cuts explicitly. A testing installation with this device is already in use in this field but details of its performance are not yet available.

The aim for the future goes still one step further: in a rolling mill where all data of interest during the entire production cycle are entered on punched cards, it is desirable to let the computer, which is given all the test information, also make the necessary decisions on alternatives. If the test discloses that a given plate is no longer suitable for its intended purpose, the computer should then select a new purpose on the basis of the orders on hand for which the remainder of the plate after being cut is still acceptable. Installations incorporating this high degree of automation have already reached the planning stage.

An interesting feature of coupling via free water jets is that by this method plate can be tested at temperatures up to approximately 250 °C. In preliminary tests on 35 mm plate it was found that adequate coupling could still be achieved up to almost 300 °C (cf. 3.113).

Compared with contact testing, a testing installation using free water jet coupling has the disadvantage of high water consumption (approx. 20 l/min per test point). Part of the coupling water can, however, be recycled provided the very dirty water is adequately filtered. Small particles of less than 0.2 mm diameter – provided not too much accumulates – do not interfere; it is therefore not necessary to use drinking water.

In all installations for continuous testing in the roller bed, the test is a purely statistical one as already mentioned above. In the case of particularly long, rolled out plate there is therefore an increasing danger that long and narrow laminations may still be overlooked between the testing tracks. In some instances therefore it will be necessary to carry out an additional test along the transverse edge at the top and bottom ends which later have to be welded. Similarly, the problem of track-accurate longitudinal tests along the edges of the plates, required e.g. for longitudinally or spirally welded pipeline pipes, cannot be solved satisfactorily by an installation for testing whole panels as described above, because the scanning of plates along rigidly specified tracks – particularly simultaneously along both edges – cannot be guaranteed during the transport through the roller bed of the testing installation. Special installations have been designed to solve this problem (see 3.242).

For plates where the absence of flaws along the edges is of particular interest, e.g. for the manufacture of large-diameter pipes from plates approximately 6 to 20 mm thick, a so-called "plate edge testing installation" has been constructed which works in combination with the lateral trimming shears. A group of 3 TR probes completely tests a track approximately 70 mm wide which borders on the edge to be cut. The sensitivity characteristic of these probes is such that flaws approximately 2 to 16 mm deep are indicated by approximately the same amplitude. The probes are coupled by flowing water. To be on the safe side a few millimetres of the testing track are located in the "scrap", i.e. in the portion cut off by the trimming shears immediately after the test. Such a combination of probes – automatically actuated and lowered and raised by the transported plate – is mounted on both sides and possibly also at the splitting shears. The problem of correct monitor gate adjustment for each plate, even if the plate gauges change, is solved in the following manner: during the interval in which the plate is straightened before it reaches the shears a holder with 3 additional probes is lowered; this produces for each of the 3 testing tracks a backwall echo at the correct distance. With the aid of these echoes the monitor gates are moved automatically into the correct position. This measurement is immediately followed by the test in front of the shears on the moving plate. Defects in the plate which are located in a given testing track actuate a paint-marking device which makes it easy to find the flaws on the trimmed plate. The usual testing speed is 0.5 to 0.8 m/s (= cutting speed at shears). This installation detects flaws of 10 mm diameter and larger. The entire testing process is automatic – except for the measuring process initiated by the roller bed operator pressing a pushbutton. In another design the correct position of the monitor gates is adjusted for each plate manually as required for the gauge concerned.

When comparing the results of the ultrasonic test obtained on heavy plate with other tests, including destructive ones, it should be mentioned that, as in the case of forgings, no agreement can be expected with a Baumann or a sulphur print because closed segregations are not indicated by ultrasound. Sometimes however a notch bend test also contradicts the ultrasonic test, the notch bend test tearing open smooth segregations which produced no flaw indications. On a plate with approximately 1% Mn it was found that the plate showed a pronounced banded structure and produced no echoes although the transverse strength was greatly reduced. Subsequent heat treatment revealed that this in fact was not a true lamination because now the result of the notch bend test was likewise negative. In this connection another observation made on a thick plate with 13% Mn is recalled. During a preliminary test while the plate was still hot (approx. 80 °C) only a few indications appeared, but considerably more showed up after cooling. These new flaws resulted from burst segregations, in contrast to true laminations which produced indications even while still hot.

The above-mentioned results are not directly applicable to the testing of *light metals*. First of all, light metal slabs can readily be tested even in the cast stage. The sometimes wrinkled surface is preferably removed by milling, as is customary before rolling out. However, since

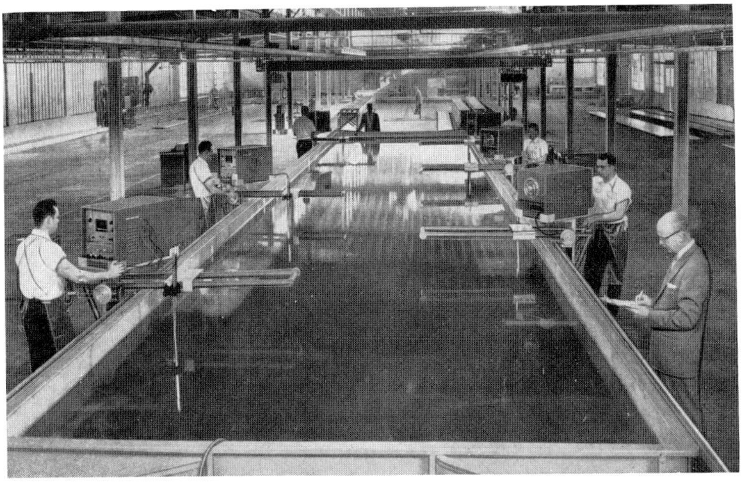

Fig. 3.109 Testing installation with 6 manually operated Immerscopes, using the immersion technique.

the demands made in respect of flawless finished products, such as thick plate, sheet bars and extruded sections required for airplane construction, are considerably higher than in the case of heavy steel plate, much more sensitive and more complete tests are required, specifically on the finished product of the rolling mill. Especially in the USA very impressive testing installations using the immersion technique have been constructed, of which Fig. 3.109 shows one for the simultaneous operation of 6 pulse-echo instruments with manual probe control. Fig. 3.110 shows a device with remote control of the probe which can be moved in 2 horizontal, 1 vertical and 2 angle co-ordinates. At the control panel the echo display can be observed and recorded on a B-scan instrument, a conventional pulse-echo instrument, and a recorder, while a twin monitor sounds an alarm when flaws are indicated. The probe can be moved by remote control in both horizontal co-ordinates automatically and by hand, at a max. speed of 450 mm/s. The tank, measuring up to 4 × 16 m, can handle, with the aid of hydraulic lifting devices, test specimens weighing up to 20 t.

The specimens are first scanned automatically at a rate of, e.g., 2 to 3 square metres per minute. For this purpose a broad-beam probe is used which scans a strip 120 mm wide, using a guiding device which keeps the probe constantly in a position normal to the surface even if the latter is undulated. If echoes of a selected minimum height appear, the location of the flaw is marked on the plate under water by means of a pneumatically operated lipstick. Subsequently, using a smaller probe,

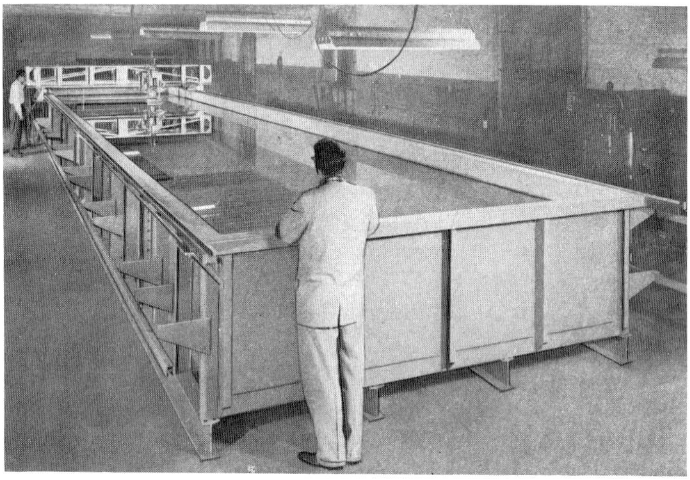

a

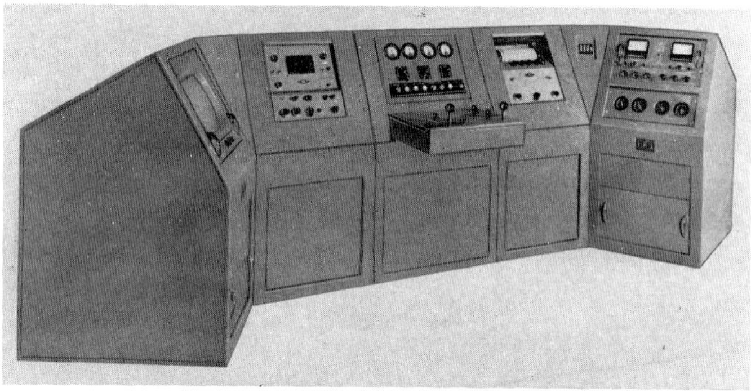

b

Fig. 3.110 Testing installation using the immersion technique (Curtiss & Wright) for automatic scanning and remote control. a) Tank with bridge supporting probes and motor-driven probe manipulator; b) control stand, from left to right: B-scan instrument, pulse echo instrument (Immerscope), remote probe control. Recording instrument for A, B and C-scan, twin monitor.

both the position and the size of the flaws are determined more accurately, making use of the echo height of test blocks with known flat-bottomed holes. A remote-controlled probe manipulator (Fig. 3.111) is used for this purpose; in this manipulator the crystal transducer can be tilted around two horizontal and the one vertical axis by means of one motor for each axis and in addition can be moved up and down. The position of the probe at any moment is remotely indicated at the control desk. This device therefore also permits measuring obliquely orientated flaws.

The test pieces concerned are high-quality light-metal products used in airplane construction which contain only few and small flaws. Consequently in spite of every single flaw being checked, the testing times are still acceptable.

An acceptance agreement exists on the permissible size of flaws (cf. 3.7).

3.242 Strip and Sheet

The testing problems and their solutions differ greatly according to the requirements. An example in which an incomplete test which covers only a few tracks in the longitudinal direction is sufficient, is the *edgetest of strip*. In the manufacture of pipes from sheet by automatic longitudinal or spiral welding, no laminations may occur in the edge, even if they penetrate only a few millimetres. Testing along the edge, however, is much more difficult than in the body of the sheet. If the strip, prior to welding, passes through trimming shears which prepare the edges and in addition cut off a narrow strip, it is recommended that a preliminary test on a slightly wider track in which the subsequent edge will be located is made (Fig. 3.112). In this case also TR probes are used for the test, as described in 3.241 for testing plate edges. In the case of strip the test conditions are more favourable because the length of the strip which is usually considerably greater, requires a re-adjustment of the installation to match other strip dimensions only at long intervals, so that this adjustment can easily be made by hand.

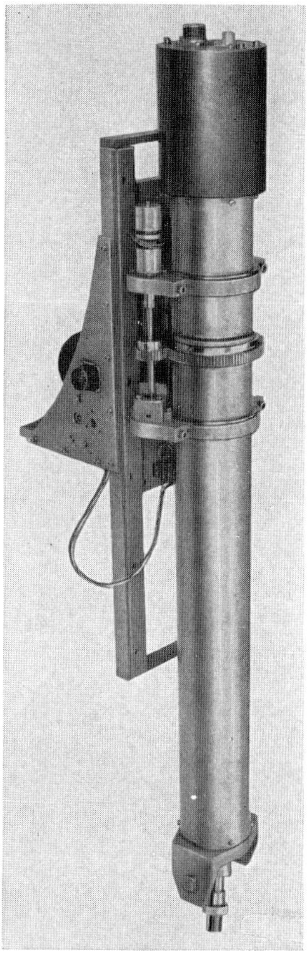

Fig. 3.111 Probe manipulator with remote control for immersion technique (Curtiss & Wright Corp.).

The TR probes mounted in sled-like holders are usually lowered on to the strip from the top and coupled by flowing water. Monitors announce the appearance of flaw echoes by means of signals. In this case there is no point in applying position-true colour markings to the top of the strip because flawed strip sections cannot be cut out in this continuous production process. Therefore the strip is usually marked from the bottom, preferably as permanently as possible (e.g. by grinding), so that the flaws can be found after bending and after welding on the outside of the finished pipes. Flaws at the edges of the strip usually cause a defective welded seam; this seam is therefore rechecked at the points marked on the strip whereupon it can be decided whether or not the affected pipe section should be cut out and rejected.

A previously used testing installation by means of which the strip was checked by the single-probe echo method and a water gap for coupling, furnished suitable echo pictures on the CR screen in the case of sheet down to 3 mm thickness, which could, however, be evaluated only by careful observation of the CR screen at low testing speeds. Efforts made to record the disappearance of the "multi-echo tail" by means of monitors at high continuous testing speeds, failed because of the brief coupling interruptions which were then still being encountered and which invariably simulated flaws. This method therefore proved to be unacceptable in practice.

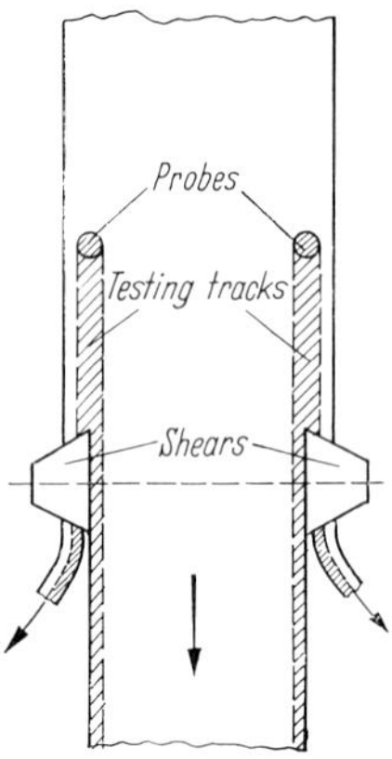

Fig. 3.112 Testing the edges of strip, diagram of probe positions.

In the case of sheet less than 5 mm thick – which is the lower limit when using TR probes – it is necessary to apply the sound transmission method and the immersion technique. Since, compared with heavy plate, the widths of the strips are relatively narrow – maximally approximately 1.6 m – and since frequently only the edges or certain tracks of the total strip width are tested, a pulse transit time method with sound transmission (Fig. 3.113) is used instead of pure intensity measurement with sound transmission and coupling by free water jets (cf. testing of heavy plate, 3.241). If the probes are staggered it becomes possible to display on the CR screen the sound transmission indications of several tracks next to each other, and to evaluate them automatically by means of several monitors. A so-called "double sound transmission" (Fig. 3.113d) in which the echo height of a reflector mounted under the sheet is used for intensity measurements, proves to be much more sensitive for locating small flaws than the simple sound transmission of Fig. 3.113c. It is advisable to incline the pair of probes and the probe-reflector assembly relative to the surface of the sheet in order to avoid broadening of the echoes due to multiple echoes returned from the sheet. Several testing tracks monitored on a CR screen by adjacent indications can be recorded separately in this way. The maximum number of tracks which can be checked simultaneously by a single instrument in the case of the "single sound transmission" is approximately 10, and in the case of the "double sound transmission" approximately 5 because of the more critical reflection conditions which in turn depend on the track density.

In practice the immersion technique described is applied by passing the strip through a "transit testing tank". This tank contains the probes and possibly also the reflector mounted in a frame which is inclined relative to the strip. The entrance and exit slots of the tank have suitable flexible seals so that the loss of water is reduced to a minimum and submersion of the probes ensured.

A complete test by means of closely spaced tracks using this method is, in the case of strip and sheet, still less economical than in the case of heavy plate. More favourable for this purpose is the *zig-zag* or *plate wave method* in which, according to Fig. 3.103, the entire plate can be covered merely by testing along one edge. Against this advantage must be counted the shortcoming that the flaw echo is then no longer correlated quantitatively with the size of the flaw, as when tested normal to the surface: it is possible to state accurately the distance of a given flaw on the basis of the echo, but it cannot be stated whether this concerns a 2 mm or a 20 mm wide lamination band or band of inclusions. The end echo or edge echo, however, is usually weakened more by a broader flaw. However, the same effect can also be produced by several smaller flaws located one behind the other in the sound beam.

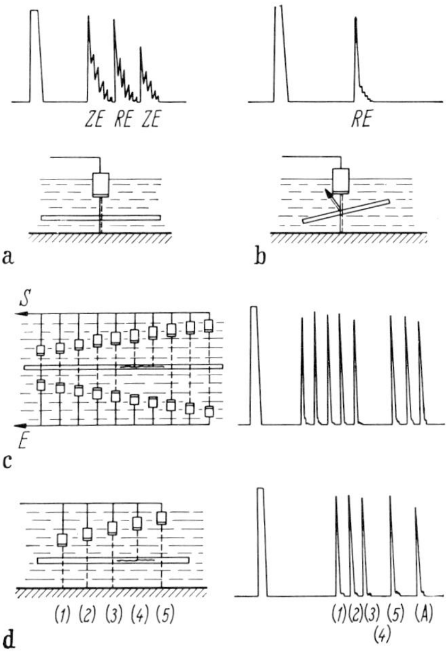

Fig. 3.113 Testing of strip and sheet by the pulse transit time method and sound transmission, using the immersion technique.
a) "Double sound transmission", sound beam normal to plate, intermediate echoes (*ZE*) and reflector echo (*RE*) broadened by multiple echoes; b) "double sound transmission" with inclined plate: the intermediate echoes which interfere in the case of a) and the broadening of the echo are avoided; c) "single sound transmission" with 10 parallel tracks, lamination indication with 2 tracks; d) "double sound transmission" with 5 parallel tracks, lamination indication on track (*4*). (*A*) = first repetition echo of reflector indication on track (*1*).

Basically, any beam entrance angles may be used. In the case of thinner plate, however, where the zig-zag reflections in the cross-section of the plate overlap increasingly (as in Fig. 3.103 towards the right), it is found that maximum testing ranges like those obtained with separate zig-zag reflections are obtainable only at definite beam entrance angles. One then speaks of plate waves. Fig. 3.114 shows the echo of a plate edge at different beam entrance angles. One should always expect that at sufficiently high gain several such wave modes may appear simultaneously. If their velocity exceeds that of the wave with the predominating amplitude, they might easily be mistaken for flaw echoes, which arrive before the edge echo. Two possibilities are given for the test: In the case of frequencies of 2 MHz and higher, plate waves can be damped by the fingertip test. Thus, if a doubtful echo can be damped in this way along its entire path right to the edge of the plate, this is merely the edge echo of an undesirable wave. In addition, in this case the distance of the echo from the end echo does not remain constant if the probe is shifted towards the edge, in contrast to a true flaw echo.

Since the speed of propagation of the plate waves is also a function of the frequency (cf. Table 9 in Appendix), the echoes of some of the plate waves are distinctly broadened and

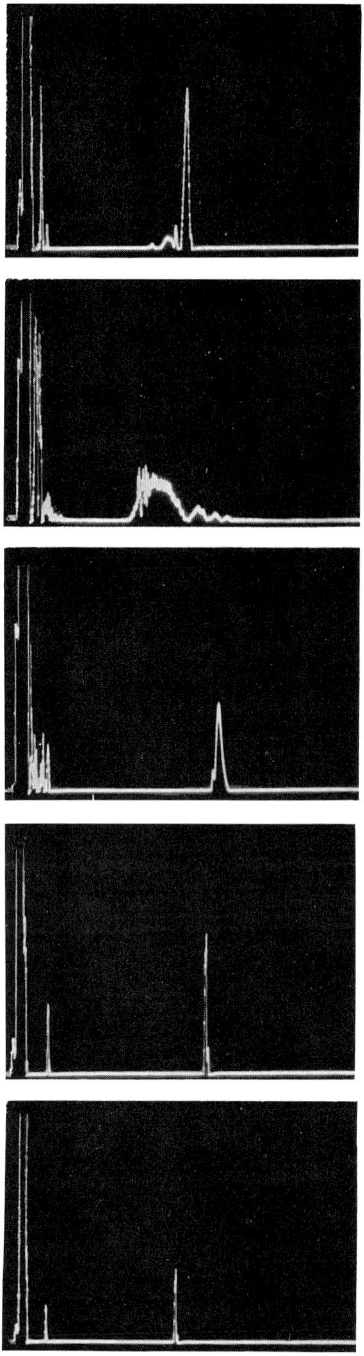

a b c d e

Fig. 3.114 Plate waves of 4 MHz in 1.1 mm thick steel sheet. Echoes of edge at different angles of transverse waves (cf. Table 9 in Appendix): a) $\alpha = 20°$ (types s_2); b) $\alpha = 34°$ (type s_1); c) $\alpha = 43°$ (type a_1); d) $\sin\alpha = 1.05$ (type s_0); e) $\sin\alpha = 1.1$ (type a_0). Compared with the diagram of Table 9, small deviations of the propagation speed caused by differences in texture may occur. The test parallel and transverse to the direction of rolling may therefore require slightly different angle adjustments.

bell-shaped, but not split (Fig. 3.115). This broadening depends on the sound path. The frequency-dependence also explains the phenomenon that the individual high-frequency oscillations of these echoes are not shifted simultaneously with the echo as a whole if the probe is shifted, but they merely wander over its peak.

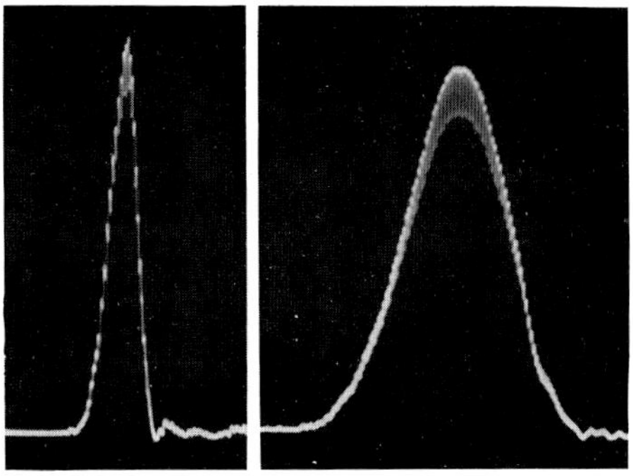

Fig. 3.115 Edge echo of a plate wave. a) After a path of 100 mm, b) after a path of 500 mm, on the same scale.

Fig. 3.116 illustrates the various plate wave testing methods. They are grouped according to the position of the sound beam relative to the direction of rolling, which atter is also the preferred

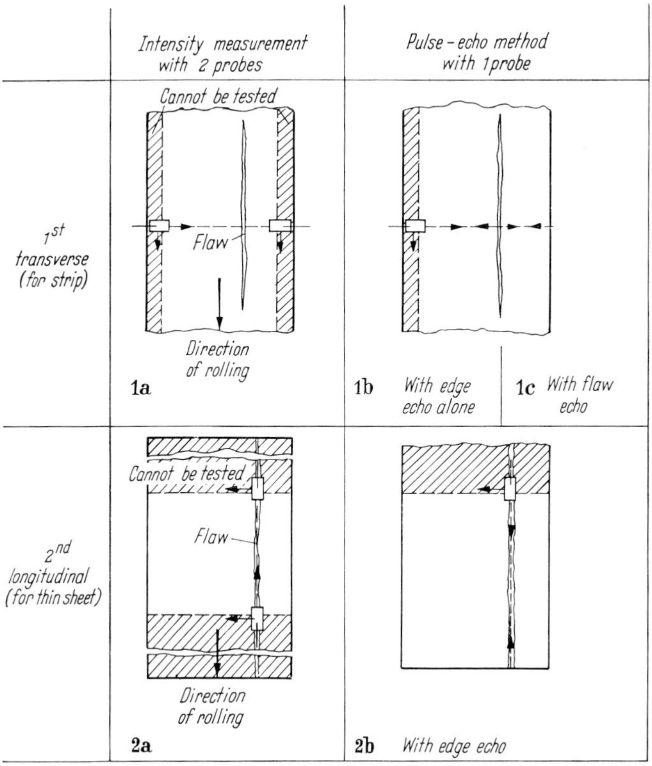

Fig. 3.116 Plate wave test of strip and sheet, schematic, top view, with flaws indicated.

direction of the extension of the flaws, i.e. the transverse and the longitudinal methods.

The *transverse test* is particularly suitable for automatic strip testing because the probes can then remain stationary while the strip travels past. In the case of methods 1a and 1b, both of which are basically identical intensity methods, a noticeable weakening can be expected only in the case of flaws several times larger than the thickness of the strip. Inclining the beaming direction of the sound relative to the rolling direction does not increase the sensitivity markedly in the case of narrow bands of flaws. On the other hand the echo method 1c is sensitive also for such flaws without, however, making it possible to relate the echo height quantitatively to the width of the flaw or similar quantities. Thus even the echo method functions more in the sense of a go/no-go indication.

If the detection of larger flaws is all that is required it will be advisable for a stationary automated testing installation, to choose method 1a with continuous sound transmission at unmodulated frequency because standing waves are hardly expected. The pulse method according to 1b, apart from the saving of one probe offers no advantages; on the contrary, it requires more expenditure, especially for recording. For sensitive testing this expenditure in the case of echo method 1c with alarm monitor, colour marking or recording must be accepted. It also permits the indications of flaw bands narrower than the thickness of the plate.

The *longitudinal tests* 2a and b can also detect such very narrow flaws provided they follow the direction of the sound beam, because they then disturb the propagation of the sound over the full length.

The disturbance caused by a flaw which is much narrower than the width of the sound beam can be explained in the same way as in Fig. 3.18. The change of the sound beam produced by artificial flaws (grooves) and bands of slag in sheet 0.75 to 2 mm thick has been investigated by KOPINECK and SOMMERKORN [189]. Beaming in the direction of the bands according to method 2a or 2b, they observed a definite splitting of the main maximum of the lobe of the sound into two lobes.

On a continuously moving strip method 2a would require a very rapid reciprocating motion in the transverse direction of the probes while 2b could not be used at all in the absence of a transverse edge. They are therefore mainly used for testing individual thin sheets. There the probe remains stationary and the sheet is moved transverse to the direction of rolling.

No satisfactory answer has yet been found regarding the optimal beaming angle to be used. In practice any angle which *serves the purpose* is tried. In longitudinal testing this also seems to be less critical than in transverse testing. It is then found that a given flaw may react very differently to different waves in respect of echo height and weakening of the waves which are let through [336]. Different types of flaws also react differently to a given wave, even if they have the same width, which is readily understandable if one considers that this may concern genuine narrow laminations with all their transitions up to loose chains of beaded or flaky inclusions (see Fig. 3.121). So far it has not been found possible to derive any practical rules from these influences.

It can readily be proved, however that the sensitivity of the plate wave method decreases rapidly if the plate thickness becomes great compared with the wave length, e.g. in steel plate thicker than 4 to 5 mm and at 2 MHz (transverse wavelength approx. 1.5 mm). In the case of heavier plate it is therefore necessary to use lower frequencies, which, however, will then permit only detection of larger flaws. In the case of sheet up to 2 mm it is therefore recommended to use a frequency of 4 to 5 MHz, and up to 5 mm approximately 2 to 3 MHz.

The usual testing lengths according to methods 1a and 2b are approximately 400 to 600 mm, so that several testing tracks must be arranged one behind the other for a complete test of wider strips or separate sheets, transposed relatively to each other to ensure complete testing. To avoid cross-interference between tracks the frequencies are changed. In the testing of separate sheets the test result obtained along one track is often regarded as valid for the entire sheet in view of the fact that a given flaw usually extends over the entire length of the sheet. On the other hand, in the case of strip, most defects usually occur in the middle zone so that the tracks along the edge can possibly be omitted.

The probes used in all methods can consist of the usual angle probes with plastic body as in the echo method. Adjustment of the angle sometimes is unnecessary, because the indication of a fixed angle probe for 35 to 80°, or for surface waves, is completely adequate for rough testing, also in the case of sound transmission. The probe which seems to be best suited is tried. Otherwise adjustable angle probes should be given preference. In the case of contact testing the coupling liquid, e.g. a little water, oil, cutting emulsion or diesel oil, should be fed sparingly so as not to wet the sound track, or alternatively the entire surface should be wetted uniformly. Naturally, wetted spots at the back also interfere, and a sheet should never be tested on a contaminated support.

For testing from one edge by the echo method, a guiding and holding device as shown in Fig. 3.117 is practical. This moves on 3 rolls over the sheet and on 2 rolls along the edge. A narrow gap between contact face and sheet is adjusted which, when the device is in use, is filled continuously with liquid, thus ensuring uniform contact and minimum wear.

For sound transmission by continuous excitation probes with a plastic body are unpractical. The heat generated by high-frequency in the crystal transducer is difficult to dissipate, and this, particularly in the case of barium titanate, can easily cause heating above the Curie point. Sound transmission through a liquid space is preferable. When the transducer is placed on the sheet, the liquid space must first be filled and, as it is also easily drained again, it is preferable to apply the transducer to the sheet from the bottom, feeding liquid continuously with a little overflow

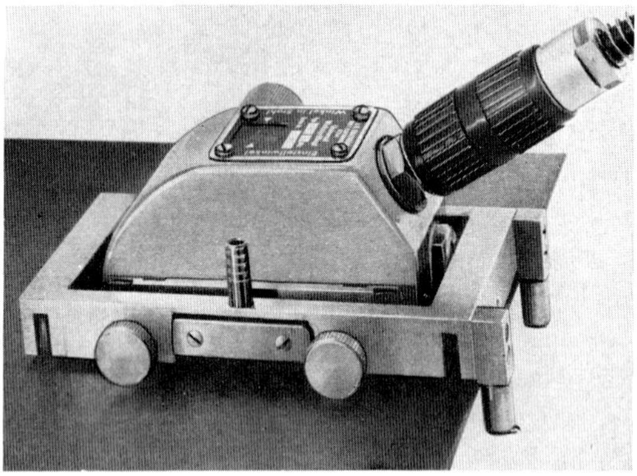

Fig. 3.117 Holder for angle probes suitable for testing plate from the edge, according to the zigzag or plate wave method in echo testing.

which makes direct contact with the entering sheet. A soft plastic gasket at the edge compensates for small differences in the height of the sheet provided the latter is not strongly undulated. Instead of swinging the crystal transducer and the connection cable around, it is simpler to

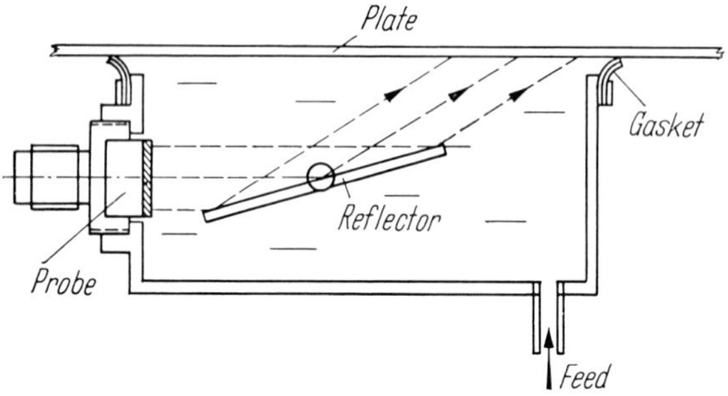

Fig. 3.118 Probe for generating plate waves, design Krautkrämer.

adjust the angle by means of a rotatable reflector, e.g. a metal plate (Fig. 3.118).

Up to the present only the method according to Fig. 3.116, 1c is being used for continuous strip testing. The probe is arranged as in Fig. 3.118 in a liquid chamber for oblique beaming by means of an adjustable water wedge. In this case, however, the probe itself can be swung around because, with the reflection method used here, it is necessary to reduce the interfering echoes from the liquid chamber to a minimum by making the distance from probe to strip as short as possible. At the top the liquid chamber has an exchangeable rim of steel or plastic. This rim slides along the surface of the strip, the entire probe assembly being pressed from the bottom against the strip. Because of the waviness of hot-rolled strip, the probe assembly is cardanically suspended. By adjusting the water feed a "water mushroom" is produced which bridges the narrow gap between sliding shim and strip.

In practice the test is usually combined with the continuous pickling process. Although the condition of the strip surface both before and after pickling is adequate for the test, preference is given to testing after the pickling. The speed of the strip here is usually 40 to 150 m/min. Normally this speed remains constant. This relatively high testing speed requires special measures to ensure sufficiently constant coupling and new methods for presenting and evaluating the test data. Observation of the CR screen cannot be considered, nor simple monitor-controlled flaw signalling. No use has yet been made of the possibility of marking flaws on the strip or on its edge – which would indicate the flaws also on coiled strip. Installations at present in operation have recording devices which display the test result in compressed form: in one installation the flaws in the longitudinal direction of the strip are recorded on a scale of 1 : 2000, while another testing installation is equipped with a tape printer which presents the result in digital form. Both evaluation methods are based on a subdivision of the strip length into recording sections which in turn are again subdivided into a given number of further subsections (Fig. 3.119a). The recording produced by the recorder is obtained as follows: the chart is fed step by step in accordance with the lengths of the recorded sections concerned. The pointer deflection indicates how many subsections in a recorded section are flawed. The counting of the flawed subsections always start from zero again for each recorded section. However, since a given flaw which is shorter than a subsection, can declare this entire subsection flawed, and since on the other hand several shorter flaws in a given subsection only declare this one subsection flawed, a second pointer is used to record the individual flaws occurring in the entire recorded section, on a second recording track of the same recorder. This track always sums the individual flaws up to a preselected maximum and then starts counting again from zero. The two adjacent, scale-true recording tracks of different meaning furnish much information on the nature and distribution of the defects in the longitudinal direction of the strip, in spite of the very concise form of the data.

The printer records the test results in the form of lines of figures. Each line is assigned to a definite, flawed recorded section. Recorded sections without flaws are not printed, so that the length of the printed tape alone already furnishes certain information on the "defectiveness" of the whole strip. The individual printed lines contain the following numerical data:

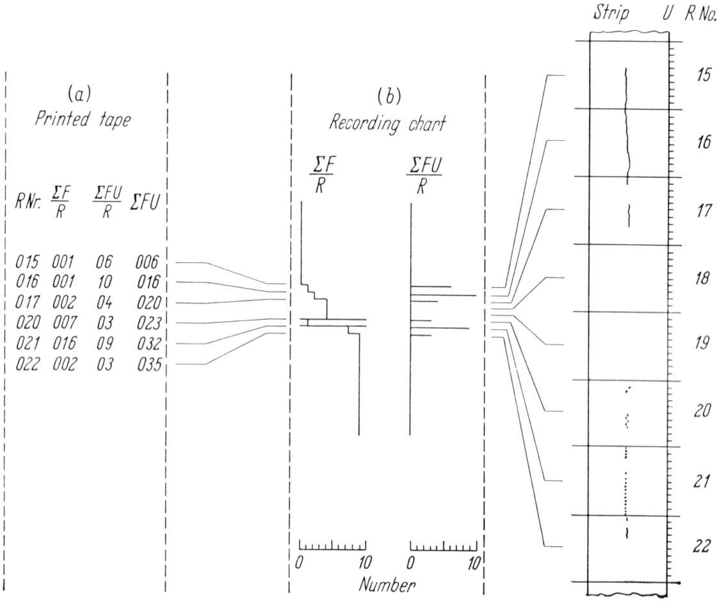

Fig. 3.119a Strip test – recording by printer (*a*), and recorder (*b*). *R* recorded sections; *U* subsections; *F* flaws (number); *FU* flawed subsections (number).

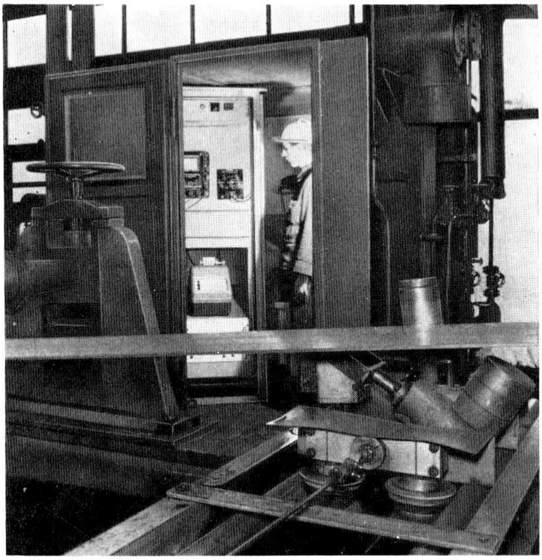

Fig. 3.119b Strip-testing installation with printer (works photo Messrs. Hoesch, Hohenlimburg).

1. The number of the flawed recorded section, which in this way gives the position of the strip in the longitudinal direction;
2. The sum of the flawed subsections in the recorded section concerned;
3. The sum of the individual flaws in the recorded section;
4. The sum of all flawed subsections preceding the recorded section concerned.

The numerical values for the end of the strip are printed in red. This last line of numbers thus permits a general statement on the quality of the strip (aggregate length of flaws in relation to the total length of the strip).

In the case of either recording method a pulse generator coupled to the strip carriage is used for a length-true division of the strip into recorded sections and subsections, irrespective of the speed of the strip. The length of the recorded sections and the number of the subsections composing this recorded section are adjustable within wide limits. Fig. 3.119a shows an example of the two recording methods. Fig. 3.119b shows a strip-testing installation equipped with printer.

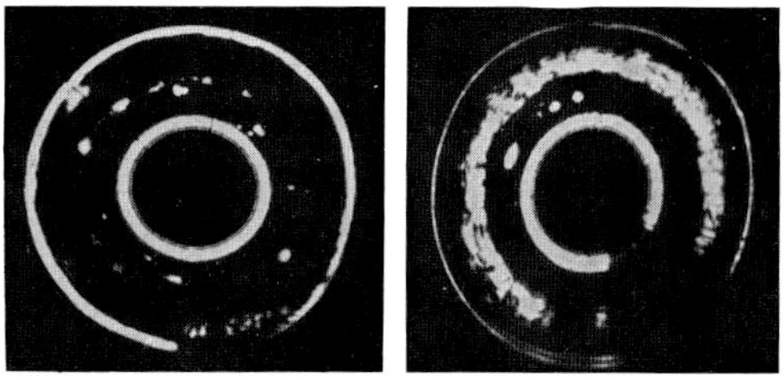

Fig. 3.120 B-scan of flawed sheets tested by the plate-wave echo method (according to BEAUJARD and HUSAREK).

Another possibility of data presentation in the application of the echo method has been exploited by BEAUJARD and HUSAREK: presentation by a B-scan [36]. For better utilization of the CR screen the display was coiled to form a ring (Fig. 3.120). As in the case of the testing methods described above, the gain was increased electronically simultaneously with the distance of the flaw (so-called "depth compensation"), to counteract the attenuation.

Thin sheets are already being tested on a larger scale, although no attempt has as yet been made, neither by the manufacturer nor the consumer, to test the entire production, in view of the enormous production and consumption figures involved. In Germany the first installation was designed by Volkswagenwerk Wolfsburg [46] in co-operation with Lehfeldt. Another installation is shown in Fig. 3.121a, designed by and used at Westfalenhütte, Dortmund [187]. In these installations the probes are placed on and lifted off from the top. In another installation by Krautkrämer for Thyssenhütte Duisburg the probes are coupled from the bottom according to the principle of Fig. 3.117, involving no mechanical motion.

Figs. 3.121b and c show two recorded bands of slag as indicated by an X-ray photo according to KOPINECK [187] and a recording of the ultrasonic intensity in the longitudinal direction of the flaw.

Further bibliographic references: [107, 108, 391, 221, 222, 188].

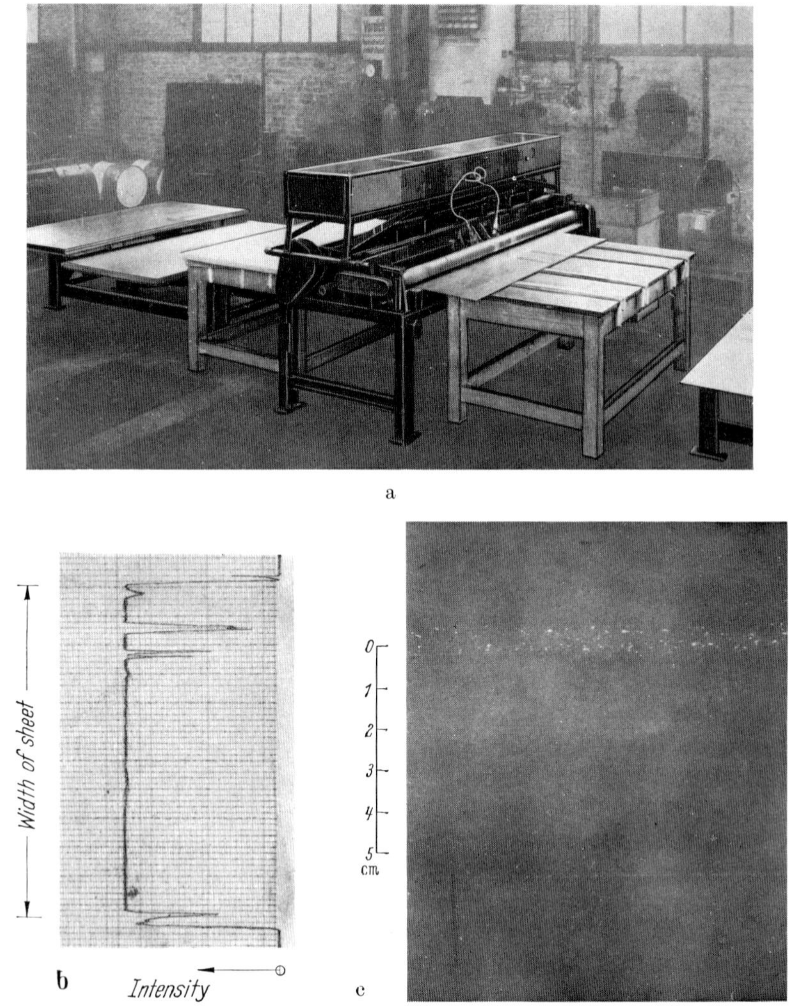

Fig. 3.121 Testing installation for sheets (according to KOPINECK, Westfalenhütte Dortmund). a) General view; b) recording of a flawed sheet by method Fig. 3.116/2a; c) X-ray recording of flaw, viz. a wide and a very narrow band of slag (compared with recording b enlarged approx. 10 times).

3.25 Semi-finished Products: Rods, Billets and Wires

Manufacturing defects occurring in such semi-finished products can either be internal defects or surface defects. Internal defects originate either from ingot defects elongated during rolling or drawing, namely shrinkage cavities and inclusions, mainly in the core; others are rolling and drawing defects, such as piping, particularly in the case of non-ferrous metals, and cracks in the core, which in cross-section appear flat or star-shaped. Surface defects, e.g. on rods, usually result from drawing defects such as radial incipient cracks or spills which penetrate to the surface at a flat angle. Since all flaws extend in the longitudinal direction, this requires that the axis of the sound beam lies in a cross-sectional plane (Fig. 3.122), either normal or oblique to the surface. Also used are surface waves in the circumferential direction.

3.251 Rod Material

In the case of drawn steel rods, testing for internal defects on material thicker than 30 mm is one of the oldest applications of the pulse-echo method. It makes the usual pickle test superfluous. To find defects in the core, it is sufficient to scan along a few longitudinal tracks using a normal probe, at least on two tracks being transposed 90° in order to obtain an echo with sufficient probability even where cracks are unfavourably orientated. The stationary rod is coated with viscous oil and scanned continuously with the protected probe. Usually the testing frequencies are 2 to 6 MHz, the higher frequencies and a small probe diameter being used on thin material in view of the better close-range resolution. Testing conditions being equal, the width of the flaw can be estimated roughly from the ratio between flaw echo and bottom echo [52]. Pohl [287] has made detailed studies with artificial and natural flaws in rods in order to determine the influence of the orientation of the flaw and of eccentrically located flaws on the height of the echo. For estimating the order of magnitude of the size of flaws, he found that the ratio of flaw echo to backwall echo alone is not sufficient to draw up evaluation statistics, but that the depth of the flaw, the diameter of the rod and – if different probes are used – also their frequency and diameter should be taken into consideration for this evaluation. In all instances it is of course necessary to adjust the echo height to maximum by scanning in the circumferential direction. In the case of smaller diameters and rough surfaces the close-range resolving power is frequently insufficient for observing the first flaw echo, and instead its repetition behind the first bottom echo is used.

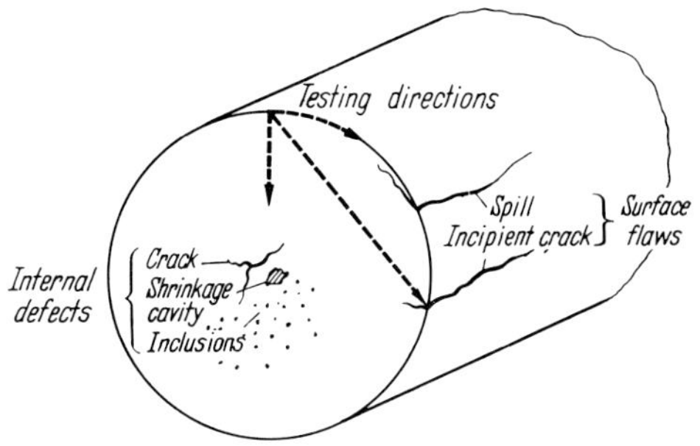

Fig. 3.122 Types of defects in round stock, and main directions of testing.

There the sensitivity of the probe is usually also improved in view of its near-field fluctuations. Of course care should be taken to avoid mistaking triangle echoes for flaw echoes (cf. 3.133).

Thin, bright rods, down to approximately 5 mm diameter, are preferably tested with a TR probe (Fig. 2.42). The probe is applied with its separation line transverse or at 45° to the rod, and it can also easily be ground in cylindrically for better guiding. A device for guiding the probes on rods greatly facilitates these tests. Usually two TR probes are placed on the circumference displaced 90° from each other and mounted in a guiding device which presses the probes by spring action against the continuously moving specimen, a flow of water being used for coupling.

In the case of rod material other than round stock, e.g. square, hexagonal or flat, testing is successful even at diameters less than 5 mm because of the higher sensitivity with plane coupling.

For a go/no-go test it is then sometimes sufficient to observe only the disturbance of the echo sequence between the flat boundary faces. In the case of more complex sections, both the method and the possibility of testing depend entirely on the shape and the probable position of the flaws.

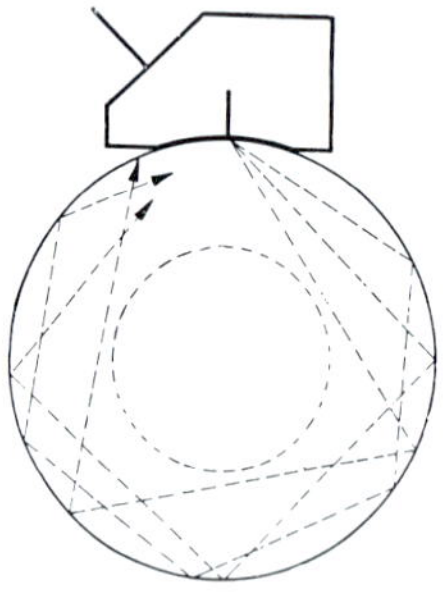

Fig. 3.123 As a result of the divergence of the beam at entrance in round material, the oblique beam of transverse waves can cover a zone up to 1/5 of the diameter, depending on the latter and the entrance angle.

Surface defects are found with oblique transverse waves or with surface waves according to Fig. 3.122; the latter can, however, be used only on very smooth surfaces, making furthermore any quantitative differentiation between deeper and shallower cracks impossible. If an angle probe with 45 or 60° is suitably ground as shown in Fig. 3.123, the broad beam after a few reflections fills a zone under the surface fairly completely up to a depth of approximately 1/5 of the diameter. This therefore covers also internal defects in addition to true surface defects, which latter can only be distinguished by the finger-tip test. The surface defects produce considerably stronger echoes than inclusions of comparable size, so that even the minutest surface defects, such as die lines interfere with the test.

The waves travelling around once or several times in the round rod, however, arrive at the probe at such unfavourable angles that at best an indistinct *revolving echo* is obtained. A revolving echo, however, can be of interest as substitute for a backwall echo, e.g. for checking the degree of coupling and for evaluating flaws. A second probe mounted homologously next to the first probe furnishes a distinct revolving echo if the second probe is simply connected to the instrument in parallel with the first probe. Such a *twin angle probe* where each probe is both transmitter and receiver for its own echoes as well as for the pulses of the other probe, has gained a certain importance for testing pipes, cf. 3.26, Fig. 3.138.

Since the sensitivity of oblique transverse waves drops after several reflections, the flaw should as far as possible be encountered in the first third to one half of the circumference. Thus, in the case of stationary rods, the test should be carried out along 2 to 3 longitudinal tracks, or better still, the probe should be advanced along a zig-zag path on the circumference. Flaw echoes then travel back and forth on the CR screen and can be detected and distinguished very much more easily from spurious interfering echoes from the probe. For the same reason it is recommended that the rod be allowed to rotate slowly at a few r.p.s. Since spills are indicated with greater sensitivity in one revolving direction of the wave (as in Fig. 3.122) than in the other, the test should be carried out in both directions, successively or better simultaneously by using a twin angle probe.

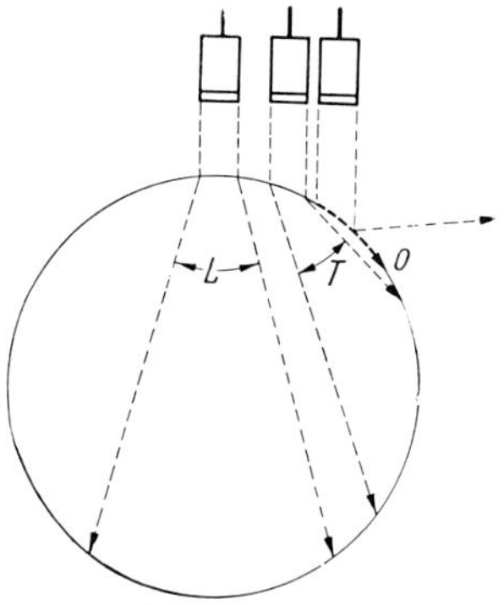

Fig. 3.124 Testing round stock by the immersion technique, path of beam shown for steel in water.

The immersion technique has already been used for some time for diameters below approx. 80 mm. According to Fig. 3.124 all types of waves and testing directions can be obtained by using a movable probe, including a surface wave (boundary wave). In the case of a broad sound beam, several waves can sometimes be obtained simultaneously. If the surface is not perfectly smooth, this may give rise to troublesome interfering echoes in a zone behind the entrance echo, which in thinner round stock may mask the echoes of core defects completely. These interfering echoes are produced by boundary waves which, although they quickly decay on the surface, still produce strong echoes from minute rough spots, foreign particles and air bubbles on the surface if they approach the sound entrance point during the rotation of the rod. Therefore narrow or focused sound beams should be used, or more simply masks with a round opening or a slot should be inserted in the sound path.

To avoid receiving interfering echoes, or worse still multiple echoes from a mask, it should be inserted either immediately in front of the probe, or at some distance obliquely to the beam. The mask can be of plastic material with good absorption, such as rubber containing fillers, or alternatively also a thin metal plate covered by a film which makes it impermeable to sound as a result of the trapped layer of air.

The relative positions of probe, mask and round stock should remain fixed, which in the case of smaller diameters of the specimen is realised most simply by the probe holder according to Fig. 3.125, which is guided by hand. The mask, which is rotatable, is mounted in front of the probe and contains two eccentric openings. Depending on the position, one then obtains two transverse waves circulating in opposite directions for detecting shallow defects, or two longitudinal wave beams through the core of the rod. By using a probe for 4 to 6 MHz (transducer material: lithium sulphate), it then becomes possible to test rod material with mill-rough, slightly oxidized surface, down to 12 mm diameter.

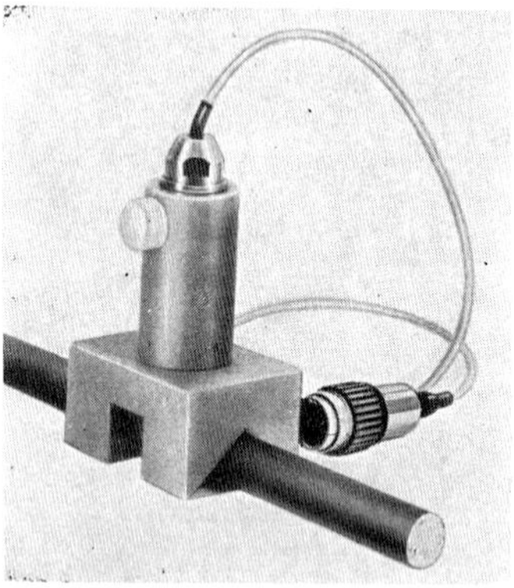

Fig. 3.125 Probe holder for testing round stock by the immersion technique.

With cylindrically curved probes (Fig. 2.46) and applying the immersion technique, the decrease in sensitivity due to the strong refraction in the rod can be compensated, or the beam can be focused at a given depth where the presence of any flaws would be particularly aggravating for the further processing. For correct adjustment, the optimal water gap is found on a section with artificial flaws. Also TR probes have a pronounced sensitivity maximum at a definite depth (see Fig. 2.44).

In order to avoid interfering echoes from the surface which occur at oblique beaming in the immersion technique when checking for longitudinal defects close to the surface, a further solution has been found: two probes – one transmitting the other receiving – are arranged in an immersion tank as shown in Fig. 3.126. Any appreciable portion of the transmitted sound beam can reach the receiving probe only if the circling direction of the sound beam travelling along a polygon is reversed at a longitudinal surface defect by reflection. If the rod is rotating, longitudinal defects are then indicated by travelling echoes. In order to detect spills reliably in the two possible directions of inclination, the test is usually carried out simultaneously in two parallel testing planes, the sound circling in opposite directions.

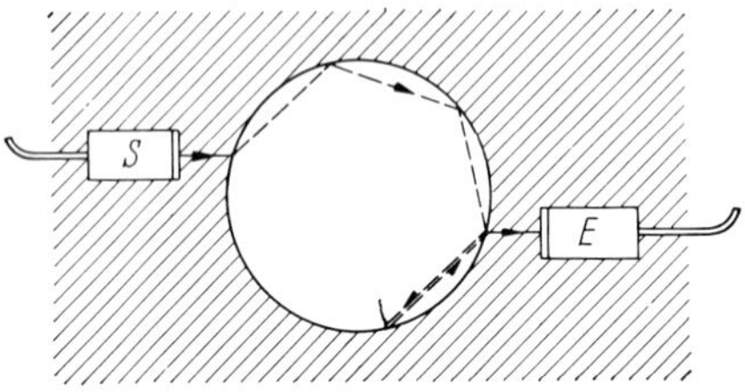

Fig. 3.126 Testing method for detecting longitudinal surface defects on rod material by the immersion technique, with separate transmitting (S) and receiving (E) probes.

Higher testing speeds and reliability are possible if these testing methods are combined with automation. This requires a suitable conveyor for moving the rod to the testing point, the rod usually also being rotated. A normal probe then scans the rod along a spiral path so that core defects are irradiated from different, radial directions. Simultaneously an angle probe can check for surface defects. Normally two instruments are used for this purpose; in the case of thicker material, where the interfering echoes of the angle probe do not mask the flaw echoes of the normal probe, the second instrument can be omitted by connecting both probes in parallel to one instrument. When the immersion technique is used, which is particularly suited for automating the testing process because of the uniform coupling, the water gaps for the two probes can be made unequal, so as to be able for instance, to display on the same CR screen the echoes from the core and from longitudinal surface defects within the same monitor gate.

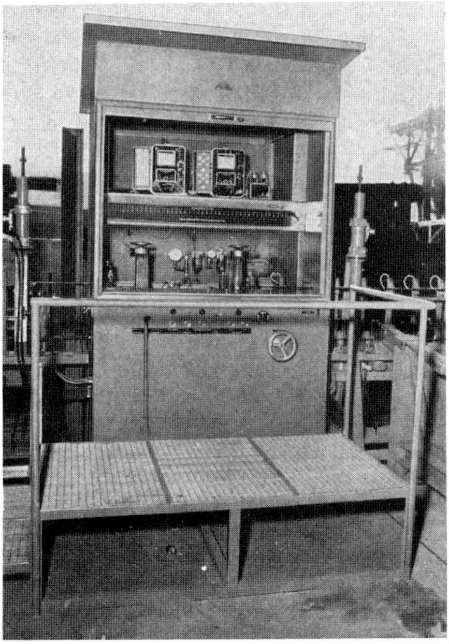

Fig. 3.127 Testing and control unit of an ultrasonic testing installation for rods up to 80 mm dia., with lamp panel (works photo Messrs. Röchling, Völklingen/Saar).

Fig. 3.127 shows an installation for testing rods of 10 to 80 mm diameter. A bundle of rods is placed on a magazine. A selector places one rod after the other on the roller bed with three oblique rollers which force the specimen to carry out a helical motion. In the centre of the testing installation the rod passes through a transit tank. A holder mounting the probes for detecting longitudinal surface defects and core defects, rides on. The probes are submerged, the water level being kept constant to compensate for the losses at the entrance and exit openings. The probes can be adjusted in the holder for correct positioning for any diameter. The roller bed on the exit side has a sorting gate which is actuated by the monitor according to the test result. The test is fully automatic: the rod which has just been sorted initiates the entrance of the next rod. To prevent the monitor from initiating a wrong operation across the open water gap while no test piece is in the tank, a second monitor blocks the flaw monitor by sound transmission until a new rod is in the tank. At 100% scanning, maximum testing speeds of approximately 4 m/min can be achieved with this installation. In the case of bright stock, surface defects having a minimum depth of a few hundredths of a millimetre can be detected, and flaws at least twice as deep as the surface roughness in the case of black rods.

The test results are indicated (at the same time as the sorting) by marking the flaws on the specimen. A paint spray gun cannot be used in this case; good results are obtained, however, with a running grinding belt which is pressed against the rod at the positions of flaws and is actuated by the flaw monitor. Since this marking has to be made outside the transit tank, a delay device makes allowance for the shift of the flaw signal from the testing point to the marking point. In one instance the same testing installation was fitted with a different flaw display, a lamp panel showing the flawed zones of the specimen. However, this luminous flaw diagram of the rod remains visible for only a short time because it has to be cleared before the next specimen enters.

Considerably higher rod testing speeds for detecting longitudinal surface defects are possible with a "rotating testing installation", as explained in Sec. 3.26 under pipe testing, which applies analogously also to rods. In this testing installation the required helical relative motion between specimen and probes is realised by means of a rotating probe assembly, the rod being transported through the installation without being rotated. In this case the maximum testing speed at 100% scanning is approximately 20 m/min.

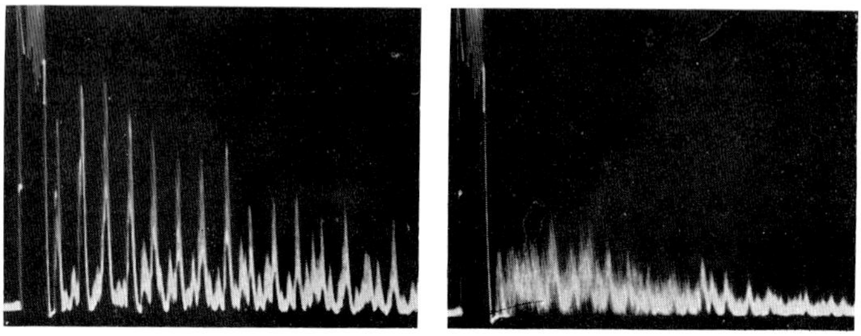

Fig. 3.128 Testing thin, bright round stock for surface defects according to GRABENDÖRFER. a) Screen trace of flawless piece (diameter 3 mm, frequency 4 MHz), b) incipient crack 0.3 mm deep.

Thin, bright round stock, down to a diameter of 1 mm, can be checked for longitudinal surface defects by dry contact with (plane) normal probes (see Sec. 3.14). It is recommended that the rod at rotational speeds up to 30 per second be allowed to move past a probe of 4 to 6 MHz protected by a plastic shoe against wear.

Fig. 3.128 shows screen pictures obtained in this way and as they appear also to the observer because of the high rotational speed. Testing speeds of 10 m/min and higher can be reached without difficulty. Cracks with a minimum depth of 0.1 mm are detectable provided they extend in longitudinal direction at least 10 to 20 mm. This testing method does away with the tiresome and time-consuming visual inspection customary hitherto. In practice, however, this method has not yet been applied to any appreciable extent.

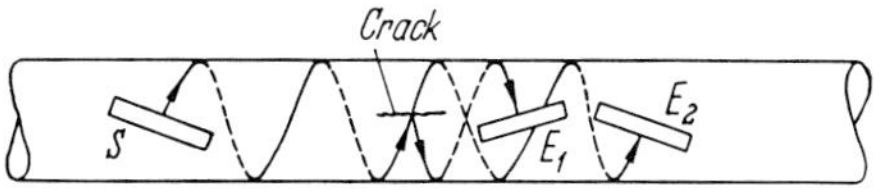

Fig. 3.129 Testing round stock by magnetostrictive excitation according to KAULE [173]. S transmitter; E_1 receiver for crack echoes; E_2 receiver for sound transmission pulse.

On the other hand, the method described in Sec. 1.105 for exciting ultrasonic pulses directly in the rod by means of the magnetostrictive effect has recently gained greater importance. For detecting longitudinal surface defects an array of several coils is mounted in such a way that the excited ultrasonic pulse spirals around the rod at a steep pitch (Fig. 3.129).

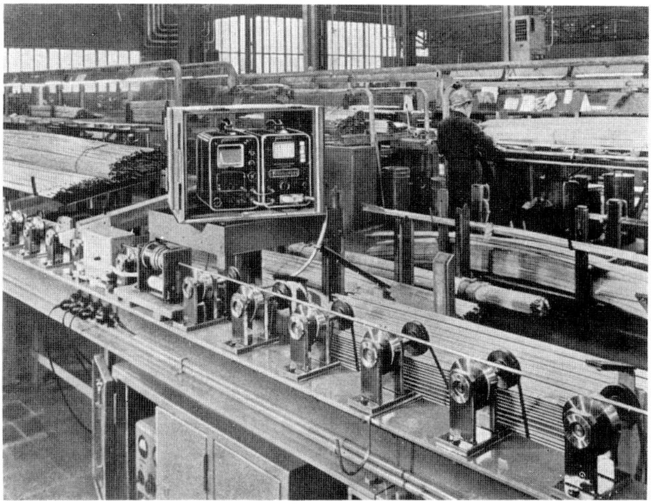

Fig. 3.130 Testing rods with the "Ferrotron" (magnetostrictive principle of excitation of sound waves; works photo Messrs. DEW, Krefeld).

Receiving coil E_1 is orientated so that it can receive part of the sound beam reflected by a longitudinal defect, thus producing a flaw echo. The other receiving coil E_2 can receive the spiralling wave directly; the sound transmission indication obtained in this way reveals, by its disappearance, the presence of large defects. Both indications are evaluated by monitors. Fig. 3.130 shows such an installation for testing rods with diameter from 2 to 14 mm, using a "Ferrotron" instrument. In this case the testing speed – the rods need not be rotated while passing through the array of probes – can be as high as a few metres per second. In the case of bright stock, longitudinal defects at least 0.05 mm deep can be detected in this way.

3.252 Billets

In order to detect core defects, rolled, round billets with diameters of approximately 50 mm and upwards are transported without being rotated on conventional roller beds, and similarly square billets of 40 mm and more. The test is usually carried out with 2 probes along 2 suitably spaced surface tracks in order to cover a wider angular range of flaw orientations (Fig. 3.131).

For the continuous testing of square billets automated testing installations have been constructed which operate at testing speeds up to 60 m/min and simultaneously discharge flawed billets into a "reject through". The billets are transported on the roller bed edgewise. In one design (Fig. 3.132 [40]) a probe holder is lowered on to the moving billet from the top. The holder rides on four rollers on the billet, thus following its movements and bends. Two probes suspended cardanically in the holder, test along the two top faces. In another design (Fig. 3.133 [160, 161]) the probes together with their holder are pressed pneumatically from the bottom against the billet, articulated with a ball and socket joint.

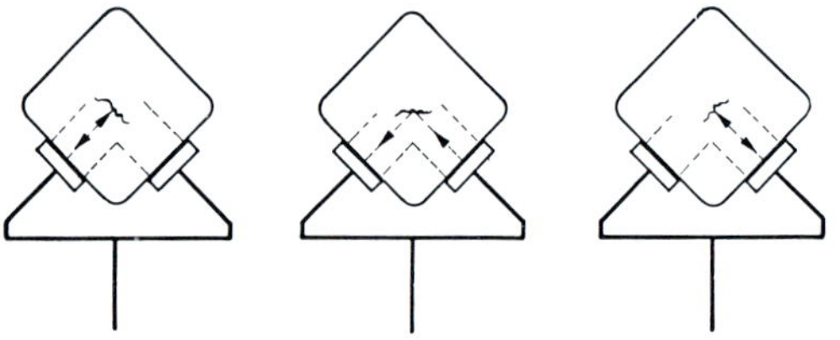

Fig. 3.131 Testing billets with two probes connected in parallel.

The testing specifications in force will determine when a specimen is "faulty" and should be rejected. Sometimes the requirements made by the management, according to which the evaluation of the test data has to be made, can only be met with the aid of a complex flaw classification requiring a data processing installation which controls a sorting gate. In addition to sorting, most installations also make provision for marking the flawed spots on the billets with colour. Automatic testing for core defects on round billets uses the same method, the riding probe holder being balanced on the round billet by means of an artificially displaced low centre of gravity.

Longitudinal surface defects, which also occur on billets, are not so easily detected by ultrasonic tests, particularly during continuous testing.

Basically, longitudinal defects in round billets can be detected by means of angle probes or pipe probes in the same way as described in 3.251 for

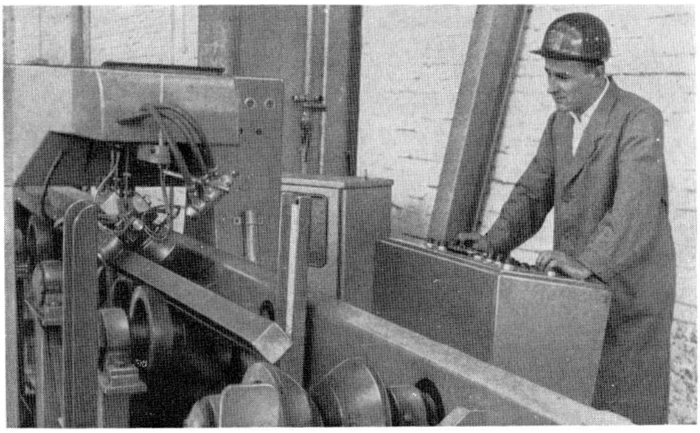

Fig. 3.132 Billet Tester, design Krautkrämer (works photo Niederrheinische Hütte, Duisburg)

drawn rods. Owing to the rough and not very uniform surface of round billets, the coupling conditions are more unfavourable. Testing by hand can therefore be considered where the requirements in respect of flaw detectability are not too high. Furthermore, in the case of continuous testing the specimen should be fed in a spiral motion, which in round billets usually meets with difficulties because they are not sufficiently straight.

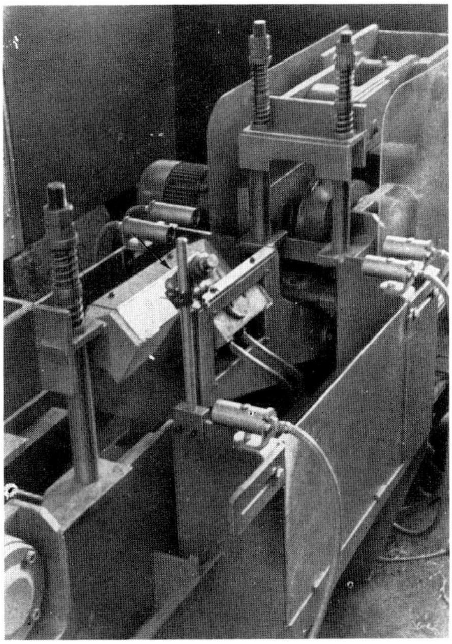

Fig. 3.133 Installation for testing billets, design Sofranel-de Wendel.

In the checking of square billets for longitudinal surface defects an additional problem arises: cracks usually start at the edges, where they cannot be detected by oblique beaming. The only possibility would be the use of surface waves radiated from the billet faces in such a way that they cover the adjacent edge. However, this is feasible only if the rounded edges of the billets are sufficiently smooth so that the flaw echoes exceed the surface noise level of the edge by a sufficient margin.

This requires testing frequencies of 2 or even 1 MHz. As far as is known, this testing method has not yet been applied in practice. Similarly, testing the billet faces for longitudinal surface defects by using 45° angle probes applied from the adjacent face, which is basically possible, has not yet found wide application in practice.

3.253 Wires

Rod waves – corresponding to the plate waves in plates – are also used occasionally for testing thin rods and wires. Magnetostrictive excitation of such waves (possible only in steel and nickel) according to Fig. 1.123 has the great advantage that no contact is required. Only a coil being pushed over the end of the rod or wire, when transverse defects and inclusions are being sought.

Where the primary object is to detect longitudinal surface defects on wires, the magnetostrictive method according to Fig. 3.129 with spirally rotating waves can be successfully applied on diameters down to approximately 2 mm. In this case also the flaw detectability starts at depths of approx. 0.05 mm, at testing speeds up to 3 to 4 m/s.

Thin wires, usually less than 1 mm, on which longitudinal and transverse cracks, shrinkage cavities, and inclusions are to be eliminated, can be checked by a number of different techniques. In the case of the inten-

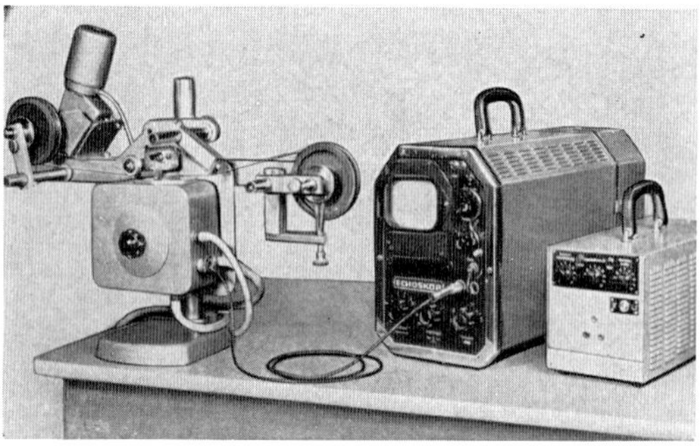

Fig. 3.134 Equipment for continuous wire tests by the pulse echo method with automatic flaw indication (Lehfeldt).

sity method with swept, or alternatively, also unmodulated ultrasound the two probes spaced approximately 100 to 200 mm touch the taut, moving wire. The small contact faces excite arbitrary types of wire waves [290, 319]. Pulsed sound transmission has the advantage that different, simultaneously excited modes of waves can be distinguished by their transit time. In a design according to Böhme [49] a buffer shoe attached to the probe makes dry contact with the wire along a very short section. This excites particularly strong bending waves which are strongly attenuated and reflected by such flaws as longitudinal cracks having a depth of more than 10% of the wire diameter, and shrinkage cracks and inclusions exceeding 10% of the cross-sectional area. In the case of frequencies of 1 to 2.5 MHz the coupling fluctuations reach only 10% of the pulse amplitude. As in the case of plate waves, the pulses are partially broadened as a result of dispersion.

In the case of the pulse echo method, one can also use the usual angle probes and probes for surface waves, the plastic contact shoe being fitted in the longitudinal direction with a small matching groove. The contact point is continuously wetted with coupling liquid, the dry wire moving in a direction opposite to the beaming direction to avoid interfering echoes by residual coupling liquid. In the case of coupling under water, as used in the device by Lehfeldt [223] (Fig. 3.134), the problem of wear and adjustability of the beaming angle is solved in a simple way. A guiding block forces the wire over a short distance under water. In bright wires of less than 1 mm diameter, even fine scratches are already clearly indicated by travelling echoes. Results of practical experience with any of these methods have so far not been published.

3.26 Pipes and Cylinders

Here again the main problems are manufacturing defects. Fatigue cracks and corrosion fatigue require the same testing technique as the manufacturing defects because they usually are in the same position. Other maintenance tests, such as determination of corrosion and wall thickness, are discussed in 3.61.

Furthermore welded pipes are not included in this group, because the only flaws they may contain are defects in the original plate and welding defects, nor cast pipes. In seamless and rolled pipes the defects which are of interest in this connection, are similar to those occurring in rod material, viz. incipient cracks and spills in the internal and external surfaces, furthermore inclusions and shrinkage cracks in the wall, which, however, appear as laminations as in plates as a result of the manufacturing process.

Generally, transverse waves beamed obliquely in circumferential directions are used as in the case of round stock, with the difference, however, that the wave is propagated along a zig-zag path in the shell of the pipe (Fig. 3.135). In the case of thin-walled pipes this usually results in oscillation forms similar to those of plate waves which, however, makes no difference from a practical point of view. Surface waves are rarely considered.

Certain cases involving unusual testing techniques will be discussed beforehand. Certain manufacturing methods may result in spills (flakes) occurring in the longitudinal direction in pipes (Fig. 3.135) which are detected by zig-zag waves in one of the two directions of the pipe. On pipes up to approximately 80 mm diameter the sound beam then broadens and is partially propagated spirally in the pipe material. This simplifies the test because it permits detection of flaws not only along the same generatrix on which the probe moves, but even on the opposite side at some distance (Fig. 3.136). Similarly also other transverse defects are found, e.g. cracks in the internal wall of steel moulds for the centrifugal casting of steel pipes, where they regularly occur next to longitudinal cracks because of the high thermal stresses, furthermore fatigue cracks in casings for boring rods.

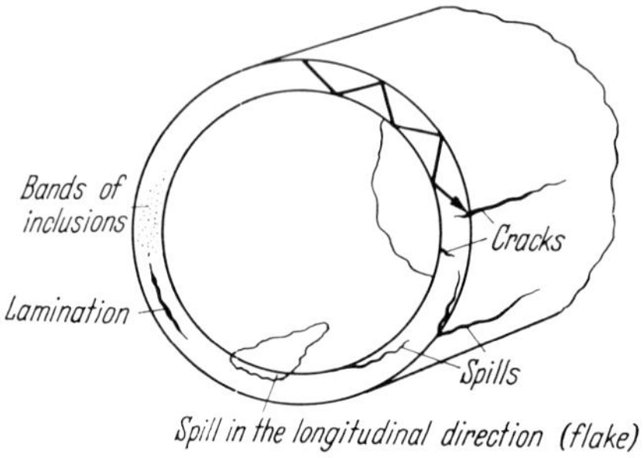

Fig. 3.135 Types of defects and main direction of testing in pipes.

Where only laminations are of interest in pipes, perpendicular beaming as in plates can be applied. In the case of thin-walled pipes it is recommended to fill the pipe with water and to utilize the wall echo of the opposite side transmitted through the water gap when applying the intensity method, either by direct contact or preferably in immersion technique.

The testing technique used for finding the usual longitudinally orientated defects in pipes mainly depends on the outside diameter (O.D.). A subdivision into the following 5 diameter groups is entirely arbitrary and is justified only because the different testing methods applied can be better correlated with these groups during tests at the manufacturing plants ("production control") or when pipes already installed are tested ("maintenance and repair"). The following classification is therefore used, the limits being transitional; "very big" pipes above 400 mm O.D., "big pipes" between 120 and 400 mm, "medium pipes" between 50 and 120 mm, "small pipes" from 25 to 50 mm, and "thin pipes" up to 25 mm O.D.

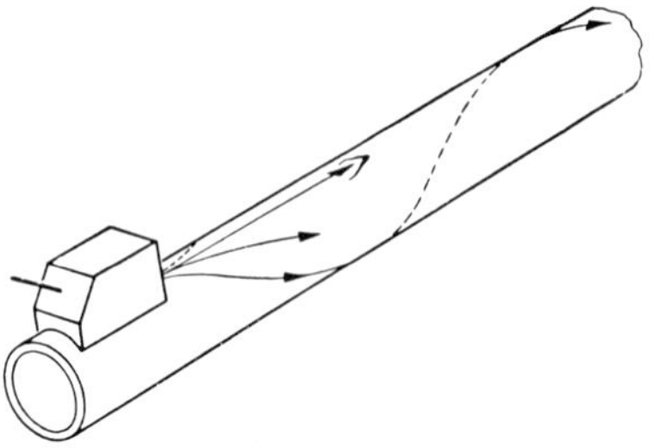
Fig. 3.136 Longitudinal test on pipes for spills and transverse cracks using zig-zag waves (only the trace of the wave on the pipe shell is shown).

In *very big pipes*, as used for gas storage tanks and accumulators for steam boilers, a zig-zag wave can always cover only a small portion of the circumference. Therefore the stationary pipe should be scanned by hand in the circumferential direction along separate tracks or along a zig-zag path using angle probes usually of 45° or 60°. Deep plug lines on the inside, which are not readily detectable by sight, may make testing rather difficult, and should therefore be avoided during manufacture as far as possible to facilitate the subsequent checking for corrosion fatigue cracks.

In the case of *big pipes* a revolving echo can be used successfully, being obtained by means of two angle probes radiating in opposite directions ("twin angle probe" or "pipe probe") according to Fig. 1.138. This echo in effect takes over the tasks which, when normal probes are used, are performed by the backwall echo: it shows immediately, even in the absence of flaw echoes, whether both the instrument and the coupling are in order, and in addition it supplements the flaw evaluation by an intensity method which makes deductions on the presence of a flaw possible even when the latter produces no echo because of oblique orientation or absorption.

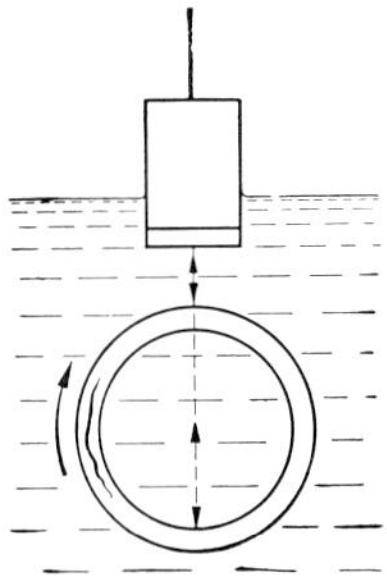

Fig. 3.137 Checking thin-walled pipes for laminations.

According to Fig. 3.138a, one usually obtains with such a *pipe probe* two indications from a single flaw, and in fact symmetrically one in front and one behind the *reference echo*. Since this echo is not a true echo but only a pulse travelling from one probe to the other and simultaneously in the opposite direction, it has the same transit time as an echo travelling from one probe to a flaw and back on the opposite side of the pipe, i.e. at 180° of the pipe circumference calculated from the centre of the probe. If it is moved to the centre of the CR screen by scale expansion, both halves of the pipe, to the left and to the right of it, are then, so-to-speak, evolved simultaneously, together with their flaw indications. Whether a given indication belongs to the right or the left half of the pipe cannot be decided if the probe is stationary, but immediately if it is moved in the circumferential direction: if the flaw echo between transmitting pulse and reference echo, both of which remain stationary, travels towards the transmitting pulse, then the probe is approaching the flaw, and vice versa. Since exact flaw location, in the testing of pipes, is usually not required, and since furthermore this is impossible because the indication is usually broad and split, the pipe probe is usually shifted in such a manner that the flaw echo is located approximately halfway between the transmitting pulse and the reference echo. The flaw is then located at approximately one quarter of the circumference of the pipe (90°) from the probe.

In contrast to the schematic drawing in Fig. 3.138a, both the flaw echoes and the reference echo are mostly composed, not of a single but of a large number of zig-zag waves which lie within the region of the angle of divergence. Consequently the indications usually are split several times.

In the case of thick walled pipes (e.g. 300 × 30, O.D. × wall thickness in mm) the envelope of a flaw echo shows distinct maxima and minima if the probe is shifted.

The positions of the maximum readings of both types of flaws can then be marked on the luminous screen with the aid of a pipe section having artificial internal and external flaws in the form of saw cuts, thus distinguishing between such flaws.

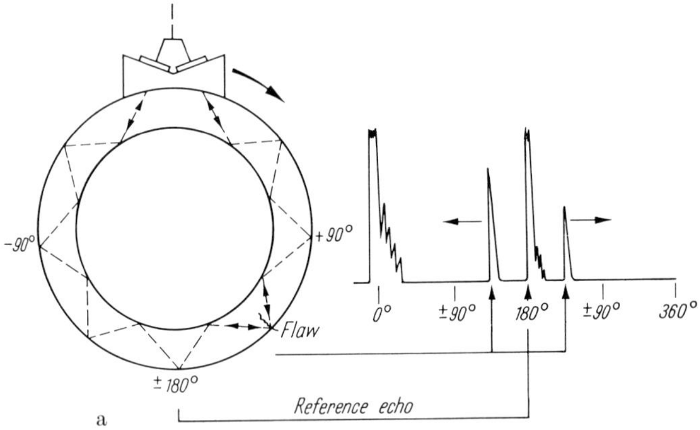

a

b

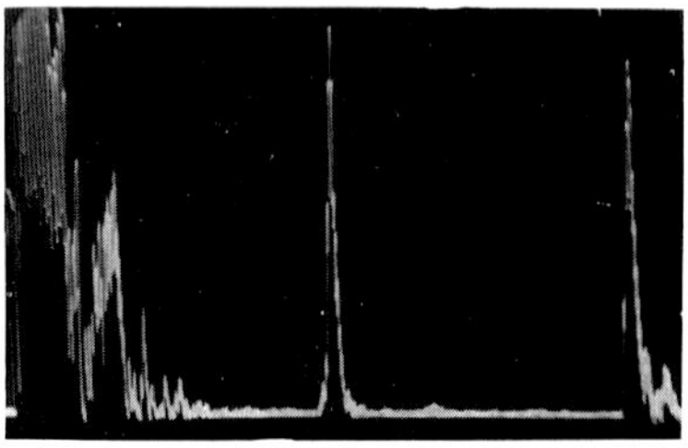

FE

c

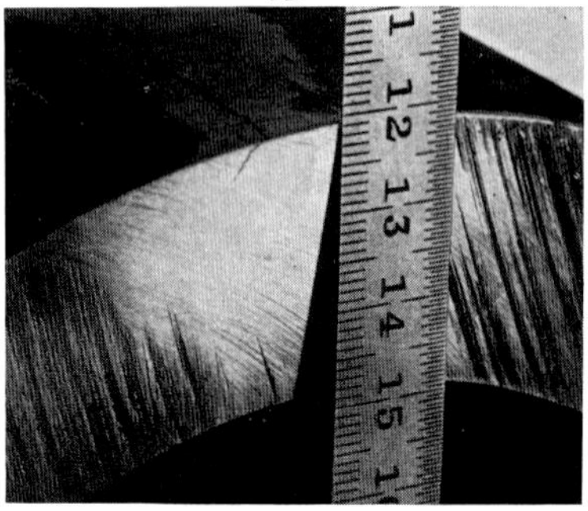

Fig. 3.138 Testing thick pipes by means of the pipe probe. a) Sound path and screen picture, schematic; b) screen picture obtained with a pipe of 30 × 300 mm showing flaw at approximately 90° position (*FE*), frequency 2 MHz; c) flaw made visible in ground section (spill 3 mm deep).

A stationary pipe should not be scanned only along a single longitudinal track because the zone below the probe will then not be checked, and because the reference echo may then mask a flaw in exact juxtaposition. For this reason, and for clearer indication of flaws by travelling echoes, the probe is moved along a zig-zag path. For the detection of spills, it may then be advantageous to observe both flaw indications simultaneously as in Fig. 3.138a. While in the case of incipient cracks the right echo with the longer sound path is usually smaller than the left echo, this may be just the other way around in the case of a spill irradiated unfavourably. Otherwise the second echo can be disregarded and the reference echo shifted to the right edge of the scale, as in Fig. 3.138b. This is particularly effective in the testing of rotating pipes because a spill always assumes a favourable orientation at one point if the pipe probe is used.

The reference echo, as implied by its name, is used for checking the coupling and the cycling of the pulse. Strong damping usually points to a defect in the pipe. In the case of new pipes this may be a lamination, which might be indicated merely by weak flaw echoes, and in the case of old pipes a corroded spot not visible from the outside which produces diffuse scattering of the waves. In the case of greater wall thicknesses, say above about 20 mm, both types of flaws can be distinguished by beaming at right angles to the surface, while in the case of pipes with thinner walls, other indirect means must be used if differentiation is essential.

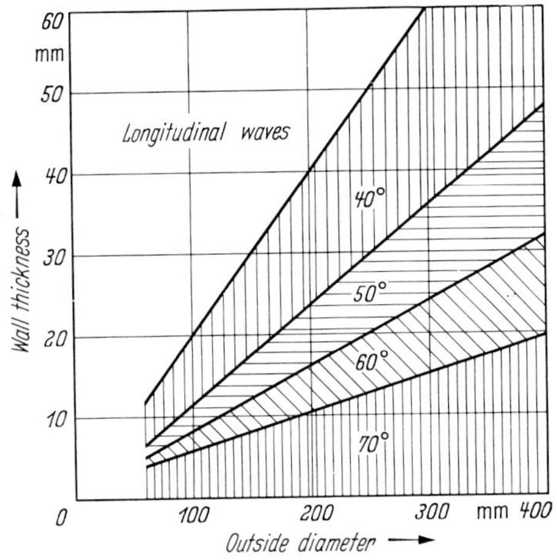

Fig. 3.139 Optimal beaming angles from 40 to 70° for testing pipes.

If a wide enough range is adjusted on the CR screen, multiple reference echoes of decreasing amplitudes are obtained, like the echo sequence from a plate. Any weakening of the pulse due to any of the causes mentioned is indicated at increased sensitivity by the multiple reference echoes.

Influence of wall thickness (d). In the case of pipes with a wall which is thin compared with the O.D., e.g. 10 × 200 mm, the waves still reach the internal wall at approximately the same angle at which they left the probe. In the case of greater wall thickness, the internal angle of incidence and thus the sensitivity for internal defects, decreases. If, however, the smallest beam angle of approximately 35° is used, too steep zig-zag paths of short range are obtained with small wall thicknesses, and excessively split echoes. Therefore, the beaming angle of the probe is adjusted in accordance with the wall thickness so that internal angles of incidence of approximately 60 to 80° are obtained. Fig. 3.139 gives for pipes of different O.D. and d the empirically found optimal beaming angles.

If pipe probes, as shown in Fig. 3.140 on the left and centre are housed in a *common* case, they can furnish optimal results only for a given range of O.D. and d, whereas the design shown in Fig. 3.140 on the right, with exchangeable and hinged inserts for different beaming angles can be adapted to both the outside diameter and the wall thickness. Feeding the coupling water through holes in the plastic body directly to the contact point ensures very uniform contact and saves time.

According to Sec. 3.14, Eq. 3.8, wall thicknesses above 20% of the O.D. can no longer be checked reliably for internal defects by means of oblique transverse waves. Then only longitudinal waves at angles up to 30° come into consideration; these are beamed through strongly ab-

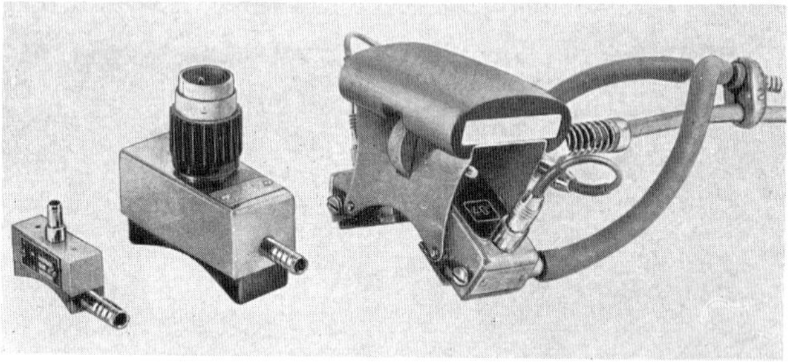

Fig. 3.140 Pipe probes for contact test and coupling by flowing water, left for pipes up to approx. 70 mm O. D., centre for pipes from 70 to 400 mm O. D., right pipe probe holder with exchangeable and hinged angle probes (design Krautkrämer).

sorbing wedges, e.g. of vulcanized rubber. This reduces the interfering echoes to a tolerable level (Fig. 3.141). Since a portion of the beam then still strikes the wall perpendicularly, an echo sequence is obtained from the wall in which flaw echoes can be distinguished readily only if they shift, e.g. if the pipe revolves.

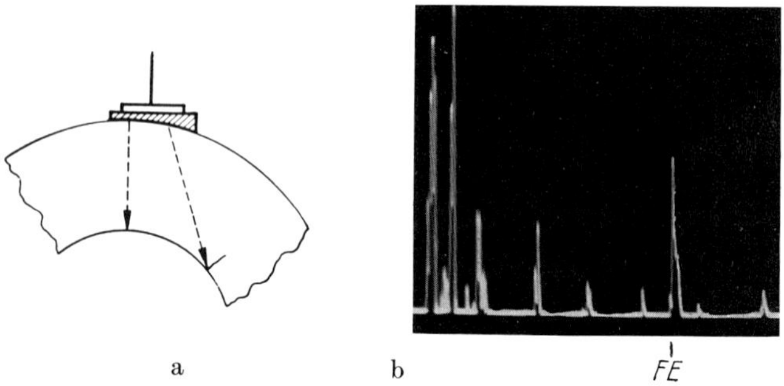

Fig. 3.141 Testing of very thick pipes with longitudinal waves, a) schematic, b) screen trace.

Testing devices for thick pipes and cylinders have been used for some time in Germany, i.e. since on the one hand a DIN specification prescribes ultrasonic tests for heat-resistant high-pressure pipes (cf. 3.7) and since the Technical Supervisory Association carries out routine tests on compressed gas cylinders cracks. In the installation shown in Fig. 3.142, the pipe, which may be up to 14 m long, passes through the test bench in a screw motion. The probes are coupled to the pipe from the bottom via a water gap (so-called "puddle technique"). For optimal detection of longitudinal defects on the external and internal surfaces the position of the probes can be adjusted to match the pipe dimensions (diameter and wall thick-

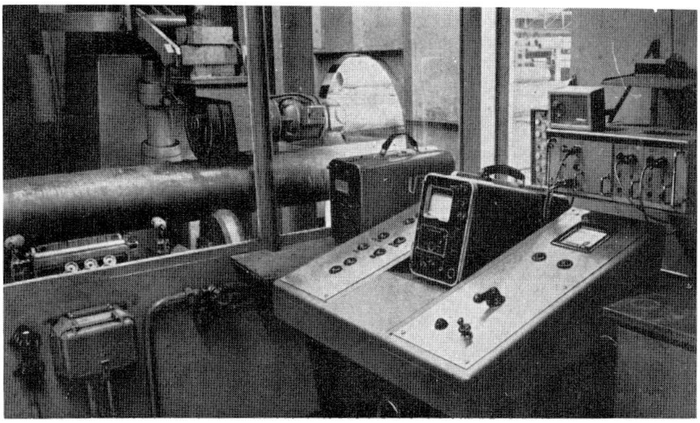

Fig. 3.142 Testing thick-walled, seamless pipes at Phoenix-Rheinrohr AG., Düsseldorf.

ness). Flaw indications actuate a marking device by means of a monitor. Pipes with diameters between 130 and 620 mm can be tested by this device. The maximum surface speed is 1.5 m/s and the feed can be adjusted to 100 mm/revolution maximally. In another testing installation (Fig. 3.143) – with a similar spiral feed of the pipe – pipe probes are used which are coupled to the pipe from the top by flowing water. To be able to attain as high a feed rate per revolution as possible, i.e. maximum

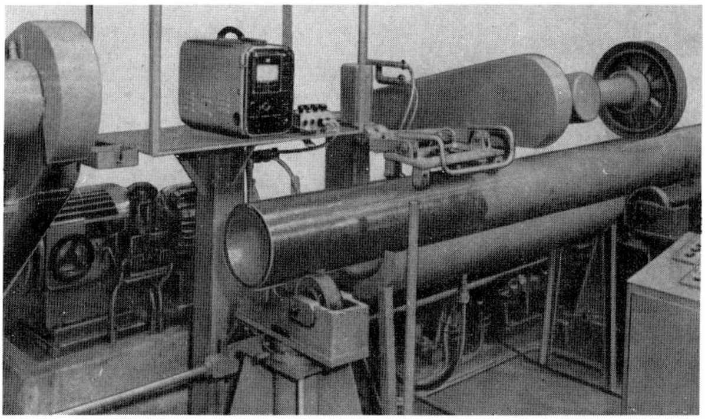

Fig. 3.143 Testing of seamless pipes for extreme-line casings of oil drilling rigs at Mannesmann AG, Düsseldorf.

testing speed with 100% scanning, 4 pipe probes connected in parallel are placed next to each other on the pipe in this installation. In the cylinder testing installation shown in Fig. 3.144 the gas cylinders also go through a spiral motion. A special feature here is the annular suction gap of the pipe probe for discharging excess coupling liquid, which has not only the advantage that after the test the cylinder is almost dry, but also that disturbances of the screen picture by water running down in the form of flickering "grass" are avoided. After filtering, the sucked-off water is recycled to the pump, so that no external water connection is required.

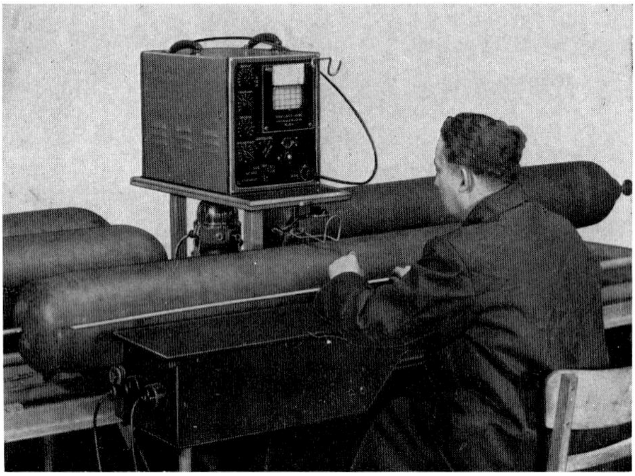

Fig. 3.144 Installation for testing compressed gas cylinders (BV Aral AG, Bochum).

In the above examples the surface of the pipes is pickled, resulting in very uniform coupling if the probes are hinged so that they can adapt themselves to any eccentricities. Gas cylinders which are returned after long use covered with rust marks and old layers of paint, are sand-blasted prior to the test and detached from their base. In all the examples mentioned above the wear of the probes is reduced by supports of hardened steel or hard metal.

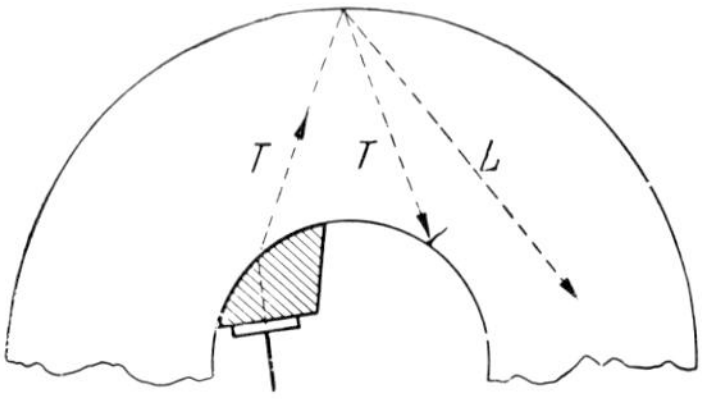

Fig. 3.145 Testing of pipes with very thick walls from the inside.

Where pipes cannot be tested from the outside or where this is not practical, e.g. on ribbed pipes with welded-on cooling fins, or drilled pipes with conical (gun barrels) or eccentric external surface, the test can also be carried out from the inside. A construction made by Sperry for testing gun barrels for internal cracks [337] uses the same device which is used for boring the barrel, the cutter being replaced by a special probe which is moved through the rotating barrel. Flaw echoes which are returned from the internal wall in accordance with their transit time, are classified by a monitor and recorded.

Purely transverse zig-zag waves can be used for internal testing only as long as $d < 0.2$ O.D. In the case of pipes with thicker walls, the transverse wave transmitted by the probe is split according to Fig. 3.145 into a weaker transverse and a longitudinal wave when reflected at the external surface at an angle smaller than 33°. Both wave modes can produce echoes which may complicate the screen picture.

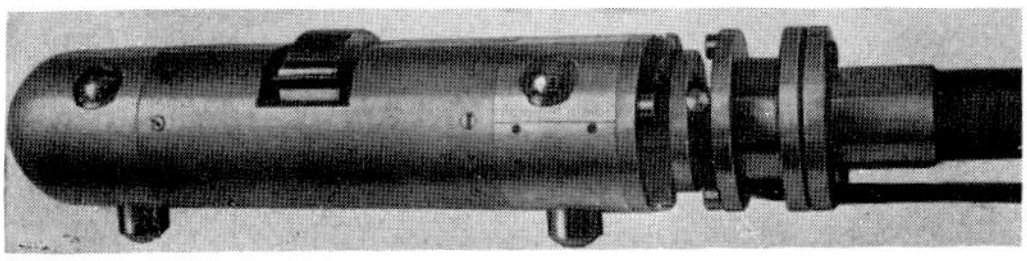

a

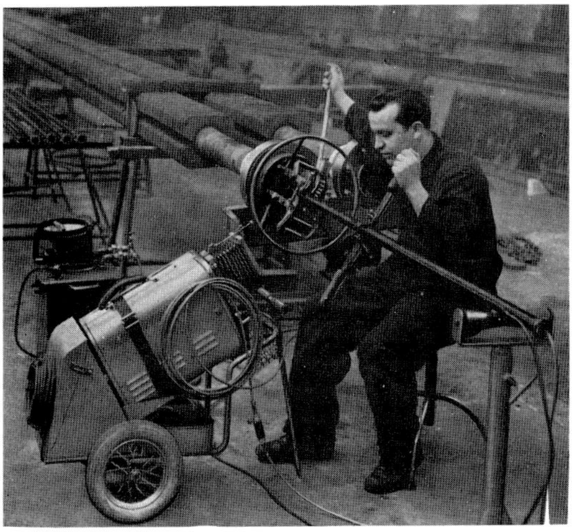

b

Fig. 3.146 Internal pipe probe used for testing hairpin pipes (according to NAGEL, BASF, Ludwigshafen). During the test the examiner actuates a probe guiding device which at the same time rotates the probe holder mounted on a rod, which may be up to 15 m long, around the axis of the pipe and which shifts it through a distance equal to the width of the probe each time.

Fig. 3.146 shows such an internal pipe probe for crack detection and its application for testing dismantled high-pressure ribbed pipes (hairpin pipes) used in the chemical industry. When combined with a normal beaming transducer these devices can also be used for measuring wall thicknesses from the inside.

The pipe probe can also be used on *medium pipes* (diameter 50 to 120 mm) by applying the same testing method. Pipe manufacturers furthermore make increasing use of the immersion technique. When medium pipes are tested by means of the pipe probe, the interfering echoes produced by the probe and the reference echo occupy too much space on the CR screen in relation to the total pipe circumference. To reduce both echoes preference is given to 4 MHz probes as against the usual 2 MHz probes provided the surface condition does not result in too much "grass" on the CR screen.

In addition to the testing installations which have been described for thick pipes, other types have been developed, covering the entire range of thick and medium pipes. One of them uses two angle probes connected in parallel to an instrument and coupled to the pipe as shown in Fig. 3.147. This produces a reference echo, as in the case of the pipe probe, with flaw indications travelling across the CR screen while the pipe is being fed with a helical motion. The angle probes are exchangeable; a pair of probes is chosen which furnishes for each pipe size (pipe diameter and wall thickness) the most suitable beaming angle. The positions of the flaws are marked with colour. Fig. 3.148 shows such an installation.

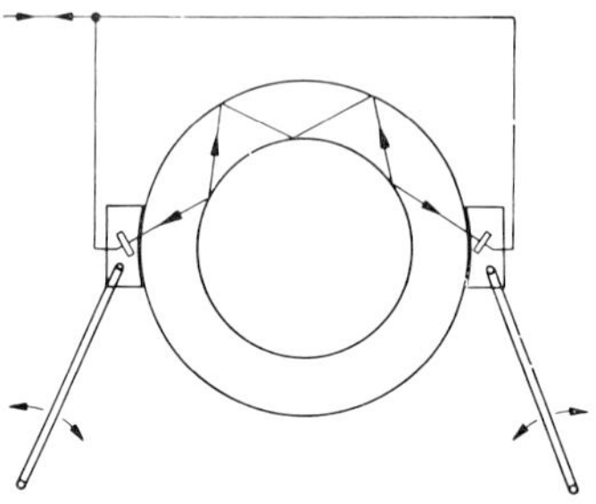

Fig. 3.147 Pipe test with 2 angle probes connected in parallel.

An installation, which has been given the name "ATLAS", was designed by Stewarts and Lloyds Ltd., Department of Research and Technical Development, Corby/U.K. (Fig. 3.149 [138]). It has four probes

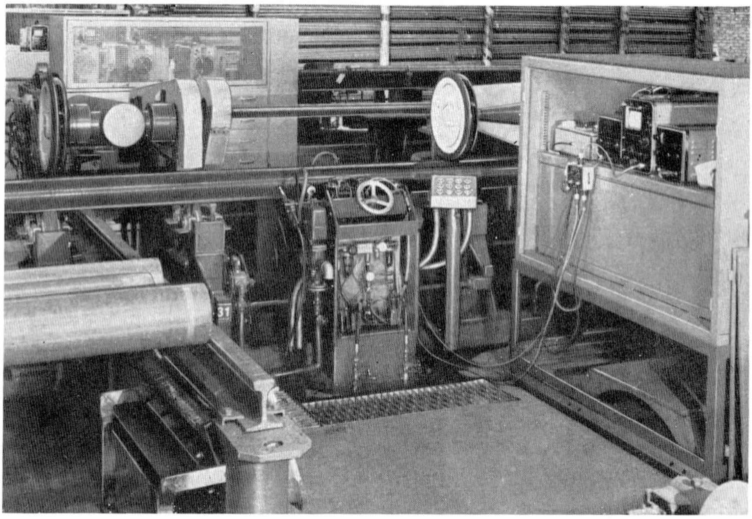

Fig. 3.148 Pipe testing installation with 2 angle probes connected in parallel (works photo Bous Saar, design Krautkrämer, model RSK 400).

transposed 90°, which rotate at a maximum speed of 150 rpm around the rectilinearly moving pipe. The guide shoes and probes, which are coupled by a water gap, are pressed against the specimen by compressed air. In the same test as for longitudinal cracks, the wall thickness is measured by the counting method (2.352), and laminations are revealed (Fig. 3.149). Incorporated in the same testing installation is also an electromagnetic diameter gauge which transmits a signal if the set tolerance limit is exceeded. A multigraph recorder records the testing

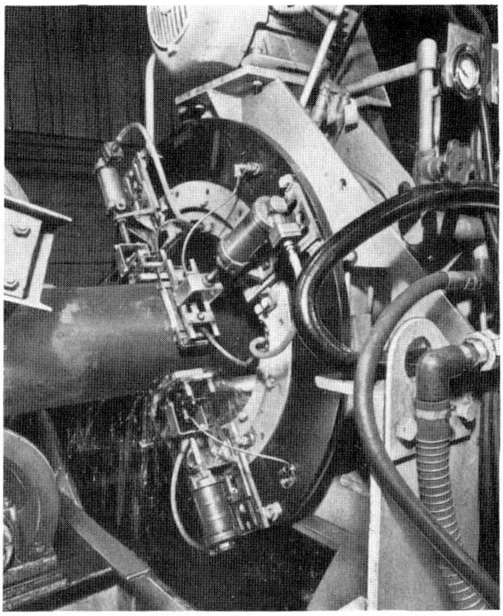

a

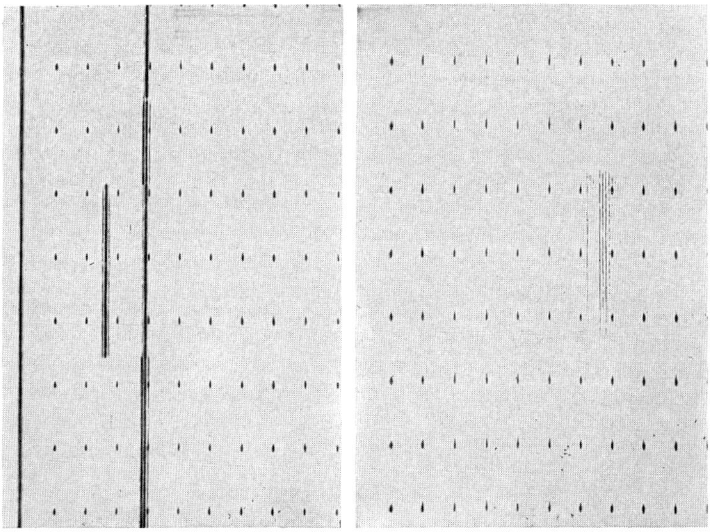

b

Fig. 3.149 Pipe testing installation "ATLAS" for pipes up to 450 mm diameter, using revolving probes (works photo Stewarts and Lloyds, U.K.). a) Probe array for longitudinal defects, wall thickness and laminations; b) recording of wall thickness (left, B-scan) and laminations (right, C-scan with evolution of pipe shell).

and measuring results by an electrochemical method. Longitudinal defects and laminations are presented as an evolution of the pipe shell by an array of 100 recording pens (C-Scan). A second array of 100 pens records the thickness variations.

Small pipes in the range from 25 to 50 mm O.D. are tested by hand with a miniature pipe probe for 4 MHz (Fig. 3.140, left). Also used are

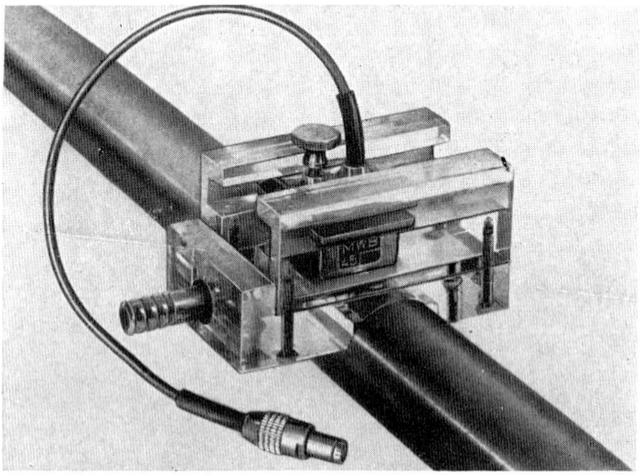

Fig. 3.150 Miniature angle probe for 4 MHz with pipe testing saddle for contact test on pipes of about 10 to 40 mm diameter.

small angle probes with contact face ground to match the pipe. Small angle probes fitted with a perspex shoe are furthermore used for production tests on new pipes of these diameters (see Fig. 3.150 "pipe testing saddle"). The contact face of the saddle matches the pipe. In this device the probe is coupled with a little oil to the internal flat face of the saddle and adjusted by trial and error on a test tube until a given flaw is clearly indicated. The beaming angle of the probe of approx. 45° is no longer important because the entrance angle of the beam can be changed as required by shifting the probe. At the test point the saddle provides only a short length of contact and does not touch the pipe at any other point along the circumference to avoid damping the wave.

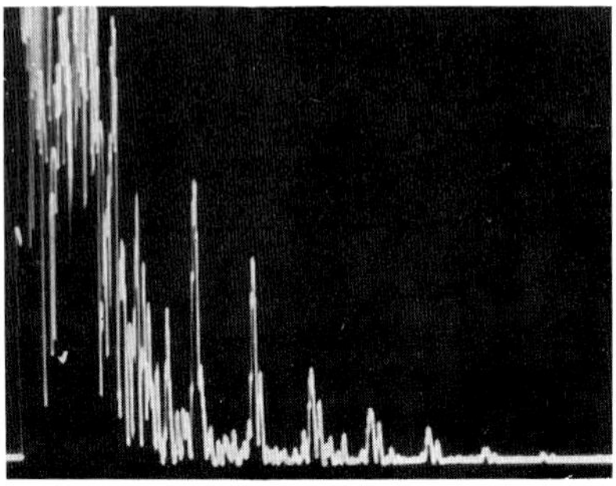

Fig. 3.151 Screen trace obtained with the device shown in Fig. 3.150 on a pipe of 15 × 3 mm containing an incipient crack. If the pipe is rotated, the sequence of flaw echoes moves and can thus readily be distinguished from stationary interfering echoes.

If the pipe is very smooth, the wave circles it many times producing no reference echo. Any flaw, however, produces an echo at every cycle.

Where the flaw echo, owing to trailing oscillations of the probe, cannot yet be observed during the first cycle, this will definitely be the case during the next cycles. In the case of incipient cracks a whole sequence of flaw echoes can frequently be observed (Fig. 3.151) which, if the pipe is rotated, are readily distinguished from any stationary interfering echoes as travelling echoes. Flaws are indicated automatically by a monitor. The test piece should contain an internal and an external flaw, so that it is possible to check whether only the external flaw is not perhaps indicated merely by surface waves. The detection of internal flaws at equal sensitivity is usually a little difficult.

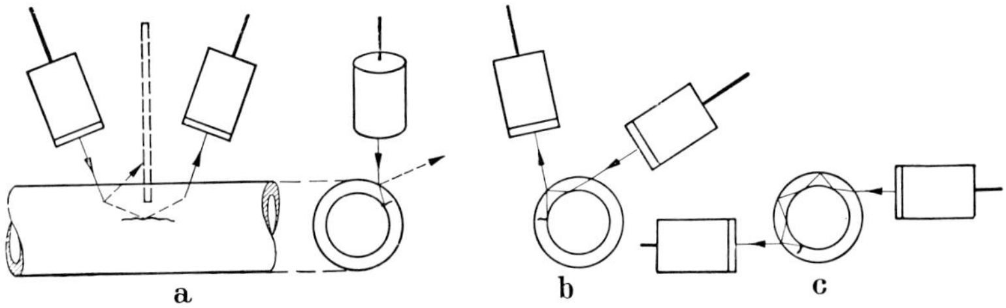

Fig. 3.152 Pipe testing by the immersion technique with separate transmitter and receiver, a) according to TERRY, b) and c) according to ZÖLLMER and GRABENDÖRFER.

It is precisely the range of the small pipes which includes a large portion of the boiler tubes and precision tubes where rapid and economic testing of large quantities constitutes the main problem. Here the immersion technique applied on a large scale has emerged as the main testing method. In order to avoid direct reflections from the surface of the pipe when oblique beaming is used in the immersion technique, separate transmitting and receiving probes are usually used. If a common probe is used as transmitter and receiver, – especially if the pipe is not very smooth – the entrance echo is broadened excessively by the echoes of boundary waves resulting from insignificant scratches, thus masking any flaw echoes. Fig. 3.152 shows some of the probe assemblies used with separate transmitter and receiver. According to a suggestion by TERRY ([399] and a private communication) (Fig. 3.152a) the probes are inclined towards each other but at the same time displaced out of the plane of the pipe axis. This prevents waves reflected homologously on the surface reaching the receiver. In the case of rough surfaces a soundproof partition which tightly borders to the pipe, has proved effective as an additional precaution. According to another suggestion by ZÖLLMER and GRABENDÖRFER [126] (Fig. 3.152b, c) the two probes are arranged in a plane normal to the pipe axis but making equal angles in the same direction relative to the radius at the point of reflection. The adjustment of the probes, particularly in the case of different pipe diameters, becomes very simple if the axes of the probes are parallel, e.g. horizontal, so that they need only be shifted vertically without changing their angles. Usually, two such probe systems are mounted one close behind the other in the longitudinal direction of the specimen, the circling direction of the sound is then opposite in both planes. Both the internal and external spills are in this way covered reliably during one test run because the sound beam of the one testing system always strikes the spill from the side most favourable for reflection.

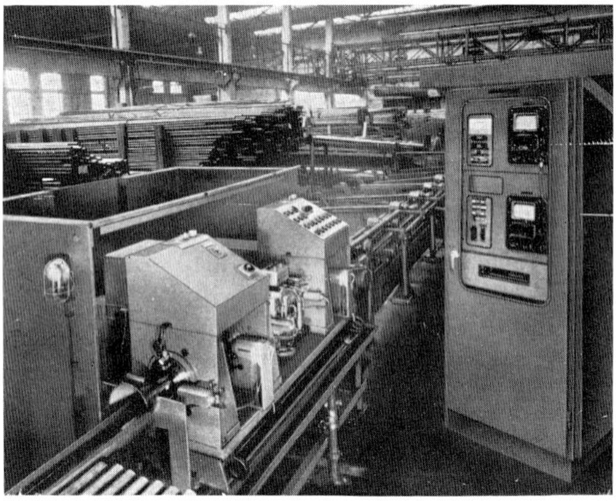

Fig. 3.153 Revolving testing installation for pipes of up to 50 mm diameter – System Reisholz-Krautkrämer – with guiding device (works photo Messrs. Hoesch-Rohrwerke, Hiltrup/Westphalia).

For practical continuous testing the immersion technique is applied in two variants: in one the pipe is fed in a spiral motion through a so-called "transit testing tank" in which the correctly adjusted probes mounted in a holder ride on the pipe; in the other version the necessary helical relative motion between pipe and probe assembly is realized by rotating the latter around the pipe which merely carries out a rectilinear motion. While in the first case the maximum revolving speed, assuming normal pipe lengths of 6 to 18 m, is about 600 rpm, the second arrangement permits considerably higher speed of up to 3000 rpm. At 100% scanning this allows testing speeds of approximately 4 m/min in the first case and 20 m/min in the second case. Fig. 3.127, p. 341, shows a testing installation with transit tank which can also be used for testing pipes. Fig. 3.153 on the other hand shows a "rotating tube tester" (system "Reisholz-Krautkrämer").

In the case of the first mentioned testing installation where the probe holder rides on the pipe while submerged in the transit tank, accurate maintenance of the chosen probe position as determined by tests on a sample tube is ensured automatically during the entire test because the probe holder can follow every motion of the pipe. In the rotating testing installation, the rotating probe assembly is coupled much more loosely to the pipe which passes through it; careful centering of the pipe is therefore essential to ensure that the geometrical relations are maintained as accurately as possible. The specimens are centered in the testing equipment automatically by means of specially designed guiding devices (Fig. 3.153). In spite of this special precaution, the flaw detectability for routine testing realizable with riding probes, is greater. The higher testing speed of the rotating testing installation is thus achieved at the cost of slightly lower testing accuracy.

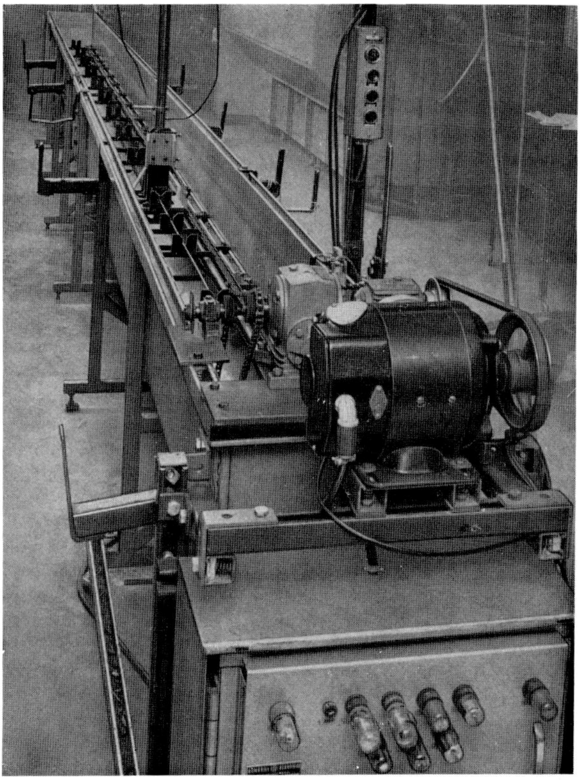

Fig. 3.154 Equipment for testing thin pipes by immersion technique (Oak Ridge National Laboratory, USA).

Thin pipes below 25 mm O.D. are almost invariably tested by the immersion technique. Only when pipes which are already installed are checked does it become necessary to use matched miniature angle probes or the pipe testing saddle. Guiding the probes by hand is, in view of the dimensions involved, difficult in both cases because no reference echo is available for checking the coupling which, especially in the case of unfavourable space conditions, would be particularly important for maintenance. The only remedy in these circumstances is a liberal application of couplant and great experience.

As previously mentioned, the immersion technique for testing pipes in its various forms is used for routine tests by the manufacturer or as an acceptance test by the consumer. As far as bright, drawn high-quality pipes of these dimensions are concerned, the rotating testing installation, as already described for small pipes, is used. The 4 MHz probes rigidly installed in the rotating testing blocks are then fitted with a cast-on lens which focuses the sound beam to improve the flaw detectability.

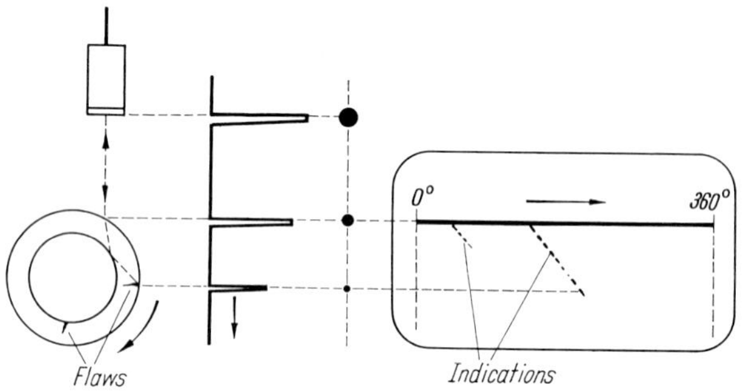

Fig. 3.155 Pipe test by the immersion technique with flaw indication according to OLIVER.

Special problems are posed by the testing of thin-walled special-purpose pipes as used in reactor construction. Very high demands are made in respect of the quality of such pipes; defects as shallow as 0.03 to 0.05 mm must be found. This in turn requires very exact placing of the probes relative to the pipe to attain this high testing accuracy.

Fig. 3.154 shows an installation for testing reactor (fuel element) tubes [278] where the tubes, measuring 5×0.6 mm and larger, are completely immersed in a long tank and rotated, a probe scanning the tube while at the same time being guided by it. As shown in Fig. 3.155 the probe is slightly off-centre in order to obtain the desired beaming angle. If required, a thin sound beam is obtained by masking part of a broader beam, to suppress multiple echoes of perpendicularly incident waves from the wall, and also boundary waves at angles which are too large. The tubes are sealed on both ends to prevent the entrance of water, resulting in both greater range and greater sensitivity of the waves propagated in the wall of the tubes. An interesting feature is the display on a long-persistence screen of TV dimensions (Fig. 3.156). Entrance and flaw echoes are recorded by luminous spots with vertical time base which, during each rotation of the tube, travels once from left to right across the CR screen. The entrance echo produces a bright horizontal line from which flaw echoes, depending on the size of the flaws, emerge as oblique branches of varying brightness and length. Fig. 3.156 shows the screen picture of a 6 × 0.6 mm tube containing a large, external incipient crack 0.2 mm deep, and 3 small incipient cracks on the inside approximately 0.04 mm deep. This sensitivity is realized by means of a 5 MHz lithium sulphate probe. At 240 rpm the testing speed is approximately 1.5 m/min.

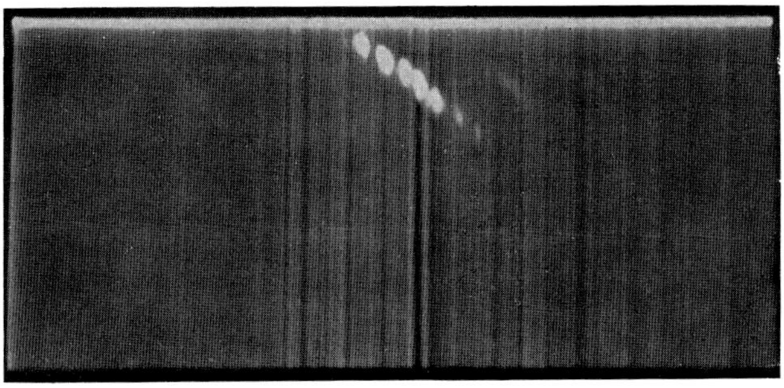

Fig. 3.156 Screen picture with flaw indication using the method of Fig. 3.155, showing four different cracks in a 6 × 0.6 mm tube, according to OLIVER et al. [278].

In another installation for the same testing problem (Fig. 3.157) the tubes are passed through the testing tank in a spiral motion. The tank contains four probes (4 MHz, with focused beam) in two testing planes according to Fig. 3.152c, arranged in such a way that the sound waves rotate in two planes in opposite directions. An additional probe during the same test run continuously measures and records the thickness of the

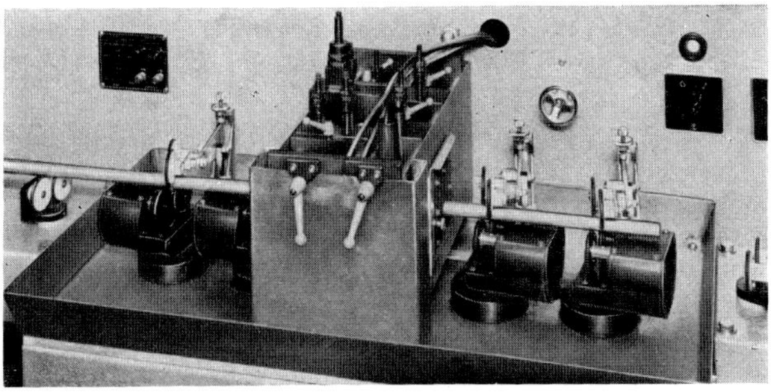

Fig. 3.157 Testing tank and device for helical feed of thin-walled canning tubes (design Krautkrämer).

tube wall according to the resonance method in the immersion technique (see Sec. 2.12). This installation permits a maximum testing speed of 4 m/min at the required 100% check.

Finally, very thin tubes (2 × 0.25 mm) are reported to have been tested according to [284] with 1 MHz angle probes in the longitudinal direction, which presumably resulted in waves similar to rod waves being excited in the longitudinal direction. In this way flaws extending in the circumferential direction, as well as holes and notches could be indicated satisfactorily by the echo method. Whether this also permits detection of longitudinal defects such as cracks is not yet known.

3.27 Castings

Here flaw detection almost exclusively concerns manufacturing defects such as shrinkage cavities and blow holes (the former with coarse, jagged, the latter with smooth surface, in smaller dimensions also as pores and porosity), furthermore inclusions (usually sand or slag) and cracks (caused by internal stresses during cooling while already solidified). Pure segregations are detected very rarely and then only by indirect means. If, in exceptional cases, a casting has to be checked for fatigue cracks, the testing technique, as in the case of forgings, mainly depends on the stresses because they determine the possible position of the flaw.

This discussion furthermore will be limited to shaped castings. Ingots have already been dealt with under forgings, and large sand castings or chill castings, such as hammers for heavy forging presses (steel casting) or pile drivers (steel or cast iron) can be tested like ingots, i.e. with normal probes at low frequency.

In the case of shaped castings ultrasonic testing methods are used, for instance to assist in the design of a new casting by quickly locating regularly occurring defects in a series of trial castings so as to be able to improve the position, number and size of sprues and risers, and furthermore for piece tests. The latter can be omitted once sound casting methods have been developed.

A number of circumstances limit ultrasonic testing in the case of shaped castings:

1. Often the shape of the surface is too complex, which on the one hand makes coupling difficult, and on the other hand is time-consuming, especially since automation is hardly possible.

2. The surface quality in the cast state is mostly unsuitable, while for economic reasons, any improvement by working is possible only to a limited extent.

3. The structure is more or less coarse-grained, causing strong attenuation of the sound in the case of anisotropic material. In addition, the structure mostly varies from the periphery to the centre, as well as between thin and thick-walled parts of the specimen. This impairs the flaw detectability.

4. Economic considerations play a considerable role because the costs of the test become too high compared with the low manufacturing costs

and because on the other hand the stresses to which the castings are subjected usually are not so critical as to induce the consumer to pay a higher price for tested pieces.

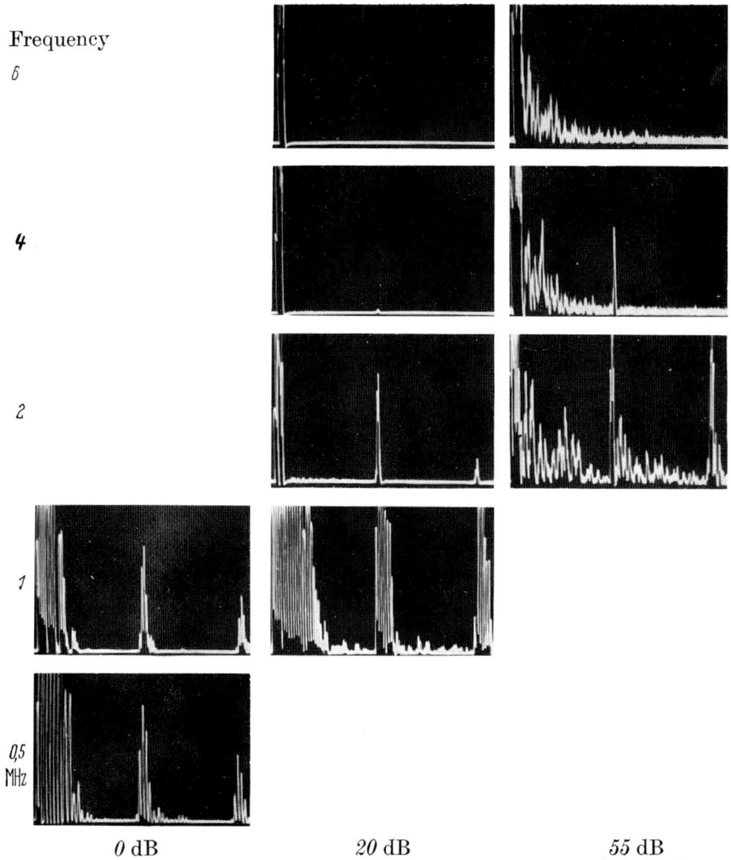

Fig. 3.158 Test on cast iron of thickness 100 mm (ASTM 3-4) at different frequencies and gain. All probes have been adjusted to the same echo height of a 30 mm steel plate at 0 dB gain. At 0,5 and 1 MHz the attenuation is of no consequence: also on cast iron a full backwall echo is obtained at 0 dB, but with 2 MHz only at 20 dB, with 4 MHz only at 55 dB and with 6 MHz none at all. At identical gain (55 dB) the scatter with 2, 4 and 6 MHz is remarkably constant. The difficulty of testing cast iron thus arises from the attenuation and not from the scattering. With 0.5 and 1 MHz the interference zone of 50 and 40 mm, respectively, prevents flaw detection near the surface; remedy: TR probe, see Fig. 2.43.

For these reasons smaller mass-produced pieces are practically excluded a priori. What remains are mostly components for heavy machinery, e.g. rolls, casings, crank shafts and heavy pipe fittings.

Defects which penetrate to the surface can usually be detected more cheaply by magnetic or penetration tests, or even by the naked eye, so that chiefly only internal defects in expensive specimens remain for ultrasonic testing.

Basically, the demand made for the absence of flaws in the testing of castings, cannot be as high as for worked components because the small shrinkage cavities and pores which are always present, produce some "grass" and small individual echoes even at 2 MHz. The acceptable limit can be determined by cutting a specimen.

In the case of thicker specimens flaws close to the surface are easily over-estimated if a backwall echo of full scale height, as normally used, is obtained by a forced higher gain (overdriving). As shown in Fig. 3.158, a frequency optimal in respect of the thickness should be chosen (here 2 MHz) which requires only moderate gain. It should not be overlooked that the phenomenon in which scatter echoes at low frequency hardly interfere at all depends less on the fact that the wave length in this case is large compared with

a
b
c

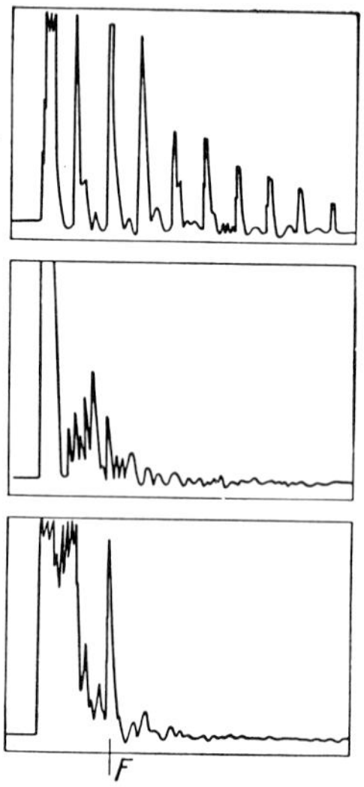

d

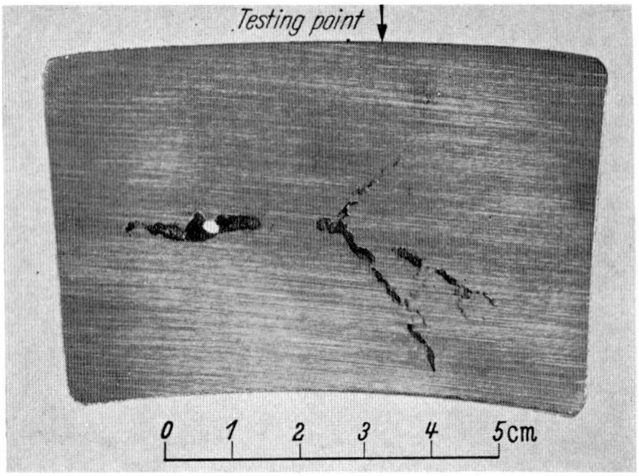

Fig. 3.159 Test on 50 mm cast steel. a) and b) screen pictures with 2 MHz, normal test at sound and flawed points, respectively; c) at flaw with 45° angle test; d) cut section of flaw showing testing point. Screen traces copied by drawing (Sulzer Bros., Winterthur).

the scatter centres (graphite flakes in cast iron), but rather that a considerably lower gain suffices to penetrate the specimen. The main role is therefore played by the attenuation. With equal gain (referred to the reference plate) the scatter interferences in Fig. 3.158 change remarkably little between 2 and 6 MHz. Quantitative evaluation of flaw echoes in castings requires a calibrated gain control, so as to be able to compensate for the attenuation.

Frequently the influence of the shape of the surface can be reduced by a design which is more suitable from the point of view of testing, e.g. by making provision for flat contact faces at certain strategic points. There the surface can then also be improved without much cost by grinding. Alternatively, testing surfaces which can be considered are first of all those which have to be machined in any case, flanges, bearings, etc. By applying normal or angle probes to such surfaces one tries to cover as large a volume as possible, particularly e.g. cross-sectional transitions between the flange and the wall on a fitting where shrinkage cavities and cracks may occur. At such improved contact faces it will also be possible to deduce the size of given flaws from the echo height, which in the case of unworked surfaces is usually impossible. Where no backwall echo for comparison is available, a plate

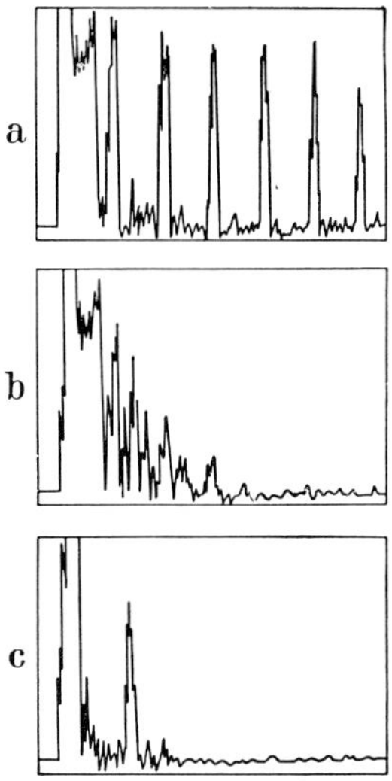

d

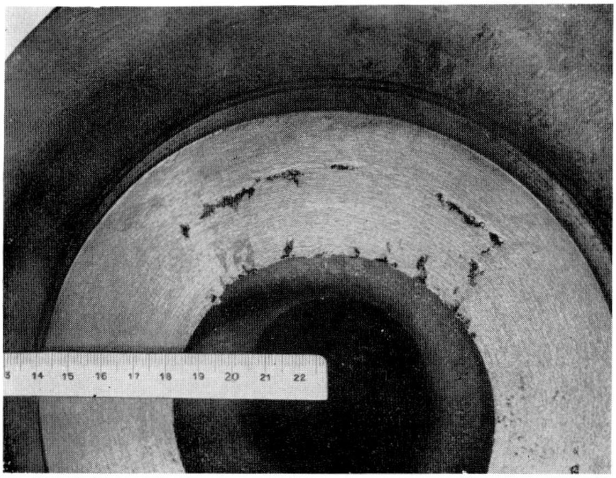

Fig. 3.160 Testing 40 mm spheroidal cast iron with rough surface. a) and b) screen traces with 2 MHz, normal testing at sound and flawed point, respectively; c) 45° angle test with 2 MHz at flawed point; d) flawed area cut open (Sulzer Bros., Winterthur).

made of the same material and with a similar surface can be used.

In the case of uneven, irregular and unworked surfaces one has to fall back mainly on a backwall echo, so that reliable statements can only be made for shell-like specimens which permit mapping the large flaw areas on the surface. The reduction of the backwall echo can be used for this purpose or better still that of its multiple echoes (Figs. 3.159 and 3.160). If both surfaces are even, although rough, any localized strong attenuation can then only be caused by flaws. Evaluation on the basis of the flaw echoes *alone* is usually unreliable because of the unfavourable shape and orientation of the casting defects: a jagged shrinkage cavity can produce echoes similar to those of a number of separate smaller pores. However, both types of defects can in certain circumstances be distinguished with the aid of the backwall echo, which in the latter case will be less suppressed. No flaw echoes at all may be obtained if a shrinkage cavity is located in an area of high porosity, i. e. sponginess, which absorbs the sound completely. Finally, the rough surfaces produce long interfering zones of the probes compared with the usual wall thicknesses of a few centimetres in which flaw echoes frequently get lost, so that one can work only with backwall echoes, or use a TR probe.

Very simple are tests on steel castings (Fig. 3.159) and spheroidal cast iron (Fig. 3.160) where even transverse zig-zag waves can be used to advantage. This permits faster testing than with normal probes because a given flaw can already be recognized from some distance by its travelling echo which contrasts with the interfering background of the structure and surface indications. On less transmissive material the use of 1 MHz transverse waves is recommended. Attention is drawn to the dependence of the beaming angle on the material (see 2.332, Table 2.1). For instance, perspex as wedge material is no longer suitable when scanning thin-walled cast iron with flat zig-zag waves. Here soft rubber proved useful in one particular case. By slightly pressing on the applied probe, it was furthermore possible to change the angle of the rubber wedge.

A difficult problem arises when castings have to be machined and small shrinkage cavities and pores may be cut open, while at greater depth such defects are of no consequence. This makes it necessary to find small shrinkage cavities and sand-spots and to determine their distance from the surface to within a few millimetres. This applies, for instance, to glazing rolls for paper manufacture whose surface must be completely free of defects, and also to toothed rims. It will hardly be possible to penetrate the material working from the back with frequencies of e.g. 4 to 5 MHz which on the other hand are necessary for locating such small flaws, and which moreover would only determine the position of the back of the defect farthest from the surface to be machined. The test is therefore made from the front using a TR probe, after preliminary tests have confirmed that the quality of the unworked surface permits this. The scanning of large areas will always remain a very time-consuming procedure.

How successful the detection of flaws can be even on coarse-laminar and thicker cast iron if TR probes and lower frequencies (2 or 1 MHz) are used has already been shown in Fig. 2.43. Generally the success or otherwise of tests on castings largely depends on the probe used. In diffi-

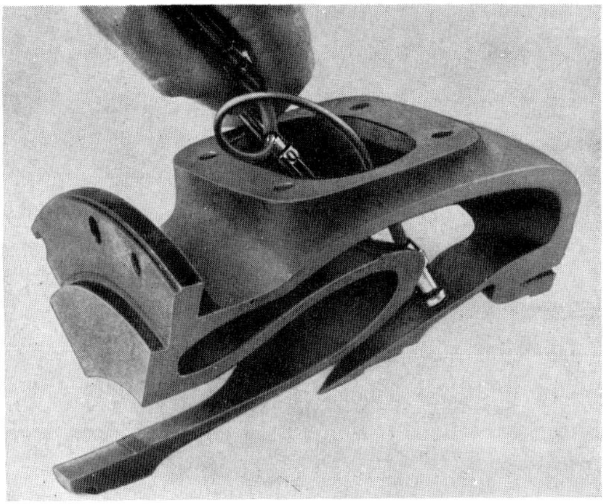

a

cult cases it is therefore recommended that different frequencies and probe designs be tried out. Since precisely here contradictory requirements are specified for the probes, e.g. small contact face, high sensitivity and resistance to wear on rough surfaces, and low frequency with short pulses, special designs will be the answer such as e.g. a 5 mm lithium sulphate probe with 4 MHz and a protective layer for wall thickness measurements on thin-walled cast-iron casings (Fig. 3.161), which are mounted in a special holder to facilitate tests at inside points difficult of access. As shown by the screen picture, both the sensitivity and the power of resolution are adequate for measuring wall thicknesses of less than 6 mm.

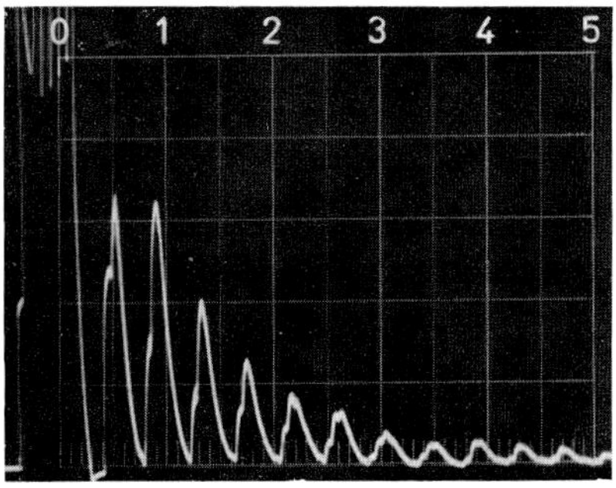

b

Fig. 3.161 Wall thickness measurement on complex, thin-walled iron castings, CR screen picture calibrated on 50 mm cast iron. Measured value 4.2 mm.

Results of wall thickness measurements made in practice on cast iron liners for motors of Diesel locomotives have been reported [260]. Since these measurements can only be made from inside the liner, special probe guiding devices must be used in view of the limited space available for testing. The measurements are made both with a normal probe of 5 mm diameter and with TR probes with matching contact shoes.

On castings one occasionally also uses the intensity method with sound transmission, either pulsed or continuous, instead of the pulse-echo method. This is indicated particularly where no echo can be obtained because of excessive attenuation. A simple calculation, or a glance at Table 10 in the Appendix, shows that at an attenuation of 300×10^{-3} dB/mm and 200 mm path one obtains an amplitude of 0.1%, but at 100 mm path 30 times greater, viz. 3%. (A very frequent mistake made is to "think" linearly instead of logarithmically, i.e. to expect only double the amplitude.) For instance, it was possible in this way to detect on a very thick-walled bell of cast bronze, areas with pronounced shrinkage cavities by using separate 1 MHz probes on the inside and outside with pulsed sound transmission, and to determine solid areas serving as striking points for the bell hammer; this would have been impossible with the echo method.

Pulsed sound transmission is also used in an installation for testing cast uranium plates [39] (approximately 18×180 mm cross-section, and up to a few metres long) with the immersion technique. The pair of probes is moved under water in a zig-zag path and the transmitted echo amplitude is recorded on Alfax paper by a spiral recorder in the form of a go/no-go recording.

Finally, the influence of the casting method and of the material which will be discussed in detail in 3.3, may be briefly mentioned. Both factors can influence the testability decisively. Experience has shown that castings of light metal, unalloyed and slightly alloyed steel, as well as spheroidal cast iron castings, can be tested also if cast in sand or moulds, provided an unfavourable shape and position of the casting do not result in porosity or a particularly coarse grain [346, 352]. In the case of the pronounced anisotropic copper alloys, the testability is nevertheless influenced by the grain size to such an extent that as a rule they cannot be tested if cast in sand or moulds, but surprisingly easily if produced by centrifugal casting, e.g. brass, aluminium bronze, red brass and German silver [347]. In the case of cast iron the main factor of influence is not the grain size but the length of the graphite flakes. Since the strength is inversely proportional to the length of these flakes, experience has shown that grades below 20 kg/mm^2 can no longer be tested. Finally, austenitic manganese steel castings as well as high-alloyed, acid and heat resistant chrome-nickel and manganese steels can usually not be tested even if produced by centrifugal casting.

The fact that a simple designation of the material, e.g. brass, even if accompanied by data concerning the chemical composition and the type of structure, does not permit any prediction concerning the testability in the absence of any additional data on the grain size or at least the casting method, will be elucidated by a brief calculation. The attenuation increases with the third power of the grain size; a three times greater mean grain size thus increases the coefficient of attenuation 27 times, e.g. from 10 to approximately 300. If these two values are looked up in Table 10, it will be found that backwall echoes of 80% and 0.1%, respectively, can be expected from a depth of 100 mm. From a practical point of view this means that in the first case the specimen can be tested very well, but in the latter not at all, unless lower frequencies can be used.

3.28 Welded joints

3.281 Butt-welded Joints

The following types of manufacturing defects can be detected in welded butt joints by ultrasonics: slag inclusions, pores, lack of fusion (cold shuts), lack of penetration (root defects, undercutting), cracks (longitudinal or transverse cracks, depending on their orientation relative to the seam).

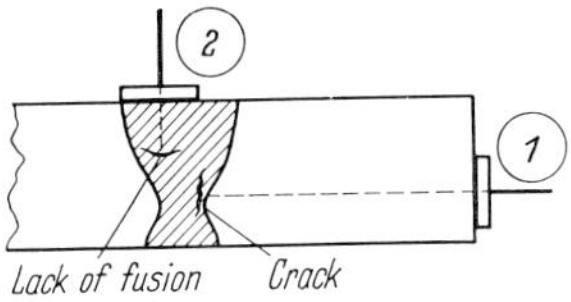

Fig. 3.162 Testing of welded joint with normal probes.

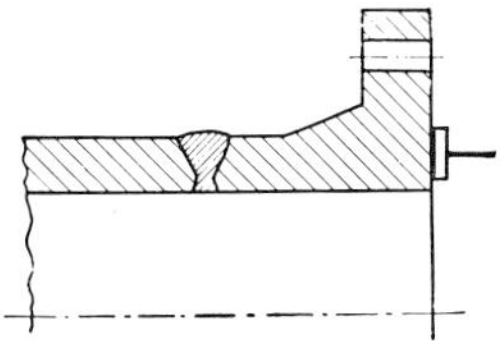

Fig. 3.163 Testing a circumferential pipe weld from the welded-on flange.

3.281.1 Testing Method, General. Obvious testing methods as shown in Fig. 3.162 with normal probes are rarely possible. Examples are flash butt welds on turned components, joining flanges to pipes or fittings (Fig. 3.163), or joining forgings (Fig. 3.164). The testing direction ② in Fig. 3.162 with direct contact on the "ground" joint is, for most defects, less useful than ①, particularly for cracks and flaws close to the surface. When testing takes place in direction according to ① in thin cross-sections interference from the walls can be expected, resulting in the splitting off of transverse waves and reduced sensitivity for defects close to one of the two surfaces.

The example illustrated in Fig. 3.164 [266] shows also how an otherwise insoluble testing problem can be solved very elegantly by a form specially modified for the test. The machined 60° reflection face (see 3.134) produces a transverse wave exactly in the direction of the critical root zone which is inaccessible from inside the specimen.

As a rule the intensity method cannot be used for butt joints and fillet welds because the dimensions of the flaws are unfavourably small in relation to the distance between probes. An exception occurs in cases where the probes for directed radiation in the pulse-echo method cannot be positioned because of their larger contact face and the small and complex shape of the specimen concerned. An example was the weld in a valve shown in Fig. 2.9. The non-directional, radiated sound energy is propagated by a mixture of wave modes and is guided away between the walls. Large defects reduce the transmittance along the propagation path.

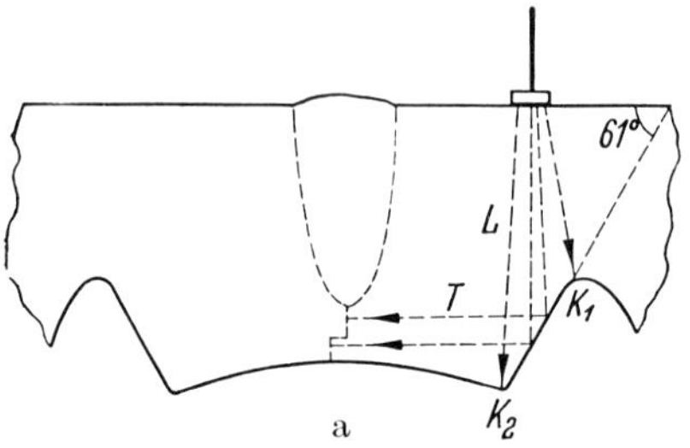

For butt-welded joints of plates and pipes the pulse-echo method

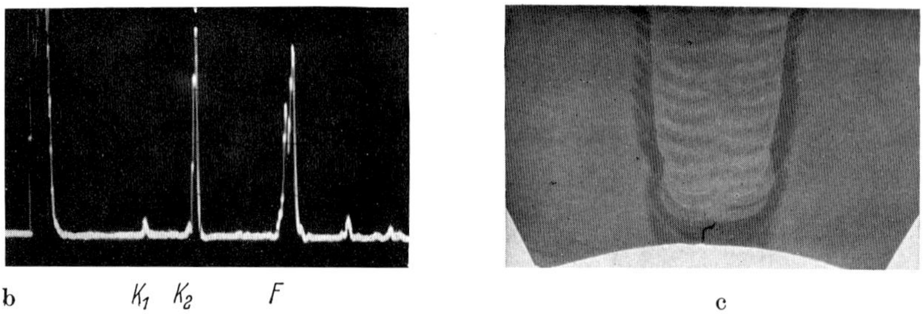

Fig. 3.164 Testing a welded joint on an assembled turbine rotor (Brown-Boveri, Baden, Switzerland) as suggested by BRUTSAERT. a) Cross-section and sound path. The stepped seat should be welded through; b) screen trace with split flaw echo F which shows that a portion of both faces of the step remains unwelded (observe double echo). The echoes K_1 and K_2 are produced by the edge of the reflection face; c) ground section showing flaw found.

using zig-zag transverse waves (Fig. 3.165) chiefly comes into consideration, the reflections between the two surfaces of the plate being utilized. A broad beam would cover a joint of low height in one pass. On heavier plates it is, however, necessary to shift the probe at right angles to the joint so as to irradiate successively the entire cross-section. According to Fig. 3.166 a shift of one half to one full skip distance is required, preferably, however, a little more in view of the width of the joint. As a check and for the sake of greater certainty, the test can be repeated from the opposite side as indicated, because some defects are indicated more favourably if irradiated from one direction than from the other. In this way practically all defects are covered, except transverse cracks.

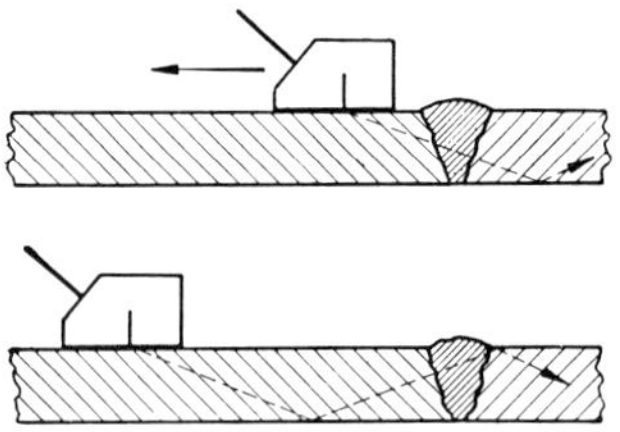

Fig. 3.165 Test of welded joint with zig-zag transverse waves.

As shown in Fig. 3.167a, it is recommended that the reciprocating motion between $s/2$ and s be combined with the longitudinal shift in the form of a zig-zag motion, on to which is superimposed a still more rapid swivelling motion, so as to strike also slightly inclined flaws at favourable angles. If transverse cracks are suspected, the method according to Fig. 3.167 b should be applied. The two angle probes are connected in parallel and mounted in a common holder and need only be shifted along the seam. The point of intersection of their axes is here adjusted to a full skip distance since only the top part of the cross-section of the joint where stress cracks mostly occur because of the greater volume of the weld need be scanned.

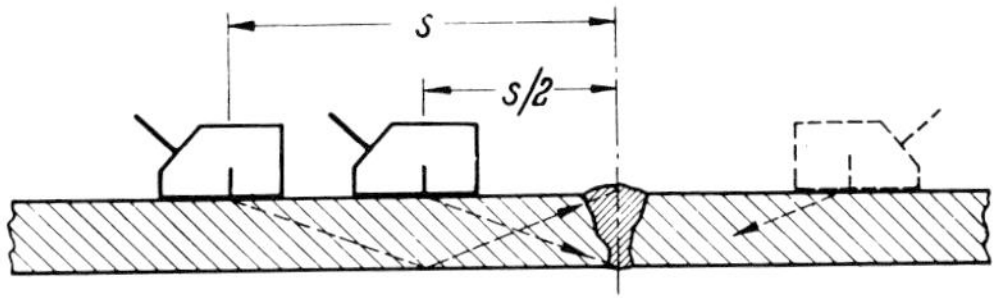

Fig. 3.166 Sound path at half and full skip distance.

Flaw echoes are detected most reliably if the CR screen is observed while simultaneously the probe carries out capering motions, i. e. by applying a dynamic testing method. If the probe is stationary the coupling may accidentally be bad or the beam be incident at an unfavourable angle or miss completely. Only when a flaw echo flashes across the screen is the motion of the probe slowed down for optimal direction finding and distance gauging until a maximum echo is obtained. The scanning can therefore be greatly facilitated by a monitor and alarm device.

If this reciprocating and simultaneous swivelling motion is to be carried out quickly and smoothly, some practice is required so as to loosen the wrist. Excessive pressure on the probe tires the examiner and causes rapid wear of the contact shoe, and if the pressure is one-sided, the shoe will be worn at an angle introducing an unacceptable change in the sound beam.

For simple flaw detection without location a beginner will find it necessary only to mark the distance lines at $s/2$ and s on the plates with chalk, reddle or quick-drying, thin paint. Later these distances will be estimated by eye, especially as it is not necessary to adhere strictly to them.

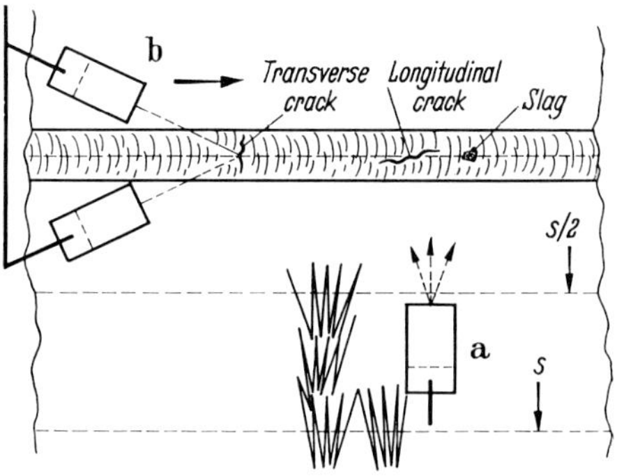

Fig. 3.167 Longitudinal scanning of a weld, a) for all defects excluding transverse cracks, b) for transverse cracks.

If large, plane crack surfaces normal to the plate surface occur in the centre of the weld, as in the case of resistance-welded thick sections or on very thick welded joints, one cannot rely on distinct indications being obtained with only a *single* probe as transmitter and receiver. The pulse is reflected away from the direction of incidence and is then better received with a second probe. For economic testing, this second probe should, however, be mounted in a common holder with the first probe, so that its angle relative to the joint remains correct, and so that if the first probe comes closer to this joint, the second moves the same distance away. Such a device has been described by LACK [212].

Only on old, corroded or paint-covered plate will it be necessary to prepare the surface thoroughly by grinding or sand-blasting. New plate requires at most, cleaning with a steel brush in order to remove a thin film of rust, or a spatula, scraper or similar tool to remove welding spatter. On a horizontal surface it is best to use water for coupling, otherwise oil or paste, particularly on vertical walls and overhead. When water and paste are used it is recommended that the surface be wet a certain distance in advance.

By far the best and most constant coupling in any position, particularly for automatic testing, is obtained with flowing water. The higher consumption of water (from a tap or a raised bucket, a bucket with a small pump or a pressure tank) is almost always worthwhile for longer testing in view of the saving of time for coating, and faster testing.

For checking the coupling it has been proposed to work with two probes facing each other from either side of the joint; these would be connected in parallel as in the case of the twin pipe probe (Fig. 3.138), and therefore would produce a double flaw indication in addition to a (sound transmission) reference echo. Although this arrangement has considerable advantages, it is unsuitable for testing by hand because the required rapid swivelling motions are not possible with this device. Also for slower scanning it requires both hands which in the long run is very tiring [192].

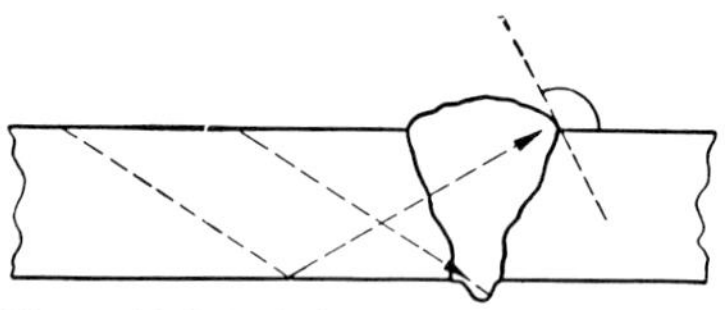

Fig. 3.168 Interfering echoes resulting from excessively steep camber of the bead and from drop formation.

In its simple application it can be expected that the method will be subject to disturbances by laminations and larger inclusions in the plate, thus preventing the beam from being propagated as desired and resulting in echoes which in the absence of at least an approximate fault location as described below, may simulate flaws in the joint. Before starting on the weld, one should therefore make a quick check of the quality of the plate and then select the more favourable of the two sides.

3.281.2 Plate Thickness, Beam Angle and Testing Frequency. The shape of the bead can affect the welding test by interfering echoes from the sharply projecting edges (Fig. 3.168), particularly if the beaming angle is chosen too small. A similar disturbance can be caused by sagging drops. On heavy plate, however, beam angles of 70 and 80° would result in excessive skip distances and much lower sensitivity. As a compromise, one may give the following values:

Plate thickness mm	Beam angle degrees	Skip distance mm
5 to 15	80	55 to 165
15 to 30	70	80 to 165
30 to 60	60	105 to 210
above 60	45	above 120

The use here of the 80° beam angle is controversial. If the shoulder of the bead starts at a sufficiently flat angle, a steeper beam angle is also more favourable here because in general it allows better flaw indication. Interfering echoes produced by the bead can also be tolerated occasionally if the shoulder of the bead and possibly the root can be inspected visually for unfavourable zones, or if the position of the suspected flaw is determined by one of the locating methods described below. In doubtful cases it is recommended that the shoulder or the root of the bead be smoothed at one point with a grinding disc while simultaneously the suspect echo is observed. Echoes from the shoulder of the bead can also be distinguished from true flaw echoes by a check test from the other side of the joint because they are obtained only from one side.

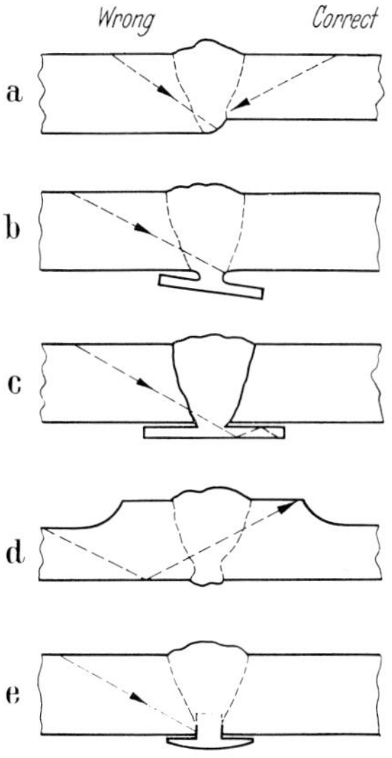

Fig. 3.169 Interfering echoes in the testing of welds, a) displaced plates of different thicknesses; b) and c) backing strip or fitting ring (circumferential welds on pipes); d) welded swaged collar; e) inserted and incompletely fused fitting ring (to be judged as a genuine flaw).

If an echo from the root of a Vee-butt joint is obtained from one side only, it can be suspected that the plates are either slightly displaced or are of unequal thickness (Fig. 3.169 a), e.g. circumferential welds on pipes. The interference then disappears if one tests from the side of the thinner plate. Other interfering echoes according to Figs. 3.169 b, c and d occur if backing strips are used or fitting rings, and in the case of welded swaged collars [137]. Such spurious echoes can usually be interpreted correctly by accurate flaw location. This of course presupposes that the construction and the shape of the joint are known accurately.

Usually a frequency of 2 to 2.5 MHz is chosen; with approximately 1.5 mm wave length this permits detecting flaws of less than 1 mm diameter in steel and aluminium. As a rule much smaller flaws should not be indicated because a weld is rarely completely free of minute pores and inclusions. Occasionally one also uses the handier probes with higher frequencies (4 MHz) which in spite of their smaller contact faces produce a narrower sound beam for propagation distances up to approximately 100 mm. This makes it possible to approach the joint more closely, so that many flaws can already be detected reliably and accurately by the direct beam. Welded joints on pipes of less than 100 mm O.D. are tested in this way down to wall thicknesses of about 5 mm. Such probes also are used for the automated testing of longitudinally or spirally welded pipes (see below). With 4 MHz, beam angles of 70 and even 60° are preferred as against 80°, even more than with 2 MHz, and also on thin walls.

Surprisingly, the cast structure of the joint seldom seems to interfere, except in the case of austenitic welds which even at 2 MHz often produce such strong interferences that they cannot be tested [392]. As far as this type of weld is concerned, it has not yet been established whether the interference indications do not in fact result from microcracks rather than from reflections in the structure, particularly because welds have occasionally been encountered which could be tested without difficulty [285]. This will be difficult to prove because in the cutting up the flaws are easily missed. Furthermore, it has not been established whether the disturbance is caused merely by the austenitic state or simply by the coarse structure of the highly alloyed material of the weld.

With longer propagation paths through the weld, the attenuation already makes itself felt even with ordinary welding and 2 MHz longitudinal waves; e.g. if welded rails are tested, not as in Fig. 3.199, but from the thread with normal probes through the full height of the rail. The attenuation is then revealed by the bottom echo. In the absence of such a reference the attenuation effect is, however, often disregarded. As a precaution, it is therefore always advisable to select a path of minimum length through the welded material.

In the case of plate thinner than 10 mm, reliable detection of smaller defects becomes increasingly difficult because of the interference by the bead unless this interference is avoided as described below (in automated testing). Plate of about 3 mm thickness with a bead projecting about the same distance, can therefore be tested reliably by neither the echo nor the sound-transmission method [379]. Naturally, if the bead is removed there is no such limitation, and plate waves can be used as in the case of sheets. For longitudinally welded pipes the same testing methods as described in the case of pipes apply, including the immersion technique for thin tubes. An example is given by the resistance-welded steel pipes of e.g. 40 to 100 mm diameter and approximately 1 to 3 mm wall thickness, on which the burr has been planed off on both sides. If this results in no sharp edges, however small, remaining, they can readily be tested. Usually, however, this is not the case, particularly on the inside. In one instance it was nevertheless possible to detect incompletely fused, small spots on the external surface by using surface waves. An automated testing installation for pipes of this type (see below) uses 1 MHz surface probes; there, however, it must be assumed that a mixture of plate waves forms in the 1.5 mm wall, which nevertheless serves the same purpose [26].

Resistance-welded joints may contain defects which cannot be detected reliably with ultrasonics, i.e. so-called cold shuts resulting from incomplete fusion. If stressed slightly, the joint cracks right through the centre, revealing crack faces with a uniformly dull appearance. If previously ground, the same section would have shown no separation, only a loose line of minute inclusions by which apparently ultrasonics, including transverse waves up to 4 MHz, are not reflected. As far as is known no reliable non-destructive testing method for this defect is as yet available.

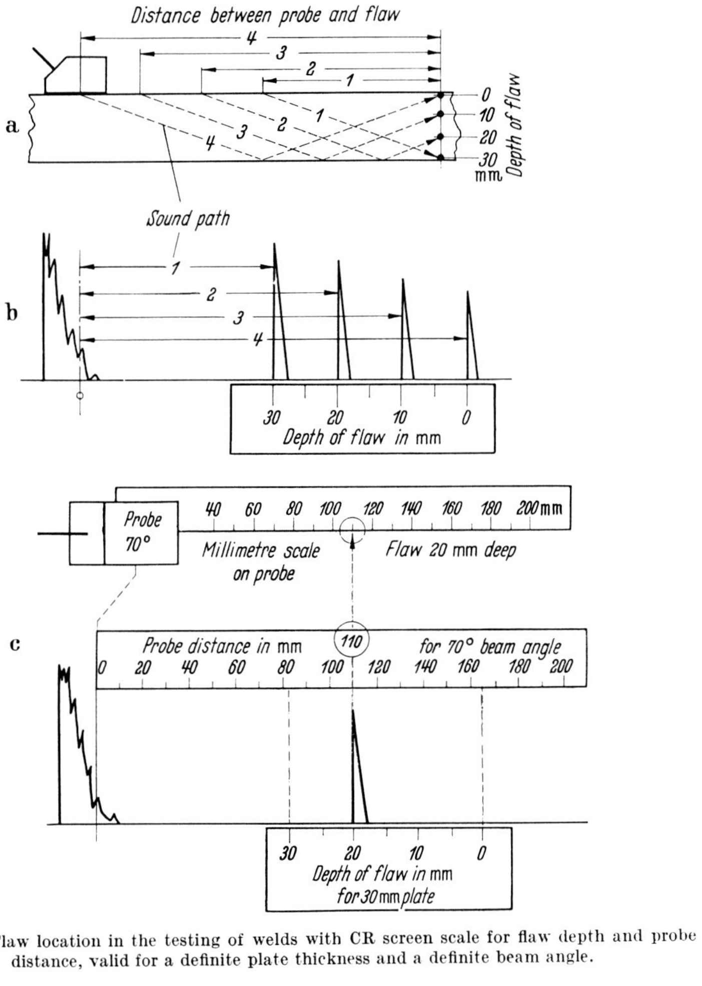

Fig. 3.170 Flaw location in the testing of welds with CR screen scale for flaw depth and probe distance, valid for a definite plate thickness and a definite beam angle.

3.281.3 Flaw-locating Methods. Determination of the depth (from the surface) and lateral position (distance from the centre of the welded joint or the probe) is desirable, not only in order to distinguish weld defects from defects outside the joint such as inclusions in the plate or interfering echoes according to Figs. 3.169a and d, but also for judging the nature of the flaw on the basis of its position within the joint, and thus its importance. The latter, however, requires long and thorough experience.

The method of location will readily be understood from the geometric configuration of the beam path as indicated in Fig. 3.170. It is assumed that only indications between one half and one full skip distance are counted and that the flaw is lined up on the axis of the sound beam by finding the maximum echo, assuming a non-directional reflection characteristic.

One first of all recognizes that a definite depth is related to a definite sound path. It is thus possible to attach to the CR screen a flaw depth scale valid for a given beam angle (e.g. 70°) and a given plate thickness (30 mm), extending from the right to the left. Where only the depth is of interest, this is then all that is necessary. For calibration the echoes from the top and bottom edge of a test plate are moved to the ends of the thickness scale by successively expanding and shifting the indication [314].

Fig. 3.170a clearly shows that every flaw depth is related to a definite distance between probe and flaw. At the beginning of the depth scale, i.e. for surface defects, this distance equals the skip distance. As indicated in Fig. 3.170c, a calculated distance scale can be placed on the CR screen. The distance in millimetres read on this scale for a given flaw echo is then transferred to a scale on the probe, so that both the flaw location and the depth can be marked directly on the plate [155]. The distance scale is valid only for a definite beam angle and the depth scale, in addition, only for a definite plate thickness. If no direct depth readings in millimetres are required, the bottom and top surface of the plate can be marked by movable pointers between which the depth of the flaw in fractions of the plate thickness is estimated, e.g. 1/4 *from the bottom* (Fig. 3.175). In this way the device is suitable for any plate thickness. Instead of using a separate millimetre scale during testing, it is more practical to attach such a scale directly to the probe with the zero mark at the sound exit point.

Since a distance scale has to be attached to the probe in any case, it is advantageous to combine this with a locating scale. This locating *rule* (Fig. 3.171) has a slider which can be adjusted to any plate thickness and which gives the flaw depth in millimetres. As indicated in Fig. 3.172, a scale for the sound path is placed in front of the CR screen. This is identical to the locating rule, but is calibrated in arbitrary units, e.g. naught to five, because the true sound path in millimetres is no longer of interest. Prior to the test this scale is calibrated with the aid of a test block by shifting and expanding it to a total distance of, for instance, 250 mm in steel. The position of the flaw echo is read in scale divisions, e.g. 2.6, and transferred to the locating rule. There the five-division scale is expanded in such a way that the true probe distance in millimetres can be read from it, or more simply, the location of the flaw is marked directly on the plate next to the edge. The oblique line starting at the

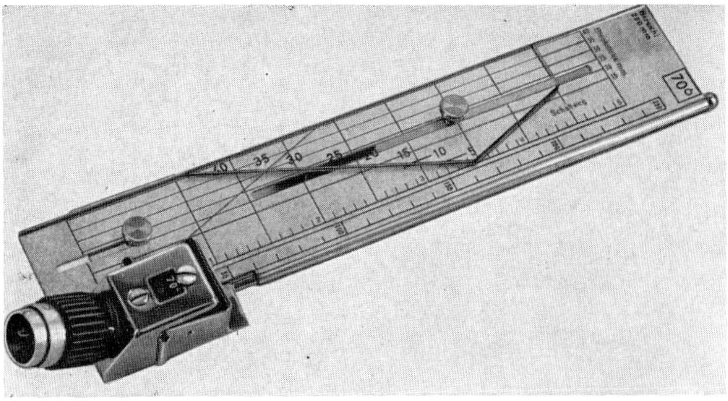

Fig. 3.171 Flaw locating rule for weld testing, design Krautkrämer.

probe, together with the oblique edges of the slider, indicate the sound path between the two surfaces of the plate, rotated 90° from its true position into the plane of the plate. Thus the depth of the flaw can be read

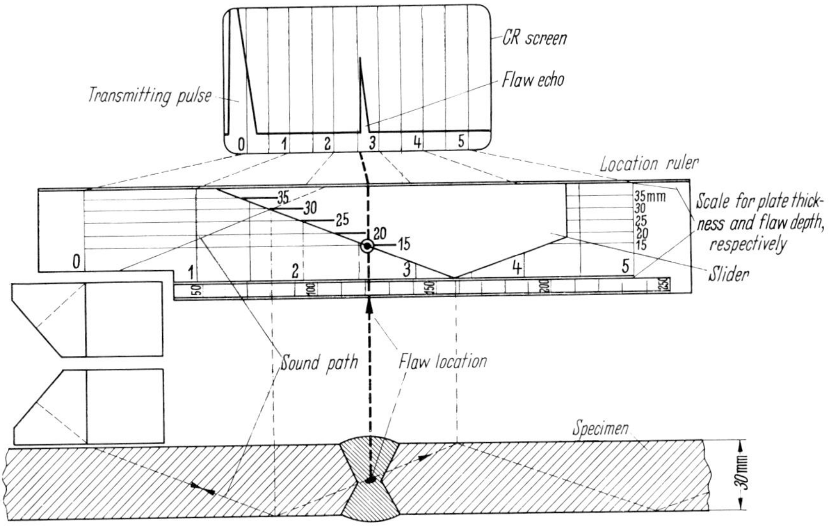

Fig. 3.172 Locating flaws with the Krautkrämer locating rule for testing welded joints.

on this line if the probe distance has been transferred to it from the CR screen. Usually the rising leg of the sound path between half and full skip distance is used, for which the flaw depth scale can conveniently be read on the edge of the perspex slider. It is, however, also possible to use the lower leg of the direct beam, or the beginning of the second skip leg.

Suitable locating rules are available for the usual beam angles of 45°, 60°, 70° and 80°. The locating accuracy for thicker plate is greater with smaller angles. In 30 mm plate and thicker, small flaws can be located accurately to within a few millimetres in all directions with the locating rule for 70° or 60° and a carefully calibrated instrument. On thin plate, say less than 12 mm, and using an 80° beam angle, flaw location is less reliable and the use of the locating rule or any other locating method questionable. In this case, however, accurate depth location is of no great importance because thin joints, in contrast to thick joints, need not necessarily be repaired from the nearest surface. According to [282] one can, however, still determine the lateral position of a given flaw, which only requires a rule for the probe distance. Penetration defects at the flanks on one side of the joint can thus be distinguished from root defects in the median plane.

Another – likewise very neat – solution determines the position of the flaw by the intersection of two straight lines in a traced cross-sectional sketch of the joint [192]. This requires reading on the scale attached to the probe its distance from the centre of the weld and transferring it to a locating map mounted above the CR screen. On this map the true cross-section of the welded seam, i.e. double Vee, Vee or bell joint, is drawn to scale by hand. The point of intersection of the normal line of the beam path with the oblique distance line gives the position of the flaw inside or outside the welded joint.

Because of its simplicity, the following locating method according to Papke [283] has found wide application in practice: an engraved per-

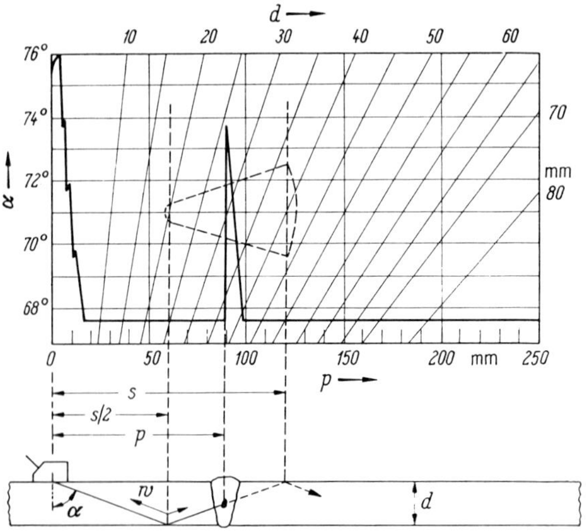

Fig. 3.173 Locating flaws with the locating scale according to Papke [283]. *s* skip distance; *p* projected distance of flaw, i.e. distance between flaw and sound exit point; *w* sound path to flaw.

spex disc is placed in front of the CR screen as "locating scale". The projected distance p which corresponds to a given sound path w is entered on the abscissa, cf. Fig. 3.173. The beaming angle α is entered on the ordinate, indicating the nominal angle of the angle probe used and a number of other adjacent angles which may occur during the test, either as a result of manufacturing tolerances of the probes, or uneven wear of the perspex contact shoe. The wall thicknesses d, which determine the reflection points at the bottom and top of the plate on the obliquely incident sound beams, are drawn as oblique parameter lines. With the aid of the auxiliary lines explained above a cross-sectional sketch of the plate can now be drawn on this transparent diagram [bottom surface = perpendicular through point of intersection between angle line and plate thickness (d), top surface = perpendicular through point of intersection between angle line and double plate thickness ($2d$); in the example in Fig. 3.173 the values $\alpha = 71°$, $d = 20$ mm have been chosen]. The shape of the joint is then drawn symmetrical to the angle line inside the cross-sectional diagram of the plate.

The instrument is then adjusted by entering the echoes of reflection points at given distances as calibration marks for the correct projection distances of the locating scale; the true sound path is then always longer by a factor of $1/\sin\alpha$ than the distance reading of the locating scale. Herewith the instrument is no longer calibrated in "sound path w" but in "projection distance p". In Fig. 3.38 this would mean that by changing the scale of the instrument the maxima of the envelopes would be moved exactly over the reflection points in the lower section of the drawing.

A (preferably flexible) longitudinal scale with millimetre divisions is then attached to the angle probe. The zero mark on the scale is adjustable and should coincide with the previously determined sound exit point.

This device greatly facilitates the location of flaws: the flaw echo, as usual, is adjusted to maximum amplitude by shifting the probe. The rising front of this echo immediately indicates the depth of the flaw below the plate surface on the plate cross-section drawn on the locating scale. In addition the projected distance of the echo is read on the locating scale in millimetres; this value is then transferred to the distance scale on the angle probe, and in this way the position of the source of reflection on the specimen is determined. If this transfer shows that the flaw is located in the welded joint, this also gives the lateral position relative to the joint while the locating scale gives the depth. In addition defects outside the joint, e.g. inclusions in the plate, can be recognized immediately as such.

One of the advantages of this method of location is that the location remains accurate even if the angle of the sound beam is changed, provided the drawing of the joint is corrected on the locating scale in accordance with the beam angle used. Furthermore little difficulty is encountered in locating a flaw in a joint between two plates of unequal thickness; for this purpose a cross-section of the thinner plate is drawn, e.g. under the angle line, and a cross-section of the thicker plate above the angle line, corresponding in each case to "half the weld profile". Naturally the "correct" side of the diagram has to be used in the test.

So far locating methods have usually been carried out at 2 to 2.5 MHz. With narrower beams and higher frequencies the accuracy could possibly be improved.

All locating methods discussed so far presuppose plane plate cross-sections. In the case of pipes these methods can therefore be applied directly only to circumferential welded joints. In the case of longitudinal joints according to Fig. 3.43 (configuration of beam in pipe cross-section) both the sound path and the skip distance are enlarged which would require special scales or rulers valid only for definite wall thicknesses and definite external diameters. It is therefore usually preferable to use a hand-drawn sketch of the pipe cross-section showing the configuration of the beam, even if this is less convenient and less accurate.

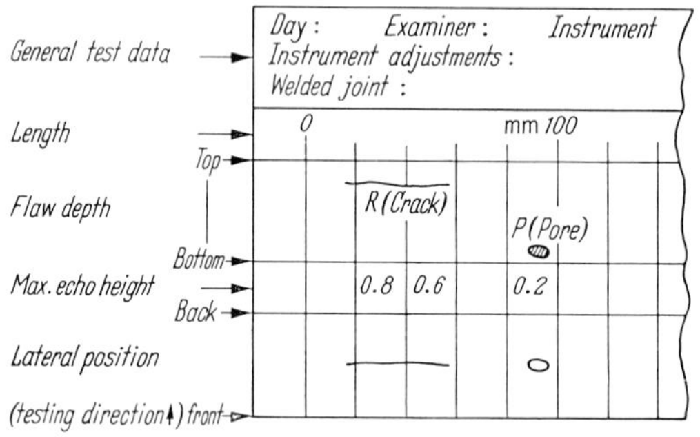

Fig. 3.174 Suggested report card for testing welds.

A form as suggested in Fig. 3.174 can be used for the test report and for documentation purposes [282]. This report gives length, lateral position and depth of the flaw, together with data on the echo amplitude and the suspected type of defect. Such a report can serve as a substitute for an X-ray film and even surpasses it in giving depth location. When comparing the two methods, it should not be overlooked that the detection of the most dangerous defects, viz. cracks, becomes questionable in welded joints thicker than 30 mm if X-rays are used, so that the test should be supplemented by the ultrasonic method. For joints thicker than 60 mm the ultrasonic method is regarded as the only acceptable one, quite apart from cost consideration (see also Hornung [153]).

3.281.4 Nature, Shape and Size of Defect. After a certain amount of experience a pronouncement regarding the nature, shape and size of the flaw can definitely be made by the application of the general method described in Sec. 3.15, at least in simple cases. For swivelling the probe around a flaw located as in Fig. 3.53, one can use the locating scale, with a pencil placed on the position of the flaw as a stop. Figs. 3.175 and 3.176 show typical screen traces of cracks and slag inclusions where the shape of the echo when adjusted to maximum indication already permits certain deductions on the shape of the flaw (see also Bastien and Evrard [34]).

Additional experience, e.g. concerning the influence of the quality of the plate and its surface, the wear of the perspex wedge and the position of the flaw, on the evaluation of the CR screen picture are quoted by Hornung [154].

In the case of flaws which are no longer very small compared to the cross-section of the sound beam, the envelope of the echo according to [282] provides some information on the shape of the flaw if the probe is shifted in direction of the weld and back. While small pores and thin bands produce a simple bell-shaped curve with a distinct maximum, the envelope of an areal defect which happens not to be orientated in the direction of the sound, shows a mountainlike structure with a broad base, and in favourable cases a structure with a plateau. The envelope can be recorded

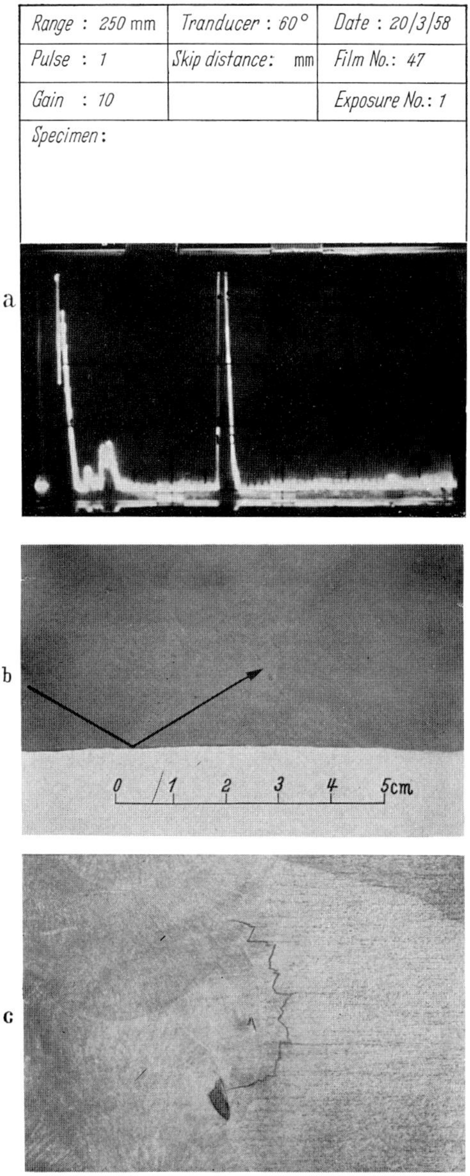

Fig. 3.175 Crack in a welded joint of thickness 38 mm (Sulzer Bros., Winterthur). a) Screen picture at 60° beam angle; b) ground section through flaw; c) same flaw as in b) but enlarged 6 times.

photographically if the probe is shifted back and forth while the shutter remains open (Fig. 3.177). This requires very steady coupling.

Complex screen pictures are obtained if the sound beam covers several flaws. When the probe is shifted, one echo *merges* into the next and the beginner finds it difficult to keep his eye on a given echo and to determine its maximum, unperturbed by the reforming of the echoes. Careful location even then frequently allows one to distinguish between several flaws, of which PAPKE [282] has furnished a very good example. Here an additional test with smaller probes of higher frequency, and possibly with smaller beam angle, often proves useful.

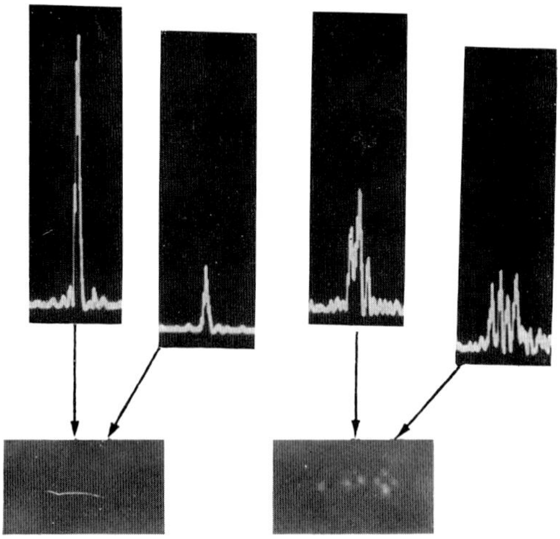

a b

Fig. 3.176 Echo traces of weld defects compared with X-ray pictures, sound in each case beamed normal and obliquely to the longitudinal direction of the joint. a) Crack in root; b) slags and pores in 50 mm Vee-joint. The picture of the crack has been retouched since it was barely discernible in the original X-ray plate. Probe 4 MHz, 70°.

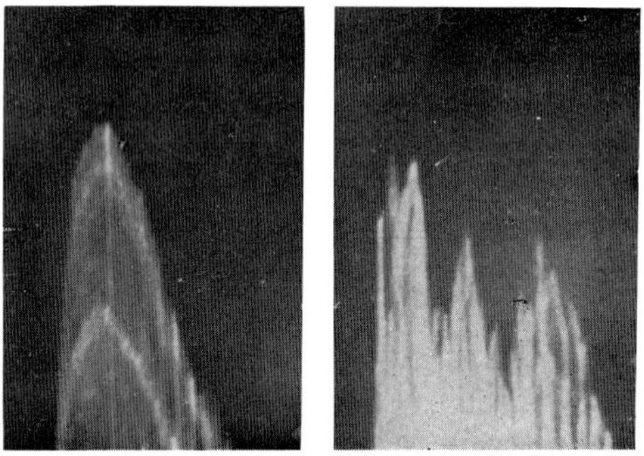

a b

Fig. 3.177 Envelopes of flaw echoes, a) 3 mm bore parallel to test surface; b) crack in a 35 mm welded joint, probe 4 MHz, 70°.

Concerning the gain to be selected and the estimation of flaw sizes exclusively on the basis of the echo amplitude (in the case of small flaws), one has so far had to rely largely on experience and practice with a given instrument. As a rough guide the echo of an edge was used, whose height as a flaw echo was assumed to be equal to that of a very large separation in the weld. Therefore the testing sensitivity would have to be so high, that the edge echo considerably surpasses the height of the screen. This introduces an uncertainty factor because a given degree of overdriving is difficult to reproduce on instruments having no calibrated gain control. The conditions are slightly better if a small hole in a plate parallel to its surface (artificial slag band) is used as reference echo for a small flaw. When testing is done on old surfaces with corrosion or deposits of scale or old paint, the sensitivity will be quite uncertain unless one accidentally encounters a hole or an edge. More reliable information will then be obtained with the twin probe method and its reference echo. If an instrument with calibrated gain control is used, rough allowance could be made for the attenuation by the surface by comparing the backwall echo of the specimen concerned with that of a plate when using a normal probe, and applying the difference in gain also to angle probes. The twin angle probe method would nevertheless be more reliable also for this purpose. If the influence of the surface is negligible or if it has been determined in one of the ways described, flaw sizes can be estimated also on welded joints according to [207], (see also Sproule [345]).

3.281.5 Recording and Automation. In the methods described for testing welds, the condition of the joint is evaluated by observing a fleeting CR screen picture. Data concerning a given test can then be accumulated only if the examiner not only marks in chalk the defects found on the joint but if in addition he enters his findings regarding nature, position and extension of a given flaw in a test report. In order, however, to obtain for acceptance or insurance purposes a document which is less dependent on the reliability and carefulness of the examiner, various methods of recording test data for testing welded joints have been developed. Recording methods have been introduced more particularly where the testing problem permits automation of the test. These conditions exist for instance if the test can be combined with automatic seam welding, or if it can be used on highly stressed, thick joints where sufficient testing time is available for using special, automatic scanning devices.

In one case the test results are recorded by a recorder even though the test is made by hand, viz. when testing joints on thin-walled boiler tubes. An interesting feature in this connection is that in spite of the usually pronounced reinforcement of the bead, a small 4 MHz angle probe with 60° beam angle gave the best results. Although echoes from the bead always produce more or less strong indications on the CR screen, important defects in the joint, such as lack of penetration, root defects and cracks, are nevertheless clearly recognized. All defects which appear when a circumferential joint is tested are recorded in proportion to amplitude by a simple recorder connected to a monitor. In this case, however, there is no correlation between the motion of the probe moved by hand and the chart feed. As a check the testing sensitivity adjusted on the instrument is recorded simultaneously with the "testing trace"; any change in the adjustment of the gain during the test is then immediately recognized on the recording chart. A switch which interrupts this "gain trace" enables the examiner to mark the beginning and the end of the test. A fixed "tolerance trace" on the recording chart separates "dangerous" indications from "acceptable" indications, exactly as in the case where the examiner ignores indications on the CR screen below a given amplitude, while he evaluates as serious only echoes exceeding this amplitude. Next to him at the testing place the examiner has only the testing instrument, the recording monitor, the probe and the marking switch, which in addition also contains the remote control for the chart feed in the recorder, while the recorder itself is mounted at a greater distance (e.g. in the test car) and out of his sight. In this way a document is obtained for each circumferential joint containing data on the echo amplitudes occurring and the testing sensitivity used.

The possibility for automating the test exists in the case of pressure-welded longitudinal joints on pipes (resistance or induction welding). In these welds the zone of the joint is very narrow. Essential for the possibility of testing is the satisfactory removal of the bead produced during welding on the internal and external surface of the pipe. Otherwise any remaining ridges may produce echoes which cannot be distinguished from true flaw echoes in the welded joint. On the other hand, if the bead is removed completely, a test, e.g. inside the cooling distance behind the welding machine, is definitely feasible. The testing method applied in this case is oblique beaming by the immersion technique, the correct beam entrance angle being readily adjustable by shifting the probe – as in the testing of pipes by the immersion technique, see Section 3.26. During the test it is not necessary to keep the distance between beam entrance point and welded joint absolutely constant. Defects in the welded joint are detected with a monitor gate which need not be adjusted very critically, the signals then being transmitted to suitable evaluation devices (e.g. via a delay line to a colour marking device). Cold shuts, however, cannot be detected in this way.

Complete removal of the reinforcement of the bead is usually successful only on the outside surface. The remaining partial or full ridge on the inside then causes difficulties. In the case of thicker walls, from approximately 5 to 6 mm, a sound beam can be transmitted through the joint in such a way that it misses the internal wall at the welded joint if certain critical, geometrical testing conditions are fulfilled [117]. Another device, designed by Sperry has been in use for some time in current production [26] in vehicle driving shafts 80 × 1.5 mm, where, however, the bead has been planed off on both sides. When the pipe enters the testing device, a limit switch actuates a compressed air cylinder via a solenoid valve which presses a 1 MHz surface wave probe with matching contact face against the pipe. The cooling liquid, distributed as required by a wiper in front of the probe, is used for coupling. A monitor gate ensures that only the zone containing the welded joint is covered. Flaw echoes actuate a compressed air operated paint gun. No failures during the test have been reported. In another installation the above-mentioned cold shuts caused difficulties.

In the case of wall thicknesses above 6 mm interferences by the bead can be eliminated in an elegant manner suggested by DE STERKE [353]. This is particularly suited to automated testing. The interfering echoes

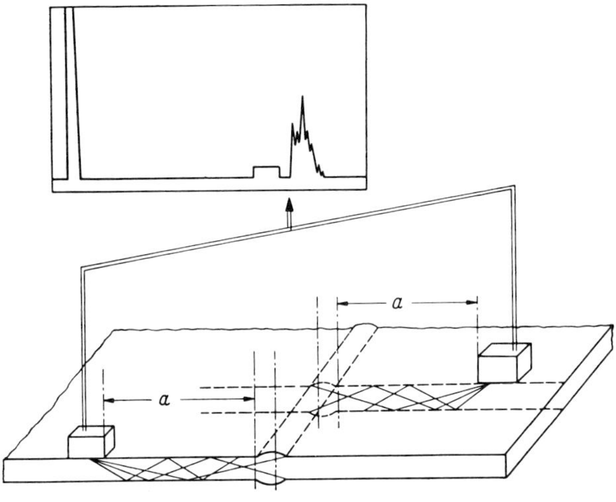

Fig. 3.178 Continuous testing of thin seams produced by automatic welding.

of the shoulder of the bead are always produced by the opposite side and consequently their sound path is slightly longer than that of echoes coming e.g. from the centre. Using zig-zag transverse waves, the entire cross-section of the joint can be irradiated with a probe from a fixed distance. If, as shown in Fig. 3.178, a monitor gate is adjusted so as to cover approximately 2/3 of the width of the seam in front of the interference zone, the interference can be avoided but, to ensure complete testing, this requires that a second, parallel-connected probe is applied at the same distance from the other side but slightly transposed in the direction of the joint. The middle zone of the joint is then covered twice while the lateral thirds of the seam are covered once only.

Where transverse defects can be expected, the device is supplemented by two additional, parallel-connected probes according to Fig. 3.167b. Although all four probes could be connected to one instrument, it is preferable to use two different monitor gates by allocating to probe pairs *3* and *4* echo transit times which differ from those allocated to probe pairs *1* and *2*, by maintaining a fixed but different distance from the joint (Fig. 3.179). Two recording tracks permit differentiation between the various types of flaws encountered (Fig. 3.180); transverse cracks, as well as cracks with a certain angle relative to the transverse direction to the joint (because each of the probes *3* and *4* also use the echo method) are indicated only by *3* and *4*, pure longitudinal defects only by *1* and *2*, and pores and slags more or less by all four probes.

The arrangement described does not permit exact correlation with the "fault-tracing" probe in the case of continuous testing where the positions of the flaws have to be marked on the specimen in colour or where the test results should be recorded. However, a novel method permits clear coordination between tested spot and flaw marking or recording. Fig. 3.181 shows such a probe combination: four angle probes irradiate the point of intersection of the two diagonals of a rectangle from its four corners. Probes S_1 and S_2 (at the two ends of one diagonal) operate as transmitters, and E_1 and E_2 at the two ends of the other diagonal as receivers. Longitudinal defects in the welded joint are indicated by probes S_1 and E_1 and simultaneously also by S_2 and E_2, whereas a transverse flaw is detected by its reflection by the combinations S_1 and E_2 and S_2 and E_1, respectively. This has the following advantage: whenever a flaw is indicated on the CR screen, this flaw will be located at the point of intersection of the sound beams.

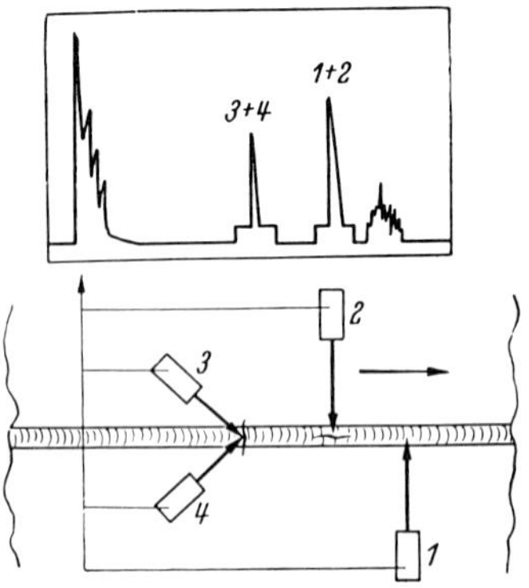

Fig. 3.179 Testing arrangement for longitudinal and transverse defects.

The method according to Fig. 3.179 is used preferably for continuous testing of welded joints in pipe sections because they can be tested with probes *1* and *2* (Fig. 3.179) right to the end. On the other hand, the test according to Fig. 3.181 comes to an end when the probes S_1 and E_2 or S_2 and E_1 drop off the specimen as soon as the end of the joint is reached. The last-mentioned testing method is therefore preferably used for testing spiral joints produced by welding machines in continuous production.

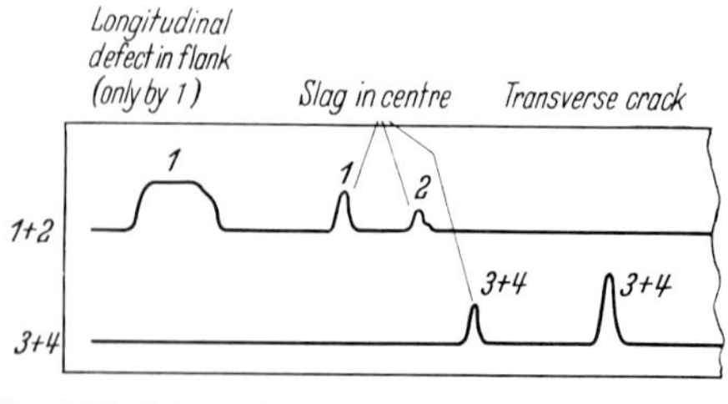

Fig. 3.180 Schematic recording diagram used with device according to Fig. 3.179.

If the test specification does not require testing for transverse defects, the arrangement shown in Fig. 3.179 is limited to probes *1* and *2* which, according to a suggestion by Schlusnus and Koch [323] can be mounted opposing each other to avoid the disadvantage of possible ambiguous marking or recording. Mutual interference of the two probes is excluded by switching over. During the first cycle probe *1* is connected which operates both as transmitter and receiver; during the second cycle the same applies to probe *2*. During the third cycle both probes are connected to the instrument in parallel, resulting in the "opposing beams" producing a reference echo whose amplitude is a measure of the coupling.

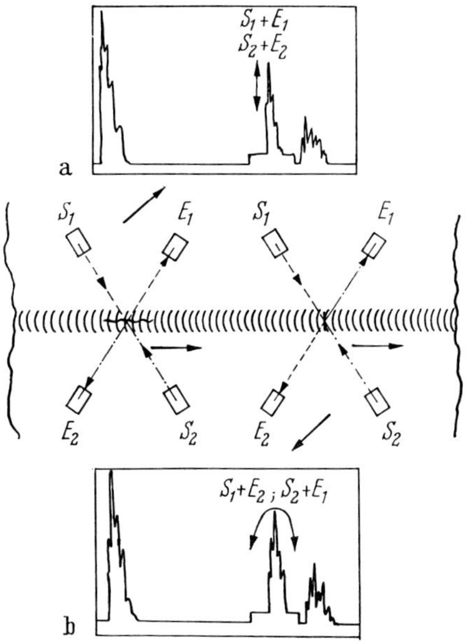

Fig. 3.181 Testing joints welded under powder, using separate transmitting and receiving probes. a) Indication of longitudinal defect; b) indication of transverse defect.

In practice longitudinal and spiral joints on pipes can be tested by the method described immediately as they leave the welding machine, the testing equipment being mounted in a fixed position. In the case of spiral joints it is even necessary to test exactly at this point because only there can the joint be guided accurately (Fig. 3.182). In the case of longitudinal joints in pipe sections it is often advisable to test only after the pipe has been expanded by hydraulic pressure and after straightening because this may still produce cracks. The pipe sections are then either moved on rollers past a stationary test bench with the welded joint on top, or the testing installation is mounted on a truck travelling on rails which moves alongside the pipe (Fig. 3.183). In this case the testing speeds for production tests are 2 to 6 m/min.

A device moved by hand is used for the semi-automatic testing of longitudinal joints, e.g. on site when laying pipelines (Fig. 3.184). The device is guided by the welding bead and track rollers. A device for testing circumferential joints has been developed by HUSAREK and RUAULT [162].

Automatic testing installations are being used in practice in large numbers only for welded joints of thin plate up to approx. 15 mm. For thick welded joints the usual hand testing has been mechanized and automated only in a few instances [212]. In addition to the obvious solution in which, as in manual testing the angle probes are guided by a mechanical device along a zig-zag path, it has been suggested that the reciprocating motion of the probe be replaced by a shifting or swivelling motion of the sound beam and to cover the welded joint by scanning only parallel to it at a constant distance with such a probe unit. A probe construction by SPERRY [372] according to Fig. 3.185, in which a slotted diaphragm in a rotating, sound-absorbing belt cuts out and periodically shifts a narrow section of the broad sound beam would limit the motion of the probe to the longitudinal direction of the joint. As far as is known, this suggestion has not yet been implemented.

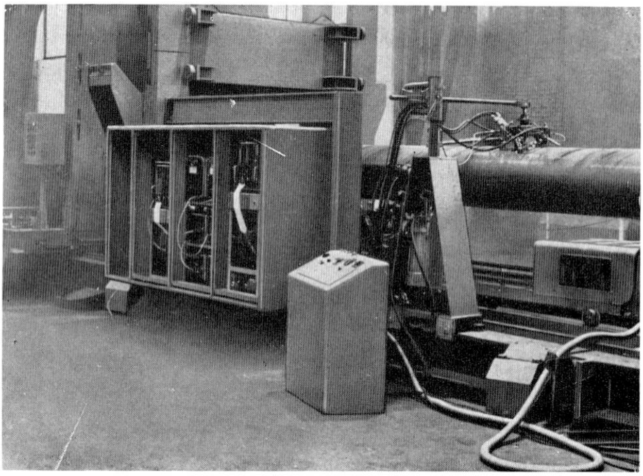

Fig. 3.182 Stationary testing device for spirally welded pipes (Salzgitter-Stahlbau, Salzgitter).

The arrangement shown in Fig. 3.186 permits scanning the camber height of the seam also when the position of the probe remains constant, by changing the beaming angle. In the Ultrasonic Weld Recorder according to KRAUTKRÄMER, the sound beam of a motor-driven angle probe periodically traverses the zone between two pre-adjusted limiting angles. The CR screen of the connected instrument reproduces the cross-section of the welded joint. Various recording instruments can be connected; one of them in simple "go/no-go" form can record the distribution of flaws in the longitudinal direction of the welded joint, independently of their position in the cross-section of the weld, while another can produce a comprehensive recording chart containing, in addition to data on the length of the flaws, also information on their position in the cross-section of the weld as determined by horizontal and vertical co-ordinates, together with a recording trace which indicates the degree of coupling (see Figs. 3.186 and 3.187b).

The beam is swept approximately 6 times per second over the desired testing sector. On the CR screen the obliquely adjusted time base is moved parallel to itself from left top to right bottom with increasing beam angle. Brightness-modulated dots are traced on the zero line instead of peaks, using a well-known technique. The transmitting pulse remains completely outside the picture. It can be seen that four

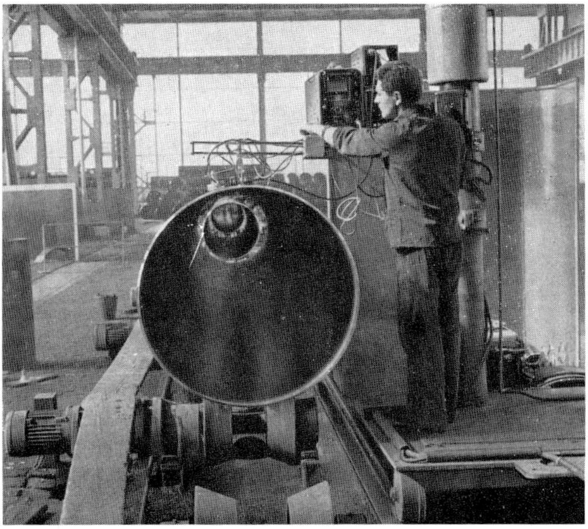

Fig. 3.183 Testing longitudinally welded pipes (Phoenix-Rheinrohr, Mühlheim) (equipment supplied by Röntgentechnische Dienst, Rotterdam, and Krautkrämer).

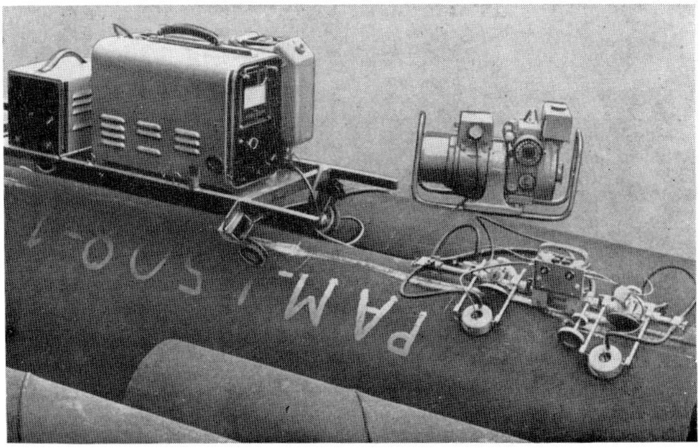

Fig. 3.184. Manual testing of longitudinally welded pipes (Gaz de France, Paris) (device designed by Krautkrämer).

artificial defects in a plate are recorded successively as four bright dots or, more accurately, as line patterns (Fig. 3.187a). This display is not completely free of distortions, which can, however, largely be compensated electronically. The four artificial flaw echoes which limit a real welding joint according to height and width, are first moved to the four corners of a transparent template of the welding joint. During the test the actual flaws then appear in this field sufficiently position-true.

Except for points *3* and *4*, all echoes must then be obtained via *one* single reflection. If in addition they are produced along the direct beam or by a double reflection, they form mirror images, below and above the picture.

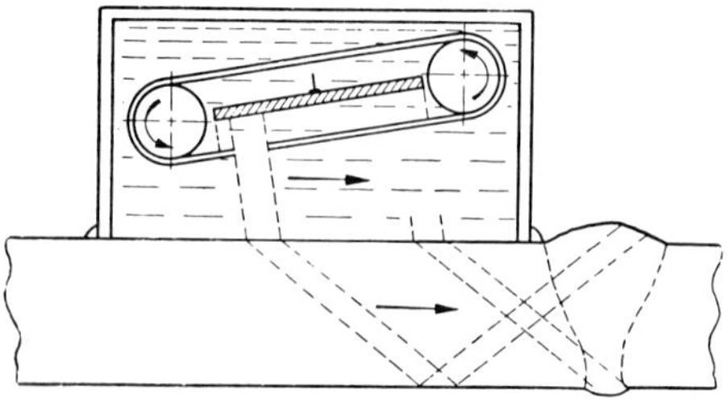

Fig. 3.185 Suggestion for a probe with rotating slotted diaphragm (Sperry).

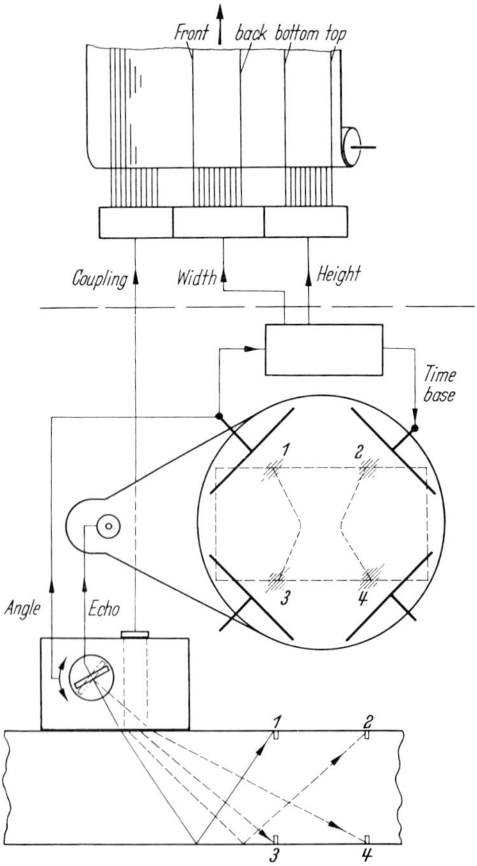

Fig. 3.186 Method for the automatic recording of tests on welded joints according to Krautkrämer with cross-sectional presentation of flaws and simultaneous recording of flaw position and degree of coupling.

For recording the deflection voltages for angle and transit time are resolved electronically and recomposed to produce voltages which are proportional only to the width and the height of the welded joint. The result appears as bright spots on two CR screens of the recording instrument, while the multiple echoes of a crystal transducer beaming perpendicularly into the plate are likewise presented as bright spots on a third CR screen (cf. Fig. 3.7). These three pictures are fed to the pens of a multirecorder via a system of photoelectric cells and after suitable amplification. The motion of the probe along the joint is synchronized with the chart feed of the recorder. The complete recording (Fig. 3.187b) thus shows flaw echoes according to position (regarding lateral orientation, depth and length) together with a continuous dotted trace as a check of the coupling.

For the routine testing of welded joints in thick-walled containers the Ultrasonic Weld Recorder is used with simple "go/no-go" recording (Fig. 3.188). Simultaneously, a second recorder records deflections which are proportional to the number of the multiple coupling echoes. A motor-driven test car guided by a rail parallel to the longitudinal joint and held in position by magnets, ensures uniform movement of the probe at the correct distance and steady coupling by flowing water. In the case of circumferential welds the container is rotated. The test car, guided by a chain fastened around the container, moves at a controlled speed so that it always remains

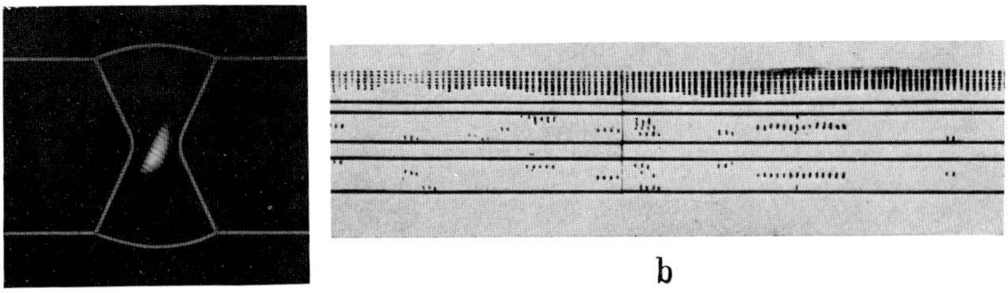

a b

Fig. 3.187 Flaw indication with the Ultrasonic Weld Recorder. a) Screen picture of root defect in a 40 mm double Vee-joint; b) recording strip of joint with different flaw indications.

at the highest point of the container. The joint is checked from each side for flaws in the longitudinal direction and, in addition, also for transverse flaws from the ground-off bead. Whenever the operator observes indications pointing to considerable welding defects which extend over a given length, he marks the position of the flaw on the recording

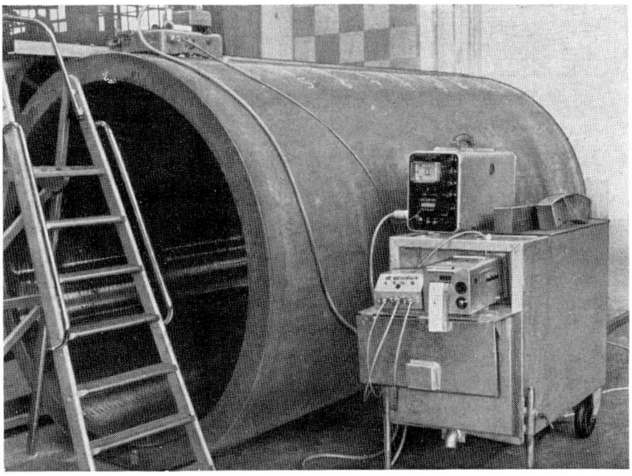

Fig. 3.188 Ultrasonic Weld Recorder used for testing the longitudinal joint on a container (works photo J. Thompson Ltd., Wolverhampton, U.K.).

chart as it appears in the cross-sectional diagram of the joint on the CR screen. Before deciding on repair or rejection, these flaw positions are checked by hand. The testing speed of this device is approximately 400 mm/min.

Another instrument for automatic testing of welded joints, with the name *Sonolog* [448], has been constructed by Röntgentechnische Dienst

N. V., Rotterdam. It uses three conventional angle probes at a fixed distance from the joint, of which one beams at right angle and the other two obliquely to the joint. This enables one to make deductions regarding the shape of the defect from the differences in the readings. Flaw location is not attempted; a single test run can cover only a thinner joint of up to approximately 20 mm along one path, or in the case of a thicker joint, only a given layer. A 7-line direct recorder records, in addition to the echoes of the 3 probes, also the reflections between probes, which is realized by using separate, alternately controlled transmitters.

Another automatic testing installation for heavy butt welds has been described by HANSTOCK [131]. Using 4 probes distributed in 2 pairs on either side of the joint and connectable in various combinations by change-over switches to 8 different amplifiers and recorders, the device gives information concerning the nature and orientation of the flaws.

Automatically guided probes are furthermore required for nozzle welds in nuclear reactor pressure vessels. HANSTEAD and MCELWEE [130] have constructed such a device which can be inserted in the water-filled nozzle and which scans the welded joint with normal probes. The result is recorded photographically in the form of 180 cross-sectional pictures per joint.

3.281.6 Main Applications and Economic Viewpoints. The testing of butt joints combined with flaw location has become practically indispensible, especially for thick joints welded automatically under powder because it was found time and again that the most dangerous defects in this type of welding, viz. stress cracks, have escaped both X-ray and gamma radiation tests as well as hydraulic pressure tests of the finished product. Some organisations therefore prescribe a 100% ultrasonic test by experienced examiners as the only method. In other organisations certain sections of the joint where the ultrasonic test produced indications are subsequently X-rayed. Where X-ray films are specified for the acceptance, these pictures are frequently taken only after the ultrasonic test and the necessary repairs. While in the workshop, the greater testing reliability and the considerably lower costs are regarded as the main advantages of the ultrasonic tests, their handy application and the absence of any danger are an additional advantage on the building site.

At the building site ultrasonics are mainly used for testing thick-walled joints subjected to stresses by pressure, e.g. in power plants, boilers, reactors and so forth. The time required for hand testing here depends largely on the accessibility of the joint, the frequency of flaws, and the specified, smallest flaw indication. This time therefore may range from approximately 5 to 20 min/m, not counting intervals for reconversion of the instrument and transportation.

In recent years the field of application for thin-walled specimens has also grown; this concerns on the one hand circumferential joints produced on site on pipelines with thin walls from approximately 6 to 10 mm, and on the other circumferential joints on boiler tubes with diameters from approximately 25 to 110 mm and wall thicknesses ranging from about 2.5 to 8 mm [378, 389]. This applies to routine tests which, because of the high costs of the alternative methods, could otherwise not be carried out at all or only at random. The problem is therefore not the detection of the minutest flaws, or for that matter of every flaw, but to be able to exclude on a more or less statistical basis a high percentage of such flaws. Consequently this allows relatively short testing times. In the case of tests on a pipeline during which many thousands of joints were tested ultrasonically, it was found that approximately 20 min/circumferential joint of approximately 2 m length could be achieved, including intervals. Moreover, examiners with only a short training period could be used.

Finally, a rare, but rather interesting application should be mentioned, viz. supervision of already known flaws while the component concerned is in use. Since in the case of pressure installations only the external surface is accessible, such checks can only be made with ultrasonics and then only if the surface is not too hot for coupling. To ensure satisfactory reproducibility, each testing point can be marked by cementing to it small plastic discs which match the contact face of the angle probe. Where the object is to keep the progress of a given crack under observation so that the component can be shut down as soon as a certain safety is exceeded, the ultrasonic beam is aimed at the end of the crack, at a point where the maximum echo has already decreased to approximately one half. Making use of several such contact points, one can, if need be, observe the defective zone over a period of years in order to check whether the crack is growing or not and in which direction.

3.282 Fillet Welds

Not all fillet welds lend themselves to ultrasonic testing. However, also in this case, as in that of butt welds, the rule applies that a joint designed correctly for high mechanical stresses, and where therefore a quality check is very important, can in general also readily be tested.

A good example is the double fillet weld in Fig. 3.189. A joint with incomplete penetration, as in Fig. 3.189a shows bad mechanical design. It is unable to absorb high stresses because the open gap produces dangerous notch effects. It is also much more difficult to test than a so-called K-joint welded through completely (Fig. 3.189b).

However, where a joint according to Fig. 3.189a has to be tested, this can be done more or less successfully on plate thicker than about 12 mm by using a sensitive probe with high near-field resolution (e.g.

4 to 6 MHz, 10 mm diameter, without protective layer) or a TR probe, by moving the probe along a zig-zag path on the butt strap over the zone of the joint. The results are improved if a guiding device is used which maintains a constant distance between probe and plate edge provided the joint runs parallel to it. As indicated in Fig. 3.189a a sequence of multiple echoes is obtained above the free plate as well as above the thwart, while it disappears completely above the weld. In this case larger defects are recognized by their direct echo. Occasionally also echoes with longer transit time are obtained via the detour through both welds.

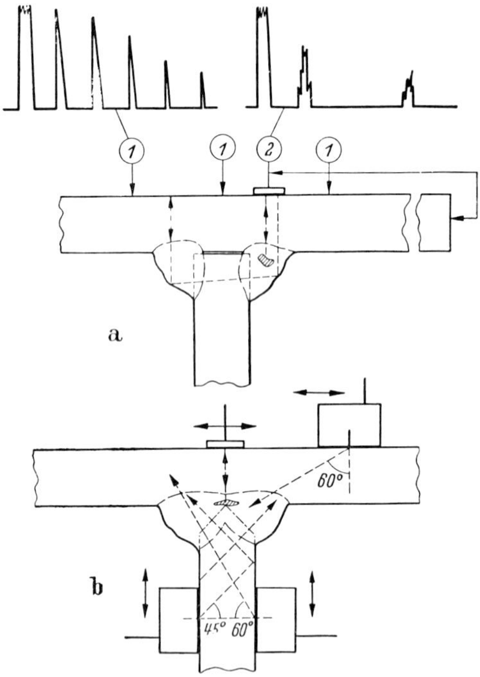

Fig. 3.189 Testing fillet welds, a) joint not welded through, b) joint welded through (K-joint).

In the case of a K-joint, containing no defects, the echo sequence should disappear over the full width. Bonding defects and zones of incomplete penetration in the centre, which are the most critical flaws, are located favourably. In practice tests can be carried out on plate as thin as 10 mm and if TR probes are used, even on thinner plate. For flaws in the welding bead, such as cracks and slag inclusions, oblique testing may bring better results, for which purpose small angle probes of 4 to 5 MHz with angles of 45 to 60° are used on plate of less than 30 mm. With some reservation the method can also be used on welds not completely welded through. From the thwart, this is the only method of testing if the strap plate is not accessible or is very much thicker, or if the thwart is attached in this way to a complex forging or casting. Only in the case of low thwarts, say up to ten times the plate thickness, is it possible to test also from the free, flat edge using normal probes, which however, cover only the middle zone of the joint welded through.

Another fillet weld which sometimes can also be readily tested is a sleeve joint according to Fig. 3.190 with wall thicknesses above 10 mm. Here handy, small angle probes of 60° and smaller likewise prove successful. Echoes from the bead can be obtained in position ① of the probe. When the probe is shifted towards the joint, a spot with incomplete penetration produces echoes with a shorter transit time, which can readily be distinguished from the echoes produced by the bead. At spots without flaws, the beam passes through the weld into the bottom plate without echo and disappears.

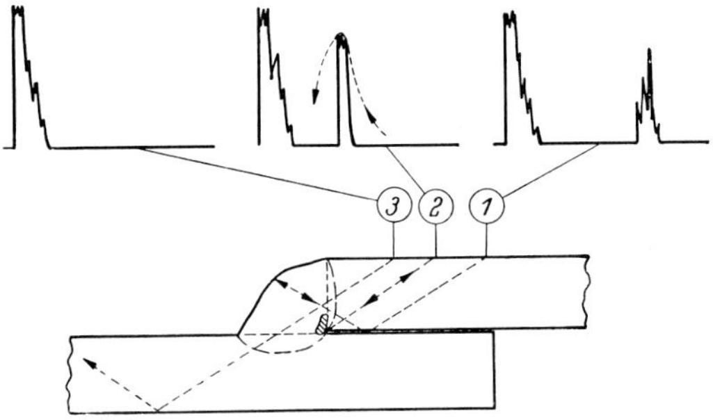

Fig. 3.190 Testing a fillet weld with lap-joint or sleeve joint (according to VON HEESEN).

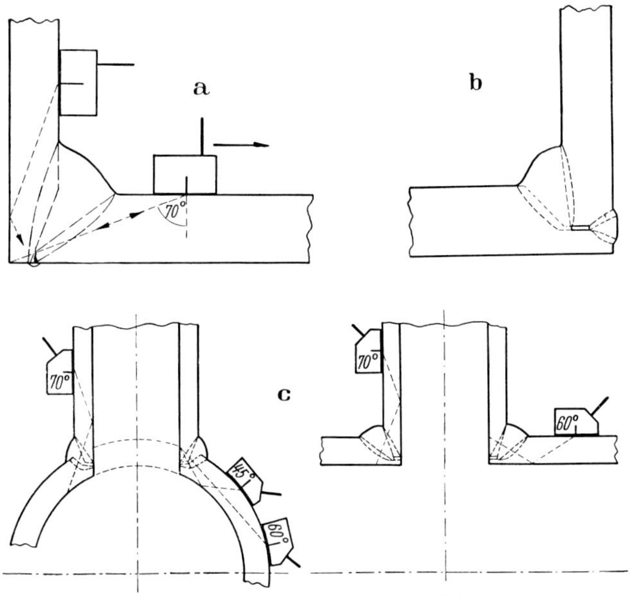

Fig. 3.191 Testing fillet welds in pipe joints.

Usually less favourable, and furthermore very much dependent on the specific shape of the joint, are tests on welded-in pipes according to Fig. 3.191. In a flat plate the joint, according to Fig. 3.191 a, has the same cross-section everywhere and can readily be tested with oblique transverse waves. The echo from the edge can serve as reference echo. Usually, however, the fitting faces show incomplete weld penetration. The point of separation can then be distinguished from adjoining flaws only in the case of thick walls and sharply focused sound beams. Here also mechanically better designed joints can more easily be tested, e.g. a thinner pipe joined by a simple circumferential butt-weld to extruded sockets of the thicker pipe.

Fig. 3.191c demonstrates how the complex penetration curve of two not very dissimilar pipes impedes the test. The sound is propagated in a plane only at 4 points of the joint (in the longitudinal and in the circumferential direction of the thicker pipe). Between these points the zig-zag path is bent and the skip distance simultaneously changes from point to point. Flaw locating is impossible here. If the test is made from the attached pipe, both the position and the shape of the joint around the circumference also changes, but at least the beam angle remains constant. The latter method is therefore usually more advantageous.

Simple sealing welds, e.g. on threaded plugs, are unsuitable for ultrasonic testing because the problem here is the determination of leaks which may occur in the form of fine, filamentary pores, but hardly cracks. Since the thread is not welded through, the resultant discontinuities cannot be distinguished from genuine flaws.

In the case of fillet welds, even more so than in other cases, a sound design which provides for testing facilities, is particularly important here, especially since other tests are impeded here by troublesome obstacles.

3.283 Spot Welds

Flaws in spot welds occur preferentially in a plane parallel to the plate surface in the form of slag inclusions and bonding defects. They are therefore best detected by perpendicular testing (Fig. 3.192). Where the total thickness is sufficient to produce clearly separated multiple echoes, which is the case with frequencies of 4 to 6 MHz and good-quality probes on approx. 3 to 4 mm steel or aluminium, flaws are recognized by their intermediate echoes, and even permit a rough estimation of their size. On thinner plate the length of the echo sequence is observed which in the case of faulty spot welds decreases. Frequently these echo bands show an irregular pattern with maxima and minima, and experience has shown that the area of the band rather than its length can serve as a measure of the quality of the spot weld. It is advantageous not to step up the gain of the echo picture at a sound spot weld, to avoid overdriving. So-called cold shuts cannot be detected in this way on a finished spot weld, because they are highly transmissive to sound.

If the surface is satisfactory, there is no objection to using a probe which is slightly larger than the spot weld, e.g. 10 mm in the case of spot welds of 6 to 8 mm. The projecting boundary area then does not yet cause interference by echoes from the top plate, and the quality of the weld can be determined by shifting the probe back and forth from the same starting point. Smaller spot welds, however, require better matched probe diameters. Because of the rapidly decreasing sensitivity, the maximum probe diameter which can still be accommodated should be determined by trial and error in the case of routine tests.

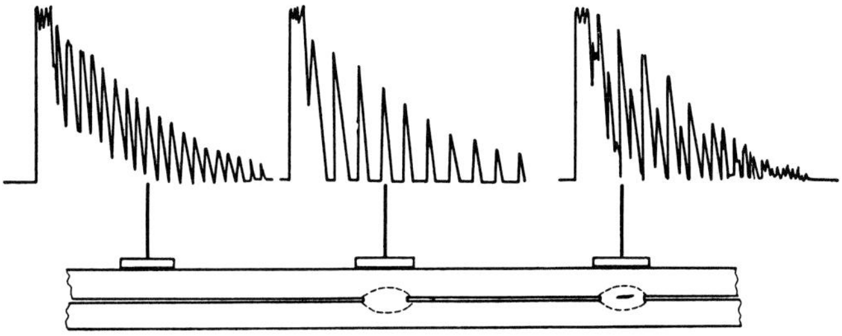

Fig. 3.192 Testing spot-welded joints.

A very annoying difficulty of this method usually arises from bad coupling caused by cup-shaped deformations of the surface. Naturally, if possible, the better of the two surfaces is chosen and protruding edges of the cup might be ground off. However, the long interference zone of the probe when placed over an oil-filled depression frequently limits the method to a rough test in the case of heavier sheets, say 3 + 3 mm. If the surface at the bottom of the cup is more or less flat and clean, smaller probes which fit in may be used.

On thicker sheets of greatly different gauges, the difference of the echo sequences from the side of the thinner sheet is more pronounced.

Also, when the intensity method is used with sound transmission, bad contact causes wrong diagnosis. If the surfaces are not deformed excessively, thin sheet of any gauge can be tested by this method. In practice, however, this is of little use because it would require that the specimen be placed between the accurately adjusted probes; in view of the usual dimensions this is impossible. The same applies also to the echo method in the immersion technique.

An interesting application of the intensity measurement in sound transmission on spot welds is at present being tried out practically. According to Wilkens [253] the probes are mounted for this purpose in the electrodes of the automatic welding machine. The cooling water for the electrodes serves as couplant between probes and electrodes and the work pieces to be joined. This makes it possible to observe the change in sound transmission on the CR screen of the instrument right from the moment when the welding begins. Pores, cracks, spatter and differences in the diameter of the spot welds can be recognized on sheets of 0.5 to 2 mm gauge with testing frequencies of 2.5 to 5 MHz. Even co.d shuts can be detected and distinguished from other types of defects. For reasons not yet fully explained the sound transmittance at such spots is approximately 10% higher than on a sound spot weld.

Only experience gathered over a long period of time will reveal whether these positive results can be obtained persistently under practical conditions of production, particularly if the shape of the electrode changes after comparatively long use.

Welded-on stud bolts can also be tested ultrasonically using a small probe provided the end face is reasonably flat. If the weld is satisfactory, the end echo will have disappeared and only the backwall echo of the plate will be obtained.

3.29 Joints Produced by Rivetting, Glueing and Shrinking

3.291 Rivet Hole Testing

Rivet joints can be tested for fatigue cracks by applying the pulse-echo method on plate 10 mm thick and heavier. The rivet itself may develop transverse cracks between head and shank which can be found by testing from the rivet head, as on screws (cf. 3.22). Smaller incipient cracks are found more reliably from the far rivet head.

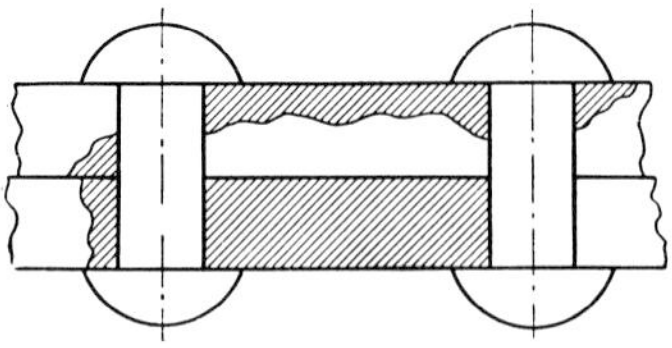

Fig. 3.193 Incipient cracks and full cracks on rivet joints.

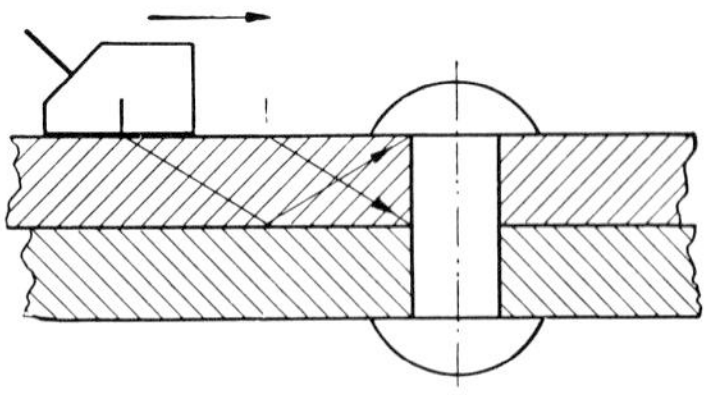

Fig. 3.194 Rivet hole testing, reference echo from top and bottom edge of rivet hole.

Incipient cracks in the rivet hole start from the wall of the hole, usually at its edge (Fig. 3.193); they may penetrate through the full width of the plate and, if the rivet joint is stressed, may extend from one rivet hole to the next. Small incipient cracks can even be caused by excessive expansion during rivetting. As a consequence of stress-corrosion they grow and lead to cracked rivet joints which in the case of steam boilers has often been the cause of explosions.

These cracks can of course be detected only from the surface of the affected plate and if three plates are rivetted together, the centre one usually cannot be checked. On plate 15 mm thick and heavier, angle probes of about 70° and 2 MHz are usually used or alternatively also miniature angle probes with 4 MHz [147]. The probes are moved in the same way as when welded joints are tested, but over a sufficiently wide angular range with the rivet hole as centre, so as to irradiate favourably at least the most dangerous cracks in the direction of the row of rivets.

When beaming towards the rivet one should in general obtain a good echo from the hole while moving the probe back and forth, particularly from the bottom and top edge, which can serve as a coupling check (Fig. 3.194) If the beam is directed slightly to one side, a given crack echo increases while the hole echo disappears (Fig. 3.195). This opposing echo build-up is a criterion for distinguishing between true crack echoes and a double echo obtained simultaneously from the top and bottom edge of the hole due to the divergence of the beam: if this is the cause of the double echo, both disappear almost simultaneously when the beam is swung. The crack echo about half a hole diameter behind the hole echo is readily recognizable if the hole diameter is 15 mm or more.

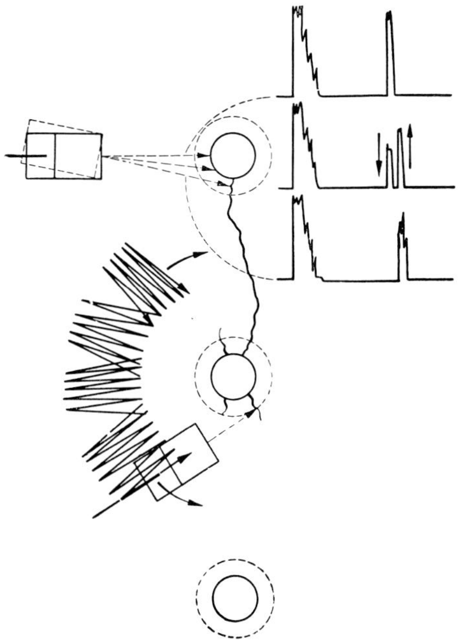

Fig. 3.195 Testing rivet holes, swing-motion of the probe and indication of an incipient crack in a rivet hole on the CR screen.

When the back row of rivets is scanned, the front row interferes so that smaller angle probes with smaller beaming angle may have to be used.

The time required for testing one rivet should be about 5 to 15 seconds under favourable conditions, provided an assistant is available for subsidiary tasks such as cleaning the surface on old boilers, applying the couplant, writing the report, etc.

Recently, the checking of rivet holes has gained greater importance for tests on aircraft. There, rapid checking of rivet holes at the joints of critical structural components is essential. The thin gauges make reciprocal motions of the angle probe unnecessary. The beam is directed at a grazing angle towards the edge of the hole and the probe, while maintaining its relative position to the rivet hole, is moved, with the rivet as centre, once completely around. Incipient cracks manifest themselves by the appearance of echoes which travel a short distance across the CR screen [419].

3.292 Laminar Joints Produced by Soldering, Brazing, Glueing, Plating, etc.

To the great diversity of laminar joints in respect of the type and the thickness of the layers and the nature of the bond, all ultrasonic methods are applicable. Fig. 3.196 gives a summary.

If the bond between two materials with identical or similar acoustic impedance is very strong, a resonance test according to Fig. 3.196a

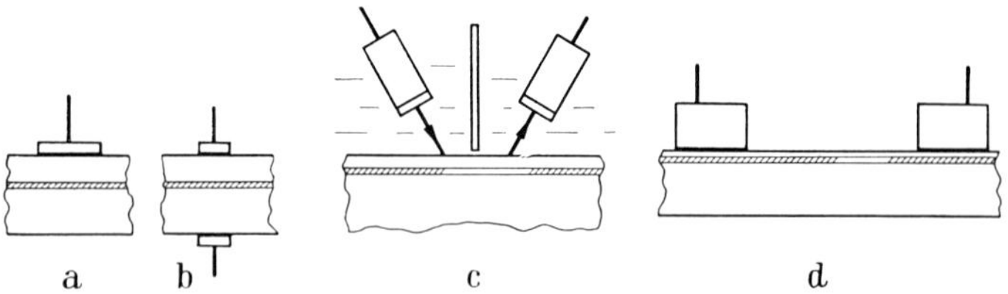

Fig. 3.196 Method for testing laminar bonds. a) Resonance or pulse-echo method with longitudinal waves; b) intensity method with sound transmission; c) intensity method with plate waves or transverse waves in one layer; d) intensity method with plate waves or surface waves in the whole layer.

amounts to measuring the thicknesses d_1 (bad) and $d_1 + d_2$ (good). The same applies to the pulse-echo method where the length of the echo sequences serves as criterion. In both methods it is preferable to measure from the thinner layer because the differences are then more obvious. When the transmission method is used, it is easier to confine the test to specific points than with the other methods where small thicknesses are concerned.

As indicated in Fig. 3.196c, the larger defects can be found with zigzag transverse waves or plate waves which can reach the receiver from the transmitter only if there is no bond, thus allowing positive flaw indication. Instead of the immersion technique where a screen excludes directly reflected waves, special probes with direct contact can also be used [391].

Conversely, a bonding defect of thin surface layers may interrupt the propagation of suitable wave modes, which can serve as indication by the reflection or transmission method. Basically, surface waves (Fig. 3.196d) or alternatively also Love waves (transverse waves parallel to the surface [129]), may be used. In both cases the wave length should be large compared with the layer thickness.

If the bonding layer contains a substance of markedly different acoustic impedance, such as an adhesive bond, a satisfactorily bonded spot can nevertheless not be equated to a solid specimen. A glued aluminium bond, for instance, furnishes a picture different from that of a solid plate of the same thickness [321]. From the frequency and the height of resonance peaks conclusions can therefore be drawn regarding the properties of the bonded layer, which furnish more information than a simple go/no-go test.

Schematic screen traces applying to the pulse-echo method are shown in Fig. 3.197. If the bonding is satisfactory, the echo trace depends on

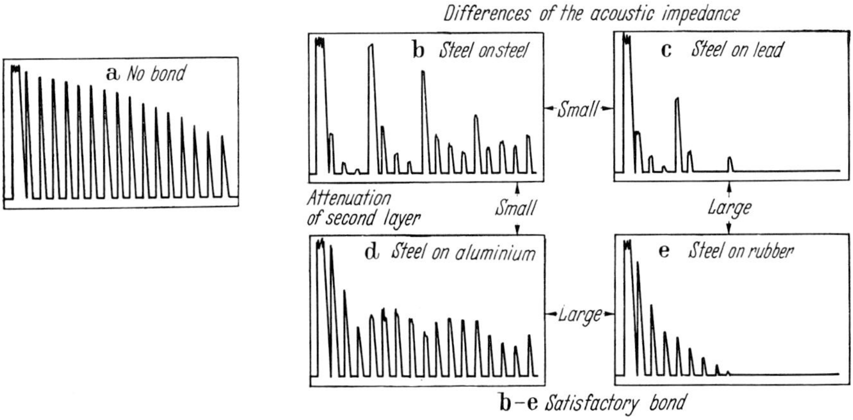

Fig. 3.197 Screen pictures when bonds are tested with the pulse-echo method. a) No bond; b) to e) satisfactory bond; b) and c) bond with small difference on acoustic impedances; d) and e) bond with large difference; b) and d) bond with small attenuation in the second layer; c) and d) bond with high attenuation.

the difference of the acoustic impedance as well as on the attenuation in the second material. In the figure it is assumed that the transit time in the second layer is several times longer than in the first layer, and that the influence of the bonding layer is nil.

Examples of the various cases are, for Fig. 3.197 b *metal-cladding*, such as special steel on steel, silver on steel, *brazing* of steel and hard-metal to steel, as well as similar bonds between heavy or light metals, furthermore *enamelling* on metal and bonding of porcelain to porcelain. Here, the echo sequence of the total layer in the picture predominates, whose transit time has been assumed four times greater than that of the first layer. If the second material is not laminar and produces no backwall echo, only weak traces of the sequence a appear. The difference between good and bad is always very clear.

Practical results concerning the testing of brazed joints between brass pipes and bronze connection sleeves are reported in [273]. A numerical value ("bonded area in %") is computed from the amplitude of the echo of the brazed bond and the amplitude of the total wall thickness, which can be used for the rapid evaluation of the quality of a brazed bond.

The case shown in Fig. 3.197c occurs in *homogeneous lead coating*. At small gain a satisfactorily bonded spot produces practically no echoes because the lead layer absorbs everything. The contrast as compared with an unbonded spot then shows up clearly. The test should be made from the lead side only if absolutely unavoidable. It is then helpful if the lead, by alloying it with antimony and tin, is harder and more transmissive than soft lead. Attention should then be paid to the echoes returned from the steel. According to [315] a lack of bonding is readily detectable even after the lead layer has been slightly heated and hammered.

Less clearly recognizable is the difference in case d. Since the two transit times are in the ratio 1 : 3, the various echo sequences partially coincide producing a picture which may be very similar to that of case a (no bond) if the coupling fluctuates. In general, however the difference can still be recognized by the mutual interference of the echo sequences. In cases b as well as d the close echo sequence may show maxima, as in Figs. 3.34 and 3.35, from which deductions can be made on the transmittance of the bonding layer. If the second material in case d is very light, e.g. foamed material on metal, and at the same time the bonding layer very thin, the test is no longer reliable.

In case e closer attention should also be paid to careful coupling in order that the difference may be recognized. Instead of observing the length of the echo sequence, it is preferable to pay attention to the decrease between successive echoes. Whether in cases c and e echoes are still being obtained from the second layer, makes little difference as far as the clarity of information is concerned. The second material therefore may also be extensive, as e.g. the copper anode of an X-ray tube, on which the brazing of the tungsten anticathode in the form of an approximately 2 mm thick small disc has to be tested.

The limit of the resolving power can be brought down to approximately 1 mm if TR probes are used. However, the echo sequence is then no longer resolved, and only the first backwall echo, whose amplitude fluctuates with the bonding, is observed.

Of particular interest are tests of vulcanized *rubber-metal bonds*. The sound transmission method according to Fig. 3.196b can be applied only rarely because it requires that both external surfaces are parallel. If at least one side is parallel to the bonding face, the echo method is used and this is done by testing from both the steel side and from the rubber side. In the first case the attenuation of the echo sequence of the steel by the rubber is observed (Fig. 3.197a). If in the second case the rubber layer is sufficiently thin or transmissive, the echo returned from the backwall of the metal can be used as a reliable criterion of the bonding. The echo sequence returned from the rubber itself is not affected much if there is no bond.

Complete non-bonding with a layer of trapped air can in this way be distinguished very easily from bonding, but this is rarely of interest. To make any statement concerning the *adhesive strength* is, however, much more difficult. In the case of rubber-metal bonds, the difference between good and only moderate bonding when tensile stresses are applied during the test should be more marked [141]. However, in this as well as in similar bonding tests, e.g. when claddings and composite castings of axle boxes are tested, the transmission of sound is not yet a sufficient indication of satisfactory adhesion.

In the chemical industry masonry or concrete *liners* of containers are checked in order to determine whether the lining still sticks to the steel shell. A bonded, dry concrete lining can readily be distinguished from one completely separated when the test is made from the outside, by the higher damping of the echo sequence in the steel, but only very unreliably if the inside is filled with liquid which has penetrated into the gap. If the concrete lining has disappeared completely, this can sometimes be recognized by a backwall echo being obtained through the liquid, e.g. on steel pipes lined with a centrifugally cast layer of concrete. In another case, viz. the linings of cellulose digesters, penetrating acid corrodes the wall. These spots can be distinguished from spots which are still protected, by the less distinct formation of the echo sequence from the steel wall.

Adhesive bonds of strongly absorbing layers on metal should be treated like rubber-metal bonds. Examples are linings for brakes or clutches. When the echo method is used, they can be tested only from the metal side because of the strong absorption in the lining. When the sound-transmission method is applied in the immersion technique, one is usually obliged to use low frequencies. An important application is the testing of adhesive bonds between thin sheets in airplane construction. There it is required to distinguish the cases of Fig. 3.198a to c (bad), from d. For the usual gauges of about 1 mm in direct contact, high frequencies above 6 MHz are required (Fig. 3.198, top). Even if the 1 mm echo sequence is no longer resolved, the indication is still clear: in cases a and b (freely oscillating top sheet) a transmitting pulse with long decay is obtained. It is strongly damped by the adhering layer of putty (c). If the sheets are properly bonded, typical beats due to interference of the waves from the glue layer and the back appear. The differences are indicated by a TR probe of 4 MHz just as clearly: if the bonding is satisfactory, the echo is low, and can also be used for automatic indication by means of a monitor. For each gauge or combinations of different gauges of the sheets, it will first be necessary to ascertain the typical screen picture as obtained with artificial flaws.

Similar satisfactory results are obtained with the resonance method. The intensity method and perpendicular sound transmission can usually

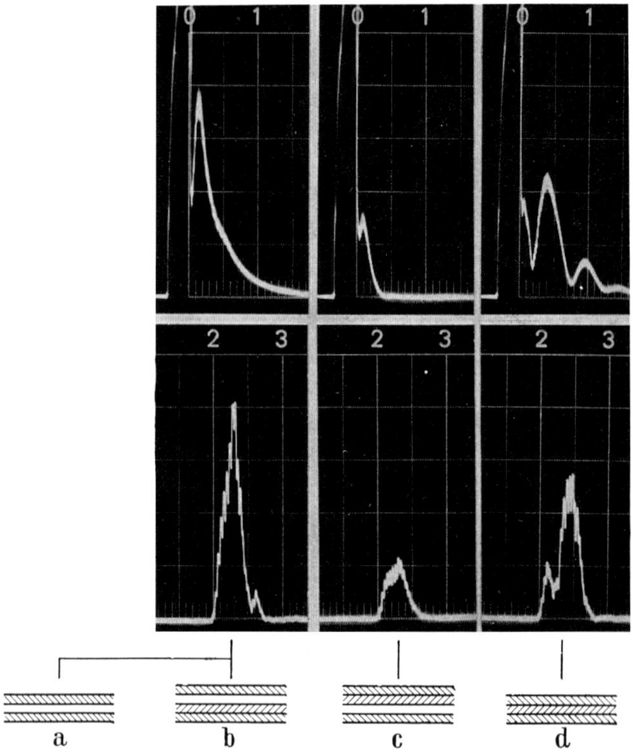

Fig. 3.198 Bonding test of glued aluminium sheets by the pulse-echo method (1 + 1 mm thick, cold-setting ethoxylin resin) top screen pictures: with direct contact at 12 MHz; centre: with TR probe and 4 MHz, range 100 mm (1 scale div. = 20 mm).

not be considered because the two surfaces are not readily accessible. In the case of overlapping adhesive joints a few centimetres wide, it is however possible to use zig-zag transverse waves to advantage with a probe arrangement as shown in Fig. 3.196d (on both sides of the joint).

The high resolving power of instruments using the shock-wave technique (Sec. 2.36) makes it possible to resolve by the echo method even total thicknesses of less than 1 mm, and to distinguish the cases a with b from c and d. With considerable expansion and a high-frequency trace, the shape of the echo can also be used as a basis for judging the quality of a given bond. However, no practical applications have yet become known.

Honeycomb structures (Fig 3.199), because of their high strength-to-weight ratio, play a considerable role in airplane and rocket construction.

They require the testing of bonds between the sheet skin (usually aluminium but also stainless steel, titanium or plastic) and the honeycomb core (usually aluminium, but also copper, steel or plastic). The bond usually consists of self-curing adhesives, and in the case of particularly strong constructions, also of brazing.

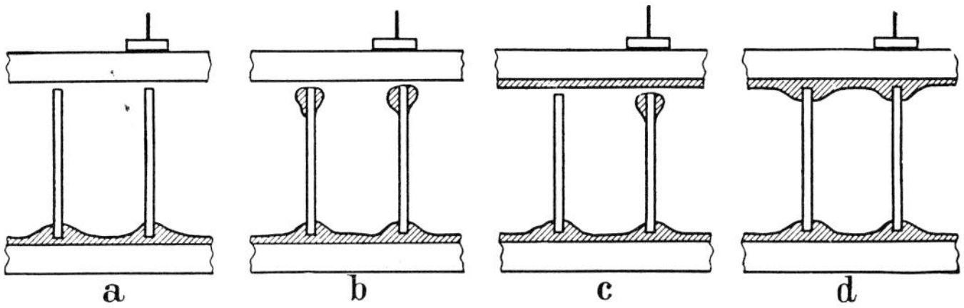

Fig. 3.199 Cross-section through honeycomb structure, schematic with faulty and good bonding.

Although the honeycomb walls usually consist of only 0.1 mm or even thinner metal strips, they transmit ultrasound of considerably greater wavelength from one side to the other, and reportedly at 0.5 and 1 MHz even better than at higher frequencies. One can thus use the immersion technique with sound transmission and still detect flawed spots of 1 to 2 cm^2.

With the echo method and the usual power of resolution, only case a with b can be distinguished from c and d (Fig. 3.199). However, since it can be assumed that flaw c occurs only rarely, this still permits safe differentiation between a good and a bad bond.

In contrast to glued layers, brazed layers damp the echo sequence from the sheet skin only very little, so that in this design it is possible to distinguish case c from d. According to [100] a carefully collimated 10 MHz beam of lithium sulphate probes in the immersion technique produces in case c a multiple echo sequence at all points, but in case d only between the honeycomb walls. Directly above a satisfactorily brazed wall the echo sequence disappears. It is possible to obtain by this method a C-scan picture on a CR screen with long after-glow (Fig. 3.200).

According to [158] probes for surface waves can be used also on bonded honeycomb structures, arranged as shown in Fig. 3.196d. The plate wave in the sheet skin produced in this way is more strongly damped along its path from one probe to the other, the more satisfactorily bonded thwart-sheets are encountered. Two probes mounted equidistantly in a common holder and using oil as couplant, are moved over the sheet in a fixed orientation relative to the thwart-sheets. After calibration by means of artificial flaws, faulty bonding and non-bonding could be eliminated on the basis of the higher transmission echoes, showing good agreement with destructive testing methods. The frequency was chosen so that the plate thickness was always less than one half of the surface wave length. Otherwise the damping effect would have been too small.

Concerning other problems in the testing of bonds in rocket and space engineering, see [410, 406].

In the case of *fuel elements for reactors*, which consist of a core of uranium or a material containing uranium, and a shell, usually of alu-

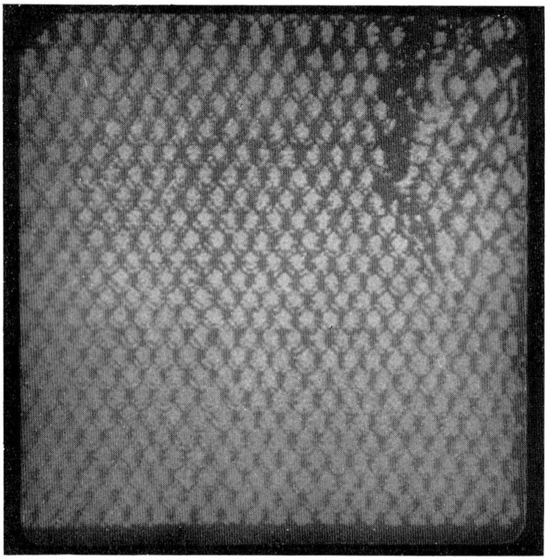

Fig. 3.200 *Ultragraph* screen picture of a honeycomb structure with defective bond (Automation Industries Inc., Pasadena Calif., USA).

minium, zirconium or its alloys, uniform heat dissipation requires satisfactory bonding between shell and core. This bond is produced by the material being rolled on, or preferably by brazing. Since the wall thickness is less than the limit of resolution for conventional pulse-echo instruments (less than 2 mm), plate-shaped elements are preferably scanned by sound transmission under water. To achieve high scanning speeds a testing equipment, made by Sperry, uses two narrow, long quartz plates as transmitter and receiver, respectively, which cover the full width of the reactor element (approximately 12 cm) (Fig. 3.201). A rotating belt of sound-absorbing material with holes, similar to the one shown in Fig. 3.185, blanks out all sound except for a narrow beam which scans the slowly fed element line by line. The result is recorded on a direct recorder as a go/no-go indication. In this way, both bonding surfaces are scanned simultaneously so that, if a flaw is detected, it is not possible to state which side is affected. A testing device according to [39] for flat fuel elements of about 6 × 100 mm cross-section and 1.35 m long, uses a mechanically moved pair of probes. A 5 MHz beam, reduced by masking to 2 mm diameter, detects bonding defects as small as 0.8 mm in diameter, using go/no-go recording. The testing time per element is approx. 7 min. Fuel elements of this type are mounted in a block each consisting of 6 elements spaced 11 mm apart. So that they may be tested also when installed, a special probe guide which fits between the elements, has been designed.

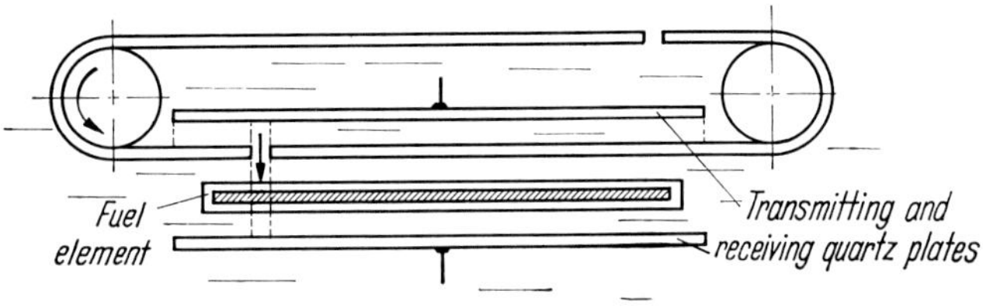

Fig. 3.201 Scanning device with sound transmission and rotating diaphragm (Sperry).

Cylindrical reactor elements are tested by sound transmission as in the immersion technique, wherein the rod is moved past the probes in a spiral motion [316]. In the case of wall thicknesses over 1 to 2 mm, one can also use a TR probe and the pulse echo method, which has the advantage that all flaws can be located by testing from one side only. For extensive flaws the method according to Fig. 3.196 using plate waves, may also be considered.

Regarding other problems of bonding tests in reactor engineering, see McClung and Cook [254].

On bearing *boxes*, the bonding of the tin or lead-bronze liner to the steel backing can be tested. If the bearing metal is *cast on*, it is readily penetrated by frequencies up to 5 MHz for the usual thicknesses of up to 10 mm. This bearing alloy has approximately the same acoustic impedance as steel, resulting in a properly bonded spot furnishing only weak echoes. *Sprayed* metal coatings are transmissive in thin layers only, e.g. silver of a few tenths of a millimetre in small bearings. Thicker layers may have such low transmittance that their bonding cannot be tested through the layer.

The bushings of small bearings usually are smooth and cylindrical, apart from oil grooves and collets. Using sound transmission, they can therefore best be tested by the immersion technique. For this purpose the bearings, or in the case of split bearings both halves assembled, are placed on a turning device and scanned spirally by an axial feed of the probe.

Layers of bearing metal thicker than 2 to 3 mm can also be tested by the pulse-echo method, smaller bearings in the immersion technique and larger bearings with layers exceeding 4 mm alternatively also in direct contact, the probe being fitted with a matching plastic contact shoe [249]. In the case of large bearings for heavy machinery, the liner backing is a complex steel casting unsuitable for sound transmission, where the pulse-echo method furnishes no uniform backwall echo. The test is made in direct contact, attention being paid only to the echo of the bond and any possible multiple echoes produced by it.

On very small bearings the probe can no longer be placed inside. It is then recommended that the immersion technique be used and a reflector which reflects the axial beam normal to the wall, at the same time focusing it.

In the case of *composite castings* the problems and their solutions are very similar, e.g. grey cast iron cylinders for internal combustion engines around which aluminium jackets with cooling fins are cast. These are tested from the inside by the immersion technique. It has been reported that in the case of larger bonding defects the method according to Fig. 3.196c, but with direct contact, has proved successful.

The bonding of *enamel coats*, e.g. in chemical equipment, can be tested from the enamel side using probes with a metallized contact face. Here the detection of cracks in the layer is also important. Since as a rule these cracks have no preferred orientation, they should be scanned with an angle probe of approximately 70°, the sound beam being swung continuously through a large arc to ensure that at one stage the cracks are irradiated perpendicularly. Either surface can be used for this purpose but preferably the convex side.

Galvanic coats are tested from the plating side for flaking, provided a backwall echo can be obtained. Specimens of a simple shape can alternatively also be scanned by means of surface waves, which is quicker where larger areas are concerned. Flaws will then reveal themselves by their echoes.

If particularly onerous demands are made in respect of the ultrasonic test results concerning any of the various types of bond mentioned and requiring more than mere determination of a complete detachment, it is strongly recommended that first the applicability of the method be checked by a larger number of subsequent destructive tests.

3.293 Shrink Fits

The transmittance of a boundary face separating identical materials with no binder between them depends on the ratio of the residual air gap to the wave length (Figs. 1.17 and 1.18). While optically plane faces, e.g. precision gauge blocks, become largely transmissive if simply placed together without external pressure being applied, a more or less high pressure is required to achieve the same result if the surfaces are less perfect. Thus, the transmission or reflection of the boundary face can be used for determining the external pressure at a given surface roughness, e.g. for general measurement of high pressures [191], or the pressure of a shrink fit [139, 140], which is equivalent to a quality test.

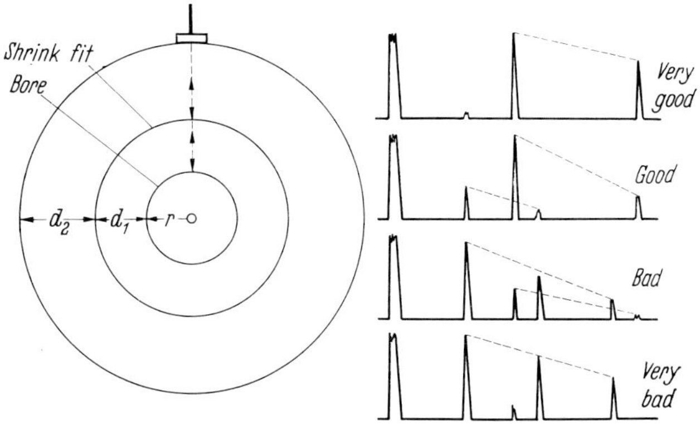

Fig. 3.202 Shrink-fit test and schematic screen pictures (combination echoes have been omitted for greater clarity).

According to Fig. 3.202 the ratio of shrink-fit echo to backwall echo in a specimen producing a backwall echo can be used for qualitative grading according to the following pattern:

1. Shrink-fit echo $\ll$ backwall echo: shrink fit very good,
2. shrink-fit echo $<$ backwall echo: shrink fit good,
3. shrink-fit echo $>$ backwall echo: shrink fit moderate to bad,
4. shrink-fit echo $\gg$ backwall echo: shrink fit very bad.

In the last case a long multiple echo sequence of the shrink fit is also obtained.

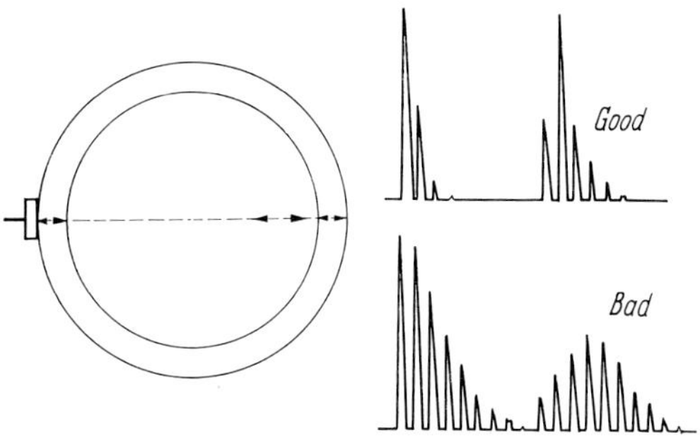

Fig. 3.203 Shrink fit on solid core and with relatively thin shell; schematic screen picture of good and bad bond respectively.

As far as any quantitative evaluation is concerned, it should be noted that both echoes are a function of the radius of curvature and the sound path. If one operates in the distant field of the probe, it is recommended that the multiplication factors be first determined from Fig. 1.47 so as to arrive at the echo amplitude for flat boundary faces. With the latter it is then possible to compare also the shrink fits of differently shaped specimens if one makes additional allowance for the dependence of the echo amplitude on the distance as in Figs.1.87 and 1.88 ($G = \infty$). For instance, using flat plates one can calibrate the echo amplitudes empirically by applying different pressures and computing the results for cylindrical shrink fits of arbitrary shape. If the surface conditions are approximately the same, the shrink-fit pressure can then be given in absolute figures. If an instrument with calibrated gain control is used, no backwall echo is required for this purpose because it can be replaced by the echo of a plate. To exclude the influence of attenuation, low frequencies are used.

In a solid specimen with cylindrical shrink fit, as shown in Fig. 3.203 the sound travels through the latter twice. The backwall echo then appears as an echo sequence which may start with small echoes as in Fig. 3.35 and which has a maximum. The further back the maximum appears in this sequence, the greater is the power of reflection of the shrink fit and the less satisfactory therefore the latter.

Any oil which has entered, as may happen in the case of old shrink fits which have become loose, greatly increases the transmittance as shown in Figs. 1.17 and 1.18, so that evaluation according to the above grading table may give wrong results. The evaluation should then be graded down by at least one step. To be on the safe side it is recommended that the oil be expelled by heating.

3.3 Metals and their Special Testing Problems

3.31 Steel

The differences in acoustic velocity of different types of steel, whether unalloyed or alloyed, are less than 5%, as shown in the following table[1]. For less exacting measurements, they can be neglected, where this concerns distance determination. However, the change in transverse velocity, which is usually in the same sense and of the same order, has a not inconsiderable influence on the beaming angle when beaming obliquely: at 70° a change of 1% already amounts to about 1.5°. For flaw locating it is therefore advisable to use the same steel as that of the specimen when calibrating the instrument.

Treatments of the steel, such as annealing, hardening and quenching can have a greater effect on the values of the acoustic velocities than the composition of the alloying elements, as indicated specifically by numbers 6 and 7 when compared with No. 1. Hardening and quenching as well as tempering always reduce these values. The attenuation, so far determined

[1] The test specimens in the form of short cylinders approximately 50 mm long were made available by courtesy of Deutsche Edelstahl-Werke, Krefeld.

No.	Type of steel, dia. in mm, composition		Condition	Strength kg/mm²	Rockwell hardness R_c	c_l	c_t
						in 10^3 m/s	
1	Unalloyed case-hardening steel 0.15 C	80	Annealed	42		5.94	3.24
2	Unalloyed structural steel 0.45 C, 0.7 Mn	50	Annealed	68		5.94	3.25
3	Tool steel 1.0 C	45	Annealed	64		5.96	3.23
4	Alloyed structural steel 0.35 C, 0.6 Mn, 1.0 Cr, 0.2 Mo	70	Annealed	65		5.95	3.26
			Quenched a. tempered	98		5.93	3.24
			Hardened	158		5.90	3.23
5	Alloyed structural steel 0.30 C, 0.4 Mn, 2.0 Cr, 2.0 Ni, 0.2 Mo	65	Annealed	67		5.93	3.22
			Quenched and tempered	117		5.87	3.21
			Hardened	137		5.89	3.21
6	Ball-bearing steel 1.0 C, 1.5 Cr	62	Annealed	71		5.99	3.27
			Hardened		65	5.89	3.20
7	High-speed steel 0.9 C, 4.0 Cr, 2.5 Mo, 2.5 Va, 3,0 W	52	Annealed	87		6.06	3.35
			Hardened		63	5.88	3.19
8	Alloyed tool steel 2.0 C, 12.0 Cr, 0.6 W	50	Annealed	79		6.14	3.31
			Hardened		62	6.01	3.22
9	Stainless steel ferritic 0.15 C, 17.0 Cr	75	Annealed	98		6.01	3.36
10	Stainless, can be hardened and tempered 0.4 C, 17.0 Cr, 1.2 Mo	75	Hardened and tempered	95		6.09	3.36

only qualitatively (not shown in the table), is, with a few exceptions, reduced by hardening as well as quenching and tempering.

On thin sheets, the influence of texture makes itself felt: for zig-zag transverse waves different acoustic velocities are obtained for directions normal and parallel to the direction of rolling. In the case of plate waves, this anisotropy makes itself evident in the fact that an excitation angle determined for the one direction is no longer optimal for the other.

As a rule in the forged and rolled condition almost all steels show satisfactory transmittance. A few high-alloy steels, however, show a tendency to form coarse grains and thus may show great differences from one spot to another, which can be explained plausibly by the fact that the scatter increases with the third power of the grain size. Some alloyed steels show exceptionally low attenuation which may likewise be a disadvantage in testing because very late multiple echoes would produce phantom echoes (2.321). To suppress this phenomenon, the repetition frequency should be reduced. It has not yet been explained whether this effect which is observed particularly in stainless nickel steels, results from the alloying or the fine-grained structure, or simply from the fact

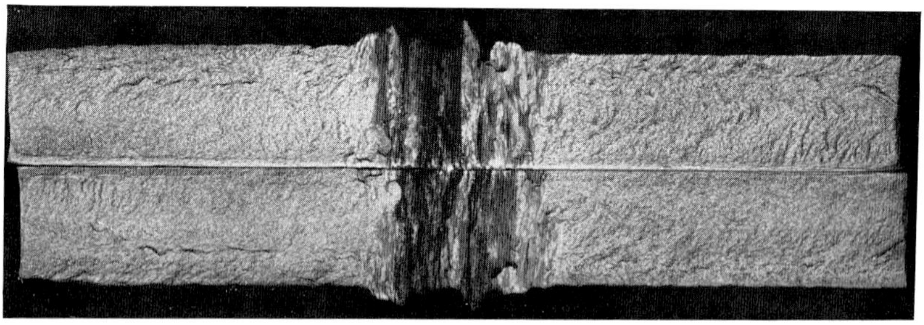

Fig. 3.204 Fracture face of a Cr-Mo steel showing fibrous structure which could not be detected by ultrasonics (according to MARIANESCHI).

that these steels are less contaminated than ordinary carbon steels because of the clean melting in electric furnaces. Re. austenitic steels, see HOLMES [149].

When testing steel, failures of the ultrasonic method are rare. Dubious cases usually arise when there are closed segregations which produce no echoes. In a few cases it was also found that the cause was a pronounced banded structure which the destructive test disclosed as flaw. However, reports have also been published concerning failures in the case of true non-metallic inclusions [244]. Among others, a so-called fibrous fracture in forged Cr-Mo steel blocks of 220 × 220 mm cross-section shown in Fig. 3.204 could not be detected even at 5 MHz. This concerned segregations of chromium (III) oxide.

3.32 Cast Steel

Little is known about differences in acoustic velocities of cast steel In the case of unalloyed and low-alloy steel castings the attenuation at 1 to 2 MHz is usually so low that specimens of thickness 1 m and more can be penetrated without difficulty. High-alloy cast steel is supposedly more difficult to test, and austenitic manganese steel not at all.

As far as any type of cast metal is concerned, it should not be overlooked that the attenuation is partially influenced also by genuine small cavities and impurities, so that the possibility of testing may depend on the purity and the casting method.

Regarding difficulties encountered in the testing of cast steel and the interpretation of the indications, see also RAUTERKUS [301]. KIPKA [176] has pointed out that measurements of sound attenuation in unalloyed cast steel permit certain deductions regarding the structure. See also [183, 359, 360].

3.33 Cast Iron

In view of the very different types of cast iron as far as its composition, casting conditions and resultant structure are concerned, it is not surprising that the acoustic velocity and the attenuation also fluctuate within very wide limits.

According to the form of the graphite, one distinguishes mainly lamellar cast-iron (with lamellar graphite, cf. Figs. 3.210a and b) and spheroidal graphite (with spherical graphite, cf. Fig. 3.210c).

Let us first mention a special form, viz. *white cast iron*, which is obtained either intentionally or unintentionally by rapidly cooling ordinary cast iron and which is characterized by great hardness and brittleness. Its acoustic velocity differs only slightly from that of steel, and its attenuation, because of its relatively fine structure (ledeburite) is much lower than that of lamellar cast iron and comparable approximately with that of cast steel. It is produced intentionally in chill castings, e.g. rolls, in the form of surface layers (see below). Work pieces which have solidified completely white are usually unsuitable and these faulty castings can then readily be sorted out on the basis of their ultrasonic properties.

In *lamellar cast iron* the length of the lamellae, i.e. the coarseness of the graphite, is expressed by code numbers from 1 to 8, corresponding to lamella length visible in micro-section, which range from 1 mm to 0.015 mm [405, 456].

The relationship between the properties of cast iron and the acoustic velocities has been investigated by ZIEGLER and GERSTNER [395, 397, 115]. The dependence of the velocity of the longitudinal waves on the *size and quantity of the graphite* is shown in Fig. 3.205, indicating that with decreasing coarseness and quantity it approaches that of steel. Since in micro-lamellar cast iron the amount of graphite is usually smaller (as a result of the mixture concerned, i.e. the additives in the melt, which produce a desired quality on a purely empirical basis), the correlation can for practical purposes be simplified as follows: the finer the graphite the higher the acoustic velocity.

According to measurements by PATTERSON and BODMER [286] the velocity of the transverse waves is related linearly to the longitudinal velocity (Fig. 3.206), even if the spheroidal cast iron discussed below is included.

According to [397] a second important correlation exists for the *saturation* of the cast iron with carbon, which can be calculated from the formula

$$S_c = \frac{C}{4.23 - 0.312\,\mathrm{Si} - 0.275\,\mathrm{P}},$$

given the percentage content of carbon (C), silicon (Si) and phosphorus (P). According to Fig. 3.207 this correlation is given by a straight line with a bend at saturation 1; it can replace chemical analysis for rapid

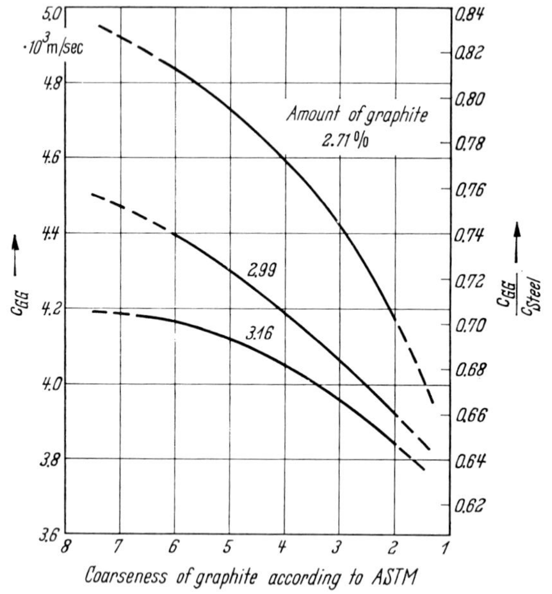

Fig. 3.205 Longitudinal acoustic velocity in lamellar cast iron containing graphite of different size and quantity according to ZIEGLER and GERSTNER, on righthand ordinate relative acoustic velocity referred to steel ($5.95 \cdot 10^3$ m/s).

determination of S_c provided the shape of the sample and the casting conditions remain constant. In this connection FRIELINGHAUS [110] has established in addition, a distinct influence of the wall thickness of the casting concerned.

Finally, the *tensile strength* is likewise a linear function of the acoustic velocity (Fig. 3.208), as long as the method of melting remains the same (electric induction furnace with medium frequency or cupola). Surprisingly, it is independent of the wall thickness although experience shows that the latter strongly influences the segregation of graphite because of the resultant cooling conditions. Clearly, however, the influences of both the size and the quantity of the graphite cancel each other. In practice, it is of great importance to be able to measure the tensile strength at various points in a casting having different wall thicknesses, by determining the true thickness d mechanically and the apparent wall thickness d_s by means of an ultrasonic instrument calibrated on steel. The ratio d/d_s (<1) is also the ratio of the acoustic velocities c_{GG}/c_{steel}[1], entered in Fig. 3.208 as ordinate on the right. However, according to [110] a slight influence of the wall thickness is detectable even here. Nevertheless, the relationship between acoustic velocity and strength when determined on similar work pieces was found to be acceptable as a quality check and even for acceptance purposes [387, 431].

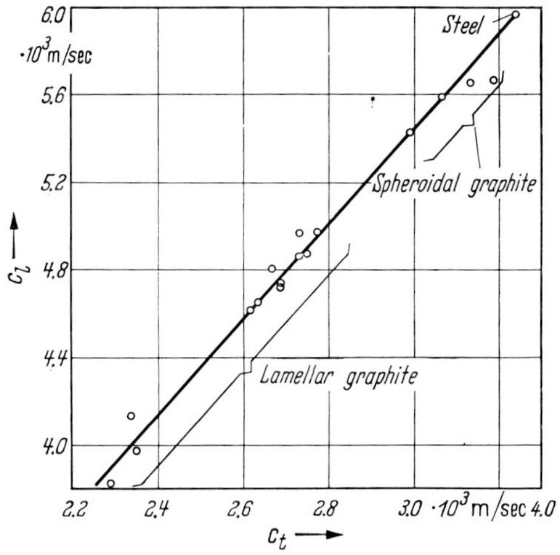

Fig. 3.206 Velocities of longitudinal and transverse waves in grey cast iron containing different amounts and forms of graphite, according to PATTERSON and BODMER.

The acoustic velocity values determined by SEEMANN [238] for cast iron of 14 to 30 kp/mm² tensile strength (quality grade GG[1] 14 to GG 30) fit the straight line for the electric furnace satisfactorily.

Also the *hardness* can be related to the acoustic velocity and determined from it empirically if the other conditions remain constant, as

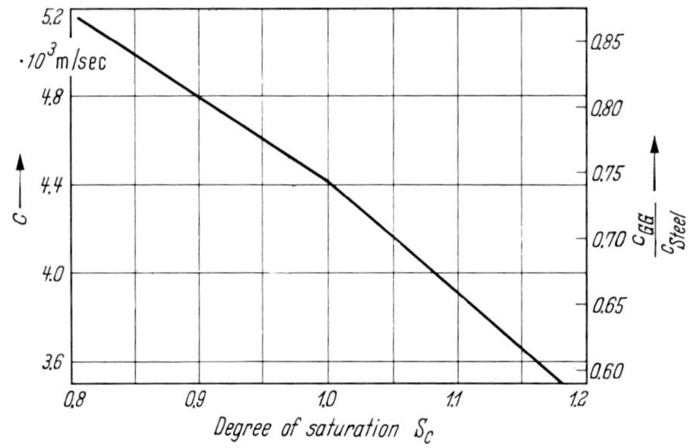

Fig. 3.207 Acoustic velocity of longitudinal waves in lamellar cast iron as a function of the degree of saturation of the carbon, according to ZIEGLER and GERSTNER.

[1] GG = cast iron.

confirmed by Thieme [365] on chilled rolls for the average hardness of the core. Allowance should be made here for the greatly differing acoustic velocity and thickness of the shell solidified white.

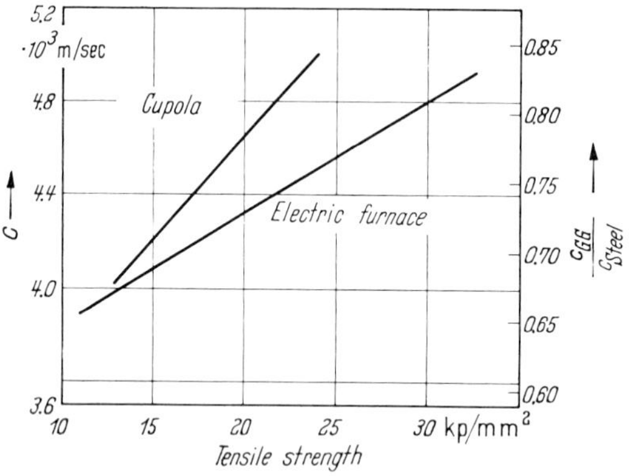

Fig. 3.208 Longitudinal acoustic velocity in lamellar cast iron as a function of the tensile strength, for melts produced in different furnaces, according to Ziegler and Gerstner.

In grey cast iron it is often important to be able to *measure the wall thickness* at mechanically inaccessible points, e.g. in motor casings. However, since the acoustic velocity in turn depends to some extent on the wall thickness, this makes the measurement difficult. According to [295] a linear relation exists (Fig. 3.209) which, however, depends also on the degree of saturation. Although the latter is constant for a given melt as well as for the whole casting, it is not always known. To overcome this difficulty, in practice one therefore measures the wall thickness mechanically at two accessible points where this thickness differs as much as possible, interpolating linearlyfor the other points. High accuracy is not possible, but also rarely required. Where an error of only about 5% is of any consequence, the influence of the wall thickness can be neglected completely if the instrument is calibrated at a mean wall thickness. Sometimes it is also only a question of determining whether the core or the bore in a cylinder is eccentric. This merely requires comparative measurements at various points with no previous calibration.

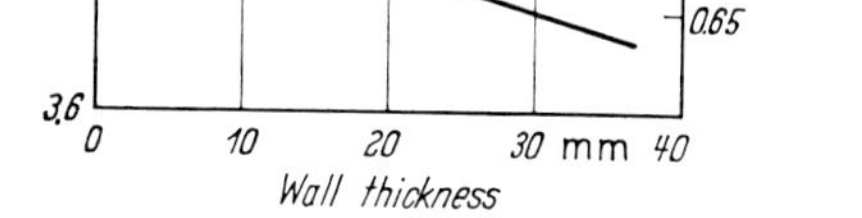

Fig. 3.209 Longitudinal acoustic velocity in lamellar cast iron as a function of the wall thickness at different degrees of saturation, according to Ziegler and Gerstner.

Spheroidal cast iron shows markedly different behaviour in respect of both ultrasonic attenuation and velocity, which becomes clear when the micro-sections (Fig. 3.210) are compared. Even at identical total graphite content, as for instance in Figs. 3.210a and c, the spheroidal form reduces the acoustic velocity of the pure matrix to a far lesser extent than the lamellar form and has also a smaller influence on the sound transmission. According to [397] the acoustic velocity is a unique measure of the ratio between spheroidal graphite and total graphite (Fig. 3.211) as long as the saturation remains constant. Since the latter is approxi-

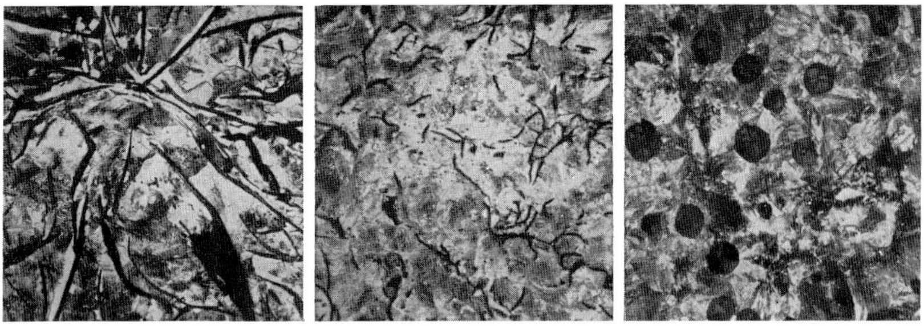

a b c

Fig. 3.210 Micrographs of cast iron with different graphite structures (PATTERSON and BODMER); a) and b) lamellar, c) spheroidal. (a) Structure A_1, 2.78% graphite; (b) A_5, 1.7% graphite; (c) 100% spheroidal graphite, 2.52% graphite.

mately known when making the mixture, the acoustic velocity can serve as a measure of quality for spheroidal cast iron. In the case of 100% spheroidal graphite the acoustic velocity is at least 96% of that of steel, irrespective of the saturation.

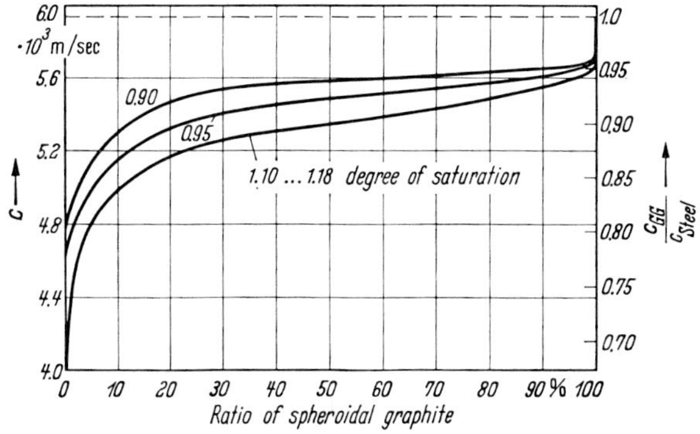

Fig. 3.211 Longitudinal acoustic velocity in spheroidal cast iron as a function of the ratio of spheroidal graphite to total graphite content, according to ZIEGLER and GERSTNER.

If it is desired to determine the tensile strength of high-quality grades of cast iron quite generally, regardless of lamellar or spheroidal, on the basis of ultrasonic measurements, it has been shown [386] that to a first approximation Young's modulus can be determined with sufficient accuracy on the basis of the longitudinal velocity alone. To deduce from this modulus the tensile strength is, however, not generally acceptable. This requires the determination of an additional quantity, e.g. the Brinell hardness. Both measurements can be made on the finished article.

The *attenuation* in grey iron castings likewise provides a useful possibility for the non-destructive determination of technological properties. Its measurement with satisfactory accuracy is, however, less simple than that of the velocity, particularly on the finished article because it requires parallel surfaces.

It has long been known that in general cast iron having tensile strength values above 20 kp/mm^2 is sufficiently transmissive for flaw detection, even at frequencies above 1 MHz [328]. Conversely, the tensile strength can be deduced approximately from the attenuation. However, satisfactory calibration is possible only if in a sample series all variables except one are kept constant, e.g. except the macro-structure of the graphite. For instance, good transmission for flaw detection with 2 MHz can be expected for lamellar cast iron with code numbers above 4 (i.e. lamellar less then 0.1 mm long).

According to [386] a correlation exists between the attenuation and Young's modulus in the case of high-quality cast iron with spheroidal graphite, which is independent of the heat treatment and the structure.

The difficulty encountered in measuring comparable, absolute values of the attenuation [206] does not prevent the establishment of quality checks on the basis of the decrease in echo amplitude of a given echo sequence, which is adequate for practical requirements. One can then either use sample blocks while keeping the conditions regarding dimensions and instrument adjustment constant [174], or alternatively one can test directly at approximately plane-parallel spots on identical castings with surfaces as cast [47]. In this way it was for instance found possible to sort out, under production conditions, brake drums for automobiles according to their strength with an accuracy of $\pm$ 2 kp/mm^2, by empirically correlating the tensile strength to the ratio of the echo amplitudes of two given echoes. Cf. [65, 168, 307].

Here it should not be overlooked that such a simply defined *attenuation factor*, in addition to the true attenuation, is affected also by the probe because spreading of the sound also changes the echo amplitude. It is therefore not permissible, e.g., to measure simply at different frequencies and deduce therefrom the frequency pattern of the attenuation. Moreover, different thicknesses of specimens may not, without more ado, be compared with each other (cf. 3.63).

Furthermore, Frielinghaus has found linear relationships between the logarithm of the coefficient of attenuation on the one hand, and the degree of saturation, the density and the tensile strength on the other. In all instances, however, the wall thickness appears as an additional parameter. Under certain conditions measurement of the attenuation, provided this can be done in a form acceptable in practice, may look more promising than measurement of the acoustic velocity [110, 111]. ZETTLER has also investigated the correlation between attenuation and elastic properties of cast iron [394].

In thick-walled castings the unavoidable different solidification times are responsible for structural differences between zones on the surface and zones in the core, which as a rule do not manifest themselves by distinct echoes during sound transmission because the zone transitions are gradual and involve longer distances. These differences are nevertheless pronounced if the specimen is tested parallel to the surface: the attenuation is lower near the surface, and the acoustic velocity higher than in the centre, because of the finer segregation of graphite during rapid cooling. Only in the case of chill castings where the choice of a given composition and rapid cooling produce a layer of white cast iron near the surface, are the transitions so abrupt and the differences of the acoustic properties so great that distinct echoes are obtained from the transition zones, if irradiated perpendicularly (THIEME [365]). This has already been exploited practically for some time for measuring the thickness of the hard shell. The high transmittance of the white cast iron makes the use of frequencies up to 10 MHz possible. In the case of thin layers, e.g. of thickness less than 10 mm, the dead zone of the probe frequently interferes. It is then recommended that a TR probe be used, e.g. for 4 MHz.

Finally, of interest from a metallurgical point of view, is the fact that pig iron under certain conditions of production shows relatively good acoustic transmission, resembling in this respect as well as in other properties, good-quality cast iron (STÄGER and MEISTER [347]).

LEHTINEN has also measured the acoustic velocity in liquid cast iron [224].

3.34 Light Metals

It is well known that in the case of aluminium and magnesium, as well as alloys of these two and their alloys with small amounts of heavy metal (less than 1%), the anisotropy is so small that the grain size has little effect on the testability of interest in practice. The tests can therefore readily be made on ingots which are continuously cast, in spite of the occasional occurrence of very large grain sizes [201]. In contrast to steel the tests during the manufacture of high-quality light metal products already begin as soon as the ingot has cooled sufficiently. At this stage the transverse and longitudinal test can reveal gross defects, such as longitudinal cracks in the core (spiders). On cut-off sections of approximately 1 m length it is possible to detect also small flaws, such as entrained slag (dross) by testing from the cut face. Customary frequencies are 1 to 2 MHz. Since the outer skin on continuously cast ingots is very uneven but metallically clean, this is sufficient for a rough test. Occasionally it may be advisable to grind a few spots or along a track. Particularly careful tests can already be made on the cast ingot after the rough-milling in preparation for rolling. However, the value of excessively accurate tests is rather questionable because some flaws are later not found again in the finished product [57].

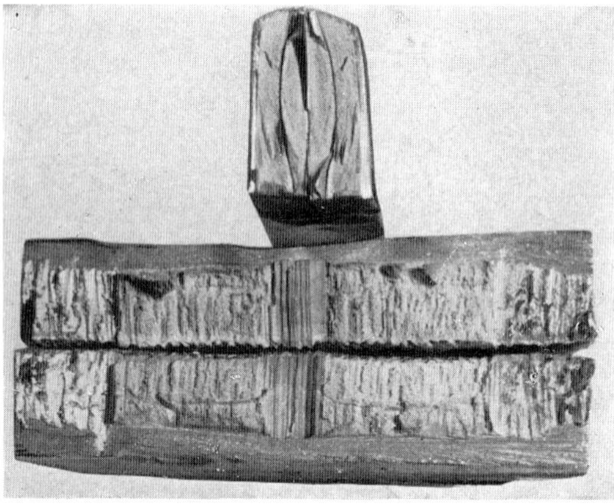

Fig. 3.212 Fracture specimens of extruded light-metal sections with flaws which cannot be reliably detected by ultrasonics. Above: rolled out shrinkage in flat material (sealed lamination); below: fibrous fracture in 60 mm round stock.

Failures of flaw tests occur in the case of worked light metal more frequently than with other metals. Firstly, some flaws in spite of favourable orientation normal to the sound beam may be considerably greater than could be expected from a comparison of the echo with that from flat-bottomed holes, which may be due to a certain transmittance of thin slag inclusions [57]. Probably for the same reason it is sometimes also possible to observe with ultrasonics rolled out shrinkages in sections only up to a certain distance, although the flaw continues and is readily revealed by a destructive test (Fig. 3.212, "fibrous fracture"). Similarly pronounced macro-segregations as in Fig. 3.213 cannot be detected with frequencies up to 5 MHz although the specimen concerned bursts even at moderate load. This particular flaw could only be detected at 10 and 25 MHz but even then only by an echo corresponding to that of a flat-bottomed hole of approximately 1 mm diameter. Higher frequencies are therefore preferable for detecting such flaws in light metal. Frequently, however, an additional preceding heat treatment proves successful.

When light metal of any given cross-section is extruded, it is of interest to find the transition from the normal, fine-grained structure to the coarser structure with its inferior mechanical properties, which is sometimes encountered during extrusion near the end of the ingot. A very simple ultrasonic method can be used for this purpose: in spite of

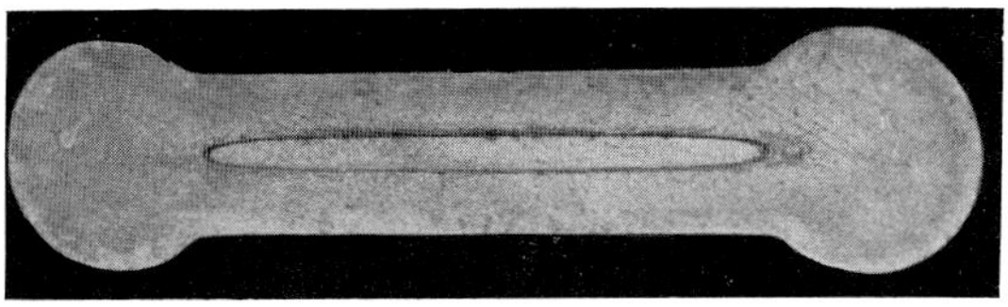

Fig. 3.213 Macro-etching of an aluminium section with a flaw which is difficult to detect (analysis 0.55 Mg, 0.80 Si, 0.33 Fe, remainder Al) (natural size).

the small cross-sectional dimensions of the section, the pulse-echo instrument is adjusted for a very long measuring range, e.g. 5 m, at high gain. The individual multiple echoes together with various transverse echoes, can then hardly be distinguished from each other (Fig. 3.214) but they form a *brush* whose length serves as a measure. As a result of the increased attenuation caused by the coarse grain, which however is very small in the case of light metals, the difference becomes very marked.

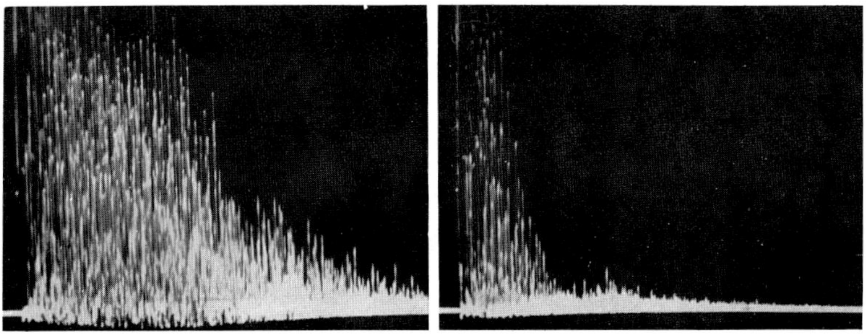

a b

Fig. 3.214 The "brush" method for comparing the attenuation in similarly shaped specimens, applied here for testing the structure in extruded round aluminium bars of diameter 80 mm, frequency 4 MHz, a) in the normal state; b) with coarsened structure.

Alloys of light metal with heavy metals differ greatly in their behaviour, particularly when cast. The casting method, viz. continuous casting or casting in sand moulds or ingot moulds, as well as the cooling conditions have likewise a great influence, which indicates that the anisotropy in some mixed crystals is no longer negligible. No measurements are available nor quantitative results of any tests on the attenuation; it is therefore only possible to draw attention to a few points.

The usual alloys produced for extruding and rolling show good to excellent transmission (at approximately 2 MHz) even if they contain several per cent of copper and manganese. According to Stäger, Schütz and Meister [346] the precipitation-hardening alloy Al-Cu-Ti (4.76 Cu, 0.27 Ti) when cast in sand shows low transmission even at 1 MHz. Strong scatter echoes may possibly result from segregations of copper, which still interfere considerably even after heat treatment. The Mg-Al-Zn-Mn alloy with 0.88 Al, 0.69 Zn and 0.17 Mn behaves similarly. In contrast, Mg-Zn-Zr with 3.93 Zn and 1.1 Zr shows good transmission, at least in a favourable casting position (upright as against flat) although some of the zirconium is deposited as insoluble zirconium oxide at the grain boundaries. After heat treatment the attenuation usually decreases slightly, but in some cases it also increases, which would seem more logical, because effective heat treatment depends on the segregation of the supersaturated mixed crystals. Since the reasons for this behaviour are as yet obscure, it is not possible to draw any conclusions concerning the hardening and tempering from the attenuation. However, since it is of practical interest to be able to check this condition by non-destructive means, the measurement of the transverse acoustic velocity may turn out to be promising. In the case of the above alloys in the cast state this velocity is increased by hardening and tempering, in contrast to the longitudinal velocity which shows no clear change [346].

The behaviour of the acoustic velocity of the longitudinal waves in light metal alloys is still puzzling in some respect. While ordinary extrusion alloys, such as Al-Cu-Mg-Mn-Si (with 4.48 Cu, 1.26 Mg, 0.74 Mn, 0.54 Si) very closely approach the value measured in pure aluminium (viz. around $6.2 \cdot 10^3$ m/s according to [346]), cast alloys show values some of which are considerably higher, while others are lower: according to [229] the longitudinal acoustic velocity in the case of Al-Mg-Si with only 0.57 Mg, 0.68 Si, 0.74 Mn and 0.20 Fe, $c_l = 6.72 \cdot 10^3$ m/s in the continuously cast ingot, while the above-mentioned precipitation-hardening alloys if cast in sand have values between 5.4 and 5.7 which in addition depend largely on the wall thickness (as in the case of cast iron).

Since, therefore, the structure can have a considerable influence on the acoustic velocity, one must be careful in attributing any change of its value to a shift in concentration of the alloying components. Lukas and Lutsch [229] have found in the above-mentioned alloy Al-Mg-Si an increase of 1.5% from the core towards the periphery of a cast ingot and they suspect that this is due to an increase of the silicon from 0.54 to 0.67%. However, this seems questionable because on the one hand this element does not change the acoustic velocity in Al-Cu-Mg-Mn-Si appreciably as compared with pure aluminium, and because on the other hand a quite considerable change of the acoustic velocity has been measured as a function of the grain size in pure aluminium, an effect which can also be assumed to be present in alloys. The change might thus also be explained by differences between the structure in the core and in the periphery.

The pronounced texture in continously cast ingots has already been suspected of being the cause of curvature in the sound beam ([74], contribution by E. STANFORD). However, this phenomenon can possibly also be explained by the sidewall effect.

3.35 Copper and Copper Alloys

Because of the anisotropy of copper, and particularly its mixed crystals with zinc, the examiner using ultrasonics is particularly wary of copper, brass and bronze in the cast state.

Single crystals and excessively coarse-crystalline material are, however, not particularly difficult to test: extruded brass plates with a thickness of a few centimetres occasionally have clearly visible crystals, having dimensions comparable with the plate thickness and the diameter of the probe. During scanning the clearly visible backwall echo jumps back and forth by a multiple of its width, in accordance with the random orientation of the crystal being irradiated at that moment. This shows that the true absorption can make only a minor contribution to the attenuation, while the main contribution in a cluster of crystals is the scattering.

As soon as the width of the sound beam has become wide enough to include several adjacent grains, the testability becomes nil where small shrinkages and pores up to about pea size have to be detected. This therefore eliminates all untreated sand castings and die castings, and even continuous casting. Only if a grain size smaller by about 2 orders of magnitude (referred to the mean diameter) is ensured by means of centrifugal casting, does the cast structure again become readily transmissive and can it be tested almost as easily as worked material of the same composition. This was confirmed by measurements of STÄGER, SCHÜTZ and MEISTER [347] on a number of copper alloys.

Reference [347] furthermore showed that suitable heat treatment for relieving residual stresses, i.e. below the recrystallization temperature, can slightly improve the transmittance of otherwise non-transmissive grades, so that such specimens can possibly be tested for coarse defects. However, if prior to working, e.g. conversion of copper into wire, or brass ingots into plate, a more accurate test is required, there is no alternative to performing this test after the first rolling pass. The improvement is astonishing. The testablity of the final product is no longer appreciably limited by the influence of the material itself. In the case of wall thickness measurements it should, however, be noted that the copper alloys have a pronounced tendency to show a rolling texture: for instance, if the calibration has been made on a section of one copper plate, and if one then measures the thickness of other copper plates, gross errors may result from the fact that the acoustic velocity of the latter can be very different because of different texture. The instrument should therefore be calibrated directly on the plate to be measured.

The testing problems encountered on centrifugal castings are the detection of clusters of pores (using frequencies up to 5 MHz and testing from the machined surface by observing the disappearance of the bottom echo), furthermore the detection of large pores and of voids; they can be found only if they are not hidden within clusters of micro-pores. The testability differs little from any of the alloys, particularly for brass (Cu-Zn 72/28, 58/42, Cu-Zn-Pb 58/40/2) aluminium bronze (Cu-Al 92/8), German silver (Cu-Zn-Ni 63/25/12) and red brass (Cu-Zn-Sn-Pb 88/4/4/4).

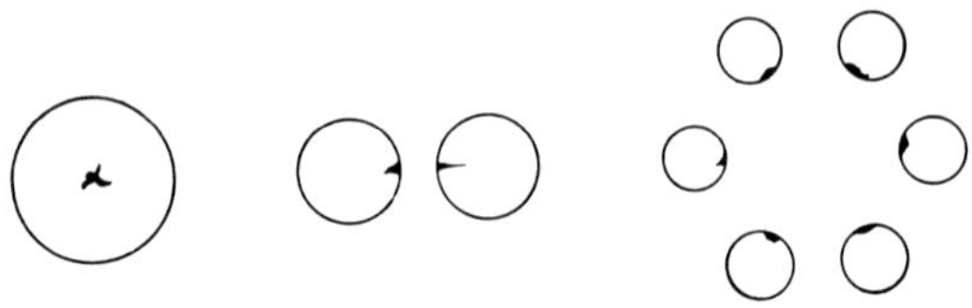

Fig. 3.215 Flaw position in piping, in cross-section of extruded brass with single, double and sextuple die.

On extruded material of copper, viz. hollow sections for water-cooled conductors, longitudinal cracks and changes in wall thickness are easily determined, furthermore transverse cracks of dove-tail pattern in laps on drawn round stock. Readily testable are also the welds of solid copper sections, using 2 MHz angle probes and a correctly designed wedge angle.

In the extrusion of brass, a longitudinal defect, viz. piping, is encountered, which is caused by core defects in the cast ingot. Depending on the extrusion die, which may be single or multiple, this defect can occur either in the centre or on the periphery of round stock (Fig. 3.215). These are separations which, e.g., in the extrusion of cartridges can lead to laminations and cracks in the wall. In the semi-finished article this defect is sometimes difficult to detect because it has been rendered partially transmissive by the vigouros working. The micro-section then shows only microscopical *discontinuous bands* of inclusions which, if stressed, burst clearly showing the nature of the defect in the fracture face. The best solution would be to test after the first working of the cast ingot, which is, however, not always possible in practice.

3.36 Other Non-ferrous Metals

Where other metals occur in ultrasonic testing they can usually readily be tested in view of the relatively small dimensions concerned.

Experience in this field is scarce. Pure *lead* has very high, true absorption. In technical alloys, particularly those with a few per cent antimony, lead is, however, harder and more transmissive. When cast into double-walled steel jackets used as shielding for reactors, it can be checked by the ultrasonic echo method if satisfactorily bonded to the steel in thicknesses of 100 mm and more and if testing is done from the outside, to detect larger voids, at a frequency of at least 1 MHz. Smaller pores, however, cannot be detected in lead linings. The bonding test on homogeneous lead claddings has been discussed in Sec. 3.292.

Uranium is markedly anisotropic; it usually has to be tested in the cast state, in the form of plates or rods. Since small defects are of little consequence, it can be tested successfully by sound transmission in the immersion technique with 1 to 2 MHz, in thicknesses up to a few centimetres. SHARPE and AVEYARD [332] have succeeded in displaying the structure of coarse-grained uranium by ultrasonic sectional pictures.

Nothing is known about the precious metals *gold, silver and platinum* in the cast state. If worked, they are readily testable with frequencies up to 5 MHz, e.g. contact rings for electrical machines of silver, regarding laminations and inclusions.

Zirconium and hafnium are used in nuclear engineering. They are already being tested during manufacture, beginning with the ingot. Zirconium ingots of 0.3 m diameter and more than 1 m long are tested by hand from the mechanically worked surface using 1 MHz, preferably with separate transmitting and receiving probes, so as to be able to detect also flaws close to the surface [101, 390]. Hafnium is obtained in smaller ingots of approximately 100 mm diameter, which can be tested in the immersion technique with 5 MHz after the surface has been worked [101]; in thin sheets both metals can be tested also with 10 MHz.

Zircalloy tubes, as used in the construction of reactors as jacket material for fuel elements, must be absolutely free of defects. However, these tubes can be tested without difficulty in the immersion technique using the method described in Sec. 3.26.

Titanium finds increasing use in aviation engineering and is tested ultrasonically both in the ingot and as a forging, e.g. landing gears of aircraft, almost as easily as light metals [380].

Zinc and its alloys are difficult to test because of its coarse cast structure. Castings made from it are usually also too complicated and of little value.

Tungsten in a dense, sintered condition, shows excellent sound transmission, but nothing is known of testing problems for which ultrasonics could be used.

Nickel and its highly heat-resistant alloys with chromium, aluminium and titanium (nimonic) can readily be tested in the microcrystalline state after being worked (cf. Sec. 3.22, turbine blades). Because of the anisotropy of the mixed crystals, the formation of coarse grains, during forging and also while in use is very troublesome. According to reference [349] this phenomenon can be observed indirectly, both by the strongly increasing attenuation and by the drop in acoustic velocity.

KLEINT and JOHNSON report on the testing of certain metals used in rocket construction ([178].

3.37 Hard Metals and Other Sintered Metals

All sintered materials have a certain residual porosity, which may either be intended and desirable (sintered iron) or unavoidable during manufacture (tungsten, hard metals), or even the result of wrong manufacturing methods (porcelain). Porosity, as a rule, increases the attenuation which sometimes, however, becomes measurable only at frequencies higher than commonly used in materials testing, the pores being no longer very much smaller than the wave length. In addition, the acoustic velocity decreases, for which presumably the total pore volume rather than the number and size of the individual pores is responsible. This effect is therefore also readily measurable at the usual testing frequencies. All other conditions remaining constant, porosity, and thus the degree of sintering, can be measured indirectly via the attenuation or the acoustic velocity.

An anomaly exists in respect of the acoustic velocity: sintered aluminium (SAP), which admittedly is practically free of porosity, with $c_l = 6.6 \cdot 10^3$ m/s has a very much higher value than normal aluminium with 6.3.

In practice this method has so far been applied only to porcelain (Sec. 3.41).

All *hard metals*, consisting of tungsten carbide in a cobalt matrix and containing also admixtures of other carbides such as titanium and tantalum, are very transmissive and can readily be tested. Occasionally internal cracks are encountered which can be clearly recognized by the greatly disturbed echo pattern of a plate in a contact test with small probes and using a high frequency. Since the acoustic velocity can vary markedly with different grades, manufacturing conditions and raw materials, valid deductions regarding porosity can be made on the basis of the velocity only in respect of a given batch. Larger pieces furthermore always have regions with distinctly higher attenuation, without the possibility that a region of higher porosity could already be regarded as a fault. The ultrasonic test has therefore not yet gained much significance. When considering echoes of seams where larger pieces are made up by sintering together several smaller pieces, one must exercise caution because of possible differences in structure which cannot be regarded as defects.

Frequently brazed joints between hard metal and steel are tested. If neither the hard metal nor the steel has a contact face parallel to the brazed face, one can with advantage use the immersion technique by irradiating the brazed face perpendicularly by means of a refracted beam.

In the case of *sintered metals* both the transmittance and the acoustic velocity depend within very wide limits on the degree of sintering. Sintered aluminium is just as transmissive as ordinary aluminium; sintered iron is still sufficiently transmissive, but carbonyl nickel, sintered intentionally in a very porous form for use in electrodes, only at the lowest frequencies.

3.4 Testing Problems on Non-metallic Specimens

3.41 Porcelain, Steatite and Glass

The raw porcelain blanks, the so-called slugs, as long as they are saturated with water, are sufficiently transmissive at frequencies of 0.5 to 2 MHz to be tested in thicknesses of a few 100 mm for larger voids and insufficiently bonded seams. In practice, however, tests are not made on specimens in this state. Dried blanks are no longer transmissive. Densely burnt porcelain, as far as transmittance and acoustic velocity are concerned, reaches values close to those for steel. Using longitudinal waves of 5 MHz and higher, lengths exceeding 1 m can be penetrated ultrasonically. Other dense ceramics show similar behaviour, e.g. steatite, whose acoustic velocity exceeds even that of steel (see below). Glass likewise has very low attenuation. In practice, however, only insulators of porcelain and steatite have so far been tested during manufacture.

Typical flaws are shrinkages, cracks, inclusions and absorptive capacity, furthermore cracks under the cap, so-called transverse core cracks as a result of *tensile tests* on cap-type insulators. Composite insulators may furthermore have bonding defects where they are joined together.

Shrinkages, when they occur in porcelain, are usually not of spherical shape but appear as gaps extending in the longitudinal direction, sometimes twisted helically (*snails*). These defects reduce both the mechanical and the dielectric strength and can be detected by the pulse-echo method using 2 to 5 MHz. On solid-core insulators the end faces prior to attaching the caps can readily be used for contact testing, especially if they are smooth and cut plane. This requires metallized contact probe faces and coupling with oil or water. As a make-shift one can also use unmetallized probes and insert a thin metal foil, or use conducting coupling paste.

The longitudinal test does in fact cover the entire core (the petticoats are not tested), but because of the long sound path of the longitudinal beam and the unfavourable position of the flaws, the transverse test is customary at least as a confirmation. This also eliminates the troublesome secondary echoes of transverse waves which somehow find their way to the screen and interfere, particularly on hollow-core insulators, with wall thicknesses of a few centimetres. In the transverse test the probe is shifted around the circumference from point to point, and is simultaneously moved back and forth as far as possible between the petticoats. Nevertheless, a small defect in the core directly under the petticoat, may occasionally be overlooked. Flat probes give sufficient contact if they are guided correctly. Curved probes are, however, more convenient to handle and are slightly more sensitive. Also the holder is preferably given an S-shape as shown in Fig. 3.216 for better adaptation to the petticoats.

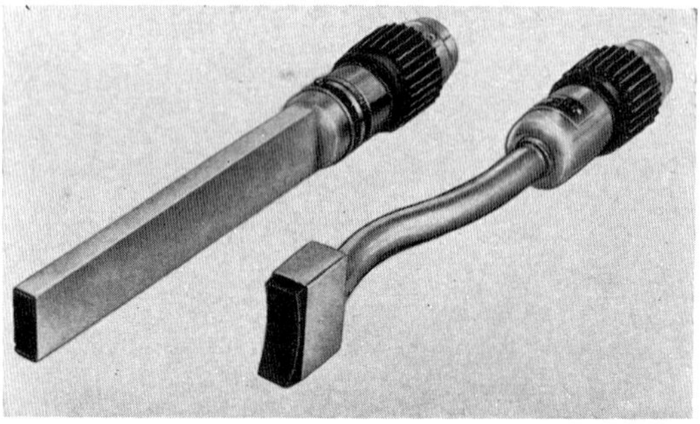

Fig. 3.216 Probes for testing porcelain insulators, left – for normal beaming, right – for oblique beaming on to transverse core cracks, with curved holder for narrow petticoat gaps.

Solid-core insulators can be mass-tested for shrinkages on a conveyor belt provided they can be rotated about their axis. Instead of using oil as couplant, which subsequently has to be wiped off carefully, one can alternatively also use flowing water fed directly to the probe. If the testing is well organised and according to size, up to 1000 insulators can be tested per day. One-piece rod-type suspension insulators and hollow insulators require more time and are preferably tested by rolling them back and forth on a table.

Absorptive capacity reduces both the mechanical and the dielectric strength as a result of the absorption of moisture while in operation. Porosity is therefore dangerous only if the pores communicate and reach the surface. Since closed porosity also occurs, the designation "hygroscopic" would be more appropriate for a defective insulator. At an early date it had already been suggested that the attenuation subsequent to a sequence of backwall echoes be used as an indication [114]. Measurement of the acoustic velocity was first suggested by KRAUTKRÄMER [452], see also [308, 31].

The absorptive capacity can readily be checked qualitatively on a plane-parallel sample using frequencies above 2 MHz, on the basis of the damping of the echo sequence. Because of the unstable coupling conditions, this is detectable only on an insulator with very strong porosity. There is also some evidence that a type of absorptive capacity is sometimes encountered which manifests itself only slightly by its effect on the attenuation but very noticeably by a change in acoustic velocity, although no quantitative observations have as yet been reported.

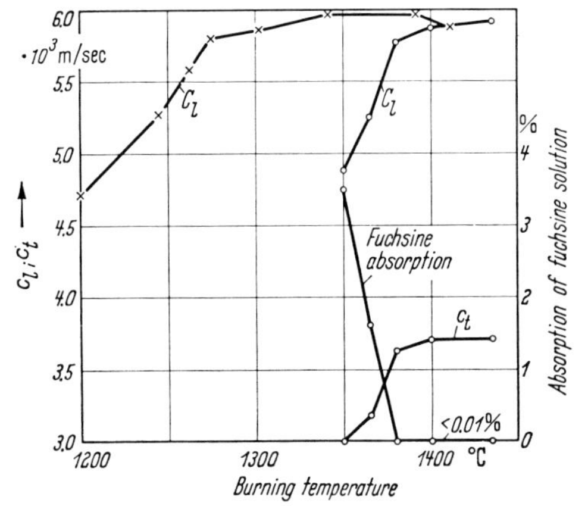

Fig. 3.217 Acoustic velocity and porosity of porcelain versus burning temperature. -o-Measurements by Stäger and Studer, -×-measurements by Ranachowski and Wehr.

Fig. 3.217 shows how according to measurements by Stäger and Studer [348] and Ranachowski and Wehr [292] the acoustic velocity increases with the burning temperature, while at the same time the porosity decreases. Absorptive capacity is observed in the range which corresponds to insufficient burning temperatures. At very high burning temperatures the acoustic velocity again decreases slightly as a result of a certain increase in porosity, which, however, concerns closed pores and is therefore harmless.

According to VDE specification [454] the fuchsine pressure test is used as a detecting method on fragments on which the effect of a methyl alcohol fuchsine solution applied under pressure is observed. For qualitative tests the fragment is then washed and again broken. Sound material should reveal no internal staining. The quantitative determination of the absorptive capacity, as in Fig. 3.217, involves measuring the increase in weight of a small test block.

According to Stüber [358] densely burnt porcelain has very different acoustic velocities which vary with the manufacturer:

	c_l transverse	c_l longitudinal	c_t longitudinal
Porcelain I	$5.60 \cdot 10^3$ m/s	5.80	3.52
Porcelain II	5.67	5.84	3.59
Porcelain III	6.11	6.18	3.68
Steatite	6.45	6.74	3.95

The permissible limit for porosity measurements can therefore be determined only for each individual case. Based on investigations by the German Federal Railways on almost 100,000 contact wire insulators [357] this limit is fixed at about 250 m/s below the values quoted above. With this object in mind it is important to measure the acoustic velocity uniformly, viz. in a direction either crosswise or lengthwise with respect to the insulator. The values show that the latter is a few per cent higher, possibly because of a certain anisotropy resulting from the working during extrusion of the mass [385]. The measurement is usually made in the transverse direction because any localized absorptive capacity, e.g. at one end of the insulator, fails to be indicated properly when the measurement is made in the longitudinal direction because of the averaging effect over the full length. For mass tests, if the cores are of uniform diameter, it is sufficient to mark on the CR screen the permissible range of the backwall echo. Otherwise the thickness would have to be measured each time. To simplify both the measurement and the calculation, devices have been suggested in the form of slide gauges or measuring calipers, one contact face of which forms the probe. When coupling has been effected, the thickness is measured and simultaneously on the CR screen, the transit time. Using a nomogram or a slide rule, which latter can also be incorporated in the calipers, the acoustic velocity can then be determined.

It is difficult to achieve an accuracy of a few per cent with a fixed scale on the CR screen. In the case of long specimens a higher accuracy is possible with electronic time markers and time base expansion; this is impossible with the usual transverse dimensions of, e.g., 100 mm, because neither the rising front nor the maximum of the echo are sufficiently distinct. Here an interferometer measurement is more advantageous (comparison of transit time with echoes of known transit path, see Sec. 3.62). Such an instrument could possibly be incorporated in the measuring calipers.

Cracks and fissures in the insulator as well as in the glazing, caused for instance by internal stresses or damage, can be detected by their echoes only by very accurate beaming at normal incidence, because of the very smooth surfaces of these faces. In the cylindrical wall of hollow insulators they can be detected as in pipes, by zig-zag transverse waves if, during scanning, the sound beam is swung through a wide angular range. Even fissures affecting only the glazing are indicated; these, however, are also readily detected by surface waves. In one case (Fig. 3.218) oblique cracks in the neck of a hollow cylinder had to be detected, the test being possible only from the end face because of the rough surface of the barrel. They remained completely invisible with narrow beams. Only after a probe of small diameter and low frequency was used could they be detected because they were then irradiated perpendicularly by part of the wide-angle beam.

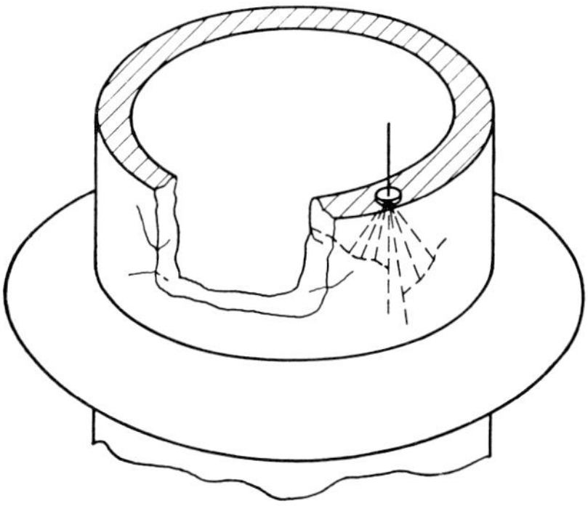

Fig. 3.218 Cracks in the neck of a hollow insulator.

Cracks under the cap occur on solid core insulators (Fig. 3.219a) or on hollow insulators under the flange (Fig. 3.219b) if they have been overloaded during the tensile test. When in use, the strain on the reduced working surface leads to further cracks and spalling and finally even to a complete break. Solid core cap-type insulators are tested with special, small angle probes from the surface between the cap and the first petticoat, or between the first and second petticoat.

If the crack in Fig. 3.219a extends only over part of the circumference, it can easily be detected as shown in Fig. 3.220 by the double echo of crack and edge which appears at the transition points when the probe is moved around the circumference, even if the crack is only a

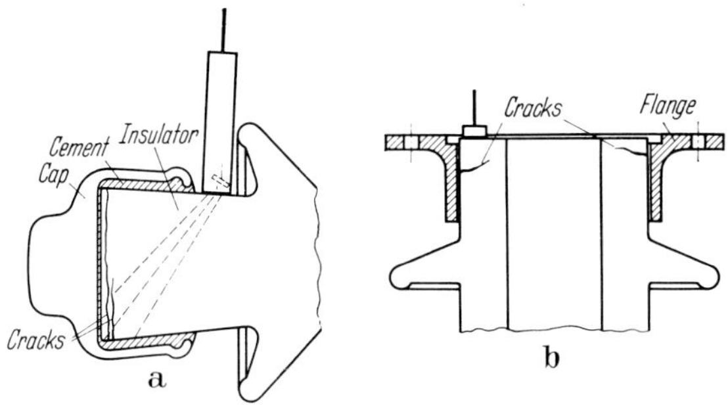

Fig. 3.219 Testing for cracks under the cap; a) on solid core insulators, b) on hollow insulators.

few millimetres from the edge. The problem becomes much more difficult if an incipient crack or a penetrating crack extends over the entire circumference; it is then very difficult to distinguish the echo of these defects from the echo of the end face of a sound insulator. This requires very accurate time base calibration of the screen picture and close tolerances in the manufacture of the insulators [32].

Large numbers of insulators for contact wires are currently checked in this way on site by the German Federal Railways on the electrified tracks [357].

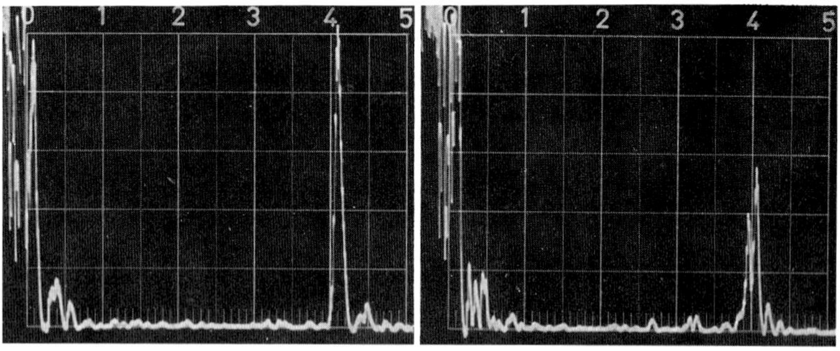

a b

Fig. 3.220 Screen pictures according to Fig. 3.219a; a) sound spot, b) transition spot towards crack.

Bonding defects at cemented spots of larger pieces can be individually detected by the echo method although the flaw echoes are often difficult to distinguish from the secondary echoes received from the petticoats. Unfortunately, cemented spots produce, on most makes, more or less pronounced echoes at points where a destructive test reveals no significant flaw. According to WEYL [385] they are caused by a pronounced anisotropy in the structure of the bonding compound; with some practice they can, however, be distinguished from true flaw echoes.

Various specifications have already been drawn up on the testing of insulators with ultrasound (cf. Sec. 3.7 [136, 434, 443, 436, 453]).

In the case of *glass*, the only testing problem encountered so far concerns the measurement of the thickness of large plates; this presents no difficulties when either the resonance or the echo method is applied, provided the glass is not too hot.

3.42 Plastics

In view of the wide range of materials which come under this collective heading, the attenuation of ultrasound which determines the testability, extends from the mean values applying to solids and materials without fillers, such as acrylic resins (perspex), ethoxylene resin (cast resin), polystyrene, polyamide and teflon, to the very high values of the soft materials, such as polyethylene and polyisobutylene (oppanol B).

The latter are excellent sound absorbers even at the lowest frequencies used in material testing. The hardness of a given plastic, unless this has been achieved by fillers, is thus an approximate measure of its testability. Plasticisers reduce the testability.

The fact that the semi-solid state shows greater attenuation than either the liquid or the solid state can be observed clearly during the curing of cast resins: after the hardener has been added, the cast resin is at first still showing good transmission; this can, e.g., be observed on the CR screen by sounding a layer with a thickness of a few centimetres. When it starts to set, the backwall echo decreases. Especially in cases where reaction heat is generated the echo can often no longer be observed even at higher gain, until it re-appears after curing, at shorter transit time as a result of increased acoustic velocity.

Among the testing problems encountered on semi-finished plastic articles, may be mentioned the detection of bubbles in extruded material, e.g. in the case of polyamides and teflon. Solid round stock of diameters up to approximately 100 mm can be tested at approximately 1 to 2 MHz by the echo method with direct contact. The limit of detectability is reached with bubbles of approximately pea size or bean size and piping in the centre of about match size. Water or oil is used as couplant. Even in the case of sliding contact the wear of metal lized probes is insignificant [124]. At 1 MHz and less it is advisable to separate transmitter and receiver for better resolution, particularly on thin material (TR probe). Compared with metals, the immersion technique here affords still better sound transmission, i.e. lower reflection losses and less deflection and splitting of the beam on curved surfaces. Longitudinal waves are used in the specimen even at oblique incidence because transverse waves are usually strongly damped. In this way it was possible for instance to check teflon tubes under water for bubbles in the wall using 1 MHz longitudinal waves, the beam being focused by a perspex lens mounted in front of the transducer. The tube was moved past the probe, while being rotated simultaneously.

Thick plates of polyethylene produced by thermoplastic pressing from granulate can be checked for homogeneity, in thicknesses exceeding 12 mm, using 1 to 2 MHz. Plastic material similarly produced from sheets is tested for laminations like metal plate. The echo method can no longer be used on insulating laminate, particularly in thin sheets. Harder plates can still be tested by transmission at frequencies above 2 MHz in the immersion technique, while wrapped insulating tubes (with resin-bonded paper) already require frequencies below 1 MHz if tested for lamination-like bonding defects [292].

Also solid-fuel rocket composition and explosives, for which the detection of voids and cracks is very important, usually require very low frequencies, so that only testing by the transmission method is possible. If the test pieces are hollow, with a circular cylindrical internal surface, one of the two probes is placed inside and the sound is passed only through one wall under water. It is recommended that pulses of such long wave length for which the first half oscillation of the received pulse is not yet disturbed by multiple reflections in the wall be used. If the pulse voltage of only this first peak is measured, this furnishes a measure of the transmittance which is independent of small changes in wall thickness and beaming direction. It can be used for flaw recording in automatic testing devices. An instrument using this principle has been designed by the Explosives Research and Development Establishment, Ministry of Supply, U.K. [444].

On material with star-shaped internal cross-section the test is limited to larger defects. The internal space can then be filled with water and two probes applied to the outside, using the immersion technique, as in the case of solid round stock.

Welded seams in plastic plates are tested in the same way as butt-welded joints in steel plate [151], but with longitudinal waves. In order to obtain large incidence angles, it is necessary to choose as wedge a material with an acoustic velocity lower than that of the material to be tested, e.g. special polyamide grades. It is then desirable to compensate the attenuation electronically by swept gain.

Ultrasonic measurements can also be used for determining the moisture content of plastics. On polyamide for instance, both the attenuation and the acoustic velocity change with the moisture content. It is, however, not recommended that the velocity be used as a criterion because differences in structure, e.g. between centre and periphery of a disc cut from round stock, affect this value. The attenuation decreases noticeably from the dry zone to the zone saturated with moisture, so that 1 MHz backwall echoes are in the ratio 1 : 10.

Materials other than fuels and those used in rocket and space engineering can also be considered for ultrasonic testing, e.g. the plastics with fillers used in the heat shield for re-entry into the earth's atmosphere. In addition to internal defects similar to laminations, the tests can also be applied to bonding defects between different types of plastics and metals. In certain cases it is also possible to assess the strength on the basis of the sound transmission which are proportional to each other [134, 146, 410].

3.43 Rubber

Vulcanized natural rubber containing no fillers can be tested in thicknesses up to a few centimetres with frequencies up to 2 MHz. The usual brands, however, contain fillers such as soot (amongst others) which greatly increase the attenuation. Here only frequencies below 1 MHz can be considered. If layers of fabric are added as in automobile tyres, frequencies around 100 kHz are used. Besides the bonding of rubber to metal, another important testing problem is the bonding between various layers of rubber and fabric in automobile tyres and transmission belts.

Suggestions for inspecting automobile tyres in a water bath by swept ultrasonic frequencies and sound transmission date back quite some

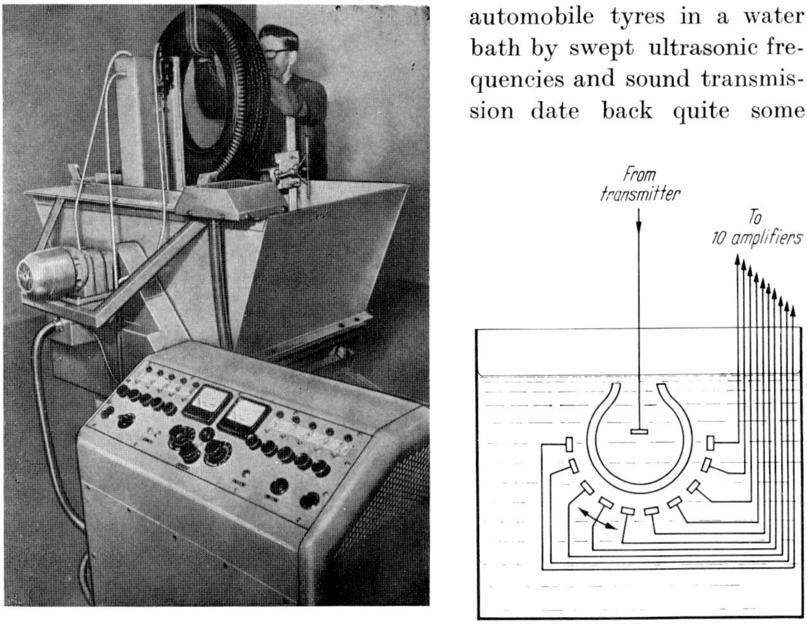

a b

Fig. 3.221 Test bench for automobile tyres (Lehfeldt); a) general view; b) arrangement of probes.

time [268, 269]. One of the two probes is placed inside the immersed tyre while the other probe is mounted in the same water tank under the tyre which is rotated around its axis. Several testing equipments have been constructed according to this design of which Fig. 3.221 shows an installation by Lehfeldt for Continental Gummiwerke, Hannover, [220]. It comprises 10 sound transmission paths evenly distributed over the cross-section of the tyre and operated simultaneously, so as to reduce the total testing time to a few minutes. This time, however, is still too long to test the entire output economically so that this method has as yet been applied only to special tyres, e.g. for racing cars, or for random tests. To improve the sound-transmission through the surface it is advisable to soak the tyre in water for a quarter of an hour, even if a wetting agent is added.

The testing of the smooth side walls of the tyre presents no difficulty in spite of their wedge shape, even if steel wire-mesh instead of cotton fabric is imbedded. It is then also possible to make random spot tests by hand with probes of low frequency and small contact face. With the long wave length of approximately 15 mm at 1 MHz it is of course only possible to detect defects larger than 5 to 10 mm diameter at a tyre thickness up to only a few centimetres. On the tread, however, the profile interferes and limits the detectability to spots of faulty bonding of rather large size. Because of the side wall effect the edges of the profile greatly reduce the transmitted intensity. This may result in smaller flaws being simulated or masked, particularly for smaller diameters of the sound beam.

Just as sound transmission is possible at lower frequencies in rubber even with dry contact, separations are transmissive to sound, i.e. difficult to detect, if their faces touch (stick to each other). Better testing conditions then result if they are made to separate, e.g. by letting the tyre run hot, before testing.

3.44 Natural Rock, Artificial Stone, Abrasive Wheels and Carbon

As far as *natural rock* is concerned, only magmatic material, such as basalt can be regarded as homogeneous and uniform throughout. In other types of rock both the acoustic velocity and the attenuation vary greatly. According to MALECKI [185] granite, for instance, depending on its grain structure, can reach values from 1.7 to $5 \cdot 10^3$ m/s. (See same source for values of many other rocks.) Moreover, samples give values which differ from those given by "in situ" tests in the stratum underground, because of the pressure effect. However, measurements of the pressure on the basis of the acoustic velocity likewise furnish unreliable values because they change from site to site.

In general, the attenuation (except in such homogeneous materials as rock salt) is so high that only frequencies below 500 kHz can be considered for ultrasonic tests. In the case of layers of sand, clay and even carbon, the frequencies have to be reduced to those of audible sound in order to reach transmission distances of 1 m. An added difficulty arises from the fact that rocks usually contain numerous small cracks and inclusions which greatly reduce the transmittance [184, 185].

Because of the poor focusing obtained with low frequencies, flaw location by the echo method is usually impossible. On the other hand, on blocks with parallel surfaces, large cracks and inclusions can be detected with separate probes by pulse transmission.

According to MALECKI (Fig. 3.222) some sort of flaw location is, however, also possible by testing from one side on a solid rock face. This presupposes that the acoustic velocity is known and that it does not depend on the direction as for instance in stratified rock. The receiving and transmitting probes are applied successively at a number of test points. If at each of these points a clear echo is obtained which can obviously be assigned to the same source of disturbance, the sound path is calculated by the transit time. Each pair of testing points is correlated to an ellipsoid of revolution on whose surface the flaw is located. The measuring points are at the focal points and the sound path there and back furnishes the main axis of the ellipsoid. If the flaw is small enough, the various ellipsoids intersect at one point,

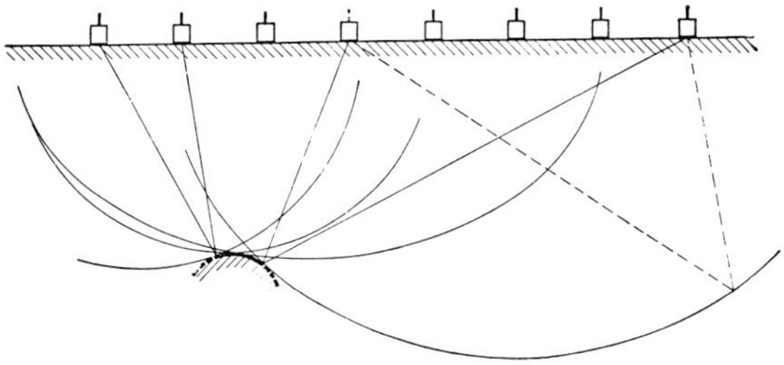

Fig. 3.222 Flaw location by to the ellipsoid method according to KOLTONSKI and MALECKI.

and if the flaw is larger, correlated enveloping surfaces are obtained. Although a strict application of the method in the space will hardly be possible in practice, it perhaps will sometimes be possible to utilize the ellipses of intersecting planes; for this purpose the measuring points on two straight lines normal to each other are taken which have the shortest distance from the flaw.

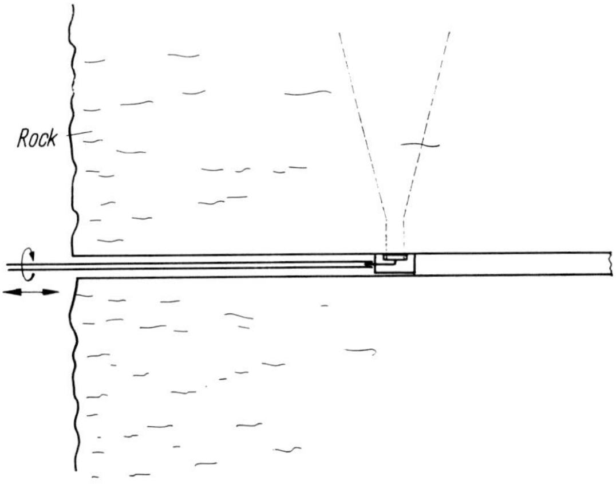

Fig. 3.223 Inspection of solid rock underground by the pulse-echo method.

LUTSCH [239] has used the pulse echo method at 0.5 MHz for testing in dense underground rock fracture zones and thus indirectly the strength of the solid rock (quartzite and reef formation) (Fig. 3.223). A special probe attached to a rod is inserted into a smooth drill hole and oil is used as couplant. It is possible in this way to inspect a volume of a few metres diameter around the hole. At depths of 1 to 2 m numerous echoes are obtained caused by cracks, but at greater depth the screen picture becomes quite clear. A drill hole of 40 mm diameter orientated parallel to the test holes and located at a distance of 1 m is still indicated very clearly by its echo. In quartzite acoustic velocities around $6 \cdot 10^3$ m/s and attenuation values around 100 dB/m were obtained at 1 MHz.

WENZEL [382] has used a pure transit time method for the same purpose and has in this way measured the acoustic velocity between two drill holes with two separate probes. The zone of reduced pressure near the surface furnishes lower velocity values and smaller, transmitted amplitudes. Assuming a given value of Poisson's ratio, Young's moduli were determined which showed good agreement with the results obtained by other methods and which were of great practical interest for the lining of tunnels. In this case the drill holes pointed obliquely downward and were filled with water to ensure satisfactory and uniform coupling. The tests were made with STEINKAMP's concrete tester (cf. Sec. 3.45) at 30 kHz frequency. In Rofna gneiss and marble the acoustic velocities were about 4.7 and $6.5 \cdot 10^3$ m/s, respectively.

Ultrasonic tests on artificial stones are occasionally used for *refractory bricks* for furnace linings. At moderate porosity they are sufficiently transmissive to permit the detection of larger internal cracks by sound transmission. Densely burnt clinkers can already be tested at frequencies above 1 MHz by the echo method, while aluminous bricks (fire bricks) with more than 50% pore volume are no longer transmissive even at 0.25 MHz in thicknesses of a few centimetres. In the case of less porous material, the acoustic velocity can serve as a measure of the porosity. For instance, in a given material where the velocity changed from 3.9 to $3.4 \cdot 10^3$ m/s the porosity rose from 20 to 30%.

Abrasive wheels bonded with silicate transmit sound in the same way as sandstone and can be tested for instance in the immersion technique by means of a fine, collimated beam of 1 MHz. Using the intensity method, defects such as cracks or unsatisfactory bonding, which reduce the transmission, can be detected. With the pulse method, it is also possible, however, to draw conclusions on the quality of the bonding from the acoustic velocity. Abrasive wheels on rubber base have low transmission. Nevertheless, using 0.2 MHz, it was possible to carry out rough tests on specimens of thickness up to 15 cm.

Pressed *carbon and graphite blocks* (electrode and reactor material) show very different transmittance. Where it was at all possible to test electrode blocks (with frequencies below 1 MHz), the acoustic velocities, normal and parallel to the main orientation of the slabs, differed greatly, viz. 1.1 to $2.3 \cdot 10^3$ m/s and 3.2 to $3.9 \cdot 10^3$ m/s, respectively. Furthermore, the transmittance changed greatly from spot to spot even in the absence of gross defects, so that flaw detection was not always possible. In another case graphite blocks could readily be tested by sound transmission in the immersion technique, using 0.5 to 1 MHz.

3.45 Concrete

Checks on defects and strength are of great interest both in large concrete structures cast on site as well as in mass production on prefabricated units. The intrinsic inhomogeneity limits the frequencies which can be used for this purpose to 100 kHz and less where probing distances exceed 1 m. This, however, no longer permits sharply collimated sound beams as is customary in the testing of metals: to obtain a collimated beam with 2 MHz probes of 25 mm in steel (angle of divergence γ_0 approximately 8°), the transducer used for concrete would have to have a diameter of approximately 350 mm at 100 kHz. A transducer of this size could of course be obtained by a mosaic of crystal plates. But uniform coupling would be very difficult, particularly where the surface of the specimen, as on metals, has to be scanned over rather large areas. In practice therefore probes which are not much larger than the customary ones are usually used and thick oil, grease, coupling paste containing water, glycerine-kaolin slurries, soft soap and similar substances are used for coupling. Occasionally the probes are also attached by means of plaster, for instance where observations over a long period are required.

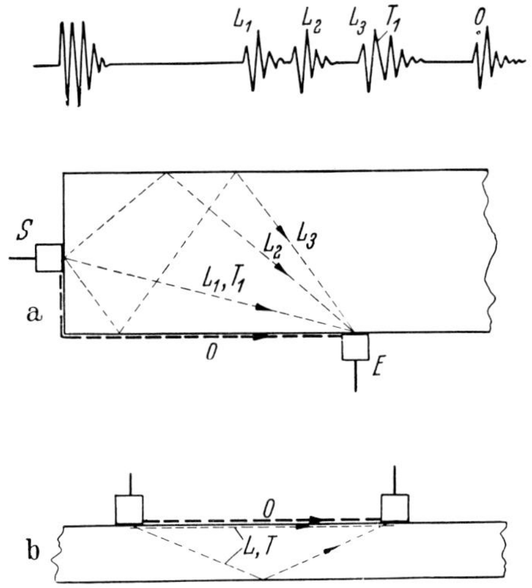

Fig. 3.224 Testing concrete by pulsed sound transmission; a) with contact on two abutting sides of a pillar, showing schematic screen pictures and the first pulses of different waves; b) with contact on the surface of a slab (road).

The contact face, which is only of the order of magnitude of the wave length, (at 100 kHz $\lambda \approx 40$ mm) naturally also radiates other wave modes besides longitudinal waves of appreciable intensity. A strong surface wave can always be assumed, which results in so many disturbing echoes of uncontrollable direction and origin being obtained with the echo method that this technique can rarely be used. As a rule one therefore uses two probes with pulse transmission. The absence of any directional effect of the probes furthermore makes it possible to couple at arbitrary points on different surfaces of the specimen inclined to each other (Fig. 3.224a). The fastest wave received in this way is then always the direct longitudinal wave. This is followed by the transverse and surface waves which, depending on the shape of the specimen, may however already be disturbed by the reflected longitudinal waves. If both probes are placed on the same surface of a given concrete structure, e.g. on a paving slab in a road (Fig. 3.224b), the direct longitudinal wave is rather weak (cf. directional characteristic Fig. 1.59).

Previously, blocks of seignette's salt were frequently used as transmitters, and magnetostrictive receivers. Now barium titanate is usually used for both. Where longer distances have to be covered, one uses, however, also electromechanical hammers and magnetostrictive receivers

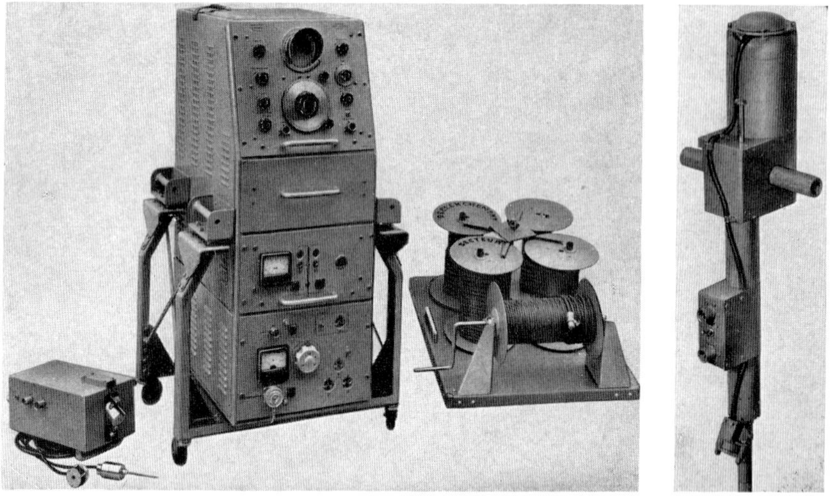

a b

Fig. 3.225 Concrete tester (Laboratoire Electro-Acoustique); a) instrument with small hammer and magnetostrictive receiving probe (left bottom); b) heavy electromechanical hammer.

with very wide frequency spectra far below 100 kHz. They represent a transition to the instruments using audible sound for soil tests, which produce shock waves by explosive charges.

The instruments with CR screen display are similar to the pulse-echo instruments as used at higher frequencies for testing other materials; however, they usually have sweep expansion and electronic time markers to be able to measure the transit time of pulses as accurately as possible. They usually have high-frequency presentation. In the United Kingdom the following instruments are regularly manufactured specifically for concrete tests: an instrument, model UCT, designed by the Road Research Laboratory, Harmondsworth, Middlesex, and constructed by A. E. Cawkell, Electronic Engineers, Southall, and a similar instrument, viz. the ultrasonic concrete tester by Mullard Ltd. Equipment Division, London. In France an instrument has been developed by Laboratoire du

Bâtiment et des Travaux Publics, Paris, marketed by Laboratoire Electro-Acoustique (L.E.A.) Rueil (S. & O.) under the name Ausculteur Dynamique, type S.B.C.4, (Fig. 3.225).

For distances of 30 cm to 20 m this instrument uses an electromechanical hammer which produces intense periodic shocks on the surface of the concrete structure concerned. A magnetostrictive receiver attached to the hammer triggers the time base and the time marker. The receiver consists of a similar magnetostrictive transducer in the form of a large pick-up. This permits differentiation between certain vibration modes of the surface if applied at an angle. With a light hammer which transmits the shock to the surface via a pin, selected wave modes can likewise be produced by inclining the pin at an angle to the surface. For measurements on smaller specimens up to approximately 30 cm thick, piezoelectric transmitters and receivers can be coupled to the instrument, and conversely for larger distances and sub-soil tests a blasting cartridge is used for excitation.

An instrument developed and constructed in Poland by the Polish Academy of Sciences, Institute for Basic Research, viz. the Concrete Tester BI 2, uses frequencies of 50 kHz to 1 MHz; for the lower frequencies barium titanate blocks with a 60 × 102 mm contact face and 30 kHz resonance frequency are used as transmitters and receivers.

Other concrete testers, which make no use of the echo amplitude, operate as pure transit time meters. The transmitting pulse either initiates simultaneously an electronic time count (e.g. the charging or discharging of a capacitor) which is then stopped by the first pulse received, or one measures in this way the time between the arrival of the pulses of 2 receivers arranged in tandem on the same face of the structure and in line with the transmitter. This is the principle of the concrete tester developed in Germany by STEINKAMP and constructed by Messrs. Phywe, Göttingen.

Regarding these and other instruments, see: [226, 170, 169, 72, 99, 351, 55, 175].

For *quality tests* on concrete one measures primarily the longitudinal acoustic velocity with the instruments described. Using formula (1.6) one can calculate from it Young's modulus if Poisson's ratio is known. The latter, however, varies greatly with the condition of the concrete: prior to setting it is usually that of liquids, viz. 0.5, after setting in the case of good-quality concrete it drops to 0.3 to 0.15 as long as it is still saturated with water. On old dry concrete it drops to 0.2 to 0.1.

In practice, however, Young's modulus is less important as a criterion of the quality of a given concrete than the compressive strength or the flexural strength. After setting, the compressive strength is proportional to the acoustic velocity, as confirmed by measurements [170]. Where only very rough measurements are of interest, it is believed that none of the many influencing factors, viz. setting time, mix (i.e. cement : sand : aggregate ratio by weight), type of aggregate (gravel, split), water-cement ratio, moisture content, etc. need be taken into consideration. The following grading can serve as a rule of thumb:

Longitudinal velocity	Quality of concrete
above $4.6 \cdot 10^3$ m/s	Very good
3.6 to 4.6	Good
3.0 to 3.6	Moderate to questionable
2.1 to 3.0	Bad
below 2.1	Very bad

Approximately 3.6 to 4.0 is regarded as the lower limit of a still acceptable quality. Fig. 3.226 gives some values measured by JONES and GATFIELD [170] on various concrete mixes with river gravel as aggregate.

By way of explanation we take a mix, e.g. the lean mix 1. If within this mix the water-cement ratio is changed, concrete of a different strength is obtained. Correlated values of acoustic velocity and compressive strength, however, always furnish a point on the straight line 1. The more water is added during mixing, the lower are both the compressive strength and the acoustic velocity in the set concrete. The specimens were measured on the 28th day after casting, saturated with moisture.

According to WEIGLER and KERN [377], both the type and the quantity of the aggregate are thought to have a decisive influence on the acoustic velocity so that deductions concerning the strength would be permissible only if the content of aggregate is constant and known.

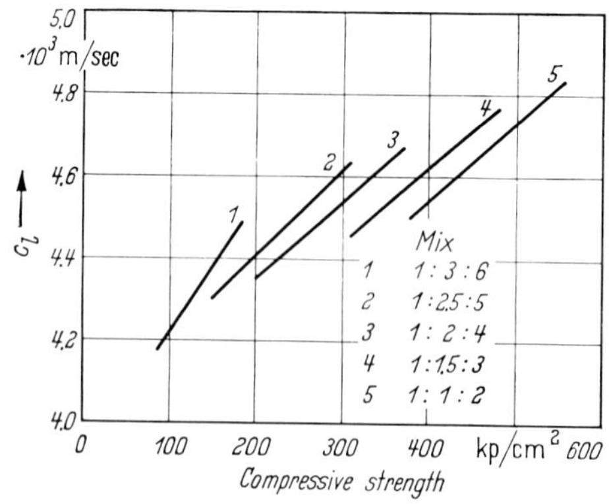

Fig. 3.226 Correlation between longitudinal velocity and compressive strength on concrete specimens with different mixing ratios and different water-cement ratios, as measured by JONES and GATFIELD.

The reinforcement has a slight influence on the acoustic velocity only if the sound beam happens to be coaxial with very thick reinforcing rods above 20 mm in diameter. This increases the velocity slightly, which may simulate a slightly greater strength.

During setting, both the velocity and the strength increase rapidly and proportionally. Measurement of the velocity thus offers a possibility, when concrete components are mass-produced, e.g. also pre-stressed components, rapidly determining the instant when the strength is high enough for the shuttering and the pre-stressing to be removed, or transporting the component. Both are of economic interest.

The velocity follows the compressive strength also where the latter has been reduced by freezing and thawing periods.

Cracks in concrete structures were determined by MEYER and BOCK [259] by means of ultrasonics as early as 1939, viz. on reinforced concrete beams by the intensity method. The disturbances by interferences while using continuous sound are now avoided by pulsed sound transmission. By this means it is possible to deduce the presence of defects from the

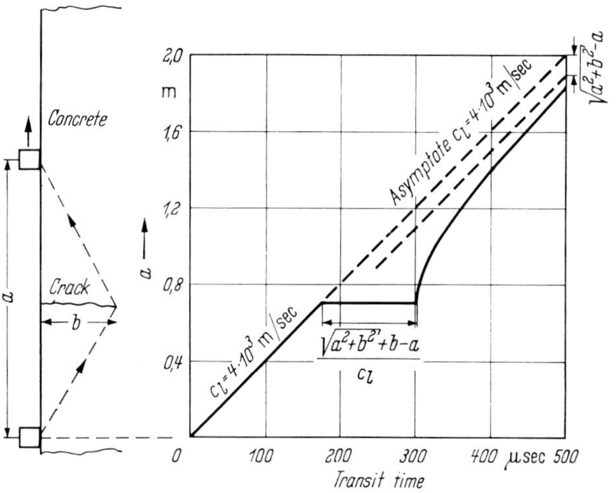

Fig. 3.227 Propagation diagram with crack in path of sound wave (according to DAWANCE and CHEFDEVILLE). Distance of probes a versus transit time, depth of crack b, crack at a = 0.7 m, with b = 0,4 m at $c_l = 4 \cdot 10^3$ m/s.

decreased intensity without, however, being able to determine their depth on large concrete structures accessible from both sides, such as dam walls and storage tanks. One cannot, however, safely conclude that these defects are cracks, shrinkages or inclusions of foreign bodies because segregation zones (areas poor in cement) likewise strongly weaken the sound. A rough determination of the position and shape of a given flaw would basically be possible with the procedure described in 3.44 (Fig. 3.222) by using the pulse-echo method on one side at different distances of the two probes. So far, however, no practical applications have been reported. If there is a defect in the sound path when sound transmission is used, the acoustic velocity is also changed because of the detour around the flaw; it is reduced, but this may also have other causes as explained above.

Surface cracks which are not visible to the naked eye or whose depth has to be measured are determined as follows. One measures the transit times between a number of measuring points on the surface arranged along a straight line from the fixed transmitter. If the distance is plotted against it as in Fig. 3.227, a sound concrete structure furnishes a straight line whose gradient corresponds to the uniform acoustic velocity. Cracks transverse to the measuring line force the ultrasonic waves to make detours. This increases the transit time the deeper the crack. The curve shows bends from whose position and shape one can deduce the position and depth of the crack. This presentation also enables one to recognize whether layers of different strength are superimposed or whether the layers are not bonded satisfactorily, e.g. as a consequence of casting errors [72].

Regarding the testing of concrete, see also [157, 166, 63, 384, 320, 376. 258, 381, 80, 169, 27].

3.46 Wood and Leather

One of the oldest applications of ultrasonic testing is the bonding test on plywood by Czerlinsky [71]. Instead of swept ultrasonic frequencies pulsed sound transmission is used today. The pulses produced by the echo method if *one* probe is used are usually too long for the required low frequencies of less than 1 MHz and the usual small testing thicknesses. A non-existent or faulty glued bond in plywood or other wood constructions is easily revealed by its lower transmittance. Since couplants containing oil or water, as well as the immersion technique, are usually undesirable, a slowly evaporating liquid has to be used which increases the cost of the test. It has not yet been applied in practice.

Of greater importance seems to be the application of ultrasonics to tests on live trees for heart rot as tried out by Waid and Woodman [375]. Since the bark is usually not transmissive, the timber must be bared on two opposite points of approximately 50 mm diameter. Glue or similar material can be used for coupling. On sound timber the thickness of tree trunks can still easily be penetrated by sound at frequencies of 0.25 to 0.5 MHz. In the case of dry beech, even 1.30 m could still be penetrated. Live, e.g. moist timber has still better transmittance.

Since timber affected by dry rot is completely sound absorbing, the intensity in a diseased tree is weakened to a varying degree. The affected zone can also be determined by scanning in the longitudinal direction. The method furthermore can be applied to telephone poles so as to be able to replace rotted poles in time to avoid service interruptions.

It is advisable to use the highest possible frequencies so that the sound beam can scan the core with sufficient sensitivity. In practice, therefore instruments suitable for this purpose are those with high sensitivity with sound transmission at 0.5 to 1 MHz; furthermore, they should be light, portable and battery-operated.

So far the acoustic velocity has not yet been used for quality tests although this may offer additional possibilities. In wood the velocity is strongly anisotropic. Fig. 3.228 shows the values found on a cube of dry beech. The attenuation at 0.5 MHz was at the same time found to be approximately 400 dB/m, which is very high compared with metals.

Quality tests by means of ultrasonics were also made on other organic materials such as leather [171]; these, however, have so far found no practical application. Here again the acoustic velocity is the measured quantity, which depends on the chemical and physical structure and on the orientation of the fibres. Numerous parameters, such as tanning method, grease and moisture content, make it difficult to follow specific variations. The correlation between velocity and tearing strength therefore furnishes reliable data only if the other conditions remain constant.

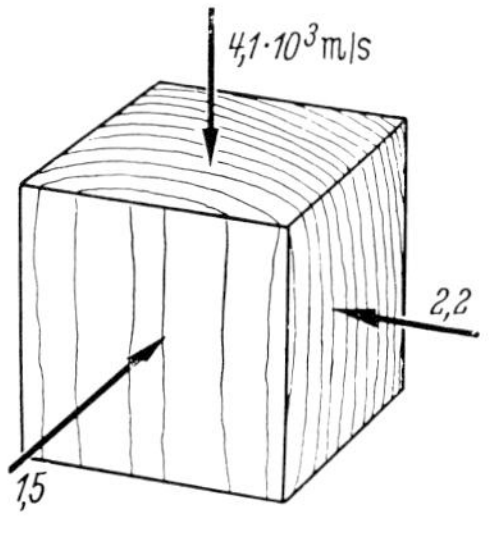

Fig. 3.228 Longitudinal acoustic velocity in a cube of beech.

In measurements by the pulse transmission method, transmitter and receiver were applied to the same side of a narrow strip. In order to radiate the energy at the low frequencies of less than 100 kHz from a narrow contact face, rochelle salt transducers were placed on its narrow side (see 1.101); for the same purpose one would today use barium titanate because of its strong coupling between thickness oscillations and transverse oscillations. The instrument used operates as a pure electronic transit time meter.

3.47 Bacon and Meat

As far as these edible "materials" are concerned, the measurement of bacon and meat thicknesses on live animals, especially pigs and cattle, has found fairly wide practical application. The method is used by animal breeding institutions, stock breeding associations and research institutes for fattened animals. It greatly facilitates the assessment of the market value of the livestock.

The animals readily tolerate the application of the probe, in contrast to the previously practised insertion of probes into pigs in order to determine the thickness of the bacon. For this purpose the animal is preferably driven into a narrow passage or cage, so as to obtain a steady display on the CR screen while the animal is stationary. Frequencies around 2 MHz offer an optimal compromise between sound transmittance and sharpness of echo. If probes of approximately 10 mm diameter are used, it is not absolutely necessary to remove the bristles on the pig. Oil, grease or water-soluble paste is used for coupling.

The reflection at the transition layer separating fat and meat results from a slight difference in acoustic impedance. In addition intermediate echoes are obtained from membranes in the bacon. At certain parts of the body echoes from bones or from the pleura are also obtained which can be used to determine the thickness of the meat in addition to the thickness of the bacon.

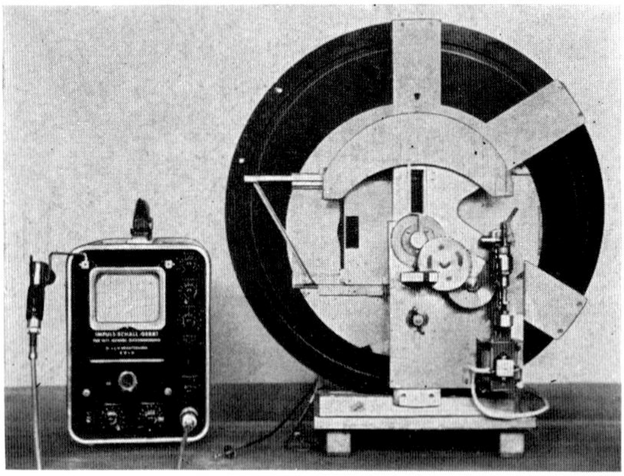

Fig. 3.229 Ultrasonic instrument with revolving cross-section recorder for meat inspection on pigs according to HORST.

According to HORST [156] the acoustic velocity in bacon of freshly killed pigs (still warm) is 1.43 to $1.51 \cdot 10^3$ m/s. As the temperature decreases the sound attenuation rises steeply so that measurements below 10 °C are difficult. In the case of pork, in the long dorsal muscles (cutlets), the velocity is $1.65 \cdot 10^3$ m/s, in the case of beef from the hind quarters about $2.04 \cdot 10^3$ m/s according to data supplied by BURGKART [60].

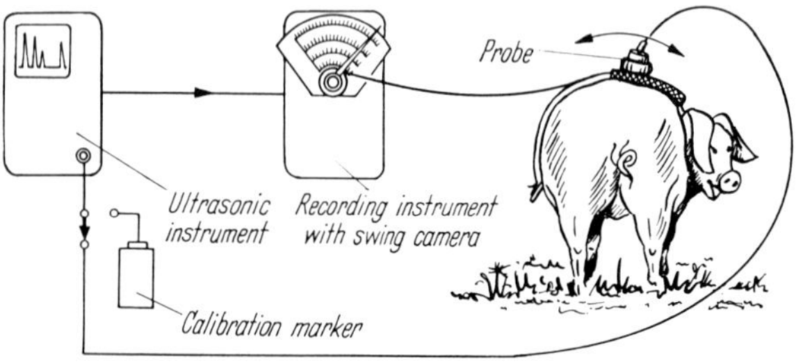

Fig. 3.230 Recording meat thickness on pigs, schematic.

When the instrument is being calibrated, one should observe that in addition to the effect of the temperature, the thickness of the bacon on the hung carcass decreases because of stretching. According to LAUPRECHT [214] the accuracy usually obtained was 1 to 2 mm on thicknesses of about 40 mm, which is quite adequate. Regarding further data on measurements on pigs see [215, 180, 62, 75].

After measurements of pure bacon thicknesses had given satisfaction until 1959, the possibility of measuring the thickness of the meat offered

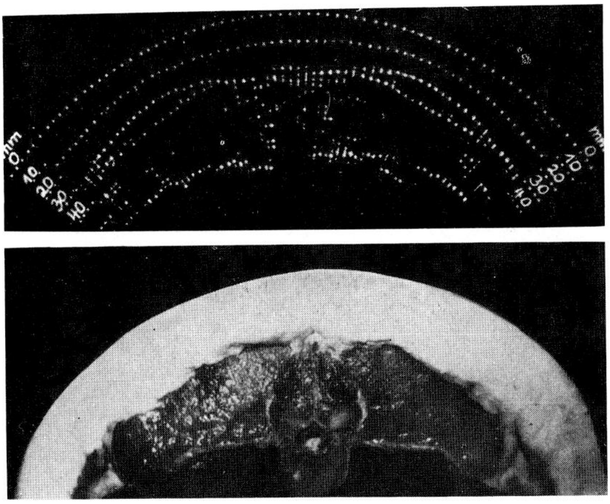

Fig. 3.231 Recording obtained by HORST with the instrument shown in Fig. 3.229 and control picture of cross-section through the back of a pig.

a new way of determining carcass values [334]. Numerical data on the carcass values are based on the ratio of the cross-sectional area of the dorsal muscle to the overlaying fat. By spot sampling by hand, plotting and integrating the areas concerned it was possible to determine the desired value, although in practice this is too time-consuming. Therefore at first a photographic cross-section recorder (see Sec. 2.353) was used for obtaining revolving cross-sectional pictures as used in the testing of materials. The probe was placed on the spine of the animal and moved laterally point by point in one or both of the two directions while simultaneously swinging the photographic plate of the camera through a corresponding angle at each measuring point. The axis of rotation thus

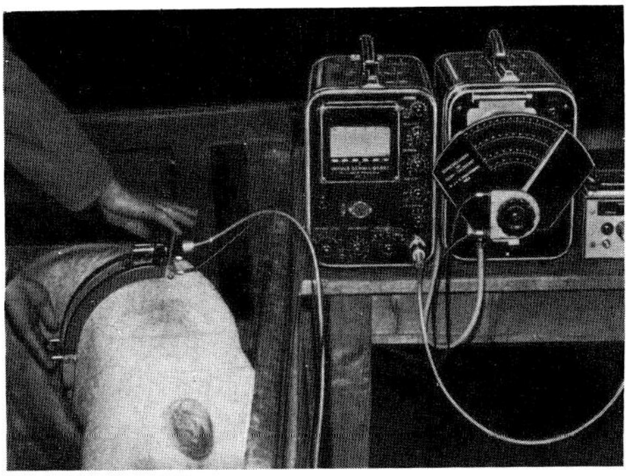

Fig. 3.232 Recording of meat thickness on a pig with the Krautkrämer recorder (photo Max Planck Institute for Stock Breeding, Mecklenhorst).

corresponded to the longitudinal axis of the animal, since a pig has a more or less circular cross-section. Since the photographic film for such a camera arrangement was utilized only very ineffectively for the cutlet sections of interest here, it became necessary to transfer the axis of rotation to a point outside the CR screen. Fig. 3.229 shows a first design of the instrument by HORST [156], and Fig. 3.230 the principle of the recording. Fig. 3.231 shows a picture produced by the instrument, together with a section through the animal after slaughter. The same principle is used by the fully automatic recording instrument by Krautkrämer (Fig. 3.232). The carrier of the probe and the recorder are both motor-driven. In addition calibration marks are recorded automatically with each picture. See also [355, 216, 217, 218, 179].

In principle it is also possible to determine the carcass value of cattle in this way on the basis of the cutlet section. In this case, however, the cross-section, because of its angular shape, is less suitable for a revolving cross-sectional picture. Branson Instruments have constructed a recording device for this purpose by means of which orthogonal co-ordinates are transferred from the probe to the CR screen. In addition Branson supplies a simplified pulse-echo instrument intended specifically for measuring the thickness of bacon and meat by hand.

3.5 Determination of Position, Shape and Level

The *testing* methods described so far (3.2 to 3.4) and the *measuring* methods discussed below in 3.6 do not cover all applications of ultrasonic diagnostics. Although ancillary to the testing of materials they shall be mentioned here briefly because they can be carried out inter alia also with the conventional instruments used for testing materials.

As far as the various applications of pure sounding methods using ultrasonics of extended frequency range of the well-known echo sounding devices for ships, or in air as guiding device for blind people are concerned, attention is drawn to the descriptions in [1, 13]. However, also in the daily applications of instruments for materials testing pure sounding problems are encountered as evidenced by the following examples.

Deep and slender holes drilled in work pieces have a tendency to wander. The problem of determining the accurate position of the hole from one side then arises, for instance in order to intercept it by an additional hole drilled at right angles to it. This happens in the case of oil holes drilled into the cylinders of heavy diesel engines in the longitudinal direction.

A similar problem is encountered in castings where the position of cast-in cooling tubes or the displacement of the core may have to be determined.

Meandering canals for hot water or steam are produced in the heating plates for plywood presses by forcing plugs into a network of holes drilled parallel to the plate at suitable points. Sometimes a plug becomes loose and shifts, thus disturbing the heating. The hole concerned is then filled with water and scanned by the echo method and the position of the plug is determined. The plug changes the echo pattern very distinctly.

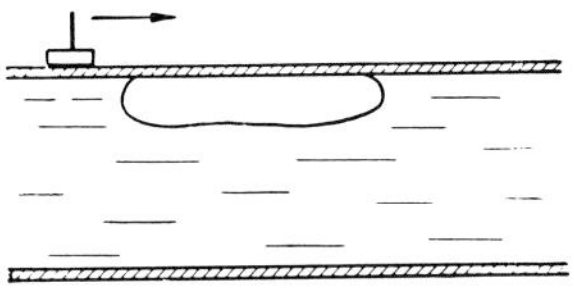

Fig. 3.233 Locating air bubbles in a pipe.

On large plate structures it sometimes becomes necessary to determine accurately the position of a piece welded to the other side, e.g. on a bridge the position of the bottom junction plates at which rails have to be laid exactly above them. The position of the fillet weld is readily determined by scanning from the top surface because the sequence of multiple plate echoes disappears at this spot.

Another problem is the determination of the shape of machine components at inaccessible spots. For instance, on a composite turbine shaft it was very important to distinguish between two externally identical parts for the purpose of repair. The differently shaped, inaccessible internal spaces could be differentiated immediately by the echo method.

On pipe lines filled with liquid, air bubbles, deposits and other foreign bodies are located by testing through the pipe wall. An air bubble (Fig. 3.233) blots out the normal bottom echo. Similarly the bubble-free filling of non-transparent containers with viscous liquids can be checked. In one practical case concerning refills for ball pens, it was found better to use sound transmission because of the small dimensions involved. For routine tests, in which this method would have to be automated, the required liquid coupling is so far still found to be an obstacle.

In order to check hydraulic lines, e.g. in control devices for aeroplanes, where air bubbles and foreign bodies can cause disturbances, ultrasonic transducers which actuate counting and alarm devices are permanently installed. Installations of this type are already in use [28].

The arrangement shown in Fig. 3.234 is used for measuring the liquid level in containers whose side walls are directly accessible, e.g. if they are not insulated nor too hot. The echo of the opposite wall, repeatedly split by the multiple echoes from both walls, appears only in the liquid space. A permanently installed probe is thus very suitable for indicating whether a given liquid level is exceeded or not reached. A monitor which monitors the backwall echo can be used for actuating a pump which maintains a constant level. Where no backwall echo can be obtained through the liquid, the attenuation or the length of the sequence of multiple echoes from the wall, which differs between the air and liquid space, can be exploited for this purpose. An array of probes mounted one above the other and co-ordinated with a selector switch, permits rough measurement of the liquid level in cases where, for instance, one of the following methods is not applicable.

The method according to Fig. 3.235 where the liquid level serves as reflector, has already found practical application (Atlas Works, Bremen,

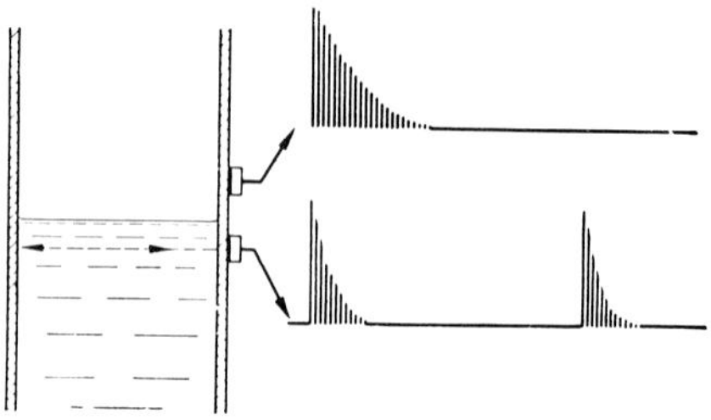

Fig. 3.234 Liquid level indication through side wall of container.

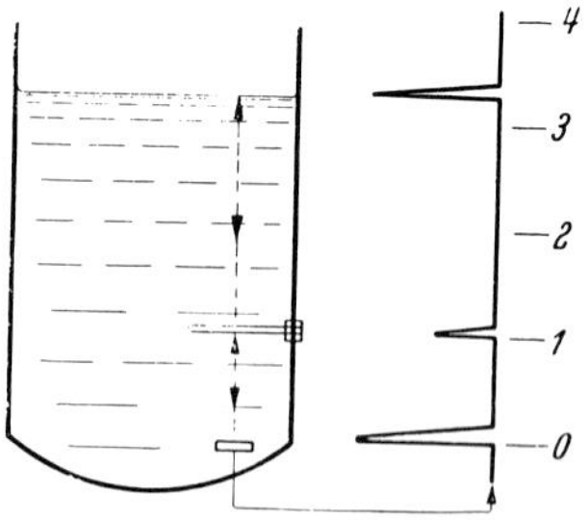

Fig. 3.235 Liquid level measurement from the bottom of the container.

cf. [364]). If the bottom of the container is flat the probe can also be coupled from the outside but if the bottom is curved it is preferable to use separate transmitters and receivers which radiate the sound pulses towards each other at an acute angle relative to the vertical. In contrast to the above methods, this requires that the acoustic velocity be known. Changes due to temperature effects or concentration can readily be taken into account during calibration by means of a reflector mounted at a known distance in the sound beam, e.g. a stick. In the case of strongly absorbing liquids, deposits on the bottom which are not transmissive to sound, or loose bulk material, the height of the air column under the lid of the container is similarly probed. Applying the same method it is also possible to measure continuously the height of bulk material on a conveyor belt, from which the volumetric conveying capacity can be computed.

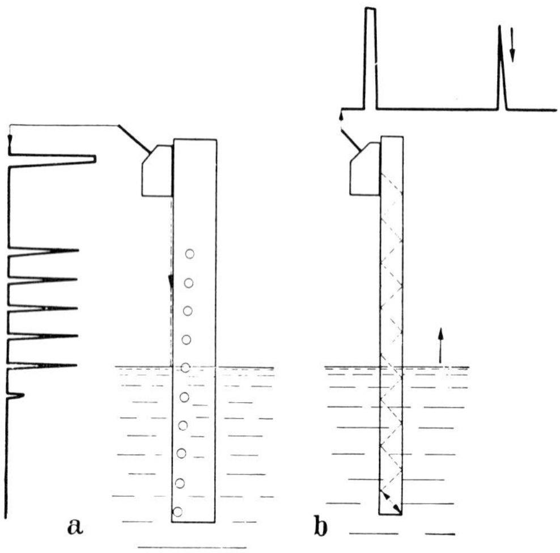

Fig. 3.236 Liquid level measurement according to Sperry, a) by means of the damping of surface waves, b) by zig-zag transverse waves in a bar.

Apart from the well known problems encountered in the chemical industry, this method can also be used for checking levels during decanting in non-transparent containers, e.g. beverages in earthen ware.

According to suggestions by SPERRY it is also possible to use the disturbance of the propagation of waves on a dipstick for level measurement, provided the liquid is non-corrosive and produces no deposits. A surface wave on a stick (Fig. 3.236a) produces echoes of calibration marks such as notches or holes immediately under the surface, only where it is not wetted by the liquid [451]. According to Fig. 3.236b a zig-zag transverse wave is damped more strongly the higher the liquid level.

3.6 Measuring Methods Using Ultrasound

This Section deals with the measurement of properties of materials and of material constants, inasmuch as they are of interest for materials testing in general and where they can be carried out by means of commercial testing instruments. This therefore excludes many scientific problems and measuring methods or permits only their brief mention.

3.61 Measurement of Wall and Layer Thicknesses

The measurement of a given wall thickness or of acoustic velocity is based on the same quantity, viz. the transit time t. The velocity being known this then furnishes the thickness, or if the thickness is known the velocity:

$$d = ct \quad \text{or} \quad c = d/t$$

The principal methods have already been explained during the description of the resonance instrument (Sec. 2.1) and of the pulse-echo instrument (Sec. 2.3) respectively. In addition we shall now discuss the pulse-resonance method of FIRESTONE [103, 107, 106] which is a combination of both. If the moderately damped probe of a pulse-echo instrument is placed on a wall with a thickness of the order of the wave length and the ultrasonic frequency is changed continuously, which the conventional instruments do not permit, the pattern of the transmitting pulse is expanded on the CR screen at the points of resonance between frequency and wall thickness, because the system consisting of transducer plate and wall then takes longer to decay. From the read difference Δf of two successive resonance frequencies the thickness is obtained according to Eq. (2.3), see Sec. 2.11. As explained in Sec. 3.62 the pulse-resonance method can also be applied as echo pulse instead of transmitting pulse. The specimen whose thickness or acoustic velocity is to be measured, can thus be coupled via a liquid or solid delay line. Based on this principle, AVEYARD and SHARPE have developed a very accurate device for wall thickness measurements [29].

Since the usual instruments permit *continuous adjustment* of the frequency only if an additional tuning element is connected between instrument and probe and only in a range of given width which depends on the design of the amplifier, this method is little used although it could extend the thickness measuring range of the pulse-echo instrument downward, into the range of the resonance instruments. Sometimes it is used in modified form for scientific purposes (see Sec. 3.62).

The "measuring" problems encountered in practice can be divided into two groups:

1. In the manufacture of pipe, containers, plate, strip, etc. continuous measurements or programmed random measurements of the wall thickness are desirable. At the measuring points of these work pieces the walls usually are parallel and the boundary faces smooth.

2. In plant supervision, e.g. in power stations, in the chemical industry, etc., the problem is the following: to check the wall thickness, or the thickness of the residual wall on installed pipes, containers, bends, etc., which are exposed to high temperatures and pressures, and to corrosive chemicals. The main problem in this case is: detection of spots of both areal and point-like corrosion, and measurement of the residual wall thickness at the critical points, i.e. precisely at spots where *no* multiple echoes can be obtained from a wall limited by parallel faces.

The measuring possibilities will be briefly summarized for both groups as follow: At the manufacturing plant of the work pieces the measurement can be made by contact and point by point, using the pulse-echo method and an auxiliary unit for wall thickness measurements, or by using the resonance method (see Sec. 2.1). A special case of the first-mentioned method is that in which the sequence of multiple echoes is produced by interposing a water gap in order to improve the coupling on rough sur faces, or if a solid, possibly liquid-cooled coupling adaptor is used for measurements on hot specimens, in order to prevent direct heat transfer to the probe. The transit time of such a delay line should here be long compared with that in the wall so that the sequences of multiple echoes no longer disturb each other (Fig. 3.237 a). Alternatively, the echo spacings can also be measured directly on the CR screen by time-base spreading (sweep expansion) or one can use a wall thickness measuring adaptor (Fig. 3.237 a). If the difference in transit time is not great enough, the individual resonance antinodes may overlap and disturb each other. Variable damping of the resonant circuit is then of advantage.

On hot walls up to approx. 500 °C the measurement can also be made by using a "water gun" [89], a sequence of multiple echoes is obtained. A short, strong jet of water transmits the ultrasonic energy to the specimen and simultaneously cools the probe. In order to obtain a neat sequence of multiple echoes, the water jet should impinge exactly at right angles on the wall. This is not so simple because the water gun with its cable and hose connections cannot be manipulated so easily. This can be remedied as follows: As soon as an optimal echo picture which is suitable for evaluation appears briefly, this is photographed and later evaluated.

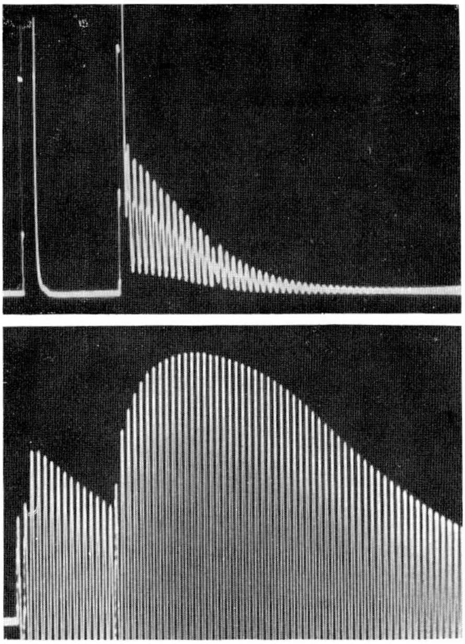

Fig. 3.237 Wall thickness measurement via a transit section, a) screen picture of echo sequence obtained on an 8 mm steel plate with a 50 mm plexiglass coupling adaptor, b) when the wall thickness meter after tuning to maximum is used (see also Figs. 2.61 and 2.62).

Direct contact between the probe and the surface of the specimen to be measured cannot be considered for continuous wall thickness measurements because of the excessive wear of the probe. This leaves either the immersion technique or coupling via a liquid film of constant thickness. The resonance method has been further developed by Branson Instruments in 1960 [132, 225] (cf. Sec. 2.11 and 2.12), so that wall thickness measurements can be made by this method also with a water delay line. Within certain limits the measuring result is here independent of the change in length of the delay line. This method is presently being successfully applied in practice as a continuous check of the thickness of thin-walled, smooth pipes (see Sec. 3.26). If a specified tolerance range is exceeded this is indicated or alternatively the actual wall thickness is recorded.

The "Atlas" pipe tester described in Sec. 3.26 measures the wall thickness continuously according to the counting method (see 2.352); it is coupled via a film of water of constant thickness. The distance between the first and the fourth multiple echo is counted electronically: the first backwall echo triggers the counter while the fourth stops it. A recorder with 100 recording pens records the result (see Fig. 3.149) [138].

With TR probes it is possible to construct a device which, by simple means, indicates any deviation from the permissible wall thickness tolerance. The only critical parameter is the constancy of the coupling gap: a change in the thickness of the film of flowing water of only 0.1 mm introduces an error in measurement of 0.4 mm (for steel, because of the unfavourable ratio ot the two acoustic velocities). The surface quality and the roundness of, e.g., precision tubes is such that an adjusted coupling gap can be maintained with an error less than 0.1 mm and better by using guiding devices for the probes, if the measuring process is automated. In the case of steel, the measuring accuracy is thus 0.4 mm

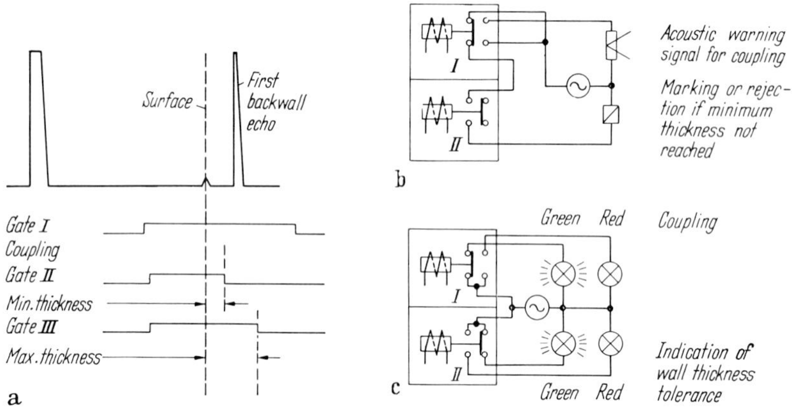

Fig. 3.238 Measurement of wall thickness tolerance with pulse-echo instrument, TR probe and twin monitor. a) Screen picture with gate curves shown below it; b) circuit diagram of the two monitor channels for continuous measurement: coupling satisfactory, wall thickness exceeds minimum thickness; c) circuit diagram for scanning by hand: coupling satisfactory, wall thickness exceeds minimum thickness.

or better. With the aid of a two-channel monitor as shown in Fig. 3.238 it is thus possible to construct a measuring device for a specified wall thickness tolerance. Monitor channel *I* with gate *I* checks the coupling. A hooter sounds an alarm as soon as the amplitude of the backwall echo drops below a set value. Monitor channel *II* produces a signal if the minimum wall thickness is not reached. The right limit of gate *II* corresponds to the minimum wall thickness. This limit is set by means of a calibrated specimen with the critical limits. If the minimum wall thickness is not reached, the backwall echo falls into gate *II* which initiates the marking of the measuring point or which rejects the specimen concerned. A third monitor (*III*) whose right limit corresponds to an upper tolerance limit can be used in a similar manner for indicating excessive wall thicknesses.

Further interesting possibilities are offered by the transit time monitor (see Sec. 2.352). If such a monitor is introduced into the above-mentioned measuring device with TR probes, the wall thickness can be recorded directly and continuously. Here again the measuring error is determined by the constancy of the coupling gap. If a normal probe produces via a water delay line a backwall echo clearly separated from the entrance echo, the transit time monitor for use with the immersion technique can be utilized for this purpose: the measuring of the transit time is started by the entrance echo. The measured value then refers to the distance between entrance echo and first backwall echo; thus this value is independent of any change in length of the delay line.

The requirements concerning wall thickness measurements on pipelines and other construction components of power plants, chemical factories, and particularly the petrochemical industry almost exclusively call for the application of the TR method. Only in a relatively few cases where uniform, areal erosion can be assumed, can the measurement be made by means of multiple echoes, e.g. with the wall thickness measuring adaptor, or by means of the resonance method. Furthermore, since only spot tests by hand can be considered the number of promising measuring methods is here reduced to a few variants of the TR technique. Fig. 3.238c shows a simple arrangement with a two-channel monitor. Two of the four monitor pilot lamps (a green – channel *I*, coupling – and a red – channel *II*, wall thickness tolerance indication) can also be mounted on the probe or in a small signal box attached to the wrist of the examiner for convenient observation. Once the instrument and the monitor gates have been accurately adjusted by means of a stepped test block, the examiner need no longer watch the CR screen for pure tolerance measurements. He can then pay full attention to the coupling of the probe. If the green pilot lamp lights up, this tells him that the coupling is satisfactory; if simultaneously the red pilot lamp lights up, this indicates that the adjusted minimum wall thickness is not reached. These measurements can be carried out very quickly, requiring only occasional checks of the calibration at approximately half hour intervals.

The same method – but used for measuring absolute wall thicknesses – was found to be reliable in practice. The thickness is measured directly on a greatly expanded time base, so that the width of the screen corresponds to 10 mm steel. The transmitting pulse is shifted far to the left, corresponding to the delay line in the probe. Once the instrument has been calibrated on a test block with 1 mm steps, thickness readings to within 0.1 mm are possible. It is recommended that the adjustment of the instrument be checked after approximately every 20 to 30 measuring points. The same method can also be used for measuring residual wall thicknesses at spots attacked by pitting.

Recently it has become possible to equip TR probes with delay lines of highly heat-resistant material. The measuring method described can thus also be used on hot specimens. With silicon high-vacuum greases, measurements can be made at temperatures of 500 to 600 °C (cf. Sec. 3.113). Sufficient acoustic contact can be established for a fraction of a second. This is quite enough to obtain a reading of the wall thickness. After each measurement the probe must again be adequately cooled.

More difficult wall thickness measurements occur for instance on pipes from the inside if the outer surface is not accessible. Special probes attached to rods are available for this purpose, similar to the inside pipe probe, Fig. 3.146, for crack tests. The examination is greatly facilitated if the pipe can be filled with water because this eliminates coupling difficulties.

In the case of non-ferrous metals there is a risk of wrong wall thickness measurements if the specimen, as a result of anisotropy, has an acoustic velocity normal to the wall different from that of the specimen used for calibration.

Water or other liquids behind the wall usually disturb the thickness measurements only very little, e.g. on filled pipelines and containers and on ships below the water line. Only in the case of lead cables where the thickness of the lead sheath has to be determined does it make much difference whether the inside is dry or filled with oil. Because of the curvature of the surface and the attenuation in the lead, the resonance or the sequence of multiple echoes is rather weak.

Deposits on the inside of pipes and containers usually have a much lower acoustic impedance than the wall, which results in the ultrasonic wave being almost totally reflected at the boundary between wall and deposit so that only the pure wall thickness is measured. There are, however, exceptions. In oil refineries it has been observed that a layer of iron sulphide forms in the fire tubes if crude oil containing sulphur is used; this layer adheres strongly and apparently has a sufficiently high acoustic impedance to simulate a considerably greater wall thickness. This disturbance was observed on pipes of (14 Cr-1 Si) steel but is suspected to occur also on other steels. Where this seems possible, e.g. if the measuring values have increased from one test to the next, an attempt can be made to spall off the layer at a few spots by strong hammer blows in order to be able to check the pure wall thickness at such spots. Naturally, this disturbance applies to both the resonance method and the pulse method.

Problems of particular importance and wide application are presented by plate thickness measurements on *ship plating*. The old trepanning method which requires dry-docking of the ship and subsequent sealing of the holes by welding, is obviated by ultrasonic tests for which the ship can remain in the water. Particularly on oil tankers the partitions and outside plates corrode rapidly because the empty tanks are filled with sea water. Tankers have already been successfully checked by using either resonance instruments [90, 91], or pulse-echo instruments, although the testing conditions here are not simple. To avoid the erection of scaffolds, the examiner is lowered in a basket by a rope. The examiner is in any case connected to the stationary instrument by a long testing cable and in addition by telephone to an assistant who operates the instrument. Grinding of the measuring points or preferably chipping with a hammer is usually unavoidable. EVANS [90] gives an interesting comparison of costs under American conditions for testing an oil tanker: a price of approximately \$4.50 per measuring point was calculated on the basis of approximately 600 readings, which corresponds to approximately 1/4 to 1/5 of the costs of the old method. To the latter must be added, however, the daily costs of \$ 1500 to \$ 2000 for the drydock. Since in addition the ultrasonic measurement is much quicker, there is a further saving of \$ 3000 to \$ 4000 for every day the ship is laid up. An Audigage was used for the thickness measurements (see Sec. 2.12). The measurements themselves could be speeded up considerably if pulse-echo instruments are used.

Measurements of layer thicknesses with ultrasonics are possible only if the acoustic impedance of the layer differs markedly from that of the base and if the layer is not too thin. The usual layer thicknesses of chromium or nickel on steel thus violate both these requirements. With pulse-echo instruments of maximum subsurface resolution, e.g. according to the shock-wave method, layers above approximately 0.1 mm of acoustically softer material on steel, e.g. copper, plastic or paint, can still be determined by the direct echo method. Thicker layers, such as rubber on steel, thicker platings of metals with markedly different acoustic impedances, and, e.g., also ledeburitic shell sin the case of chill castings (see Sec. 3.33) can also be measured with standard instruments. In general the resonance method cannot be considered as a solution to these problems, nor the multiple echo method with pulse instruments.

For measuring the *case thickness* of surface-hardened work pieces the conditions are much more favourable for case hardening than for flame or induction hardening because the former produces a greater change in the composition of the steel and thus also in its ultrasonic properties. With frequencies of the order of 40 MHz and very short pulses, the measurement was successful, even for case thicknesses of less than 1 mm (ELION [82]). Thus the boundary of the case is indicated by scatter, which, however, with the gradual transition desired in practice, does not set in abruptly enough to permit a reliable measurement.

While therefore beaming normal to the surface only rarely provides practical results, propagation along the surface still offers promising possibilities. If the transverse velocity in the layer is lower than in the base, the layer thickness will change the propagation velocity of surface waves or Love waves (HÄUSLER [129]). Investigations are still in progress with a view to determining the extent to which measurements with pulse instruments are feasible in spite of the dispersion of the phase velocity. Unfortunately, Love waves have the disadvantage that they can be excited only via a solid, or at least highly viscous, couplant.

Finally, transit time measurements according to the pulse-echo method are used for determining the length of bolts, their change when stressed, and thus the strain in the bolt. The mechanical method used so far has relied on a torque measurement at the torque spanner which is, however, not very accurate because of unknown frictional resistances. The transit time of the bottom echo is therefore measured from the accessible end of the bolt, both before and during tightening. Here, the transit time does not change exclusively as a result of the true change in length, but in addition also because of a dependence of the acoustic velocity on the stress (cf. Sec. 3.62). The calculation can therefore not be based on the normal acoustic velocity, and it is preferable to make allowance for both effects by using an empirical calibration curve for the material concerned [116, 198].

3.62 Measurement of Acoustic Velocity

Since in materials testing the main interest centres on the acoustic velocity in solids, attention is here drawn to the book by BERGMANN [1] concerning methods for measuring this quantity in liquids.

Using a resonance or pulse-echo instrument calibrated for a definite acoustic velocity c, e.g. in steel, one readily determines an unknown acoustic velocity c_x by measuring the apparent thickness d_s of the specimen. The true thickness d having been determined by mechanical measurement, we then have

$$c_x = c\,\frac{d}{d_s}\,.$$

The accuracy is determined by the calibration accuracy of the instrument; in general this will not be better than approx. 1%.

With the use of interferometers (cf. 2.35) and of pulse-echo instruments one aims at accuracies of approximately 0.1%. In the above formula the apparent thickness d_s is then replaced by the length of the reference delay line which can be measured with a micrometer, and c by the accurately known acoustic velocity of the delay line.

This requires that the temperature effect of the interferometer liquid be taken into consideration. In the case of distilled water or water which has been standing for some time, we have

$$c = 1483.1 \text{ m/s}$$

at 20 °C; this value is increased by 2.5 m/s for every degree C. If suitable mixtures of ethyl alcohol and water are used, the temperature effect can be neglected. A suitable mixture is 15 to 20% by weight alcohol for the temperature range from 5 to 30 °C. The acoustic velocity depends on the concentration. At 15.6% by weight alcohol it is very nearly 1600 m/s (according to GIACOMINI, cf. [1, p. 425]). Such mixtures can be used over

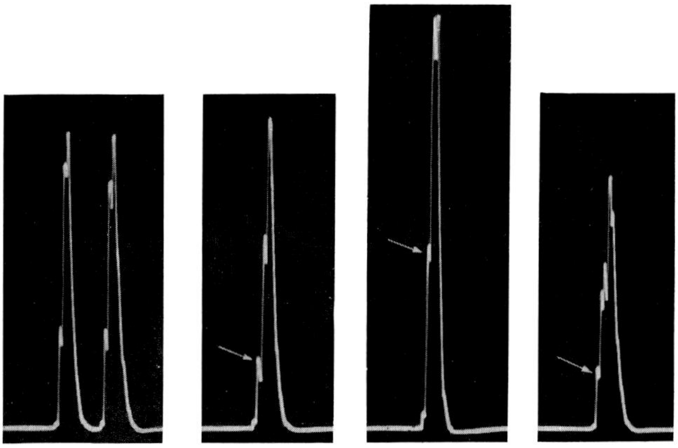

a b c d

Fig. 3.239 Interference of two echoes in different phases. a) Both echoes widely separated, the right (echo of delay line) is shifted to the left; b) first minimum of the observed high-frequency node; c) maximum; d) second minimum. Reflector shift between b) and d) 0.20 mm of water, i.e. change of sound path 0.40 mm water equals one wave length, whence frequency = 3.8 MHz. Readings reproducible within less than 0.01 mm, therefore measuring error for 15 mm water section (corresponding approximately to 60 mm specimen thickness in case of steel) less than 0.01/15 ~ 0.7%.

fairly long periods without risk of changing the concentration only if kept in closed containers. The temperature effect of metallic delay lines in dry interferometers is approximately only 1/10 of that of water and can therefore usually be neglected.

Accurate observation of the interference of two echoes on the CR screen presupposes high-frequency indication with the ultrasonic frequency, or video indication with clearly distinguishable high-frequency oscillations. Perfectly smooth echo peaks, i.e. with totally filtered high frequency, are just as unsuitable as high-frequency presentation in the intermediate frequency range in the case of heterodyne amplifiers (Fig. 3.239).

Shifting the reflector from a minimum or maximum of a high-frequency node to the minimum or maximum of the *following* node indicates exactly one half wave length in water. This makes it possible to measure the true echo frequency of the specimen which may differ from the rated frequency of the probe. Furthermore, this can be used for measuring the frequency at different points of the echo pulse.

A high frequency in the specimen gives a high accuracy, but only as long as the attenuation of the sound remains insignificant (see below). The frequency of the reference echo need not necessarily be the same. To avoid zero errors, it is recommended that the distance between transmitting pulse and first echo be not measured; and, instead, one or several distances between multiple echoes. The reference echo is successively brought to interference with the first, second and subsequent multiple echoes which then furnishes several measured values. At each echo the maximum is observed at the same high-frequency node. In the case of the sequence shown in Fig. 2.16a a given node can readily be followed from one echo to the next because its amplitude decreases little due to the shortness of the specimen. With high attenuation the multiple echoes are, however, distorted and become dissimilar. An error of one or several wave lengths is then easily made. Furthermore, the gain of the instrument should, if possible, not be changed between two measurements. The reference echo is adjusted to approximately the same amplitude as that of the echo of the specimen by means of an adjustable attenuator in the circuit of the reference probe (see Figs. 2.57 and 2.58a). The setting of this control should likewise not be changed between two measurements.

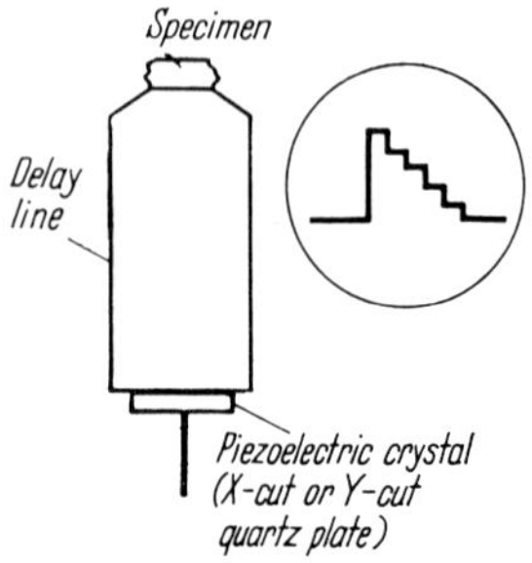

Fig. 3.240 Device for measuring acoustic velocities in small specimens according to the pulse resonance method, with schematic echo pattern according to McSkimin and Bond.

In the method described the echo of the specimen and the reference echo do not cancel each other completely or add up to double the amplitude because they are not exactly equal due to the different coupling of the probes, both to the specimen and to the liquid, as far as the build-up and decay phenomena are concerned. For scientific purposes the accuracy of the interference method can still be considerably increased if the echoes to be compared are made exactly equal. For this purpose two identical piezo-electric plates without a damping backing are cemented to accurately plane-parallel specimens. If the frequency is tuned exactly to the natural frequency of the piezo-electric plates, very uniform and long echo sequences are obtained. If initially the transit times in the two bodies are exactly the same and if one now changes the ultrasonic velocity in one of them, e.g. by changing the temperature or the pressure, then the superimposed echo sequences show beats at uniform distances, as they may occasionally appear unintentionally and irregularly in every echo sequence from a plate, e.g. in Fig. 3.31. If n echoes appear between two maxima or minima, the transit time in one of the test specimens has changed by $1/n$ of the period of one wave length. It is thus possible to observe changes of the velocity with high accuracy. (See also papers by Truell et al. [88, 350], furthermore Bradfield [2].)

If only small specimens of a given material are available, e.g. crystals, it is advisable to use a modification of the pulse-resonance method according to McSkimin and Bond [256]. As shown in Fig. 3.240, the specimen is cemented to the one end of a delay line or coupling adaptor, the other end of which mounts an X-cut or Y-cut quartz plate. To be able to use also high frequencies, the delay line consists of molten quartz which has very low attenuation. Pulses which are longer than double the thickness of the plane-parallel specimen are transmitted, so that the echo is composed of a sequence of multiple echoes, some of which overlap and interfere. If the frequency of the pulse is changed one obtains after rectification of the high-frequency pulses a staircase pattern whose steps show maxima and minima when going through the whole frequency range as shown in Fig. 3.240. The required acoustic velocity is calculated according to Eq. (2.3) from the frequency interval between two resonance peaks. This has been used to determine the elastic constants of crystals, e.g. diamonds.

Any of the methods described can be used for determining the longitudinal as well as the transverse velocity or their changes. In the latter case transverse waves are produced in the specimen by means of a Y-cut quartz plate, while in liquid reference delay lines, naturally as always, a longitudinal oscillator is used.

If a given specimen has a preferred direction, e.g. as a result of texture or mechanical stress, the transverse velocities may differ for the oscillation plane parallel and normal to this direction (Fig. 3.240). In close analogy to optics this is then referred to as double refraction and polarized ultrasonic waves (Firestone [106]). Thus, in this situation both the transmitter and the receiver for polarized waves are Y-cut quartz plates: if two such probes are applied as in straight pulse transmission, the maximum amplitude is obtained if the oscillation or polarization planes are parallel, and zero if they are at right angles to each other.

The measurement of elastic double refraction is of great practical interest. Several methods can be used for this purpose. If one uses two separate Y-cut quartz plates as in Fig. 3.241 arranged for echo operation, the pulse of the one transducer suffers only a small delay relative to the pulse of the other in the case of slight double refraction. A phase difference of one half wave length is obtained only after several transits. If the echo sequences are superimposed (parallel connection of both quartz plates), an echo sequence with maxima and minima is obtained, as shown above for longitudinal waves.

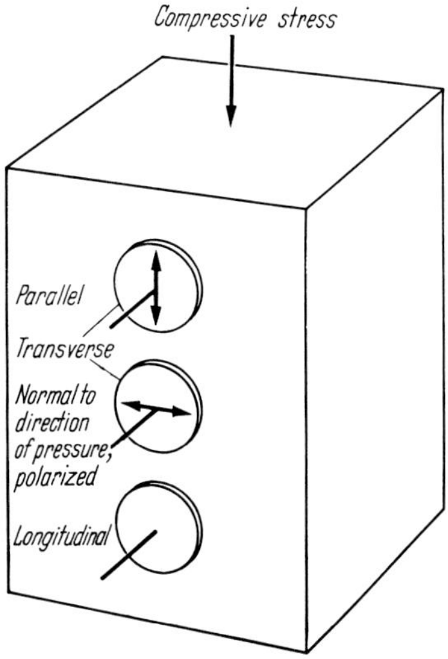

Fig. 3.241 Measurement of changes in acoustic velocity caused by mechanical stress.

Instead of using two Y-cut quartz plates, it is simpler to use only one whose direction of oscillation makes an angle of 45° with the indicated direction. The transmitted wave can then be separated into two components parallel and normal to it, which are propagated at different velocities. As in optics (cf. e.g. Pohl [16, vol. 3, para. 88]), the resultant oscillation of the particles is generally an elliptical or circular path, in special cases also a linear oscillation normal or parallel to the original, depending on the phase shift. If received by the same oscillator the elliptically and circularly polarized waves produce an electrical signal whose amplitude decreases to zero with increasing phase shift, then rises again, and so forth. The result as shown on the CR screen is then exactly the same as in the case of two separate oscillators, viz. a sequence of echoes with minima and maxima. In order to obtain distinct and numerous extreme values, the pulse should contain a reasonably large number of oscillations of equal amplitude. In order to keep the pulses short nevertheless higher frequencies are used. The sensitivity increases with the frequency and the delay line.

According to ELION [83, 81], the two Y-cut quartz plates of Fig. 3.241 could also be cemented *together*. The outer one then transmits or receives its wave through the other. Although this requires only one measuring point, the two components can be separately transmitted, and the phase shift can be measurably compensated by electrical delay lines e.g. before the receiver. With such probes it is also possible to generate arbitrary, elliptically or circularly polarized waves.

According to BENSON [44] variable double refraction, e.g. in a specimen subjected to varying loads, can be followed by the amplitude of a given echo which follows a cosine function of the phase angle; this is simpler than using the minima of the echo sequence for this purpose. Provided the double refraction is sufficiently marked, one can use the first echo for this purpose or, in the case of pulse transmission, a pulse which has travelled the distance once only. During this test it may happen that at the beginning of the application of the load, the height of the echo does not decrease immediately, but at first still increases; this can be the result of preferentially orientated residual stresses, which thus could also be measured in this way.

FIRESTONE [106, 107] has already used the pulse-resonance method on thin specimens, e.g. anisotropic plates (cf. 3.61). In the case of a Y-cut quartz oscillating at an angle of 45° to the preferred orientation, and suitably tuned frequency, the transmitting pulse decays with beats.

In order to measure the longitudinal velocity, one can also use the method of natural oscillations at ultrasonic frequencies, as has long been customary at lower frequencies (BORDONI [50]). The rod-shaped or plate-shaped specimen is then excited to natural oscillations, e.g. electrostatically, and their frequency is then measured.

Applications of the measurement of the acoustic velocity for direct materials testing are porosity tests on porcelain and other materials, determination of the tensile strength of cast iron, moisture content of plastics, and so forth. The velocity of sound can furthermore be used for measuring the velocity of flow of liquids which is added vectorially to the acoustic velocity; occasionally also for measuring the temperature of hot gases and the change of a given gas mixture.

From the longitudinal and transverse velocities and Eqs. (1.6) and (1.7) one can furthermore compute the coefficient of elasticity of materials, viz. Poisson's ratio

$$\sigma = \frac{\frac{1}{2}\, c_l^2 - c_t^2}{c_l^2 - c_t^2}, \tag{3.9}$$

the modulus of torsion or shear

$$\mu = \varrho\, c_t^2 \ \ \mathrm{N/m^2} = \varrho\, c_t^2 \cdot 1.02 \cdot 10^{-4} \ \ \mathrm{kp/mm^2} \tag{3.10}$$

(specific gravity ϱ in kg/m³) (ϱ in g/cm³)

and Young's modulus

$$E = 2\mu(1+\sigma)$$
$$= 4\varrho \frac{\frac{3}{4}c_l^2 - c_t^2}{(c_l/c_t)^2 - 1}\ \mathrm{N/m^2} = \varrho \frac{\frac{3}{4}c_l^2 - c_t^2}{(c_l/c_t)^2 - 1}\ 4.08 \cdot 10^{-4}\ \mathrm{kp/mm^2}. \quad (3.11)$$

(ϱ in kg/m³) (ϱ in g/m³, c in m/s throughout)

Measurements of the two transverse velocities can be used for determining texture (anisotropy) [107]. It can also be considered for determining internal and external stresses [45, 83, 81, 143, 44]. Fig. 3.242

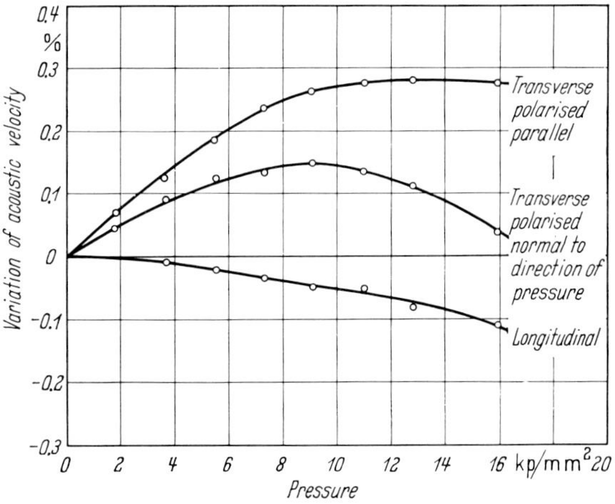

Fig. 3.242 Variations in per cent of the acoustic velocity in aluminium subjected to compressive stresses according to ELION.

shows the results of measurements obtained by ELION [83] in compression tests on aluminium of 100 × 100 mm cross-section. This shows that the longitudinal velocity decreases almost linearly. More striking is the behaviour of the two transverse velocities: the one polarized normal to the direction of pressure has a maximum, whereas the parallel polarized transverse velocity shows a linear rise in the elastic range, reaching a limit value in the plastic range. From their respective behaviour one can therefore deduce the existence of stresses without having to use zero stress for calibration. This, however, presupposes that the specimen is not double refracting due to texture (anisotropy). Not only external loads but also internal, preferentially orientated residual stresses can be indicated in this way. Such a method can be very valuable for the examination of installed structural components which can of course not be relieved to obtain zero stress. So far it has been possible to use only X-ray methods for this purpose; these, however, are limited to surface observations.

Since this method is the acoustic counterpart to the photo-elastic method used for investigating specimens in the form of transparent models, the term *acousto-elasticity,* in contrast to *photo-elasticity,* has been coined for it in the USA.

Regarding determination of Young's moduli, see also [43], and measurements of acoustic velocities at higher temperatures, [227, 242].

3.63 Measurement of the Attenuation of Sound

Absolute measurements of the attenuation are very difficult because the echo amplitude depends not only on the attenuation but also on a number of other influencing factors. Relative measurements are easier, i.e. changes of the attenuation during a given test, or also purely qualitative tests. For this purpose the shape of the specimen, the probe and the coupling are kept constant while the amplitudes of the backwall echoes are compared. On an instrument with calibrated gain control this amplitude is then adjusted to the same level on the CR screen in each case while the difference is read directly in decibels. In this way it is for instance possible to observe the effect of temperature or fatigue by means of a crystal plate cemented to a given specimen, whose shape moreover has no influence on the measurement. In the case of different specimens of identical shape any deductions on the attenuation from the backwall echo or sound transmission echo can, however, be made only if in spite of different attenuation, both have the same acoustic impedance and the same surface quality, because these quantities determine both the coupling and the reflection losses. Thus, for instance, the fact that a given aluminium block furnishes a greater backwall echo than a steel block of identical shape, does not necessarily mean that the attenuation of the aluminium is smaller. The cause usually is simply the better sound transfer in the coupling due to the better acoustic impedance matching.

For absolute measurements it is necessary to use the decrease of the echo amplitude in a given sequence of multiple backwall echoes. In addition to the attenuation of the material, the decrease is caused firstly by the energy loss of the wave due to the coupled probe when reflected at its contact surface, and secondly by the divergence of the sound beam.

According to Truell [313] the loss caused by the first factor can be made negligibly small by coupling the piezoelectric quartz plate alone, i.e. without damping body and holder, and exciting it exactly in its natural frequency. When standard probes are used, a certain loss which is not exactly known thus has to be accepted if one tests by direct contact. It is therefore usually preferable to couple via a liquid delay line, in which case the loss on reflection at the boundary can be calculated from the known ratio of the acoustic impedances.

In the case of loss due to the second cause, two procedures are possible. Either this loss can be largely neglected provided one still operates in the near field with all the multiple echoes used, or this loss can also be calculated quite simply if one uses the far field beyond say three times the length of the near field where the amplitude decreases fairly accurately inversely with the distance (Fig. 1.88).

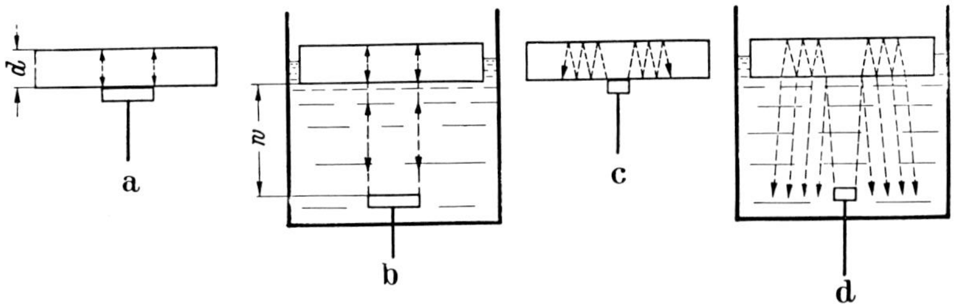

Fig. 3.243 Arrangement for attenuation measurements on the basis of multiple echo sequences. a) Direct contact, near field; b) delay line, near field; c) direct contact, far field; d) delay line, far field.

Fig. 3.243 shows schematically the arrangement for the 4 possibilities given. Accordingly, the formulas for measuring the coefficient of attenuation α in dB/mm are:

$$\text{a)}\quad \alpha = \frac{1}{2d} S_E\,, \qquad \text{b)}\quad = \frac{1}{2d}(S_E - S_R)\,,$$
$$\text{c)}\quad = \frac{1}{2d}(S_E - S_A)\,, \qquad \text{d)}\quad = \frac{1}{2d}(S_E - S_R - S'_A)\,. \tag{3.12}$$

Eq. (3.12a) follows from Eq. (1.42), if, because of the echo method used, double the plate thickness d is inserted and if S_E is the ratio of two successive echo amplitudes measured in dB:

$$S_E = 20 \log \frac{H_n}{H_{n+1}}\,.$$

If instruments with gain control calibrated in dB are used, S_E is then simply the difference of the two adjustments required to bring the echoes to a given level on the CR screen.

In the case of Eq. (3.12b), because of the incomplete reflection at the boundary between specimen and water, the loss S_R must be taken into account once for each echo:

$$S_R = 20 \log \frac{1}{R} = 20 \log \frac{W_2 + W_1}{W_2 - W_1}\,,$$

where W_1 and W_2 are the acoustic impedances of the specimen and the water, respectively [see Eq. (1.11)].

Eq. (3.12c) follows from Eq. (1.43) with the attenuation S_A due to the propagation of the acoustic beam in the far field

$$S_A = 20 \log \frac{n+1}{n} .$$

In Eq. (3.12d), the propagation correction S_A has to be subtracted in addition to the reflection loss, which, due to the path w in water, has a slightly different value:

$$S'_A = 20 \log \frac{w c_w/c + (n+1)d}{w c_w/c + n d} .$$

The path w in water enters in the distance only after multiplication by the ratio c_w/c of the acoustic velocities, both in the water and in the specimen.

In Fig. 3.243a it is assumed that the amplitude of the backwall echo remains constant over the entire near field in a material with no attenuation. According to TRUELL et al. [329] this is not strictly so, because of diffraction phenomena (cf. Fig. 1.88). Accurate measurements therefore require a correction given in [329]. This correction depends on the sound path and is approximately 2 dB at the end of the near field if the radiator oscillates like a piston.

In cases b and d of Fig. 3.243 the water can also rise above the plate. The correction for the reflection losses is then doubled, and one obtains a second relation for α which can be used in addition for determining the unknown reflection and thus the acoustic impedance of the specimen.

In such measurements the plate thickness d should be large enough to obtain good separation of the multiple echoes, but on the other hand not too large so as to be able to accommodate as many multiple echoes as possible in the near field of the oscillator. In cases c and d of Fig. 3.243 the plate diameter furthermore should be so large that the echoes used are not disturbed by lateral boundary effects. It is best to estimate the minimum diameter on the basis of double the value of divergence γ_0 instead of the simple angle (Fig. 2.41). In this respect round plates are by far more unsuitable than square or irregularly shaped plates.

According to TRUELL a rod-shaped specimen with reduced mid-section, such as a tensile test specimen, is claimed to produce a collimating effect on the sound beam so that one can work with it as in the near field although the sound paths are much longer. This would mean that it is not necessary to use the correction factor S_A for the propagation of the sound field.

The demands in respect of the plane-parallelism of a plate-shaped specimen are higher, the higher the frequency and the required accuracy. According to a calculation by TRUELL [128] the wedge angle of the plate may not exceed approximately $2.5 \cdot 10^{-3}$ degrees (= 9 s), if an attenuation of 0.5 dB/μs has to be measured with an accuracy of 10% at 300 MHz (attenuation referred to transit time instead of to path, as is customary). This already requires plane-parallelism of optical quality.

In the case of plates the arrangements shown in Figs. 3.243a and b are better suited to higher frequencies with which also sufficiently long near fields can be obtained with convenient oscillator diameters.

Only with the arrangement shown in Fig. 3.243a does the echo sequence approximately follow an exponential function. This is exploited in an attenuation measuring instrument designed by TRUELL, and produced by SPERRY called *Attenuation Comparator*. It uses the discharge of a capacitor whose voltage pattern is likewise an e-function. Simultaneously with the transmitting pulse a charged capacitor is discharged through a variable resistor. The curve appearing on the CR screen has to be matched to the echo sequence (Fig. 3.244). Since in this case both e-functions have the same exponent, the value $d\alpha$ can be read directly on the control. The instrument operates from 1 to 200 MHz. Correct measurement, however, presupposes that the multiple echoes are all in the near field and that coupling losses, as mentioned, are avoided by using a tuned, undamped crystal.

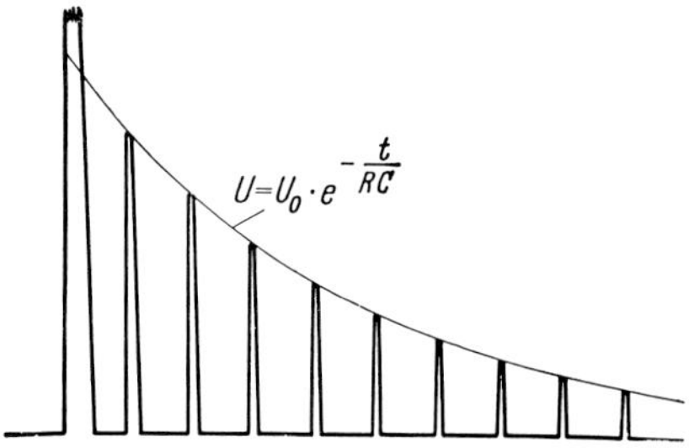

Fig. 3.244 Measurement of the exponential decay of the arrangement shown in Fig. 3.243a, by matching the discharge function of a capacitor C through a resistor R with the echo sequence.

To be able to observe rapid changes of the attenuation as well, TRUELL [369] has developed an instrument for automatic measurements, viz. the *Automatic Attenuation Readout Adapter*. By means of a logarithmic and a differential amplifier the exponent $d\alpha$ is obtained from two gated echoes of the sequence, and indicated by a pointer instrument or recorded continuously.

In a modification of the above arrangements the measurement can also be made by pulse transmission (Fig. 3.245). However, if this is used for comparing multiple echoes, and if the entire process takes place in the near field, there is nothing new in this compared with Fig. 3.243b. Sometimes, however, the signal sent through once only is used and compared with the signal of the free water section containing no test piece. Thus, if the water can be regarded as non-absorptive (only in case of high attenuation in the specimen), the difference of the two indications contains a double reflection loss and the attenuation in the specimen. Otherwise, the attenuation of the displaced water would have to be taken into consideration in addition and added to the measured value of the attenuation. This depends on the frequency and the temperature, furthermore also on the gas content (cf. BERGMANN [1, p. 465ff.]). Because of the short sound paths, this method is suitable for materials with high attenuation and where the sound path of multiple echoes would extend beyond the near field at the given values of testing thickness, frequency and transducer diameter.

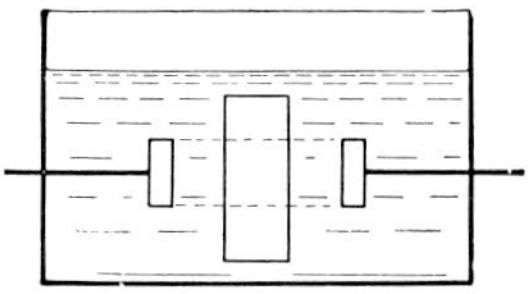

Fig. 3.245 Attenuation measurement with straight pulse transmission.

Ivens [165], using multiple echoes, has measured with a similar arrangement in the far field and in the transition zone to the near field. In this field a large receiver would have required corrections for the propagation of the sound field which cannot easily be neglected. The measurement was therefore made with a very small receiver for which the pattern of the acoustic pressure along the axis according to Eq. (1.27) applies.

Frielinghaus and Koppelmann [111, 190] have shown that accurate attenuation measurements on plate-like specimens can also be made with commercially available pulse-echo instruments if fitted with an accurate, calibrated gain control.

The methods mentioned require a specimen of the material concerned which has been specially prepared for this purpose. Frequently, however, attenuation measurements on the test piece itself are of interest, e.g. on large forgings or castings, either in order to evaluate its structure or in order to deduce the size of a given flaw from the amplitude of its echo.

This requires that the backwall of the specimen normal to the sound beam, whose echo is compared with the backwall echo of a reference plate without appreciable attenuation, is not too rough. Using the known near-field length of the probe, the ratio of the two echoes is calculated according to Sec. 1.84, or more simply, read on a diagram as shown in Figs. 1.87 and 1.88. As a result of the attenuation, the measured amplitude of the backwall echo in the specimen is lower than the calculated value. The difference gives the mean attenuation over the thickness of the specimen, which can be obtained directly in dB/mm if, instead of the echo amplitudes, the correlated gains are measured in dB or taken from Figs. 1.87 and 1.88. Corrections can be given for cylindrically curved test surfaces or backwalls [207].

Example: A specimen of 400 mm thickness with a plane backwall should furnish a backwall echo of magnitude 0.4 times that of the reference echo with a probe whose near field length is 100 mm, and in the absence of attenuation (Fig. 1.87), i.e. require a gain of 8 dB. If in fact 28 dB gain is measured, 20 dB of it is attributable to the attenuation. The mean attenuation is therefore 20 dB/800 mm $= 25 \cdot 10^{-3}$ dB/mm.

If the specimen shown in Fig. 3.243c is thicker than 3 times the near field length, the disturbance by a coupled, conventional probe (loss due to the first cause, p. 466) can be neglected for practical purposes and the attenuation can be determined according to formula (3.12c), even on the specimen itself, e.g. a forging with plane-parallel faces.

Example: Comparing the second with the first backwall echo, we have $S_A = 6$ dB, e.g. in the far field without attenuation the ratio of the amplitudes of the two echoes is 1 : 2. In the actual specimen with attenuation the difference in gain is S_E dB. Subtracting 6 dB and dividing by double the thickness immediately furnishes the attenuation α. When applying this method to thinner specimens probes with a short near field length have to be used, i.e. 4 MHz and 5 mm diameter, $N_{\text{steel}} = 4$ mm, minimum thickness to be measured in steel: 12 mm.

Also in a solid, cylindrical forging the multiple echoes behave exactly like those of a plate as a result of the focusing effect [279]. In the case of a hollow, cylindrical specimen (rotor with bore), the propagation-attenuation S_A must still be calculated on geometric-acoustic principles (see 1.47).

Naturally, the accuracy of such a routine measurement is much lower than that of the methods described above and used in laboratories. However, also in the latter case it is difficult to keep the error below a few 10^{-3} dB/mm in the frequency range used in materials testing, which, in the case of microcrystalline metals and at 2 MHz, is already of the order of magnitude of the attenuation itself. Therefore higher frequencies are usually used for scientific purposes.

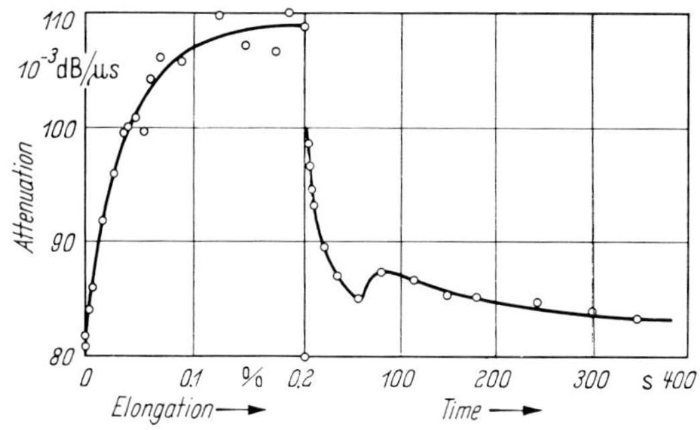

Fig. 3.246 Attenuation in aluminium during tensile test according to TRUELL [369].

Applications of quantitative attenuation measurements in the field of materials testing are still rare. Frequently, however, qualitative deductions are made on the basis of the ratio of the backwall echo of similarly shaped specimens, concerning differences, e.g. for estimating the grain size and judging the structure of cast iron. In the case of cast iron the strength can also be deduced to some extent from the attenuation, which for this purpose need not be measured quantitatively (see Sec. 3.33). In the case of steel it is reported that the hardness can be deduced from the attenuation [262]. Cf. also [194, 263].

In scientific determinations, however, the measurement of attenuation plays an important role in metal physics (cf. [144, 143, 127, 368, 369, 55, 145], the last-mentioned report quotes additional Japanese literature).

The dependence of the attenuation on the mechanical stress conditions may possibly lead to a solution of a very urgent problem of materials testing, viz. prediction of fatigue cracks under alternating stress conditions.

Fig. 3.246 explains relevant results on aluminium according to TRUELL. The left half of the diagram shows the increase of the attenuation with elongation in the non-repeated tensile test. The acoustic velocities (see Sec. 3.62) change simultaneously. On the right half the attenuation is plotted versus time, the elongation reached ultimately in the tensile test being kept constant. The decrease of the attenuation, which after some time reaches an asymptotic value, is called recovery. The change of the attenuation reached during the test depends on the load as a function of time because the recovery occurs synchronously with it. This phenomenon is explained readily by the dislocation theory in crystal lattices, likewise an irregular pattern of the recovery with maxima and minima observed occasionally.

A similar recovery of the material is observed initially after alternating stress loading, if it is interrupted. However, after a large number of alternating stress cycles this recovery is slowed down progressively and finally disappears completely. When this stage is reached the material is fatigued and failure is imminent.

In the case of magnetic materials the pattern of the attenuation during the tensile test is different and more complex. If these materials are free of residual stresses, the attenuation decreases during elongation in the elastic range. Here, the points of dislocation play a minor role in contrast to the walls of the magnetic elementary zones (Weiss' zones). The elongation reorientates the zones, resulting in improved sound transmission. The same effect, viz. a decrease of the acoustic attenuation, is therefore also observed during magnetization of the specimen. If, in the case of steel, residual stresses, e.g. by cold-working, are added, external stresses and residual stresses oppose each other so that the attenuation passes through a maximum at moderate elongation (cf. [55, 144]).

In some cases the attenuation of sound also makes possible the determination of the degree of contamination in crystals by heteroatoms, and the observation of their change during heat treatment. They reduce the attenuation because the dislocation points are pinned by the heteroatoms so that they are prevented from carrying out energy dissipating oscillations in the sound field. This has been observed in germanium, and also in titanium and copper after absorption of hydrogen [128, 393].

Little use has so far been made of measurements of the scattering as such, e.g. the laterally or backward scattered portion in the pulse-echo method. According to Elion [82] this still offers possibilities for certain practical purposes in metallurgy.

3.7 Standardization

(State 1965)

The rapid spread of ultrasonic testing has induced associations of manufacturers and consumers, as well as standardization commitees and other organisations to publish standards and specifications ranging from non-compulsory recommendations to regulations with legal standing.

Methods of a general nature were recommended at a relatively early date by the American Society for Testing and Materials (ASTM), including both the resonance method [402] and the pulse-echo method [401, 414, 412]. On the basis of preliminary investigations by Panian and van Valkenburg [281], ASTM has standardized a set of test blocks with flat-bottomed holes for the pulse-echo method [408]. Originally they had been intended by CLINE and MORGAN [64] especially for the aluminium industry, and became known as Alcoa blocks. This also forms the basis of the acceptance specification for lightmetal forgings, plate and extruded material foı the aircraft industry [450], prepared by a committee of the American Society for Nondestructive Testing (SNT).

The International Institute of Welding (IIW/IIS) has standardized the reference block of Sec. 2.333, Fig. 2.55. It is used for calibrating and checking instruments and probes by the pulse-echo method. In a similar form it was taken over by the German Standards Association as Test Block 1 [403], which also has a further Test Block 2 for miniature angle probes under consideration. The published DIN drafts furthermore contain a collection of concepts of ultrasonic testing [429] which in similar form have already been published trilingually by the IIW [437]. In the United Kingdom this corresponds furthermore to the British Standard Institute's (BSI) Glossary of Terms [422], and similar publications in India [435], Poland [445, 446] and Hungary [453]. The BSI has furthermore standardized a special British reference block, British standard number 2704 (1956), (see also [345, 421]). France has standardized a reference block similar to the IIW reference block (Association Française de Normalisation, AFNOR) [417]. In Japan the method is standardized by the Japanese Industrial Standard (JIS) [441]. At present an ASTM committee is engaged in standardizing also properties of instruments [415]. Test blocks are furthermore dealt with in the papers [25, 303, 271].

For forgings, ASTM has standardized both the testing of heavy forgings generally, as well as specifically of turbine and generator rotors [403, 404]. The last-mentioned tests are based on investigations by RANKING and MORIARTY [294], cf. Sec. 3.21. No standardized recommendations for testing heavy forgings have so far been published in Europe. The possibilities for determining the attenuation of sound and the size of the flaw quantitatively [279, 208] form the basis of a numerical characterization of the test results [302] which is at present under discussion and which could serve as a basis for an acceptance specification.

Standards exist in various countries for testing heavy plate: in Germany the Association of German Ferrous-Metallurgists (VDEh) has prepared a classification on the basis of statistical tests [457]. This was taken over in France [442, 416] and Italy [433] in a similar form. In the USA, ASTM has likewise published a standard [407].

In the field of pipe testing there is in force in Germany [432], a specification for heat-resistant pipes, which for quality grade III and diameters above 102 mm require testing by ultrasonics. Ultrasonic tests on thin boiler tubing are still under discussion [458]. Also available are specifications for pipe tests by ASTM [411], BSI [425] and API (American

Petroleum Institute) [400]. These specifications also deal with the preparation of a test flaw, discussed, inter alia, in [459].

Furthermore, the German Committee for Compressed Gases has decided to test compressed gas cylinders after a certain period of use, if there is a risk of stress-corrosion cracking, or quenching cracks. According to a decree of the Federal Minister for Works, the test shall be carried out by industrial supervisory associations [426]. In addition, the Committee for Compressed Gases has instructed the owners of tank cars for compressed gases to check them ultrasonically at spots where they are endangered by welds joining them to the supporting structure.

As far as finished products of the steel industry are concerned, a recommendation exists for ultrasonic tests on load hooks in metallurgical industries [455].

The British Steel Casting Research Association has published recommended procedures for the ultrasonic examination of steel castings [420]. DIN specification 21.501 mentions a possibility for using measurements of ultrasonic velocities to evaluate the strength of cast iron tubbings [431].

Specifications concerning the testing of porcelain or steatite insulators are available in various countries, e.g. in Germany in the VDE (Association of German Electrical Engineers) regulation [454], Austria [443], France [434], the International Electrotechnical Commission (I.E.C.) [436]. The acceptance conditions of the German and the Swiss Federal Railways prescribe ultrasonic tests [428, 429].

ASTM standards [409, 413] and BSI standards [424, 423] exist for the testing of any welded joints as well as for the testing of welded pipes, most of which, however, are as yet only available as drafts. The Central Institute for Welding in Halle (ZIS) has published binding rules for Eastern Germany [461]. The difficulty to incorporate ultrasonic tests in acceptance specifications for welded joints results, of course, from the fact that no document as such can be produced unless this concerns automated processes with recording. These, however, are still more or less being used on a trial basis. Provided the reliability of the examiner has been established, or that a check by random is acceptable, some organizations prescribe ultrasonic tests or accept them as being of equal validity. This applies for instance to the Dutch Boiler Association for Welded Joints on Steam Boilers, and the Norske Veritas for welded joints in ship plate. Some of the industrial supervisory associations in Germany (TÜV and ZIS) make the training and the successfull passing of an examination a precondition for the acceptance of an inspector. So far only the Union of the Industrial Supervisory Associations in Germany (VdTÜV) has in its memorandum on pressure vessels [460] for spherical gas tanks expressly prescribed the ultrasonic testing of the joints as a supplement to X-ray or gamma ray tests.

No regulations concerning ultrasonic measurements of wall thicknesses are yet available. In practice, however, the Industrial Supervisory Associations already use ultrasonic tests for this purpose and recognize them if the owner of a given installation carries them out reliably. Marine insurance associations, such as, e.g., the American Bureau of Shipping, recognize the checking of wall thicknesses, e.g. on oil tankers. This likewise requires that both the inspector and the inspection method are recognized on the basis of comparative trepanning tests [90, 91].

The field of standardization for the ultrasonic testing of materials is still wide open; this has also come to light at the various conferences in recent years on non-destructive testing of materials, the Symposium on "Standardization and non-destructive testing" of the British National Committee for Non-destructive Testing in Harrogate, 1962, and at the International Conference for Nondestructive Testing of Materials in Tokyo, 1960, and in London, 1963.

Table A 1

Specific gravities, acoustic velocities and acoustic impedances of some materials

Material	Spec. gravity in 10^3 kg/m³	Acoustic velocities in 10^3 m/s long. c_l	transv. c_t	Acoustic impedance in 10^6 kg/m²s $W = \varrho c_l$
Metals				
Aluminium	2.7	6.32	3.08	17
Lead	11.4	2.16	0.70	25
Iron (steel) (cf. 3.31)	7.85	5.90	3.23	46.5
Gold	19.3	3.24	1.20	63
Cast iron (cf. 3.33)	7.2	3.5 to 5.6	2.2 to 3.2	25 to 40
Hard metal	11 to 15	6.8 to 7.3	4.0 to 4.7	75 to 110
Cadmium	8.6	2.78	1.50	24
Constantan	8.8	5.24	2.64	46
Copper	8.9	4.70	2.26	42
Manganese	8.4	4.66	2.35	39
Magnesium	1.7	5.77	3.05	10
Brass	8.5 to 8.6	3.83	2.05	33
German silver	8.4	4.76	2.16	40
Nickel	8.9	5.63	2.96	50
Platinum	21.4	3.96	1.67	85
Mercury	13.6	1.45	—	20
Silver	10.5	3.60	1.59	38
Bismuth	9.8	2.18	1.10	21
Tungsten	19.3	5.46	2.62	105
Zinc	7.1	4.17	2.41	30
Tin	7.3	3.32	1.67	24
Non-metals				
Ethoxylin resin (araldit casting resin)	1.15 to 1.3	2.5 to 2.8	1.1	2.8 to 3.7
Aluminium oxide	3.7 to 3.9	10		37 to 39
Ice	0.9	3.98	1.99	3.6
Glass, flint	3.6	4.26	2.56	15
Glass, crown	2.5	5.66	3.42	14
Rubber, soft	1.3 to 2.1	1.48		1.9 to 3.1
Rubber, vulcanized	1.1 to 1.6	2.3		2.5 to 3.7
Paraffin wax	0.86 to 0.92	2.2		1.9 to 2.0
Perspex (plexiglass)	1.18	2.73	1.43	3.2
Polyamide (nylon, perlon)	1.0 to 1.2	1.8 to 2.2		1.8 to 2.7
Polystyrene	1.05	2.67		2.8
Porcelain (see 3.41)	2.4	5.6 to 6.2	3.5 to 3.7	13 to 14
Quartz glass	2.2	5.57	3.52	12.3
Teflon	2.2	1.35		3.0
Liquids				
Glycerine	1.26	1.92		2.4
Methylene iodide	3.33	0.98		3.3
Diesel oil	0.88 to 1.02	1.25		1.1 to 1.3
Motor car oil (SAE 20 a. 30)	0.89 to 0.96	1.74		1.5 to 1.7
Water (at 20 °C)	1.0	1.483		1.5

Table A 2. Reflection at boundaries and normal incidence

Upper figures: reflection factor of amplitude in %.
Lower figures: reflection loss in dB (gain of echo).

	Aluminium	Lead	Iron (steel)	Hard metall	Copper	Brass	Nickel	Silver	Tungsten	Glass (crown and ordinary)	Rubber, soft	Rubber, vulcanized	Perspex	Porcelain	Glycerine	Methylene iodide	Oil (motor car oil SAE 20 to 30) a. water	Mercury
Aluminium	0	18 15	46 6.8	71 3.0	41 7.8	29 11	49 6.1	38 8.4	72 2.9	10 20	85 1.4	72 2.9	68 3.3	13 18	74 2.6	68 3.3	84 1.5	7 23
Lead		0	30 10	60 4.4	26 12	12 19	34 9.5	21 14	62 4.2	27 11	89 1.0	80 2.0	77 2.3	31 10	82 1.8	77 2.3	89 1.1	11 19
Iron (steel)			0	37 8.6	4 27	19 14	4 28	9 21	39 8.2	53 5.5	94 0.5	88 1.1	87 1.2	56 5.1	88 1.2	87 1.2	94 0.6	40 8.1
Hard metal				0	41 7.8	53 5.6	33 9.6	45 6.9	2 34	75 2.4	97 0.2	95 0.5	94 0.6	77 2.3	95 0.4	94 0.6	97 0.3	67 3.5
Copper					0	15 17	8 22	5 26	43 7.4	50 6.0	94 0.6	87 1.2	86 1.3	53 5.6	89 1.0	86 1.3	93 0.6	36 8.9
Brass						0	23 13	10 20	54 5.4	38 8.5	91 0.8	83 1.6	81 1.8	41 7.6	85 1.4	81 1.8	91 0.8	22 13
Nickel							0	13 17	35 9.0	56 5.0	94 0.5	89 1.0	88 1.1	58 4.7	90 0.9	88 1.1	94 0.5	33 9.5
Silver								0	47 6.6	46 6.8	93 0.7	86 1.3	84 1.5	49 6.2	88 1.2	84 1.5	92 0.7	31 11
Tungsten									0	76 2.4	97 0.2	95 0.5	94 0.5	78 2.2	95 0.4	94 0.5	97 0.2	68 3.3
Glass (crown and ordinary)										0	82 1.8	67 3.5	63 4.0	4 29	70 3.1	63 4.0	81 1.9	17 15
Rubber, soft											0	50 6	40 8	80 2	30 11	40 8	3 30	87 1.2
Rubber, vulcanized												0	7 23	65 3.8	6 25	7 23	30 10	75 2.5
Perspex													0	60 4.4	10 20	0 ∞	40 9	72 2,8
Porcelain														0	70 3	60 4	80 2	20 14
Glycerine															0	10 20	25 12	78 2.2
Methylene iodide																0	40 9	72 2.8
Oil (motor car oil SAE 20 to 30) and water																	0	86 1.3
Mercury																		0

Collection of formulas relevant to 1.6 and to Tables 1 to 9

The following formulas give reflection and transmission coefficients for the acoustic pressure as a function of the angle of incidence, calculated for plane waves on plane boundaries and disregarding absorption. The notation of the formulas is based on that of Schoch [20], where, however, they refer not to the acoustic pressure but to the particle displacement. Fig. 1.20ff and the Tables only give numerical values, i.e. without regard to phase.

a) *Free boundary of a solid* (see Figs. 1.20, 1.21 and Table 1). Symbols: the angles of the longitudinal and transverse waves are α_l and α_t respectively. Thus for example $R_{l/t}$ signifies the reflection coefficient of the acoustic pressure for a reflected longitudinal wave referred to an incident transverse wave. For the reflected *longitudinal wave* we have:

$$R_{l/l} = \frac{(c_t/c_l)^2 \sin 2\alpha_l \sin 2\alpha_t - \cos^2 2\alpha_t}{N} \tag{A 1}$$

with the abbreviation for the denominator

$$N = \left(\frac{c_t}{c_l}\right)^2 \sin 2\alpha_l \sin 2\alpha_t + \cos^2 2\alpha_t,$$

for the reflected *transverse wave:*

$$R_{t/l} = \frac{2\,(c_t/c_l)^2 \sin 2\alpha_l \cos 2\alpha_t}{N}, \tag{A 2}$$

with incident transverse wave (oscillation plane parallel to plane of incidence) (cf. also Fig. 1.21) for the reflected *longitudinal wave:*

$$R_{l/t} = -\frac{\sin 4\alpha_t}{N}, \tag{A 3}$$

for the reflected *transverse wave:*

$$R_{t/t} = \frac{(c_t/c_l)^2 \sin 2\alpha_l \sin 2\alpha_t - \cos^2 2\alpha_t}{N} \equiv R_{l/l}. \tag{A 4}$$

b) *Interface liquid/liquid.* Symbols: the angles of the incident, reflected and transmitted longitudinal waves are α_e, α_r and α_d respectively. The acoustic velocities and densities of materials 1 and 2 are c_1, ϱ_1 and c_2, ϱ_2 respectively. The reflection coefficient of the acoustic pressure

$$R = \frac{\cos\alpha_e - \varrho_1 c_1/\varrho_2 c_2 \sqrt{1 - (c_2/c_1)^2 \sin^2\alpha_e}}{\cos\alpha_e + \varrho_1 c_1/\varrho_2 c_2 \sqrt{1 - (c_2/c_1)^2 \sin^2\alpha_e}}, \tag{A 5}$$

the transmission coefficient of the acoustic pressure

$$D = \frac{2\cos\alpha_e}{\cos\alpha_e + \varrho_1 c_1/\varrho_2 c_2 \sqrt{1 - (c_2/c_1)^2 \sin^2\alpha_e}}. \tag{A 6}$$

c) *Interface liquid/solid and solid/liquid.* Symbols: angle of longitudinal wave in liquid α, angles of longitudinal and transverse waves in solid α_l and α_t respectively, specific gravity and acoustic velocity in liquid, ϱ and c respectively, in solid ϱ_f, c_l and c_t respectively.

In the case liquid/solid (i.e. incident longitudinal wave in liquid) (see Fig. 1.22 and Table 2) we have:

$$R = \frac{1}{N}\left\langle\left(\frac{c_t}{c_l}\right)^2 \sin 2\alpha_l \sin 2\alpha_t + \cos^2 2\alpha_t - \frac{\varrho c}{\varrho_f c_l}\,\frac{\cos\alpha_l}{\cos\alpha}\right\rangle \tag{A 7}$$

with the abbreviation

$$N = \left(\frac{c_t}{c_l}\right)^2 \sin 2\alpha_l \sin 2\alpha_t + \cos^2 2\alpha_t + \frac{\varrho c}{\varrho_f c_l}\,\frac{\cos\alpha_l}{\cos\alpha}\,.$$

$$D_{l/l} = \frac{2}{N}\cos 2\alpha_t\,, \tag{A 8}$$

$$D_{t/l} = -\frac{2}{N}\left(\frac{c_t}{c_l}\right)^2 \sin 2\alpha_l\,. \tag{A 9}$$

In the case solid/liquid (see Figs. 1.23, 1.24 and Tables 3 and 4) with incident longitudinal wave, we have for the reflected *longitudinal wave:*

$$R_{l/l} = \frac{1}{N}\left\langle\left(\frac{c_t}{c_l}\right)^2 \sin 2\alpha_l \sin 2\alpha_t - \cos^2 2\alpha_t + \frac{\varrho c}{\varrho_f c_l}\,\frac{\cos\alpha_l}{\cos\alpha}\right\rangle, \tag{A 10}$$

for the reflected *transverse wave:*

$$R_{t/l} = \frac{2}{N}\left(\frac{c_t}{c_l}\right)^2 \sin 2\alpha_l \cos 2\alpha_t \tag{A 11}$$

and for the transmitted *longitudinal wave* in the liquid:

$$D_{l/l} = \frac{2}{N}\,\frac{\varrho c \cos\alpha_l \cos 2\alpha_t}{\varrho_f c_l \cos\alpha}\,. \tag{A 12}$$

In the case solid/liquid with an incident transverse wave:

$$R_{t/t} = \frac{1}{N}\left\langle\left(\frac{c_t}{c_l}\right)^2 \sin 2\alpha_l \sin 2\alpha_t - \cos^2 2\alpha_t - \frac{\varrho c}{\varrho_f c_l}\,\frac{\cos\alpha_l}{\cos\alpha}\right\rangle, \tag{A 13}$$

$$R_{l/t} = -\frac{1}{N}\sin 4\alpha_t\,, \tag{A 14}$$

$$D_{l/t} = \frac{2}{N}\,\frac{\varrho c}{\varrho_f c_l}\,\frac{\cos\alpha_l \sin 2\alpha_t}{\cos\alpha}\,. \tag{A 15}$$

The echo transmittances (see Fig. 1.26 and Tables 5 to 8) for both cases, solid/liquid and liquid/solid are identical. If in both materials the longitudinal wave is used, we have

$$E_{ll} = \frac{4}{N^2}\,\frac{\varrho c}{\varrho_f c_l}\,\frac{\cos\alpha_l \cos^2 2\alpha_t}{\cos\alpha}\,, \tag{A 16}$$

but if the transverse wave is used in the solid,

$$E_{lt} = \frac{4}{N^2}\left(\frac{c_t}{c_l}\right)^2 \frac{\varrho c}{\varrho_l c_l} \frac{\cos\alpha_l \sin 2\alpha_t \sin 2\alpha_l}{\cos\alpha}. \tag{A 17}$$

d) *Interface solid/solid.* The values in Tables 7 and 8 were calculated electronically (KÜHN and LUTSCH [211, 3]). For the case of coupling through a thin liquid layer, and using the above symbols, the following reflection and transmission formulas apply [211]:

Abbreviations: denominator N (index 1 for material 1, index 2 for material 2)

$$N = 2\cot\alpha_{1t} + \frac{c_{1l}}{2c_{1t}}\frac{\cos^2 2\alpha_{1t}}{\cos\alpha_{1l}} + \frac{2\varrho_2 c_{2t}^4}{\varrho_1 c_{1t}^4}\cot\alpha_{2t} + \frac{\varrho_2 c_{1l} c_{2t}^3}{2\varrho_1 c_{1t}^4}\frac{\cos^2 2\alpha_{2t}}{\cos\alpha_{1l}}. \tag{A 18}$$

For the incident longitudinal wave in material 1:

$$R_{l/l} = 1 - \frac{\cos^2 2\alpha_{1t}}{N\cos\alpha_{1l}}, \tag{A 19}$$

$$R_{t/l} = -\frac{2c_{1l}^2\cos 2\alpha_{1t}}{c_{1t}^2\sin^2\alpha_{1l}N}, \tag{A 20}$$

$$D_{l/l} = \frac{2\varrho_2 c_{2l} c_{2t}^2 c_{1l}\cos^2 2\alpha_{2t}\cos 2\alpha_{1t}}{\varrho_1 c_{1t}^4\cos 2\alpha_{1l}\sin\alpha_{1l}N}, \tag{A 21}$$

$$D_{t/l} = -\frac{2\varrho_2 c_{2t}^3 c_{1l}\cos 2\alpha_{1t}}{\varrho_1 c_{1t}^4\sin 2\alpha_{1l}N}. \tag{A 22}$$

For the incident transverse wave in material 1:

$$R_{l/t} = \frac{4c_{1l}\cos\alpha_{1t}\cos^2 2\alpha_{1t}}{c_{1t}\sin 2\alpha_{1l}N}, \tag{A 23}$$

$$R_{t/t} = \frac{4c_{1l}\cos\alpha_{1t}}{c_{1t}\sin\alpha_{1l}N} - 1, \tag{A 24}$$

$$D_{l/t} = -\frac{4\varrho_2 c_{2t}^2 c_{2l} c_{1l}\cos^2 2\alpha_{2t}\cos\alpha_{1t}}{\varrho_1 c_{1t}^4\sin 2\alpha_{1l}N}, \tag{A 25}$$

$$D_{t/t} = \frac{4\varrho_2 c_{2t}^3 c_{1l}\cos\alpha_{1t}}{\varrho_1 c_{1t}^4\sin\alpha_{1l}N}. \tag{A 26}$$

Note: For incident wave in material 2, the indices 1 and 2 must be interchanged.

Speed of propagation of Lamb waves. Referring to Table 9: Optimal sound propagation occurs if for the angle α between the transverse wave and the perpendicular of the plate, the following equation is fulfilled:

$$F_{1,2} = G \tag{A 27}$$

with the abbreviations:

$$a = \pi \frac{d}{\lambda_t}\,; \quad q = \frac{c_t}{c_l}\,; \quad s = \sin\alpha_t\,; \quad T_1 = \tanh\sqrt{s^2 - 1}\,a\,; \quad T_q = \tanh\sqrt{s^2 - q^2}\,a\,;$$

$$F_1 = \frac{T_1}{T_q} \quad \text{for symmetric Lamb waves,}$$

$$F_2 = \frac{T_q}{T_1} \quad \text{for antimetric Lamb waves,}$$

$$G = \frac{4\,s^2\sqrt{s^2 - 1}\sqrt{s^2 - q^2}}{(2\,s^2 - 1)^2} \quad \text{for both.}$$

The correlated velocity of propagation (group velocity) then is [291]:

$$u_p = \frac{c_t}{s + a\dfrac{\mathrm{d}s}{\mathrm{d}a}}\,. \tag{A 28}$$

The differential $\mathrm{d}s/\mathrm{d}a$ calculated from (A 27) is:

$$\frac{\mathrm{d}s}{\mathrm{d}a} = \frac{\dfrac{\partial F_{1,2}}{\partial a}}{\dfrac{\partial G}{\partial s} - \dfrac{\partial F_{1,2}}{\partial s}}\,, \tag{A 29}$$

and explicitly for the symmetric wave modes:

$$\frac{\partial G}{\partial s} = s\,\frac{8\,(q^2 - 1)\,s^4 + 4\,(3 - q^2)\,s^2 - 8\,q^2}{(2\,s^2 - 1)^3\sqrt{s^2 - 1}\sqrt{s^2 - q^2}}\,,$$

$$\frac{\partial F_1}{\partial s} = \frac{a\,s}{T_q^2}\left\{\frac{T_q\,(T_1^2 - 1)}{\sqrt{s^2 - 1}} + \frac{T_1\,(1 - T_q^2)}{\sqrt{s^2 - q^2}}\right\},$$

$$\frac{\partial F_1}{\partial a} = \frac{1}{T_q^2}\left\{\sqrt{s^2 - 1}\,T_q\,(1 - T_1^2) + \sqrt{s^2 - q^2}\,T_1\,(T_q^2 - 1)\right\}.$$

For the antimetric forms the tanh function should be replaced by the coth function.

Table 1. Reflection coefficients at free boundary of steel

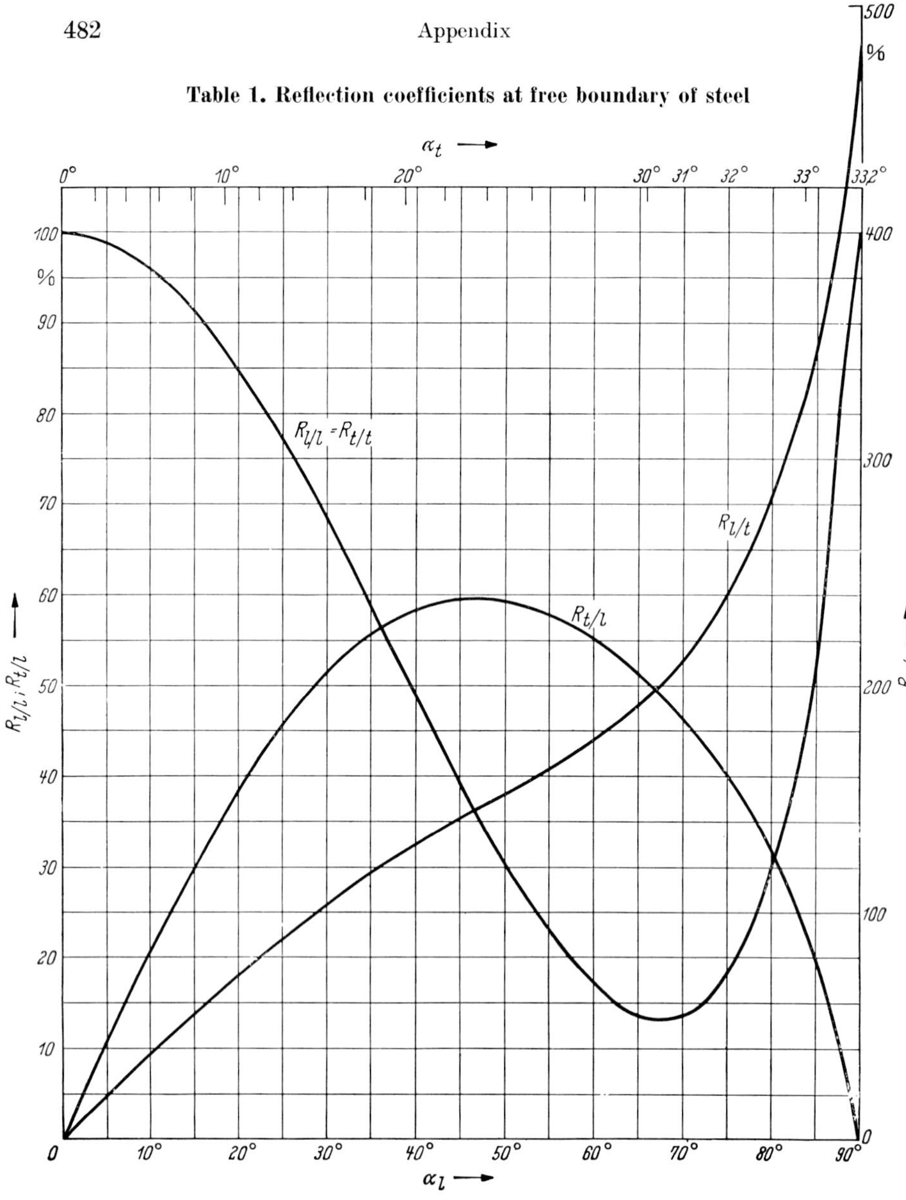

With incident longitudinal wave	Reflected longitudinal wave $R_{l/l}$ versus angle of incidence α_l [according to Eq. (A 1)]. Reflected transverse wave $R_{t/l}$ versus angle of reflection α_t (top scale) [according to Eq. (A 2)].
with incident transverse wave	Reflected transverse wave $R_{t/t}$ versus angle of incidence α_t, identical with $R_{l/l}$ according to Eq. (A 3)]. Reflected longitudinal wave $R_{l/t}$ versus angle of reflection α_l [according to Eq. (A 4)].

Table 2. Interface water/aluminium

Longitudinal wave incident in water at angle α furnishes longitudinal wave in aluminium with angle α_l and transverse wave with α_t. Calculated from Eqs. (A 7) to (A 9) with the constants

$$c_t/c_l = 0.488; \qquad c_l/c = 4.26; \qquad \frac{\varrho c}{\varrho_l c_l} = 0.0888.$$

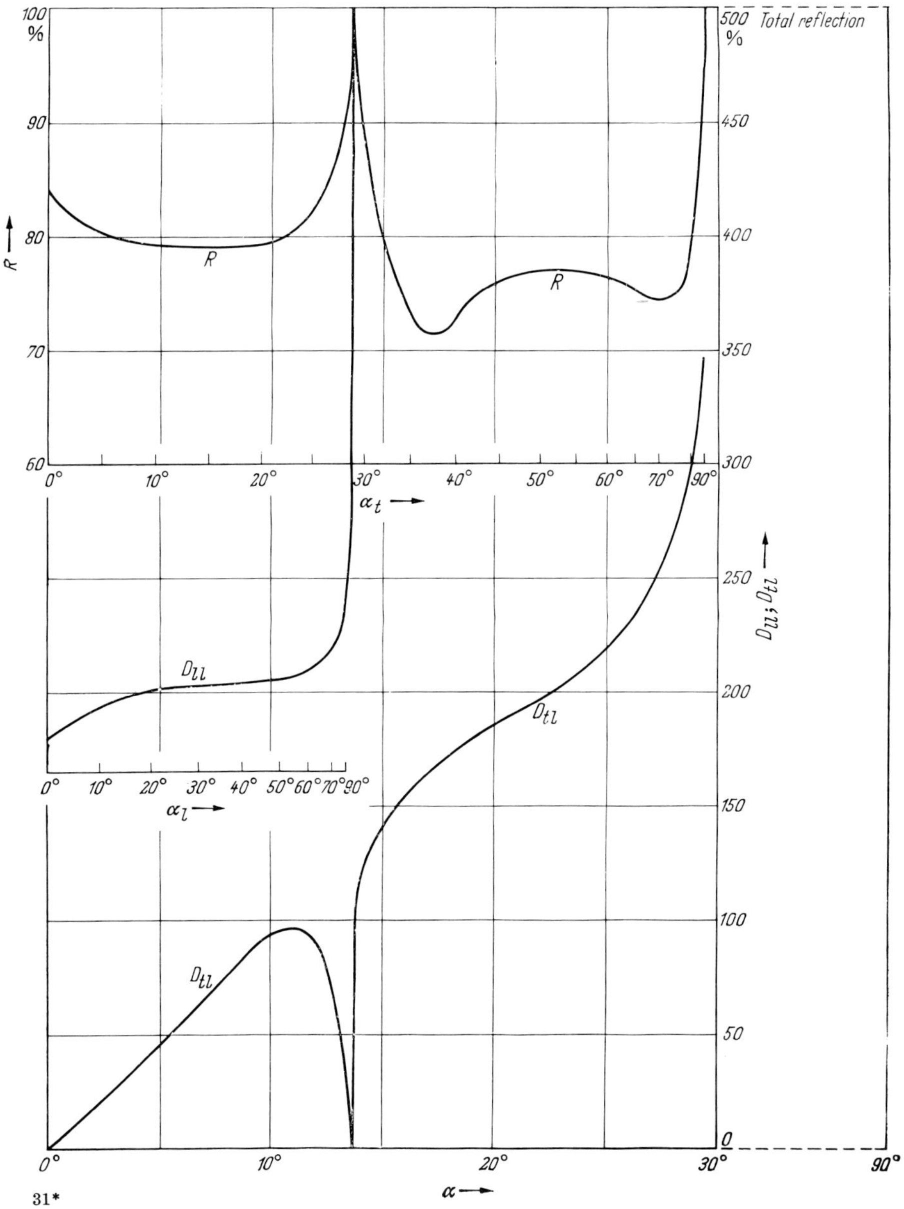

Table 3. Interface aluminium/water

Longitudinal wave incident in aluminium at angle α_l furnishes reflected longitudinal wave in aluminium with angle α_l, reflected transverse wave in aluminium with angle α_t and transmitted longitudinal wave in water with angle α (re. constants, see Table 2)

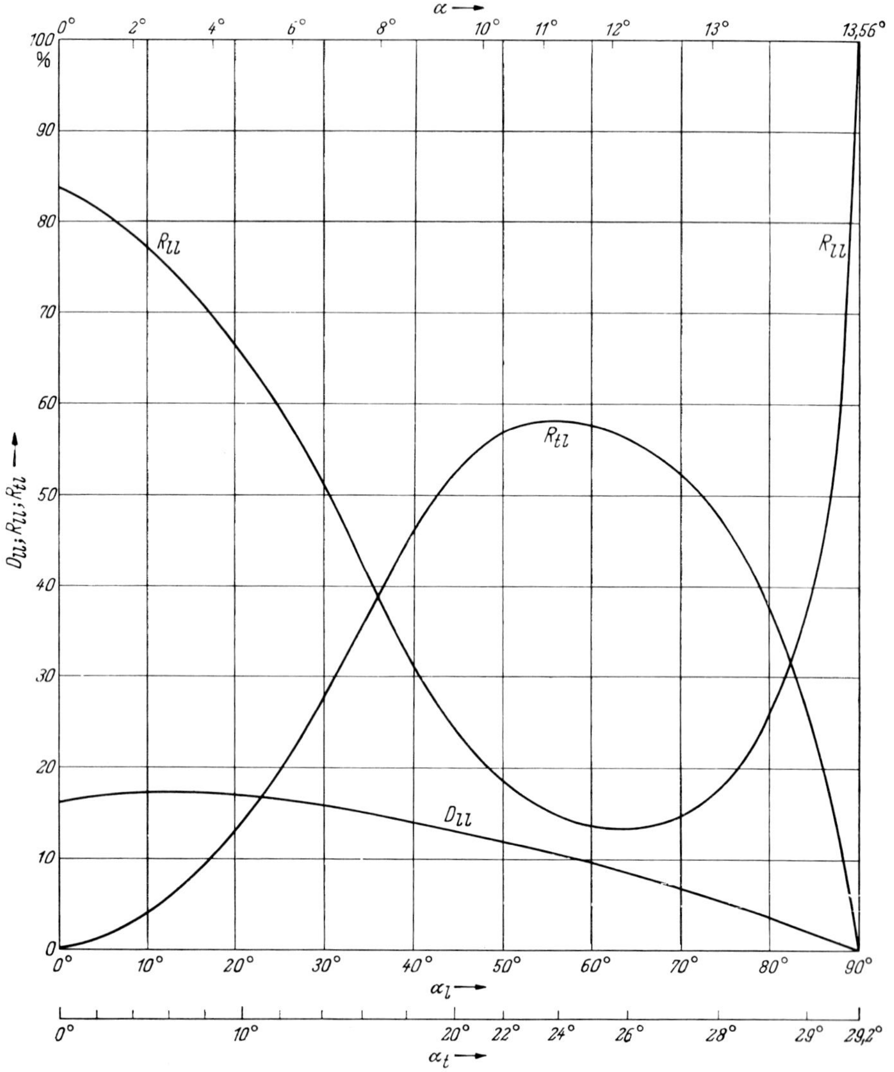

Table 4. Interface aluminium/water

Transverse wave incident in aluminium at angle α_t furnishes reflected transverse wave with α_t, reflected longitudinal wave with α_l and transmitted longitudinal wave in water with angle α (re. constants see Table 2)

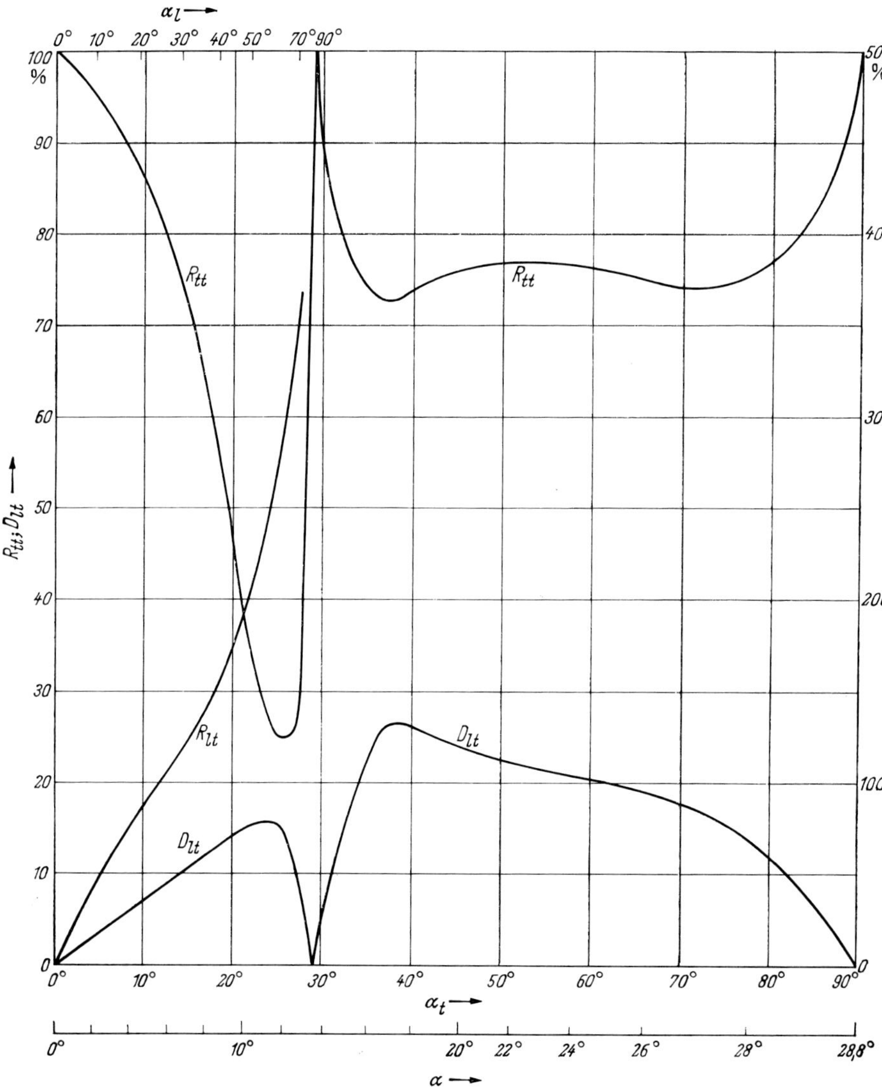

Table 5. Interface water/aluminium

Echo transmittance E_{ll} and E_{lt} versus angles of waves in aluminium α_l and α_t respectively

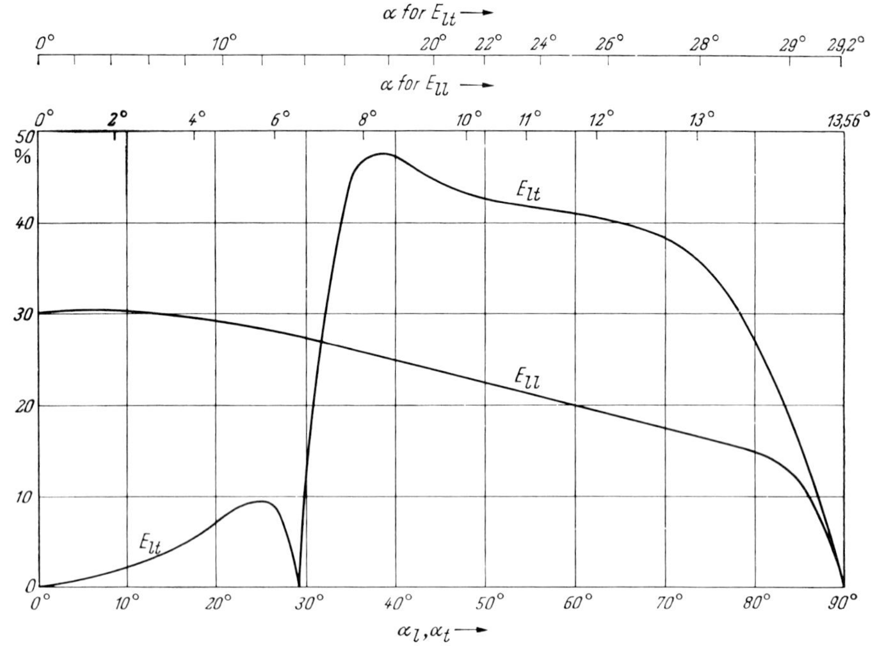

Table 6. Interface water/steel

Echo transmittance same as in Table 5

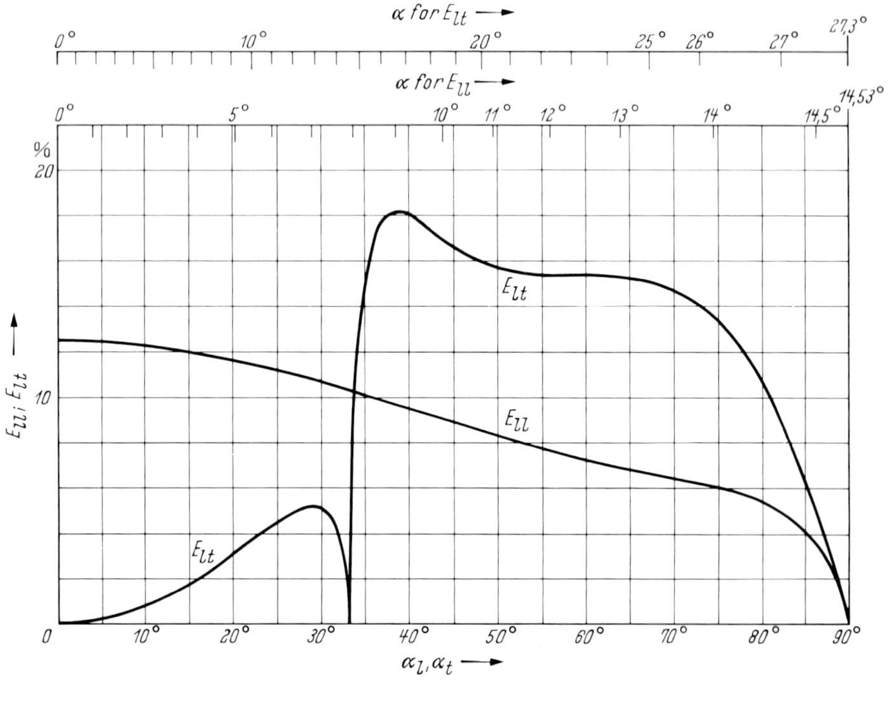

Table 7. Interface perspex/steel

Echo transmittance E_{lt} for liquid contact and solid contact (dotted line)

Perspex: $c_l = 2730$ m/s; $c_t = 1430$ m/s; $\varrho = 1180$ kg/m^3
Steel: $c_l = 5900$ m/s; $c_t = 3230$ m/s; $\varrho = 7700$ kg/m^3

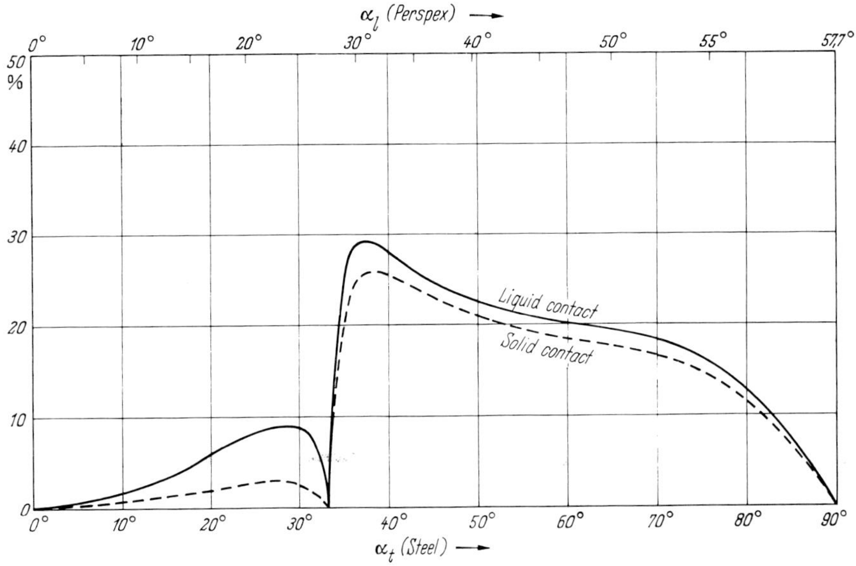

Table 8. Interface perspex/aluminium

Echo transmittance E_{lt} for liquid contact and solid contact (dotted line)

Perspex: $c_l = 2730$ m/s; $c_t = 1430$ m/s; $\varrho = 1180$ kg/m^3
Aluminium: $c_l = 6320$ m/s; $c_t = 3130$ m/s; $\varrho = 2700$ kg/m^3

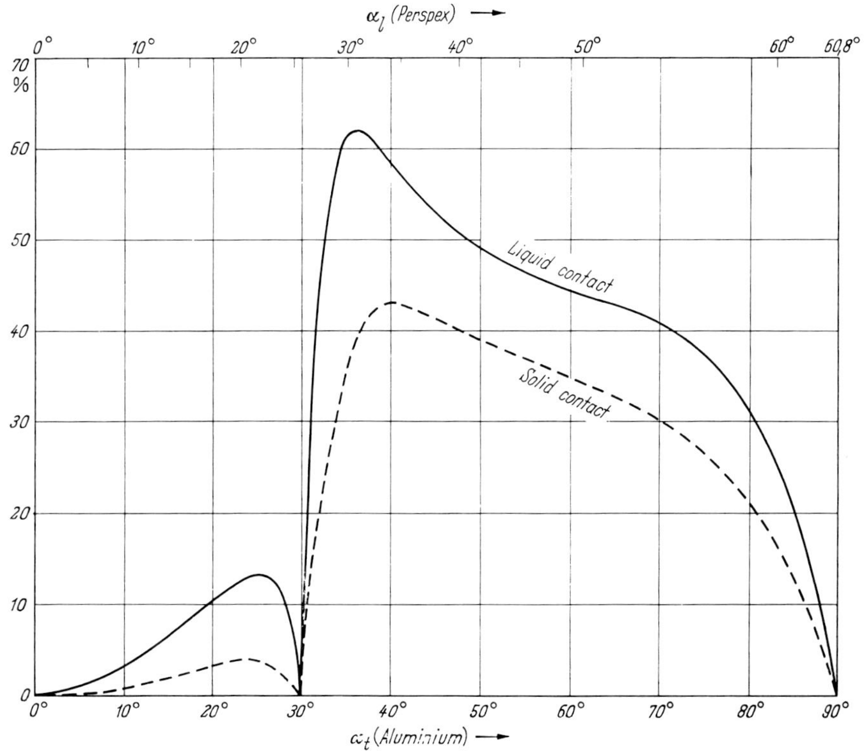

Table 9. Velocity of propagation of Lamb waves in steel

$c_l = 5.96 \cdot 10^3$ m/s; $c_t = 3.26 \cdot 10^3$ m/s

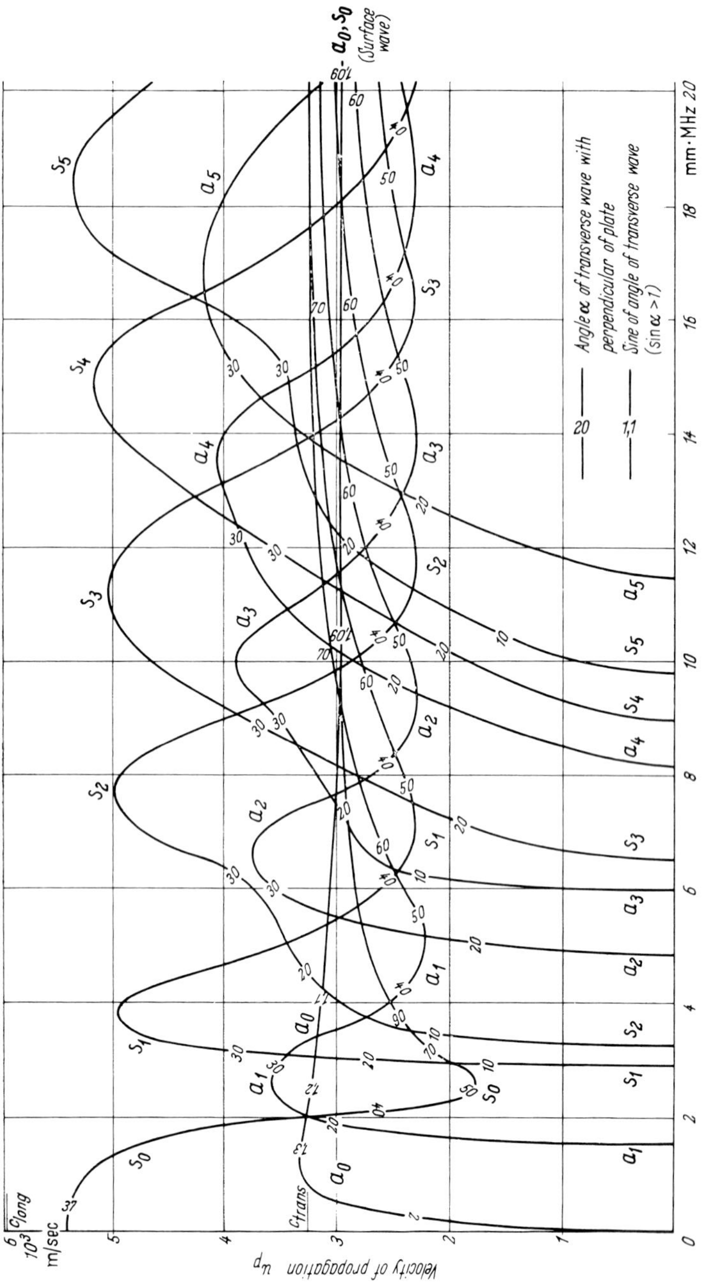

Table 10. Attenuation of a plane wave

Various attenuation coefficients and layer thicknesses according to formula $p/p_0 = e^{-\alpha d}$. Scale on right side: attenuation in dB, scale on left side: acoustic pressure amplitude and echo amplitude respectively in per cent

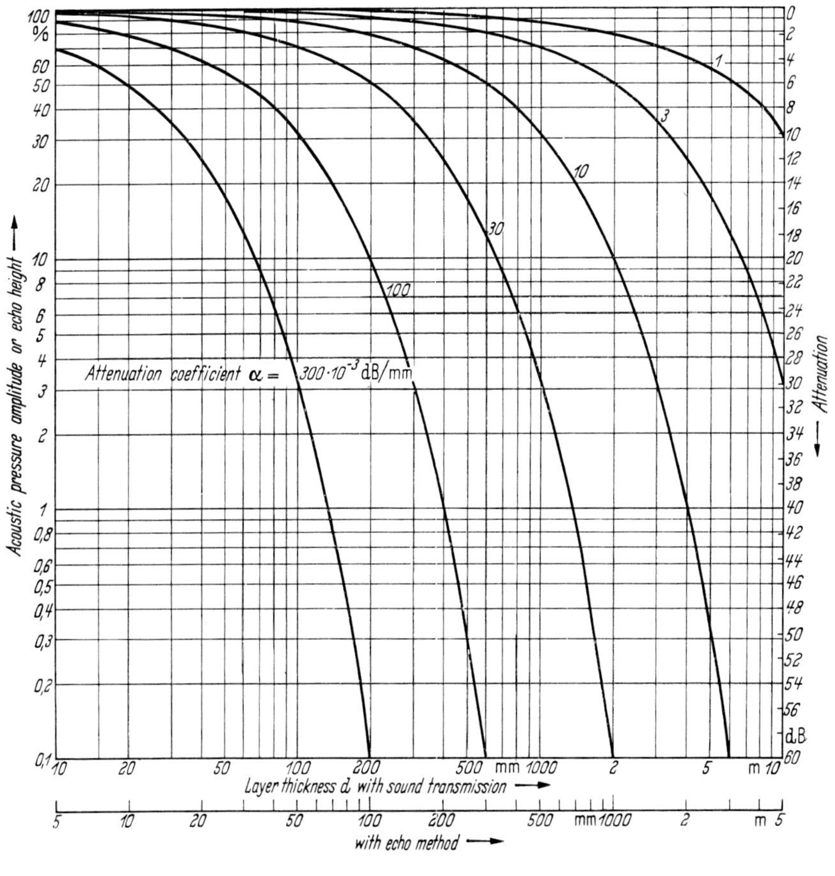

Bibliography

Textbooks and Handbooks

[1] BERGMANN, L.: Der Ultraschall, 6th Ed., Stuttgart: Hirzel 1954.

[2] BRADFIELD, G.: Ultrasonic flaw detection in metals. Chapter 12 in B. CHALMERS and A. G. QUARREL: The physical examination of metals ..., 2nd Ed., 1960.

[3] BREKHOVSKIKH, L. M.: Waves in layered media, London/New York: Academic Press 1960, pp. 61–70.

[4] CADY, W. G.: Piezoelectricity, New York: McGraw-Hill 1946.

[5] CARLIN, B.: Ultrasonics, New York: McGraw-Hill 1949.

[6] FILIPCZYNSKI, L., Z. PAWLOWSKI and J. WEHR: Ultrasonic testing of materials (in Polish), Warsaw: Panstwowe Wydawnictwa Techniczne 1959.

[7] HIEDEMANN, E.: Grundlagen und Ergebnisse der Ultraschallforschung, Berlin: deGruyter 1939.

[8] HINSLEY, F. J.: Nondestructive testing, London: MacDonald & Evans 1959.

[9] HUETER, T. F., and R. H. BOLT: Sonics, New York: Wiley & Sons 1955.

[10] MCMASTER, R. C. (Ed.): Nondestructive testing handbook, 2 Vols., New York: Ronald Press 1959.

[11] MASON, W. P.: Piezoelectric crystals and their application to ultrasonics, New York: Van Nostrand 1950.

[12] MASON, W. P.: Physical acoustics and the properties of solids, New York: Van Nostrand 1958.

[13] MATAUSCHEK, J.: Einführung in die Ultraschalltechnik, 2nd Ed., Berlin: VEB Verlag Technik 1962.

[14] MORSE, P. M.: Vibration and sound, New York: McGraw-Hill 1948.

[15] MÜLLER, E. A. W.: Handbuch der zerstörungsfreien Materialprüfung, München: Oldenbourg 1959.

[16] PIGNET, J. L.: Méthodes non destructives pour l'étude et le contrôle des matériaux, Paris: Editions de la Revue d'Optique 1957.

[17] POHL, R. W.: Einführung in die Physik, 3 Vols., Berlin/Göttingen/Heidelberg: Springer 1962/64.

[18] RAYLEIGH, LORD: Theorie of sound, London 1926.

[19] REDWOOD, M.: Mechanical waveguides, Oxford: Pergamon 1960.

[20] SCHOCH, A.: Schallreflexion, Schallbrechung und Schallbeugung. Ergebnisse der exakten Naturwissenschaften, Vol. 23, Berlin/Göttingen/Heidelberg: Springer 1950, pp. 127–234.

[21] SKUDRZYK, E.: Die Grundlagen der Akustik, Wien: Springer 1954.

[22] SOKOLOW, W. S.: Testing of materials (in Russian), Moscow: Gosenergizdat 1957.

[23] STENZEL, H., and O. BROSZE: Leitfaden zur Berechnung von Schallvorgängen, 2nd Ed., Berlin/Göttingen/Heidelberg: Springer 1958.

[24] VAUPEL, O. (Ed.): Bildatlas für die zerstörungsfreie Materialprüfung. Berlin: Verlag Bild und Forschung 1954.

2. Separate Publications

Arranged alphabetically according to the names of the authors; papers not published under the authors' names appear at the end of the list. In the case of patents the name of the inventor is given as the author where stated; the year mentioned is the year of the application.

[25] ADAMS, C. J., and J. W. MORRIS: Ultrasonic standards for the evaluation of missile materials and components. ASTM Spec. Publ. Bull. A-273 (1959).

[26] ADAMS, L. J.: Ultrasonic inspection speeds drive-tubing output. Metalworking Production 1955, pp. 1905–1907.

[27] AKROYD, T. N. W., and R. JONES: Non-destructive testing of structural concrete by the ultrasonic pulse technique. Proc. 4th Intern. Conf. Non-destr. Test. London 1963. London: Butterworths Sci. 1964, pp. 230–234.

[28] ALBERTSON, C. P., and H. E. VAN VALKENBURG: Ultrasonic detection, sizing and counting of sub-sieve particles. Proc. 4th Intern. Conf. Non-destr. Test. London 1963. London: Butterworths Sci. 1964, pp. 147–149.

[29] AVEYARD, S., and R. S. SHARPE: Applications of ultrasonic pulse interference. Proc. 4th Intern. Conf. Non-destr. Test. London 1963. London: Butterworths Sci. 1964, pp. 150–154.

[30] BACKHAUS, H., and F. TRENDELENBURG: Über die Richtwirkung von Kolbenmembranen. Z. techn. Phys. 7 (1926) pp. 630–635.

[31] BARTHELT, H.: Erfahrungen über die Anwendung des Ultraschallverfahrens in der keramischen Fertigung. ETZ A 75 (1954) pp. 69–71.

[32] BARTHELT, H., and W. BÖHME: Die zerstörungsfreie Prüfung der armierten Enden von Langstabisolatoren nach dem Ultraschall-Echo-Verfahren. Siemens-Z. 29 (1955) pp. 206–208.

[33] BASTIEN, P., J. BLETON and E. DE KERVERSAU: Etude d'anomalies de réflexion et de transmission se produisant lors du sondage par les ultra-sons des métaux. Rev. Métall. 46 (1949) pp. 277–286.

[34] BASTIEN, P., and M. EVRARD: Comportement des ultrasons en présence de divers types de défauts pouvant apparaître dans les soudures. Soudage et Techniques Connexes 1959, No. 10, pp. 11–19.

[35] BEAUJARD, L., V. HUSAREK and A. VASSET: Signalisation, comptage ou enregistrement des défauts des produits métallurgiques au moyen du sondage ultrasonore automatique par échos. Rev. Métall. 52 (1955) pp. 240–248.

[36] BEAUJARD, L., and V. HUSAREK: Einige neue Geräte für kontinuierliche Materialprüfung. Schweisstechnik 12 (1958) pp. 39–43.

[37] BEAUJARD, L., and V. HUSAREK: Applications pratiques des ultrasons au contrôle des produits sidérurgiques, possibilités et limites. Mém. Sci. Rev. Métall. 56 (1959) pp. 221–223.

[38] BEAUJARD, L., G. COLLETTE and C. DROUET: The effect of dispersion and the velocity of progation of Lamb waves during the ultrasonic testing of mild steel sheet. Brit. J. Non-destr. Test. 1 (1959) pp. 7–11.

[39] BECK, W. N.: An ultrasonic scanner and recording system. Nondestr. Test. 15 (1957) No. 1, pp. 42/43; Symposium on nondestructive tests in the field of nuclear energy. ASTM Spec. Techn. Publ. No. 223 (1958) pp. 246–258.

[40] BECK, H., and R. SPECHT: Automatische Ultraschallprüfung von Stahlknüppeln auf Innenfehler. Paper read at the conference of the Gesellschaft zur Förderung zerstörungsfreier Prüfverfahren in Vienna, April 1965.

[41] BECKMANN, G.: Zur Prüfung schwerer Schmiedestücke mit Ultraschall. Neue Hütte 2 (1957) pp. 169–178.

[42] Beckmann, G., and K. Spiegelberg: Über den Nachweis nichtmetallischer Einschlüsse in Walzmaterial mit Ultraschall. Neue Hütte 6 (1961) pp. 316–321.

[43] Beckmann, G., and K. Spiegelberg: Über die Bestimmung von Elastizitätsmoduln mittels Ultraschall-Impulsen. Die Technik 17 (1962) pp. 81–88.

[44] Benson, R. W., and V. J. Raelson: Acoustoelasticity. Product Engng. (July 1959) pp. 56–59.

[45] Bergman, R. H., and R. Shahbender: Effect of statically applied stresses on the velocity of propagation of ultrasonic waves. J. appl. Phys. 29 (1958) pp. 1736–1738.

[46] Beuse, H., and H. Hartwig: Industrielle Prüfung von Feinblechen mittels Ultraschall. Z. VDI 98 (1956) pp. 1057–1061.

[47] Bierwirth, G.: Zerstörungsfreie Prüfung von Gussstücken durch Ultraschall. Giesserei 44 (1957) pp. 477–485.

[48] Binczewski, G. B.: Standardization and application of ultrasonic surface-wave inspection. Nondestr. Test. 15 (1957) No. 1, pp. 36–40.

[49] Böhme, W.: Ultraschallprüfung von Drähten. Materialprüfung 1 (1959) pp. 111/112.

[50] Bordoni, P. G., and M. Nuovo: A tuned capacitive detector for high frequency vibrations. Acustica 8 (1958) pp. 351–362.

[51] Bradfield, G.: Improvements in ultrasonic flaw detection. J. Brit. Inst. Radio Engng. 14 (1954) pp. 303–308.

[52] Brandt, H. G.: Überschallprüfung von Rundstahl auf Innenfehler. Stahl u. Eisen 73 (1953) pp. 1717–1720.

[53] Branson, G. N.: Portable ultrasonic thickness gage. Electronics 21 (1948) pp. 88–91.

[54] Branson, G. N.: Metal wall thickness measurement from one side by the ultrasonic method. Electr. Engng. 70 (1951) pp. 619–624.

[55] Bratina, J.: Investigations of deformation processes in armco iron by means of internal friction at megacycle frequencies. Canad. J. Phys. 37 (1959) pp. 579–590.

[56] Bratt, M. J., and V. I. E. Wiegand: Detection of flaws in jet engine parts by ultrasonics. Nondestr. Test. 13 (1955) No. 5, pp. 45–47.

[57] Bresson, Y., and J. P. Pouget: Utilisation pratique du contrôle par ultrasons dans une usine productrice de demi-produits d'alliages légers. Mém. Sci. Rev. Métall. 56 (1959) pp. 81–90.

[58] Brown, T. G., A. B. C. Rankin and R. W. G. Haslett: Improvements in or relating to the ultrasonic testing of materials. Brit. P. 808274 (1955).

[59] Buchanan, R. W., and C. H. Hastings: Ultrasonic flaw plotting equipment – a new concept for industrial inspection. Nondestr. Test. 13 (1955) No. 5, pp. 17–25.

[60] Burgkart, M., D. Maucic and H. Ch. Ritter: Eine Methode zur Ermittlung der Geschwindigkeit von Ultraschallwellen im lebenden Rindermuskel. Bayr. Landwirtsch. Jahrbuch 40 (1963) pp. 567–571.

[61] Chilowski, C.: Piezoelectric plastic material and method of making same USA-P. 2420864 (1947).

[62] Claus, A.: Die Messung natürlicher Grenzflächen im Schweinekörper mit Ultraschall. Die Fleischwirtschaft 1957, No. 9, pp. 552–554.

[63] Clausen, H.P.: Zerstörungsfreie Betonkontrollen. Beton Zement Markt 5 (1955) pp. 360/361.

[64] Cline, C. W., and J. B. Morgan: Standardization in ultrasonic testing. Nondestr. Test. 13 (1955) No. 4, pp. 23–27.

[65] Cola, G.: Influenca della segregazione grafitica sulla capacita smorzanti della ghisa. La fonderia italiana 1955. No. 3, pp. 113–148.

[66] Cook, E. G.: Transient and steady-state response of ultrasonic piezoelectric transducers. IRE Convention Record 1956, Part 9, pp. 61–69.

[67] Cook, E. G., and H. E. van Valkenburg: Surface waves at ultrasonic frequencies. ASTM-Bull. 84, May 1954.

[68] Cook, E. G., and H. E. van Valkenburg: Thickness measurement by ultrasonic resonance, J. A. S. A. 27 (1955) pp. 564–569.

[69] Cook, G. G., and W. D. Walker: Ultrasonic testing of gas turbine discs and heavy rotor forgings. Proc. 4th Intern. Conf. Non-destr. Test. London 1963. London: Butterworths Sci. 1964, pp. 215–217.

[70] Czerlinsky, E.: Zerstörungsfreie Lagerprüfung mit Ultraschall. Dtsch. Luftfahrtforschung, Unters. u. Mitt. No. 1069 (1943).

[71] Czerlinsky, E.: Zerstörungsfreie Sperrholzprüfung mit Ultraschall. Dtsch. Luftfahrtforschung, Unters. u. Mitt. No. 1042 (1943).

[72] Dawance, G., and M. J. Chefdeville: Schallmessungen an Beton. Schweiz. Archiv 21 (1955) pp. 223–234 and 313–325. German translation and discussion: Bulletin No. 15 (August 1953) of Réunion des Laboratoires d'essaies et de recherches sur les matériaux et les constructions.

[73] DeLano, R. B.: Means of inspecting materials by wave trains. USA-P. 2507854 (1945).

[74] Desch, C. H., D. O. Sproule and W. J. Dawson: The detection of cracks in steel by means of supersonic waves. J. Iron Steel Inst. 153 (1946) pp. 319 to 352.

[75] Diekmann, A.: Erkennung von Fettauflage und Muskelbildungsvermögen am lebenden Schwein durch Messung mit Ultraschall. Die Fleischwirtschaft 12 (1960) pp. 447–448 and 451–452.

[76] Dory, J.: Vorrichtung zur Entfernungs- und Dickenmessung nach dem Echolotprinzip. DBP[1] applic. inspection document No. 1012467 (1956).

[77] Drake, H. C.: Shield and light cell pickup for oscilloscopes. USA-P. No. 2603966 (1950).

[78] Egelkraut, K.: Schienenprüfung mit Ultraschall. ETR 14 (1965) pp. 49–59.

[79] Eisenmann, K., and G. Steinkamp: Messung der Tiefen und Weiten von Betonrissen mittels Ultraschall. Beton- u. Stahlbetonbau 49 (1954) pp. 36–38.

[80] Eisenmann, K., and G. Odewald: Untersuchung der elastischen Eigenschaften von Beton mittels Ultraschall. Beton- u. Stahlbetonbau 54 (1959) pp. 156 to 158.

[81] Elion, A. H.: Recent advances in new areas of nondestructive testing. Nondestr. Test. 18 (1960) pp. 180–182.

[82] Elion, H. A.: Metallurgical structure analysis by ultrasonics. Proc. Nat. Electronics Conf. Chicago 1957, Vol. 13.

[83] Elion, H. A.: Recent advances in stress measurement by ultrasonics. Proc. 3rd Intern. Congr. Acoustics Stuttgart 1959. Amsterdam: Elsevier 1960.

[84] Elonka, St.: Nondestructive Testing. Power (March 1958) pp. 115–137. Reprinted in Nondestr. Test. 16 (1958) No. 3.

[85] Erdman, D. C.: Ultrasonic inspection using automatic recording and frequency modulated flaw detector. Nondestr. Test. 11 (1953) No. 8, pp. 17–31.

[86] Erdman, D. C.: Ultrasonic flaw detector. USA-P. 2593865 (1950).

[87] Erwin, W. S.: Supersonic measuring means. USA-P. 2431233 (1944).

[88] Espinola, R. P., and P. C. Waterman: US-Interferometer for the measurement of the temperature dependence of elastic constants. J. appl. Phys. 29 (1958) pp. 718–721.

[1] DBP = Deutsches Bundespatent (Pat. German Fed. Rep.).

[89] EVANS, D. J.: New ultrasonic techniques for the chemical and petroleum industries. Materials Evaluation (April 1964) pp. 164–168.

[90] EVANS, J. D.: Ultrasonic inspection in the oil refining and related industries. Nondestr. Test. 15 (1957) No. 3, pp. 156–160.

[91] EVANS, J. D.: Corrosion-rate data can be exact. Marine Engineering/Log (May 1958).

[92] EVRARD, M.: Intérêt des blocs d'étalonnage dans le contrôle non-destructif par les ultrasons. Mém. Sci. Rev. Métall. 56 (1959) pp. 111–123.

[93] FARROW, C.: Supersonic testing of hot articles. USA-P. 2697936 (1954).

[94] FILIPCZYNSKI, L.: Properties of the X-cut quartz transducer loaded with a solid medium. Proc. 2nd Conf. Ultrasonics Warsaw 1956, pp. 35–47.

[95] FILIPCZINSKI, L.: Measurement of mode conversion of ultrasonic waves on a solid-solid boundary. Proc. of Vibration Problems 4 (1963) pp. 255–263.

[96] FILIPCZINSKI, L.: Scattering of a plane longitudinal wave on a free surface of a disc in a solid medium. Proc. of Vibration Problems 2 (1961) pp. 41–56.

[97] FILIPCZINSKI, L.: Measurements of longitudinal and transverse waves radiated by a compressional source into elastic semispace. Proc. of Vibration Problems 5 (1964) pp. 89–93.

[98] FILIPCZYNSKI, L., and Z. PAWLOWSKI: Apparatur für Ultraschallmesstechnik in Polen. Feingerätetechnik 7 (1958) pp. 295–299.

[99] FILIPCZYNSKI, L., and I. GRZENKOWICZ: Ultrasonic concrete tester BI-2. Proc. 2nd Conf. Ultrasonics Warsaw 1956, pp. 251/252.

[100] FILIPPI, F. J.: Qualitative analysis of brazed sandwich. Nondestr. Test. 17 (1959) No. 1, pp. 39–45.

[101] FINK, E. W.: Ultrasonic testing as a method of determining variables in processing zircaloy and hafnium. Symposium on nondestructive tests in the field of nuclear energy. ASTM Spec. Techn. Publ. No. 223 (1958) pp. 175–179.

[102] FIRESTONE, F. A.: Flaw detecting device and measuring instrument. USA-P. 2280226 (1940).

[103] FIRESTONE, F. A.: Resonance inspection method. USA-P. 2439131 (1943).

[104] FIRESTONE, F. A.: Surface and shear wave method and apparatus. USA-P. 2439130 (1943).

[105] FIRESTONE, F. A.: Supersonic reflectoscope, an instrument for inspecting the interior of solid parts by means of sound waves. J.A.S.A. 17 (1945) pp. 287 to 299.

[106] FIRESTONE, F. A., and J. R. FREDERICK: Refinements in supersonic reflectoscopy. Polarized sound. J.A.S.A. 18 (1949) pp. 200–211.

[107] FIRESTONE, F. A.: Tricks with the supersonic reflectoscope. Nondestr. Test. 7 (1948) No. 2. pp. 5–19.

[108] FIRESTONE, F. A., and D. S. LING: Method and means for generating and utilizing vibrational waves in plates. USA-P. 2536128 (1951).

[109] FREITAG, W., and H. J. MARTIN: Ergebnisse beim Aufbau eines elektronischen Ultraschall-Bildwandlers. Acustica 8 (1958) pp. 197–200.

[110] FRIELINGHAUS, R.: Ultraschallmessungen an Grauguß. Thesis Braunschweig 1963.

[111] FRIELINGHAUS, R., and J. KOPPELMANN: Genaue Schallschwächungsmessungen mit handelsüblichen Ultraschall-Impulsecho-Geräten. Materialprüfung 6 (1964) No. 10, pp. 337–342.

[112] GERICKE, O. R.: Determination of the geometry of hidden defects by ultrasonic pulse analysis testing. J.A.S.A. 35 (1963) pp. 364–368.

[113] GERICKE, O. R.: Dual-Frequency ultrasonic pulse-echo testing. J.A.S.A. 36 (1964) pp. 313–322.

[114] GERLACH, M.: Porositätsuntersuchungen an Hochspannungsisolatoren mit Ultraschall und ihre Bedeutung für die Energieversorgung. Silikattechnik 2 (1951) pp. 371–374.

[115] GERSTNER, R.: Die Ultraschallprüfung von Gusseisen. Materialprüfung 3 (1961) pp. 213–217.

[116] GERSTNER, R.: Dehnungsmessung mit Ultraschall. Materialprüfung 6 (1964) pp. 43–46.

[117] GERSTNER, R.: Die automatische Prüfung von widerstandsgeschweissten Rohren mit Ultraschall. Materialprüfung 6 (1964) No. 9, pp. 320–322.

[118] GÖTZ, J.: Über den Schalldurchgang durch Metallplatten in Flüssigkeiten bei schrägem Einfall einer ebenen Welle. Akust. Z. 8 (1943) pp. 145–168.

[119] GOLDMAN, R. G., and M. E. AUGER: Improved ultrasonic instrumentation for the quality control of turbine-generator components. Lecture No. 204 given at the 3rd Int. Conf. Nondestr. Test. in Japan, 1960.

[120] GOLDMAN, R. G., and M. E. AUGER: Automatic ultrasonic examination of large rotor forgings. IRE Convention Record 9 (6) (1961) pp. 316–326.

[121] GOODMAN, G.: Ferroelectric proporties of lead metaniobate. J. Amer. ceram. Soc. 36 (1953) pp. 368–372.

[122] GRABENDÖRFER, W.: Über die Bedeutung des Testfehlers bei automatischen Ultraschall-Prüfanlagen. Materialprüfung 6 (1964) pp. 261–265.

[123] GRABENDÖRFER, W.: Untersuchung von dünnen runden Werkstoffen mit Überschall-Oberflächenwellen. Stahl u. Eisen 75 (1955) pp. 1273–1275.

[124] GRABENDÖRFER, W.: Untersuchung an Kunststoffen mit Ultraschall nach dem Impulsverfahren. Gummi u. Asbest 10 (1957) pp. 544–548.

[125] GRABENDÖRFER, W., and J. KRAUTKRÄMER: Über Impuls-Echo-Prüfung an plattenförmigen Körpern. Z. Metallkde. 49 (1958) pp. 22–26.

[126] GRABENDÖRFER, W., and H. WEBER: Ultraschallprüfung von Blechen, Schweissnähten und Rohren. Industrie-Anzeiger 50 (1960) pp. 775–780.

[127] GRANATO, A., and K. LÜCKE: Theorie of mechanical damping due to dislocations. J. appl. Phys. 27 (1956) pp. 583–593.

[128] GRANATO, A., and R. TRUELL: Frequency dependence of ultrasonic attenuation in germanium. J. appl. Phys. 27 (1956) pp. 1219–1226.

[129] HÄUSLER, E.: Die Anwendung elastischer Oberflächenwellen in der zerstörungsfreien Materialprüfung. Materialprüfung 2 (1960) pp. 51–55.

[130] HANSTEAD, P. D., and I. MCELWEE: Automatic ultrasonic inspection of nozzle welds in nuclear reactor pressure vessels. Proc. 4th Intern. Conf. Nondestr. Test. London 1963. London: Butterworths Sci. 1964, pp. 255–260.

[131] HANSTOCK, R. F.: Development of radiographic and ultrasonic methods of inspecting nuclear reactor pressure vessels. Proc. 4th Intern. Conf. Non-destr. Test. London 1963. London: Butterworths Sci. 1964. pp. 249–254.

[132] HARRIS, R. V.: Resonance testing without contact. Ultrasonic News (Journal of Messrs. Branson Instruments), Ed. winter 1960, pp. 10–15.

[133] VON HASELBERG, KL., and J. KRAUTKRÄMER: Ein Ultraschallstrahler für die Werkstoffprüfung mit verbessertem Nahfeld. Acustica 9 (1959) pp. 359 to 364.

[134] HASTINGS, C. H., S. A. LOPILATO and L. C. LYNNWORTH: Ultrasonic inspection of reinforced plastics and resin-ceramic composites. Nondestr. Test. 19 (1961) pp. 340–346.

[135] HATFIELD, P.: An ultrasonic phase lag method for measuring the thickness of rubber. Brit. J. appl. Phys. 3 (1952) pp. 326–328.

[136] HECHT, A.: Ultraschallprüfung keramischer Isolatoren. Stemag-Nachr. 1963, No. 37, pp. 1002–1013.

[137] HEISTERKAMP, W.: Erfahrungen bei der Ultraschallprüfung geschweisster Tankböden. Techn. Überwachung 4 (1963) No. 8, pp. 304–306.

[138] HETHERINGTON, M. J.: Continuous and complete testing of tubes. Engineering (June 1964) pp. 845–846.

[139] HETZLER, M., and A. MICHALSKI: Ultraschallprüfung von Presspassungen. Werkstattstechnik 43 (1953) pp. 321–325.

[140] HETZLER, M., and A. MICHALSKI: Ultraschall-Schrumpfsitzprüfung von Blockaufnehmern für Strangpressen. Z. Metallkde. 46 (1955) pp. 5–11.

[141] HEUGHAN, D. M., and D. O. SPROULE: Non-destructive examination of flat bonded rubber mountings. Trans. Inst. Rubber Ind. 29 (1953) pp. 255–265.

[142] HIEDEMANN, E.: Wellenausbreitung in festen Körpern. Ultraschall. Fiat-Review of German Science 1939–1946, Physics of Solids. Part I, pp. 154 to 178. Wiesbaden: Dieterichsche Verlagsbuchhandlung W. Klemm 1948.

[143] HIKATA, A., R. TRUELL, A. GRANATO, B. CHICK and K. LÜCKE: Sensitivity of ultrasonic attenuation and velocity changes to plastic deformation and recovery in aluminium. J. appl. Phys. 27 (1956) pp. 396–404.

[144] HIKATA, A.: Ultrasonic attenuation in polycrystalline steel. Government Mechanical Laboratory Bulletin (Japan) 1954, No. 1.

[145] HIRONE, T.: Quality inspection of materials by ultrasonic methods in Japan. 3rd Intern. Conf. Nondestr. Test. Tokio 1960, Keynote paper No. 34.

[146] HITT, W. C., and J. B. RAMSEY: Ultrasonic inspection and evaluation of plastics materials. Ultrasonics 1 (1963) pp. 9–13.

[147] HÖGSTRÖM, K. E.: Schwedische Erfahrungen bei der Ermittlung von Nietlochanrissen an Kochern mittels Ultraschall. Das Papier 14 (1960) No. 11, pp. 671–673.

[148] HÖLLER, P., W. DICK and E. LECHKY: Ultraschallprüfung von Grobblechen im Herstellungsfluss. Stahl u. Eisen 81 (1961) pp. 1116–1122.

[149] HOLMES, E.: Ultrasonic behaviour of austenitic stainless steel. Appl. Mat. Res. 2 (1963) pp. 181–184.

[150] HOMÈS, G. A., and I. H. OTS: Contrôle non destructif des matériaux par les ultrasons. Bull. Sci. AIM Belg. 62 (1949) pp. 23–54.

[151] HOMÈS, G. A.: Die Prüfung der Schweissungen im Kunststoff. Paper read at the conference of the Gesellschaft zur Förderung zerstörungsfreier Prüfverfahren and of the Verein Deutscher Eisenhüttenleute in Düsseldorf on 9/10/1959.

[152] HORN, C. H.: Ultrasonic testing device. USA-P. 2846874 (1958).

[153] HORNUNG, R.: Erfahrungen bei der Fehlersuche mit Ultraschall und Röntgenstrahlen. Stahl u. Eisen 83 (1963) pp. 298–304.

[154] HORNUNG, R.: Erfahrungen mit der Ultraschallprüfung von Schweissnähten. Konstruktion 14 (1962) No. 2, pp. 41–46.

[155] HORNUNG, R.: Examen supersonique des joints soudés. Schweiz. Arch. angew. Wiss. Techn. 1959, pp. 334–338.

[156] HORST, P.: Entwicklung eines Verfahrens zur Durchführung von Ultraschallmessungen beim lebenden Schwein. Z. Tierzüchtung u. Züchtungsbiologie 80 (1964) pp. 341–364.

[157] HÜTTER, A.: Methoden zur Prüfung des Betons mit Ultraschall. Bauplanung-Bautechnik 9 (1955) pp. 385–389.

[158] HUGHES, E. T., and F. B. BURSTEIN: The evaluation of bond quality in honeycomb panels using ultrasonic surface wave techniques. Nondestr. Test. 17 (1959) No. 6, pp. 373–377.

[159] HUSAREK, V.: Automatische Prüfung von Knüppeln mit elektromagnetischen und Überschall-Verfahren. Stahl u. Eisen 77 (1957) pp. 1483–1487.

[160] Husarek, V.: Neue Erfahrungen der automatischen Knüppelprüfung in Frankreich. Paper read at the conf. of the Gesellschaft zur Förderung zerstörungsfreier Prüfverfahren, Vienna. April 1965.

[161] Husarek, V.: Etat actuel du contrôle automatique par ultrasons des billettes en France. Rev. Métall. 62 (1965) pp. 711–719.

[162] Husarek, V., and P. Ruault: Emploi des méthodes de contrôles non-destructifs pour la vérification des soudures des canalisations de transport de gaz. Materialprüfung 6 (1964) pp. 37–42.

[163] Ivanov, F. I., and M. A. Akulin: Measuring the size of internal flaws in metal by an ultrasonic method (in Russian). Zavodskaya Laboratoriya 23 (1957) pp. 309–311. English translation: Brutcher[1] No. 3968.

[164] Ivens, G.: Einfluß von zylindrischer Krümmung der Prüfoberfläche auf die bei der Ultraschallprüfung eingestrahlte Energie. Works report No. 4733 of Stahl- und Röhrenwerke Reisholz AG, Düsseldorf 1958 (unpublished).

[165] Ivens, G.: Eine Methode zur Messung der Schwächung von Schallimpulsen in Stahl (will be published in „Materialprüfung").

[166] Jaburek, F.: Werkstoffprüfung mit Ultraschall unter besonderer Berücksichtigung des Betons. Österr. Bauztg. 10 (1958) pp. 37–41.

[167] Jaffe, H.: Piezoelectric ceramics. J. Amer. ceram. Soc. 41 (1958) pp. 494–498.

[168] Jarvis, J.: Ultrasonic in the foundry. Brit. Foundrym. (August 1957) pp. 400–406.

[169] Jones, R.: The ultrasonic testing of concrete. Ultrasonics 1 (1963) pp. 78–82.

[170] Jones, R., and E. N. Gatfield: Testing concrete by an ultrasonic pulse technique. Department of Scientific and Industrial Research. Road Research Laboratory, Hammondsworth, Middlesex. Road Research Technical Paper No. 34 (1955) 48 pages.

[171] Kanagy, J. R., and M. Robinson: Studies on leather by means of a sonic technique. J. Amer. Leather Chemist's Assoc. 51 (1956) pp. 174–197.

[172] Kassem, M. A.: Echo phantoms. Iron Steel (November and December 1956) pp. 503–509 and 547–549.

[173] Kaule, W.: Magnetostrictive ultrasonic testing of materials. Proc. 4th Intern. Conf. Non-destr. Test. London 1963. London: Butterworths Sci. 1964, pp. 291–294 and 316–318.

[174] Keller, G.: Attenuation power of cast iron measured by ultrasound (in Hungarian). Öntöde 7 (1956) pp. 73–84.

[175] Kesler, C. E., and T. S. Chang: A review of sonic methods for the determination of mechanical properties of solid materials. ASTM-Bull. (October 1957) pp. 40–46.

[176] Kipka, S.: Dämpfungsmessungen an Stahlguss mit Impuls-Schall-Gerät. Giessereitechnik 9 (1963) No. 6, pp. 176–178.

[177] Kleint, R. E.: Relationsship between defect orientation and ultrasonic indications. Nondestr. Test. 15 (1957) No. 1. pp. 30–36.

[178] Kleint, R. E., and C. H. Johnson: Ultrasonic inspection of liquid propellant socket motor components. Nondestr. Test. 19 (1961) pp. 418–421.

[179] Kliesch, J., and P. Horst: Untersuchungen zur Methode der Ultraschallmessungen am lebenden Schwein unter Verwendung eines Schnittbildgerätes. Züchtungskde. 34 (1962) p. 350.

[180] Kliesch, J., U. Neuhaus, E. Silber and H. Kostzewske: Versuche zur Messung der Speckdicke am lebenden Tier mit Hilfe des Ultraschalls. Z. Tierzüchtung u. Züchtungsbiologie 70 (1957) pp. 29–32.

---

[1] H. Brutcher, P. O. Box 157, Altadena, Calif., USA.

[181] Kloth, E.: Untersuchungen über die Ausbreitung kurzer Schallimpulse bei der Materialprüfung mit Ultraschall. Forschungsbericht Wirtschafts- u. Verkehrsministerium Nordrhein-Westfalen Nr. 216, Köln: Westdeutscher Verlag 1956.

[182] Knorr, W., and H. G. Ricken: Untersuchung zur Messung der Schallschwächung und Ermittlung der Fehlergrösse mit Ultraschall. Arch. Eisenhüttenwes. 33 (1962) pp. 317–326.

[183] Kolorz, A.: Zerstörungsfreie Werkstoffprüfung von Stahlguss mit Ultraschall. Giesserei 48 (1961) pp. 109–114.

[184] Koltonski, W.: Investigation of rock and raw materials of rock by means of ultrasonics. Proc. 2nd Conf. Ultrasonics Warsaw 1956, pp. 155–161.

[185] Koltonski, W., and I. Malecki: Ultrasonic method for the exploration of the properties and structure of mineral layers. Acustica 8 (1958) pp. 307 to 314.

[186] Kondo, H.: Investigation by ultrasonic inspection of the relations between flaw pattern on flaws in steel forgings made for marine vessels. Proc. 4th Intern. Conf. Non-destr. London 1963. London: Butterworths Sci. 1964, pp. 235–242.

[187] Kopineck, H. J., and H. Hoff: Prüfung von Feinblechen mit Überschall. Stahl u. Eisen 77 (1957) pp. 727–734.

[188] Kopineck, H. J., H. Krächter and W. Rauterkus: Ultraschallprüfung von Erzeugnissen der Eisen schaffenden Industrie in der laufenden Fertigung. Stahl u. Eisen 79 (1959) pp. 786–797.

[189] Kopineck, H. J., and G. Sommerkorn: Zur Physik der Ultraschallprüfung von Feinblechen mit künstlichen und natürlichen Fehlern. Materialprüfung 6 (1964) No. 6, pp. 196–200.

[190] Koppelmann, J.: Schallgeschwindigkeits- und Schallschwächungsmessungen mit handelsüblichen Ultraschallimpulsgeräten an Platten mit sehr hoher Schallabsorption. PTB-Mitt. 1964, No. 6, pp. 531–533.

[191] Krächter, H.: Ein neuartiges Verfahren zur Messung von Druckkräften mit Ultraschall. Werkst. u. Betr. 1958, No. 5, pp. 246–248.

[192] Krächter, H., and J. a. H. Krautkrämer: Schweissnahtprüfung mit Ultraschall. Schweissen u. Schneiden 5 (1953) pp. 305–314.

[193] Krainer, E.: Experience with the assessment and interpretation of ultrasonic indications in the testing of forgings. Mat. Res. 1 (1962) pp. 47–54.

[194] Krainer, E.: Messung der Ultraschall-Schwächung als Mittel der Qualitätskontrolle. Materialprüfung 4 (1962) No. 12, pp. 463–469.

[195] Krainer, H., and E. Krainer: Überschallprüfung nach dem Durchschallungs- und Impuls-Echo-Verfahren. Arch. Eisenhüttenwes. 24 (1953) pp. 229–236.

[196] Krainer, H., and E. Krainer: Zur Fehlerdeutung bei der Ultraschallprüfung. Schweisstechnik 12 (1958) pp. 28–32.

[197] Krainer, H., and E. Krainer: Influence of geometric factors on results of ultrasonic testing of heavy forgings. ASTM Spec. Techn. Publ. No. 231 (1958).

[198] Krautkrämer, H.: Application of the ultrasonic pulse echo method for direct measurement of distance, length and wall thickness. Proc. 4th Intern. Conf. Non-destr. Test. London 1963. London: Butterworths Sci. 1964, pp. 155–158.

[199] Krautkrämer, H.: Aufgabe und Ausbildung des Ultraschallprüfers. Paper read at the 3rd Congress for Materials Testing Budapest 1964.

[200] Krautkrämer, J., and H. Krautkrämer: Verfahren und Gerät zur Messung von Wandstärken mit Ultraschallimpulsen. DBP 920515 (1951).

[201] Krautkrämer, J., and W. Roth: Werkstoffprüfung mit Ultraschall in der Leichtmetall-Halbzeugindustrie. Z. Metallkde. 44 (1953) pp. 198–205.

[202] KRAUTKRÄMER, J., and H. KRAUTKRÄMER: Blechprüfung mit Ultraschall. Mitt. Forsch.-Ges. Blechverarb. 1955, No. 8, pp. 97–103.

[203] KRAUTKRÄMER, J.: Ultrasonic weld testing in Europe and the attitude of technical control authorities. Nondestr. Test. 20 (1962) pp. 319–324.

[204] KRAUTKRÄMER, J.: Datenverarbeitung bei der Ultraschallprüfung. Materialprüfung 6 (1964) pp. 279–282.

[205] KRAUTKRÄMER, J.: Determination of the size of defects by the ultrasonic impulse echo method. Brit. J. Appl. Phys. 10 (1959) pp. 240–245.

[206] KRAUTKRÄMER, J.: Die Messung der Ultraschall-Schwächung nach dem Echolot-Verfahren. Giesserei, techn.-wiss. Beih. 1958, No. 20, pp. 1067–1075.

[207] KRAUTKRÄMER, J.: Fehlergrößenermittlung mit Ultraschall. Arch. Eisenhüttenwes. 30 (1959) pp. 693–703.

[208] KREITZ, K., and G. IVENS: Routinemäßige Prüfung von Schmiedestücken mit Ultraschall. Materialprüfung 2 (1960) pp. 240–244.

[209] KRUSE, F.: Zur Werkstoffprüfung mittels Ultraschall. Akust. Z. 4 (1939) pp. 153–168.

[210] KRUSE, F.: Untersuchungen über Schallvorgänge in festen Körpern bei Anwendung frequenzmodulierten Ultraschalls. Akust. Z. 6 (1941) pp. 137–149.

[211] KÜHN, G. J., and A. LUTSCH: Elastic wave mode conversion at a solid-solid boundary with transverse slip. J. A. S. A. 33 (1961) pp. 949–954.

[212] LACK, B. J.: Ultrasonic examination of welds in thick plate using a double probe incline technique. Brit. Weld. J. (Febr. 1962) pp. 54–60.

[213] LAMB, H.: On Waves in an elastic plate. Proc. Roy. Soc. London, Ser. A 93 (1916) p. 114.

[214] LAUPRECHT, E., J. SCHEPER and J. SCHRÖDER: Messung der Speckdicke lebender Schweine nach dem Echolot-Verfahren. Mitt. Dtsch. Landwirtschaftsges. 72 (1957) pp. 881/882.

[215] LAUPRECHT, E.: Bericht über Ergebnisse von Messungen mit dem Ultraschall-Echolot an Schweinen. Züchtungskde. 32 (1960), pp. 441–449.

[216] LAUPRECHT, E., E. WALTER and T. SAATHOFF: Beitrag zur Messung der Querschnittsfläche des langen Rückenmuskels und der darüber liegenden Fettschicht von lebenden Schweinen mit dem Ultraschall-Echolot. Züchtungskde. 32 (1960) pp. 450–464.

[217] LAUPRECHT, E., E. WALTER and T. SAATHOFF: Beitrag zur Messung der Querschnittsfläche des langen Rückenmuskels am lebenden Rind mit dem Ultraschall-Echolot. Züchtungskde. 34 (1962) pp. 211–215.

[218] LAUPRECHT, E., and W. VON SCHUTZBAR: Ein Beitrag zur Messung der Querschnittsfläche des langen Rückenmuskels am lebenden Schwein mit Hilfe des Ultraschall-Schnittbildgerätes. Schweinezucht u. Schweinemast 12 (1964) No. 6.

[219] LEHFELDT, W.: Zerstörungsfreie Materialprüfung mittels Ultraschall. Maschine u. Werkzeug 55 (1954) No. 6, pp. 5–8.

[220] LEHFELDT, W.: Reifenprüfung mittels Ultraschallwellen. ATZ 56 (1954) pp. 134–136.

[221] LEHFELDT, W.: Ultraschallanlage zur Blechprüfung. Blech 2 (1955) No. 9, pp. 50–55.

[222] LEHFELDT, W.: Methoden der Blechprüfung mittels Ultraschall. Das Industrieblatt, Stuttgart (Oktober 1958) pp. 425–433.

[223] LEHFELDT, W.: Drahtprüfung durch Ultraschall. Draht-Welt 46 (1960) pp. 156–159.

[224] LEHTINEN, A.: Eine neue Untersuchungsmethode zur Qualitätskontrolle des Gusseisens mittels Ultraschall. Lecture No. 7 at the Intern. Casting Congr. Zurich 1960.

[225] LEIJSEN, W.: Ultraschallresonanz-Wanddickenmessung über eine Flüssigkeitszwischenstrecke. Materialprüfung 4 (1962) pp. 407–410.
[226] LESLIE, J. R., and W. J. CHEFSMAN: An ultrasonic method of studying deterioration and cracking in concrete structures. J. Amer. Concr. Inst. 21 (1949) pp. 17–36.
[227] LEVITT, A. P., and A. G. MARTIN: Ultrasonic determination of elastic constants of metals at elevated temperatures. Nondestr. Test. 18 (1960) pp. 333 to 336.
[228] LINHARDT, F.: Über den Einfluss der Schallfeldinterferenzen auf den Fehlernachweis in Festkörpern. Thesis Braunschweig 1957. – Metall 12 (1958) pp. 1085–1092; 13 (1959) pp. 1133–1138.
[229] LUKAS, G., and A. LUTSCH: Bestimmung der Seigerungszone im Gussblock einer Aluminium-Magnesium-Silizium-Legierung mit dem Ultraschall-Reflexionsverfahren. Z. Metallkde. 45 (1954) pp. 158–160.
[230] LUND, S. A.: Application of ultrasonics for non-destructive testing of materials (in Danish). Ingeniøren (1954) No. 41, pp. 794–803.
[231] LUTSCH, A., and G. J. KÜHN: Generation and reception of elastic waves via a plane boundary. J. A. S. A. 36 (1964) pp. 428–436.
[232] LUTSCH, A., and E. A. W. MÜLLER: Anordnung zur Prüfung von Stoffen mit Ultraschallimpulsen. DBP 971891 (1952).
[233] LUTSCH, A.: Zerstörungsfreie Prüfung der Werkstoffe nach dem Ultraschall-Impuls-Echoverfahren. Arch. Eisenhüttenwes. 23 (1952) pp. 57–65.
[234] LUTSCH, A.: Grundlagen und Verfahren zur zerstörungsfreien Werkstoffprüfung mittels Ultraschall-Wellen. ATM-Blätter V 91193-1 to 4 (1953–54).
[235] LUTSCH, A.: Ultraschallschwingeranordnung zur zerstörungsfreien Werkstoffprüfung mittels Ultraschallimpulsen. DBP 1013898 (1954).
[236] LUTSCH, A.: Ultraschall-Schwingeranordnung zur zerstörungsfreien Werkstoffprüfung mittels Ultraschall-Impulsen. DBP 929153 (1953).
[237] LUTSCH, A., and W. BÖHME: Dickenmessung mittels Ultraschallwellen. ATM-Blatt V 1124–1126 (1957).
[238] LUTSCH, A.: Ultrasonic reflectoscope with an indicator of the degree of coupling between transducer and object. J. A. S. A. 30 (1958) pp. 544–548.
[239] LUTSCH, A.: The experimental determination of the extent and degree of fracture of rock faces by means of an ultrasonic pulse reflection method. J. South African Inst. Mining and Metallurgy 1959, pp. 412–429.
[240] LUTSCH, A.: An apparatus for measuring and recording the velocity of sound and temperature versus depth in sea water. Acustica 8 (1958) pp. 387-391.
[241] LUTSCH, A.: Bariumtitanate adhesion- and paste-transducers; ultrasonic generators for the analysis of solids. Proc. 3rd Intern. Congr. Acoustics Stuttgart 1959. Amsterdam: Elsevier 1960 and Nature 184 (1959) pp. 1458–1492.
[242] LYNNWORTH, L. C. et al.: Ultrasonic measurement of elastic moduli at elevated temperatures using momentary contact. J. A. S. A. 36 (1964) pp. 1678–1684.
[243] MACKENZIE, J. K.: The elastic constants of a solid containing spherical holes. Proc. phys. Soc. B 63 (1) (1950) pp. 2–11.
[244] MARIANESCHI, E.: Alcune considerazioni sull'interpretazione degli esami ultrasonori per la ricerca dei difetti nell'acciaio. La Metallurgia italiana (April 1957). German discussion: Industrielle Organisation 26 (1957) pp. 271–284.
[245] MARTIN, E.: Überschalluntersuchungen an Achsen von Schienenfahrzeugen. Stahl u. Eisen 72 (1952) pp. 176–185.
[246] MARTIN, E., and K. WERNER: Fehleraufzeichnung beim Überschall-Impuls-Laufzeit-Verfahren. Arch. Eisenhüttenwes. 27 (1956) pp. 579–594.
[247] MARTIN, E., and K. WERNER: Schienenprüfung mit Ultraschall und der Ultra-

schall-Schienenprüfwagen der Deutschen Bundesbahn. Eisenbahntechn.Rundschau 5 (1956) pp. 487–505.

[248] Martin, E., and K. Werner: Statistische Auswertung von Ultraschall-Reihenuntersuchungen an Achswellen von Schnellzug-Dampflokomotiven. Glasers Annalen 78 (1954) pp. 1–8 and 31–35.

[249] Martin, E., and K. Werner: Prüfung verwickelt geformter Teile mit Überschall. Arch. Eisenhüttenwes. 24 (1953) pp. 411–422.

[250] Martin, E., and K. Werner: Einrichtung zur Schwächung von störenden Nebenechos bei dem Ultraschall-Impulsverfahren der zerstörungsfreien Werkstückprüfung. DBP 934504 (1953).

[251] Mason, W. P., and J. H. McSkimin: Attenuation and scattering of high frequency sound waves in metals and glasses. J. A. S. A. 19 (1947) pp. 464–473.

[252] Mason, W. P., and H. J. McSkimin: Energy losses of sound waves in metals due to scattering and diffusion. J. appl. Phys. 19 (1948) pp. 940–946.

[253] Matting, A., and G. Wilkens: Die Prüfung von Punktschweissungen durch Ultraschall. Bd. 35 der Fachbuchreihe Schweisstechnik, Düsseldorf: Deutscher Verlag für Schweisstechnik 1963.

[254] McClung, R. W., and K. V. Cook: Ultrasonic detection of non-bond in clad structures. Proc. 4th Intern. Conf. Non-destr. Test. London 1963. London: Butterworths Sci. 1964, pp. 267–271.

[255] McGonnagle, W. J., St. McLain and E. C. Wood: Application of nondestructive testing to fuel elements for nuclear reactors. Nondestr. Test. 15 (1957) No. 2, pp. 86–90.

[256] McSkimin, H. J., and W. L. Bond: Elastic moduli of diamond. Phys. Rev. 105 (1957) pp. 116–121.

[257] Mesh, W. E.: Variable angle ultrasonic transducer. USA-P. 2602101 (1950).

[258] Meyer, E., and G. Buchmann: Über einfache Werkstoffprüfungen mit magnetostriktiven Ultraschallgeräten. Akust. Z. 3 (1938) pp. 132–136.

[259] Meyer, E., and E. Bock: Hörschall- und Ultraschalluntersuchungen von Betonbalken mit Rissen. Akust. Z. 4 (1939) pp. 231–237.

[260] Meyer, H. J.: Ultraschall-Wandstärken-Messungen an Grauguss-Laufbuchsen von Fahrzeug-Dieselmotoren. Materialprüfung 5 (1963) pp. 293–297.

[261] Michalski, A.: Procédé de prise de photographies des images-coupes obtenues par le contrôle ultrasonore. Circulaire d'Information Technique (CIT) No. 9 (1959) pp. 2029–2046.

[262] Midecke, P.: Über die Ultraschall-Schwächung in austenitischen Chrom-Nickel-Stählen. Materialprüfung 3 (1961) No. 1, pp. 1–4.

[263] Mikhailov, J. G., and V. A. Solovlev: A simple method for measuring the absorption of ultrasonic waves in strongly absorbing solids (in Russian). Doklady Akademii NAUK SSSR 78 (1951) pp. 245–248. English translation: Brutcher No. 2904 (see footnote p. 497).

[264] Minton, W. C.: Inspection of metals with ultrasonic surface waves. Nondestr. Test. 12 (1954) No. 4, pp. 13–16.

[265] Mochol, N. L., R. E. Peterson, J. D. Conrad and D. W. Gunther: Large rotor forgings for turbines and generators. Trans. ASME 1956, pp. 1585–1601.

[266] Mohr, W.: Über die zerstörungsfreie Prüfung von Schweissnähten, insbesondere von Rotorschweissungen. BBC-Mitt. (Aug.-Sept. 1961) pp. 475–484.

[267] Mohr, W.: Unpublished, private communication.

[268] Morris, W. E.: Method and apparatus for ultrasonic testing. USA-P. 2378237 (1945).

[269] Morris, W. E., R. B. Stambaugh and S. D. Gehmann: Ultrasonic method of tire inspection. Rev. Sci. Instrum. 23 (1952) pp. 729–734.

[270] MÜHLHÄUSER, O.: Verfahren zur Zustandsbestimmung von Werkstoffen, besonders zur Ermittlung von Fehlern darin. DRP[1] 569598 (1931).

[271] MUNDRY, E.: Über die Anwendung verschiedener Kontrollkörper zur Justierung von Ultraschall-Impulsecho-Geräten. Materialprüfung 5 (1963) pp. 298 to 306.

[272] MUNDRY, E.: Über das Verhalten teildurchlässiger Zwischenflächen bei der Materialprüfung mit Ultraschall. Teil I: Theorie. Materialprüfung 8 (1966) No. 12, pp. 433–444. Teil II: Modellversuche und Anwendungsmöglichkeiten. Materialprüfung 9 (1967) No. 4, pp. 120–130.

[273] NANDA, M. M., N. A. SINCLAIR and J. F. LOVELACE: Ultrasonic inspection of brazed pipe joints. Materials Evaluation 22 (1964) No. 7, pp. 315–320.

[274] NAUMANN, F.: Messanordnung zur Messung von Schall an der Oberfläche von festen Körpern. DBP 1097721 (1959).

[275] NIKLAS, L.: Eine neue Methode der Dicken- bzw. Schallgeschwindigkeitsmessung. Z. Metallkde. 49 (1958) pp. 152–155.

[276] NIKLAS, L.: Plattenwellen. Materialprüfung 4 (1962) No. 1, pp. 12–20.

[277] NIKLAS, L.: Gruppenlaufzeit und Bündelversetzung bei der Schrägreflexion. Auswirkungen auf die praktische Werkstoffprüfung mit Ultraschall. Materialprüfung 7 (1965) No. 8, pp. 281–288.

[278] OLIVER, R. B., R. W. MCCLUNG and J. K. WHITE: Immersed ultrasonic inspection of pipe and tubing. Nondestr. Test. 15 (1957) No. 3, pp. 140–144.

[279] OPEL, P., and G. IVENS: Fehlergrößenermittlung mit Ultraschall an Schmiedestücken. Arch. Eisenhüttenwes. 33 (1962) pp. 311–316.

[280] OSTERHAMMEL, K.: Optische Untersuchungen des Schallfeldes kolbenförmig schwingender Quarze. Akust. Z. 6 (1941) pp. 73–86.

[281] PANIAN, F. C., and H. E. VAN VALKENBURG: Development of ASTM reference blocks for ultrasonic inspection. Nondestr. Test. 19 (1961) pp. 45–57.

[282] PAPKE, W. H.: Schweissnahtprüfung mit Ultraschall. Schweissen u. Schneiden 10 (1958) pp. 131–135.

[283] PAPKE, W. H.: Vorschlag zur dokumentarischen Erfassung des Befundes von Ultraschall-Schweissnahtprüfungen. Schweissen u. Schneiden 13 (1961) No. 10 pp. 457–463.

[284] PARDUS, A. J.: Ultrasonic testing used for small diameter tubing. Iron Age (January 1953) pp. 110–113.

[285] PARKER, F. C.: Ultrasonic examinations of weldments and the etablishment of safe acceptable limits for defects. Nondestr. Test. 11 (January 1953) pp. 12 to 20.

[286] PATTERSON, W., and E. BODMER: Ultraschalluntersuchungen an Gusseisen mit lamellarer und kugeliger Graphitausbildung. Giesserei, techn.-wiss. Beih. 1957, No. 17, pp. 909–917.

[287] POHL, D.: Ein Beitrag zur Ultraschallprüfung von Rundstahl. Stahl u. Eisen 82 (1962) pp. 97–106.

[288] POHLMANN, R.: Verfahren zum bildmäßigen Sichtbarmachen und Messen einer Energieverteilung von thermischer, elektrischer, Schall- oder Ultraschallenergie. DRP[1] 710413 (1937).

[289] POHLMANN, R.: Über die Möglichkeit einer akustischen Abbildung in Analogie zur optischen. Z. Phys. 113 (1939) pp. 697–709.

[290] PRINGLE, F. E.: SIMAC – Sonic inspection, measurement and control. Nondestr. Test. 14 (1956) No. 3, pp. 22–25.

[291] PURSEY, H.: The launching and propagation of elastic waves in plates. Quart. J. Mech. Appl. Math. 10 (1957) Part I.

[1] DRP = Deutsches Reichspatent (German Patent).

[292] Ranachowski, J., and J. Wehr: Application of ultrasonic methods to tests of some high voltage insulating materials. Proc. 2nd Conf. Ultrasonics Warsaw 1956, pp. 187–193.

[293] Rankin, A.W., C. J. Boyle, C. D. Moriarty and B. R. Seguin: Thermal cracks in turbine and generator rotor forgings. Mech. Engng. (July 1955) pp. 559–566.

[294] Rankin, A. W., and C. D. Moriarty: Acceptance guides for ultrasonic inspection of large rotor forgings. ASME Paper No. 55 A. 194 (1956) (Amer. Soc. Mech. Engng.).

[295] Rankin, C. A.: Autosonics – Problems and experiences in automatic production testing. Materialprüfung 2 (1960) No. 11, pp. 421–428.

[296] Rankin, C. A., H. C. Brooks and A. W. Brown: Ultrasonic inspection of the Nimrod power plant alternator rotors. Proc. 4th Intern. Conf. Non-destr. Test. London 1963. London: Butterworths Sci. 1964, pp. 196–202.

[297] Rasmussen, J. G.: Ultrasonic inspection of turbine and compressor rotor blades for cracks and other flaws. Nondestr. Test. 16 (1958) No. 3, pp. 228–236.

[298] Rasmussen, J. G.: Prediction of fatigue failure using ultrasonic surface waves. Nondestr. Test. 20 (1962) pp. 103–110.

[299] Rassweiler, G. M., and W. S. Erwin: Automatic sonic measuring means. USA-P. 2431234 (1944).

[300] Rath, R., and M. Thivin: Some examples of nondestructive test methods used by Electricité de France. Proc. 4th Intern. Conf. Non-destr. Test. London 1963. London: Butterworths Sci. 1964, pp. 222–229.

[301] Rauterkus, W.: Schwerer Stahlguss in der Ultraschallprüfung. Giesserei 47 (1960) pp. 475–486.

[302] Rauterkus, W.: Vorschlag zur zahlenmäßigen Kennzeichnung von Ergebnissen der Ultraschallprüfung an Schmiedestücken. Arch. Eisenhüttenwes. 34 (1963) pp. 601–604.

[303] Rawding, H.: Ultrasonic testing standards. Ultrasonics 1 (1963) pp. 35–38.

[304] Read, T. A.: The internal friction of single metal crystals. Phys. Rev. 58 (1940) pp. 371–380.

[305] Redwood, M.: A study of waveforms in the generation and detection of short ultrasonic pulses. Appl. Mat Res. 2 (1963) pp. 76–84.

[306] Redwood, M.: Ultrasonic waveguides – a physical approach. Ultrasonics 1 (1963) pp. 99–105.

[307] Reti, P.: Gütekontrolle von kugelgraphitischem Gusseisen mit Ultraschall. Wiss. Z. Hochsch. Schwermaschinenbau Magdeburg 3 (1959) pp. 195–202.

[308] Reverey, G.: Die zerstörungsfreie Prüfung von Isolatoren. ETZ A 73 (1952) pp. 451–455.

[309] Richter, H. U., and D. Linke: Automatische Ultraschallimmersionsprüfanlage mit A- und B-Bild sowie Digitalanzeige für schwere Schmiedestücke. Neue Hütte 9 (1964) pp. 455–460.

[310] Rieckmann, P.: Über den Nachweis von Fehlstellen bei der Reifenprüfung nach dem Ultraschall-Durchstrahlungsverfahren. Z. angew. Phys. 8 (1956) pp. 386–391.

[311] Rocha, H. A. F.: A new nondestructive test tool: The ultrasonic micrometer. Nondestr. Test. 14 (1956) No. 6, pp. 32–34.

[312] Roderick, R. L.: The radiation pattern from a rotationally symmetric stress source on a semi infinite solid. Metals Research Report Brown University 1950 (USA).

[313] Roderick, R. L., and R. Truell: The measurement of ultrasonic attenuation in solids by the pulse technique and some results in steel. J. appl. Phys. 23 (1952) pp. 267–279.

[314] RODEWALD, H. J.: Die Schweissnahtprüfmethode der AIAG – Die Ultraschallprüfung von Vertikal-, insbesondere Rundschweissnähten. Reports Nos. 247 (1958) and 246 (1959) of Aluminium Industrie AG, Neuhausen, Schweiz.

[315] ROLL, K. H.: Inspection and testing lead linings Nondestr. Test. 16 (1956) No. 1, pp. 20–24.

[316] ROSS, J. D., and R. W. LEEP: Ultrasonic transmission tester for detection of unbonded areas. Symposium on nondestructive tests in the field of nuclear energy. ASTM Spec. Techn. Publ. No. 223 (1958) pp. 246–258.

[317] ROTH, W.: Scattering of ultrasonic radiation in polycrystalline metals. J. appl. Phys. 19 (1948) pp. 901–910.

[318] ROTH, W.: Piezoelectric transducers. IRE 37 (1949) pp. 750–758.

[319] RÜB, F.: Prüfverfahren bei der Herstellung und Verarbeitung von Draht; II: Zerstörungsfreie Prüfverfahren. Draht 14 (1963) pp. 650–654.

[320] SAWCZUK, A.: Application of ultrasonic techniques to concrete quality testing. Proc. 2nd Conf. Ultrasonics Warsaw 1956, pp. 201–207.

[321] SCHIJVE, J.: Ultrasonic resonance testing of glued metal joints. Aircraft Engineering 30 (1958) pp. 269–271.

[322] SCHINN, R., and U. WOLFF: Einige Ergebnisse der Überschallprüfung schwerer Schmiedestücke mit dem Impuls-Echo-Verfahren. Stahl u. Eisen 72 (1952) pp. 695–702.

[323] SCHLUSNUS, K. H., and F. O. KOCH: Prüfung von Spiralrohren. Bänder, Bleche, Rohre 6 (1963) pp. 282–286.

[324] SCHMAUCH, H.: Über ein neues Verfahren zur Messung von Schallgeschwindigkeit mit hoher Genauigkeit. Ann. Univers. Sar. 3 (II) (1953) pp. 257–269.

[325] SCHRODT, H.: Werkstoffprüfung mit Ultraschall bei der Deutschen Bundesbahn, insbesondere in der Anwendung bei Fahrzeugachsen. ETR 1960, No. 6, pp. 245–255.

[326] SCHUBRING, N. W., and J. E. STEVENS: Multichannel swept sonic tester for casting quality control. IRE Transactions on Industrial Electronics 8 (1959) pp. 46–58.

[327] SCHUSTER, K.: Ultraschall-optische Abbildung nach dem Reliefbild-Verfahren. Jenaer Jahrbuch 1951, pp. 217–228.

[328] SEEMANN, H. J.: Versuche zur ultraakustischen Prüfung von Gusseisen. Giesserei, techn.-wiss. Beih. 1952, No. 9, pp. 403–408.

[329] SEKI, H., A. GRANATO and R. TRUELL: Diffraction in the ultrasonic field of a piston source and their importance in the accurate measurement of attenuation. J. A. S. A. 28 (1956) pp. 230–238.

[330] SERABIAN, ST.: Influence of geometry upon an ultrasonic defect size determination in large rotor forgings. Nondestr. Test. 14 (1956) No. 4, pp. 18–21.

[331] SETTE, D.: Ultrasonic lenses of plastic materials. Ric. Sci. 18 (1948) pp. 831 to 842.

[332] SHARPE, R. S., and S. AVEYARD: The visualization of an ultrasonic extinction network in coarse grained uranium. Appl. Mat. Res. 1 (1962) pp. 170–175.

[333] SHRAIBER, D. S.: Problems of flaw testing with ultrasonics (in Russian). Zawodskaya Laboratoriya 11 (1945) pp. 1051.

[334] SIEBURG, H.: Methoden zur Bestimmung des Schlachtwerts am lebenden und geschlachteten Schwein. Thesis Göttingen 1957.

[335] SILBER, F. A.: Entwicklung einer Ultraschall-Anlage zur automatischen Prüfung vorgewalzter Brammen. Berg- u. hüttenm. Monatsh. 108 (1963) pp. 8–14.

[336] SIPEK, M.: Die Anwendbarkeit des Plattenwellen-Verfahrens bei der Ultraschallprüfung im Stahlwerk. Materialprüfung 8 (1966) No. 8, pp. 294–297.

[337] Smack, J. C.: Immersed ultrasonic inspection with automatic scanning and recording or warning signal. Nondestr. Test. 12 (1954) No. 3, pp. 29–33.

[338] Sokolow, S. J.: Zur Frage der Fortpflanzung ultraakustischer Schwingungen in verschiedenen Körpern. ENT 6 (1929) pp. 454–461.

[339] Sokolow, S. J.: Ultrasonic waves and their application (in Russian). Techn. Phys. (in Russian) 2 (1935) pp. 522–544.

[340] Sokolow, S. J.: Ultrasonic methods for determining internal flaws in metal objects (in Russian). Zavodskaya Laboratoriya 4 (1935) pp. 527 and 1468 to 1473.

[341] Sokolow, J. S.: Means for indicating flaws in materials. USA-P. 2164125 (1937).

[342] Sokolow, S. J.: Ultrasonic methods for determining the properties of heat-treated steel and for determining internal flaws of metal objects (in Russian). Techn. Phys. (in Russian) 11 (1941) pp. 160–169.

[343] Sokolow, S. J.: Topical problems of the application of ultrasonics (in Russian). Uspekhi Fiz NAUK SSSR 40 (1950) pp. 3–39.

[344] Sproule, D. O.: Improvements in or relating to apparatus for flaw detection and velocity measurement by ultrasonic echo methods. Brit.P. 774675 (1952).

[345] Sproule, D. O.: Ultrasonic testing of welds. Brit. Weld. J. 6 (1959) pp. 470 to 479.

[346] Stäger, H., E. Schütz and R. Meister: Untersuchungen mit Ultraschall an aushärtenden Leichtmetallgusslegierungen. Techn.Mitt. 47 (1954) pp. 149–157.

[347] Stäger, H., E. Schütz and R. Meister: Untersuchungen mit Ultraschall an verschieden hergestellten Kupferlegierungen. Techn. Mitt. 48 (1955) pp. 34–45.

[348] Stäger, H., and H. Studer: Untersuchungen an elektrotechnischem Porzellan mit dem Elektronenmikroskop und mit Ultraschall. Techn. Mitt. 49 (1956) pp. 170–178.

[349] Stäger, H., and R. Meister: Der Ultraschall als Mittel der Werkstoff-Forschung. Berg- u. hüttenm. Monatsh. 105 (1960) pp. 60–74.

[350] Stein, F., N. G. Einspruch and R. Truell: Temperatur dependence of fractional velocity changes in a silicon single crystal. J. appl. Phys. 30 (1959) S. 820–825.

[351] Steinkamp, G.: Ultraschall-Impulsgerät für Beton. Thesis Braunschweig 1953. – Elektron. Rdsch. 10 (1956) pp. 172–173.

[352] de Sterke, A., and A. Bordes: Experiments with ultrasonics on test pieces of s. g. iron. Paper read at the 21st Intern. Casting. Congr. 1954.

[353] de Sterke, A.: Inspection of welds by means of ultrasonics. In: L. van Ouwerkerk: The relative advantage and limitation of nondestructive testing methods. Nondestr. Test. 15 (1957) No. 5, pp. 298–312.

[354] Stoll, H.: Wanddickenmessung an heissen, korrodierten Rohren mit dem Impulsechoverfahren. Paper read at the conference of the Gesellschaft zur Förderung zerstörungsfreier Prüfverfahren in Vienna, April 1965.

[355] Stouffer, J. R., M. V. Wallentine, G. H. Wellington and A. Dieckmann: Development and application of ultrasonic methods for measuring fat thickness and rib-eye area in cattle and hogs. J. Anim. Sci. 20 (1961) pp. 759.

[356] Strassburger, Ch.: Beitrag zur Ultraschallprüfung von Vormaterial für Breitband nach dem Impuls-Echo-Verfahren. Stahl u. Eisen 81 (1961) No. 13, pp. 885–893.

[357] Stüber, C.: Zerstörungsfreie Untersuchung von Hochspannungsisolatoren mit Hilfe des Ultraschall-Impulsverfahrens (Paper read at the 3rd Intern. Congr. for acoustics in Stuttgart 1959). Proc. 3rd Intern. Congr. Acoust. Amsterdam: Elsevier 1960.

[358] STÜBER, C.: Private communication of the Testing Bureau of the German Federal Railways, Munich.

[359] SULLY, A. H., and J. D. LAVENDER: Fehlernachweis in Stahlguss mit Ultraschall. Giesserei 48 (1961) pp. 571–579.

[360] SULLY, A. H., and J. D. LAVENDER: Correlation between destructive and nondestructive testing of a large steel casting. Engineering Materials and Design (May 1963) pp. 354–357.

[361] TARNOCZY, H.: On the propagation of Ultrasonic energy through thin air layers. Proc. 2nd Conf. Ultrasonics Warsaw 1956, pp. 91–94.

[362] TARNOCZY, T., and A. ILLENYI: Akustische Zonenlinsen. Proc. 3rd Intern. Congr. Acoust. Amsterdam: Elsevier 1960.

[363] TEUTONICO, L. J., A. GRANATO and R. TRUELL: Effect of copper on ultrasonic attenuation in germanium. Phys. Rev. 103 (1956) pp. 832–833.

[364] THIEDE, H., and G. DANIEL: Behälterstandsmessungen mit Hilfe von Echolotungen. Erdöl u. Kohle 6 (1953) pp. 554–556.

[365] THIEME, J.: Untersuchungen von Proben zur ultraakustischen Prüfung von Hart- und Walzenguss. Giesserei 46 (1959) pp. 552–558.

[366] TIMMERMANS, F. D.: Ultraschallbehandlungsgerät. DBP 910466 (1939).

[367] TROST, A.: Nachweis von Werkstofftrennungen in Blechen durch Ultraschall. Z. VDI 87 (1943) pp. 352–354.

[368] TRUELL, R., and A. HIKATA: Fatigue and ultrasonic attenuation. ASTM Spec. Techn. Publ. No. 213 (1957).

[369] TRUELL, R., B. CHICK, A. PICKER and G. ANDERSON: The use of ultrasonic methods to determine fatigue effects in metals. WADC Techn. Rep. 59-389 (Wright Air Development Center Wright-Patterson Air Force Base, Ohio, USA).

[370] VAN VALKENBURG, H. E.: Ultrasonic inspection device. USA-P. 2667780 (1951).

[371] VAN VALKENBURG, H. E.: Transducer Control. USA-P. 2651012 (1952).

[372] VAN VALKENBURG, H. E., and E. G. COOK: Vorrichtung zur Materialprüfung mittels Ultraschall. DBP 1057356 (1959).

[373] VIKTOROV, I. A.: Rayleigh waves on cylindrical surfaces (in Russian). Akust. J. Akad. SSSR 4 (1958) pp. 131–136.

[374] VIKTOROV, I. A.: The effect of roughness on the propagation of Rayleigh waves (in Russian). Doklady Akademia NAUK SSSR 119 (1958) pp. 463–465.

[375] WAID, J. S., and M. J. WOODMAN: A nondestructive method of detecting diseases in wood. Nature 180 (1957) p. 47.

[376] WALZ, H.: Resonanzverfahren und Laufzeitmessung zur Prüfung des Betons. Beton 8 (1958) pp. 35–37.

[377] WEIGLER, H., and E. KERN: Über die Anwendungsmöglichkeiten des Ultraschallverfahrens zur Beurteilung der Betongüte. Betonstein-Zeitung 1965, No. 5, pp. 279–286.

[378] WEISE, H. D.: Erfahrungen bei der zerstörungsfreien Prüfung von Schweissnähten in Rohren. Schweissen u. Schneiden 8 (1956) pp. 355–363.

[379] WELLINGER, K., and S. SCHARSCHMIDT: Prüfung von Schweissnähten an dünnen Blechen mit Ultraschall. Schweissen u. Schneiden 8 (1956) p. 469–476.

[380] WENK, S. A.: Survey of ultrasonic methods and techniques. Symposium on nondestructive tests in the field of nuclear energy. ASTM Spec. Techn. Publ. No. 223 (1958) pp. 29–43.

[381] WENZEL, K.: Über die Möglichkeiten einer Betonuntersuchung mittels Ultraschall. Dissertation Braunschweig 1950.

[382] WENZEL, K.: Die Bestimmung elastischer Eigenschaften von anstehendem Fels durch Ultraschall-Sondierung. Schweiz. Bauztg. 77 (1959) pp. 479–484.

[383] WERNER, K.: Fortschritte der Schienenprüfung mit Ultraschall bei der Deutschen Bundesbahn. ETR 10 (1961) pp. 417–437.

[384] WESCHE, K. H.: Möglichkeiten für die Anwendung von Ultraschall bei der Betonprüfung. Bautechn. 32 (1955) pp. 151–155.

[385] WEYL, D.: Möglichkeiten der Prüfung von Porzellanisolatoren mit Ultraschall. ATM V 8242/43, No. 257 (June 1957).

[386] WIEGAND, H., and H. HENTZE: Bestimmung von Werkstoffkennwerten an Eisen-Graphit-Werkstoffen mit Ultraschall. Metall 13 (1959) pp. 1110–1113.

[387] WILD, H. W.: Die Ultraschallprüfung von gusseisernen Tübbingen. Glückauf 98 (1962) No. 4, pp. 231–235.

[388] WILLARD, G. W.: Ultrasound waves made visible. Bell. Labor Rec. 25 (1947) pp. 194–200.

[389] WINTER, H.: Schweissen und Schweissnahtprüfung beim Bau der Rohölleitung Wilhelmshaven-Köln. Schweissen u. Schneiden 11 (1959) pp. 270 bis 279.

[390] WOOD, F. W., and J. O. BORG: Ultrasonic inspection of arc-cast zirconium and its alloys. U.S. Bureau of Mines, Report of Investigation 5126, March 1955.

[391] WORLTON, D. C.: Ultrasonic testing with Lamb waves. Nondestr. Test. 15 (1957) No. 4, pp. 218–222.

[392] WULFF, F., and W. RECHNER: Die Ultraschallprüfung von Schweissverbindungen an Chrom-Nickel-Stählen. ZIS-Mitt. 4 (1962) No. 4, pp. 644–664.

[393] YING, C. F., and R. TRUELL: The effect of hydrogen on ultrasonic attenuation and velocity measurements in titanium. Acta Metallurgica 2 (1954) pp. 374 to 379.

[394] ZETTLER, E.: Ermittlung elastischer Kenngrössen von Gusswerkstoffen mit Hilfe von Ultraschallgeschwindigkeits- und Schwächungsmessungen. Paper read at the 3rd congress for materials testing, Budapest 1964.

[395] ZIEGLER, R., and R. GERSTNER: Die Anwendung des Ultraschall-Impuls-Verfahrens zur Wanddickenmessung bei Grauguss. Giesserei, techn.-wiss. Beihefte 1956, No. 16, pp. 829–835.

[396] ZIEGLER, R., and R. GERSTNER: Verfahren zur zerstörungsfreien Ermittlung der Zugfestigkeit von Gusstücken aus Grauguss. DBP Nr. 1074290 (1957).

[397] ZIEGLER, R., and R. GERSTNER: Die Schallgeschwindigkeit als kennzeichnende Grösse für die Beurteilung von Grauguss. Giesserei 45 (1958) pp. 185–193.

[398] ZOTTMANN, W.: Beitrag zur Fehlergrössenermittlung beim Ultraschall-Impuls-Echo-Verfahren. Arch. Eisenhüttenwes. 35 (1964) pp. 353–358.

[399] Accles and Pollock, Ltd.: An improved method for testing tubes by ultrasonics. Brit.P. 24663 (1958).

[400] American Petrol Institute, API Standard 5 AX, 3rd edition (March 1964): High String Casing and Tubing.

[401] American Society for Testing and Materials (ASTM): Ultrasonic testing by the reflection method using pulsed longitudinal waves induced by direct contact. ASTM-Designation E 114-55T.

[402] ASTM: Ultrasonic testing by the resonance method. E 113-55T.

[403] ASTM: Ultrasonic testing and inspection of heavy steel forgings. A 388-59.

[404] ASTM: Tentative method for ultrasonic testing and inspection of turbine and generator steel rotor forgings. A 418-57T (1957).

[405] ASTM: Recommended practice for evaluating the microstructure of graphite in gray iron. A 247–47.

[406] ASTM: Nondestructive testing in the missile industry. ASTM Spec. Techn. Publ. No. 278 (1959).

[407] ASTM: Tentative method and specification for ultrasonic testing and inspection of steel plates of firebox and higher quality. A 435-59T (1959).

[408] ASTM: Tentative recommended practice for fabricating and checking aluminum alloy ultrasonic standard reference blocks. E 127-61T (1961).

[409] ASTM: Tentative methods for ultrasonic contact inspection of weldments. E 164-62T (1962).

[410] ASTM: Symposium Recent developments in nondestructive testing of missiles and rockets. ASTM Spec. Techn. Publ. No. 350 (1963).

[411] ASTM: Tentative method for ultrasonic inspection of metal pipe and tubing for longitudinal discontinuities. E 213-63T (1963).

[412] ASTM: Tentative recommended practice for immersed ultrasonic testing by the reflection method using pulsed longitudinal waves. E 214-63T (1963).

[413] ASTM: Tentative method for the ultrasonic inspection of welded pipe and tubing. Draft 1963.

[414] ASTM: Tentative recommended practice for ultrasonic contact inspection by the reflection method using angle projection of the sound beam. Draft 1964.

[415] ASTM: Tentative recommended practice for evaluating performance characteristics of a pulse echo ultrasonic testing system. Draft 1964.

[416] Association Française de Normalisation AFNOR FD A 04-305: Contrôle des tôles fortes aux ultrasons.

[417] Association Française de Normalisation AFNOR FD A 04-311: Blocs d'étalonnage, examen par ultrasons de pièces en acier (1964).

[418] Ateliers de Constructions Electriques de Charleroi (ACEC): Übertrager für elastische Wellen. DBP 966392 (1950).

[419] Boeing Service Bulletin No. 1995 (R-2) A 1964.

[420] British Steel Castings Research Association: Recommended Procedure for the ultrasonic examination of steel castings (1964).

[421] British Standard Institution (BSI): British standard specification for ultrasonic reference standards and recommendations for their use. Draft. Document No. D 64/7194 (1964).

[422] BSI: Draft British standard. Glossary of terms used in non-destructive testing, Part 4 – Ultrasonic flaw detection (B. S. 3683: Part 4) Doc. No.: D 64/1456 (1964).

[423] BSI: Draft British standard methods for automatic ultrasonic examination of welded seams. Draft. Doc. No. D 64/9636 (1964).

[424] BSI: Code of practice for automatic ultrasonic examination of welded seams. Draft. Doc. No. D 64/6372 (1964).

[425] BSI: The non-destructive testing of pipes and tubes, Part 1 – Ultrasonic Testing – Section A – Ferrous pipes and tubes. Draft. Doc. No. D 64/7645 (1964).

[426] The Federal Minister of Labour: Druckgasverordnung. Ultraschallprüfung der durch Spannungsrisskorrosion oder Härterisse gefährdeten Stahlflaschen. Bundesarbeitsblatt, Ed. December 1955, pp. 1110–1111.

[427] German Federal Railways, testing bureau for mechanical tests of materials, Minden: Vorläufige Richtlinien für die Untersuchung von Radsätzen der Dampflok und sonstigen Lok mit Stangenantrieb auf Querrisse in den Achswellen mittels Ultraschall.

[428] German Federal Railways: Technische Lieferbedingungen No. 91995 mit Ergänzungen. Isolatoren für Fahr- und Fernleitungen (1954).

[429] DIN 54119 (preliminary standard Jan. 1964): Zerstörungsfreie Prüfung – Ultraschallprüfung – Begriffe.

[430] DIN 54120 (preliminary standard Dec. 1964): Kontrollkörper 1 und seine Verwendung zur Justierung und Kontrolle von Ultraschall-Impulsecho-Geräten.

[431] DIN 21501: Schachtausbau aus gusseisernen Tübbingen (1963).

[432] DIN 17175: Nahtlose Rohre aus warmfesten Stählen (1959).

[433] Ente Nazionale Italiano di Unificazione UNI 5329: Prove non distruttive dei materiali metallici, controle con ultrasuoni delle lamiere di acciaio con spessore maggiore di 15 mm, metodo a reflessione di impulsi (1963).

[434] French specification: C-66-300/1958: Isolateurs en porcelaine à fut massiv pour lignes de traction électrique alimentées en courant alternatif de tension supérieur à 1000 Volts.

[435] Indian standard: IS SMDC 3 (292); 1962: Glossary of terms relating to ultrasonic testing.

[436] International Electrotechnical Commission, draft 36: I.E.C. Recommendations for solidcore insulators for overhead traction lines at a voltage greater than 1000 Volts.

[437] International Institute of Welding (IIW/IIS): Nomenclature des termes utilisés dans le contrôle par ultrasons en trois langues. Paris: Publishers Publication de la Soudure Autogène 1959.

[438] IIW/IIS: Report of Commission V, No. IIW/IIS 23-59, chairman Prof. G. A. Homès, University of Brussels.

[439] Second Intern. Conf. for non-destructive testing of materials in Chicago 1957, lectures. Nondestr. Test. 16 (1958) No. 2, pp. 84–174.

[440] IRSID (Institut de Recherches de la Sidérurgie): Dispositif de correction automatique des conditions variables de sondage ultrasonore par échos des matériaux. French.P. 1147106 (1956).

[441] Japanese Industrial Standards: JIS Z 2344: Method of ultrasonic flaw detection test for metals (1958) (in English).

[442] Marine Nationale Française Etablissement d'Indret: Instruction relative a l'examen des tôles aux ultra-sons, No. 102 (revue 1959).

[443] Austrian specification: ÖVE-L 30/1956.

[444] The Physical Society (England): Handbook of Scientific Instruments and Apparatus, Exhibition 1956, London.

[445] Polish standard: PN-61, M-70050 (US test, concepts).

[446] Polish standard: PN-61, M-70051 (US test, test blocks).

[447] Réalisations Ultrasoniques: Perfectionnements aux appareils de mesure des épaisseurs par échos ultra-sonores. French.P. 1105631 (1954).

[448] Röntgen Technische Dienst N.V. Rotterdam: Trade prospectus Sonolog.

[449] Swiss Federal Railways, division power stations: specification for the supply of rod-type suspension insulators models L 75/8 and L 85/8 for installation in 66 and 132 kV transmission lines. 1st Ed. 1959 (in German).

[450] Society for Nondestructive Testing (SNT), Airframe Committee. Recommended ultrasonic acceptance standards for airframe aluminium alloy plate, forgings and extrusions. Report No. 1, SNT-Nr. NA 57-1277, also in Nondestr. Test. 15 (1957) No. 6, pp. 368–370.

[451] Sperry Products Inc.: Ultraschall-Höhenstandsmesser. DBP 960318 (1954).

[452] Studiengesellschaft für Höchstspannungsanlagen Berlin: Zerstörungsfreie Isolatorenprüfung mit Ultraschall. Technical Report No. 157 of 25/2/1952.

[453] Hungarian Standard: MSZ 7863 (draft, ultrasonic test, basic concepts).

[454] VDE-Bestimmung 0446 (Freileitungsisolatoren) of March 1955, para. 11: Prüfung des Isolierkörpers mit Ultraschall.

[455] Verein Deutscher Eisenhüttenleute (VDEh): Stahl-Eisen-Betriebsblatt 66010.55. Düsseldorf: Verlag Stahl-Eisen.

[456] VDEh: Stahl-Eisen-Prüfblatt No. 1560-57.
[457] VDEh: Technische Lieferbedingungen für überschallgeprüfte Grobbleche (geprüft nach dem Impuls-Echo-Verfahren). Stahl-Eisen specifications 072-57 (October 1957).
[458] Ultrasonic tests on tubing. Stahl-Eisen test specification 1915 (proposal, Aug. 1964).
[459] Verein der Grosskessel-Besitzer (VGB), Bericht über die 22. Sitzung des Ausschusses für Materialfragen: Die zerstörungsfreie Prüfung von Kessel- und Überhitzerrohren. Mitt. d. VGB No. 88, Febr. 1964.
[460] Verein der Technischen Überwachungsvereine in Deutschland VdTÜV: Merkblatt Druckbehälter No. 309 (1961).
[461] Zentralinstitut für Schweisstechnik, Halle/Saale (ZIS): ZIS Richtlinien für die Prüfung von Schweissverbindungen mit Ultraschall ZIS R 63-59.

Subject Index